D0221446

Administrative
Medical Assisting

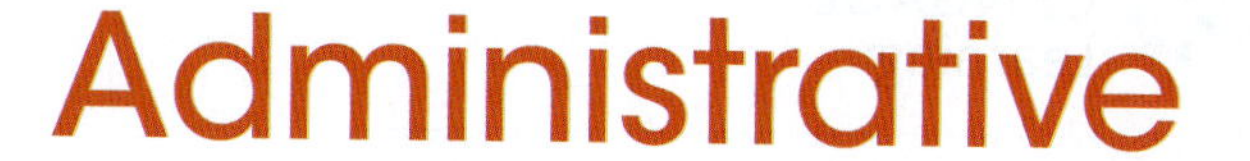

Administrative Medical Assisting

WILBURTA Q. LINDH, CMA (AAMA)

CAROL D. TAMPARO, CMA (AAMA), PHD

BARBARA M. DAHL

JULIE A. MORRIS, RN, BSN, CBCS, CCMA, CMAA

CINDY CORREA, AHI (AMT)

Sixth Edition

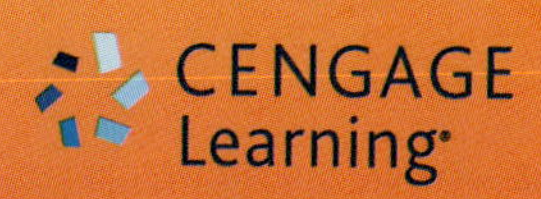

CENGAGE Learning

Australia • Brazil • Mexico • Singapore • United Kingdom • United States

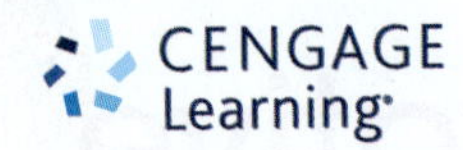

Administrative Medical Assisting, Sixth Edition
Wilburta Q. Lindh, Carol D. Tamparo, Barbara M. Dahl, Julie A. Morris, Cindy Correa

SVP, GM Skills & Global Product Management: Jonathan Lau

Product Director: Matthew Seeley

Product Team Manager: Stephen Smith

Senior Director, Development: Marah Bellegarde

Product Development Manager: Juliet Steiner

Senior Content Developer: Lauren Whalen

Product Assistant: Mark Turner

Vice President, Marketing Services: Jennifer Ann Baker

Marketing Manager: Jonathan Sheehan

Senior Production Director: Wendy Troeger

Production Director: Andrew Crouth

Senior Content Project Manager: Thomas Heffernan

Senior Art Director: Jack Pendleton

Media Producer: Jim Gilbert

Cover image(s): My Portfolio/Shutterstock.com
Vikpit/Shutterstock.com
Svetlana_Okeana/Shutterstock.com

WCN: 01-100-101

Library of Congress Control Number: 2016953587

ISBN: 978-1-305-96480-8

Cengage Learning
20 Channel Center Street
Boston, MA 02210
USA

Printed in China
Print Number: 02 Print Year: 2017

TABLE OF CONTENTS

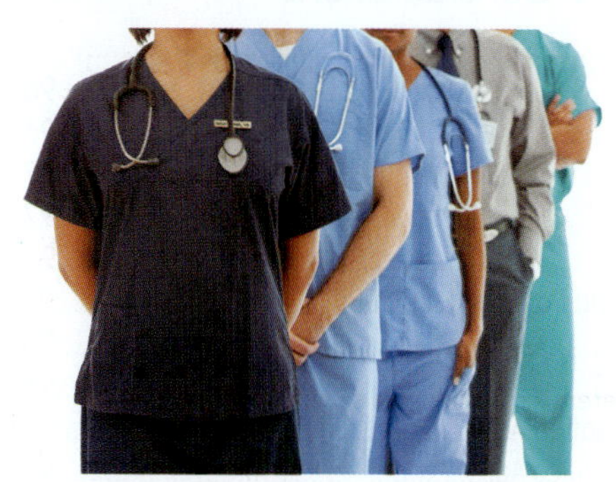

UNIT II: **THE THERAPEUTIC APPROACH** 38

UNIT III: **RESPONSIBLE MEDICAL PRACTICE** 92

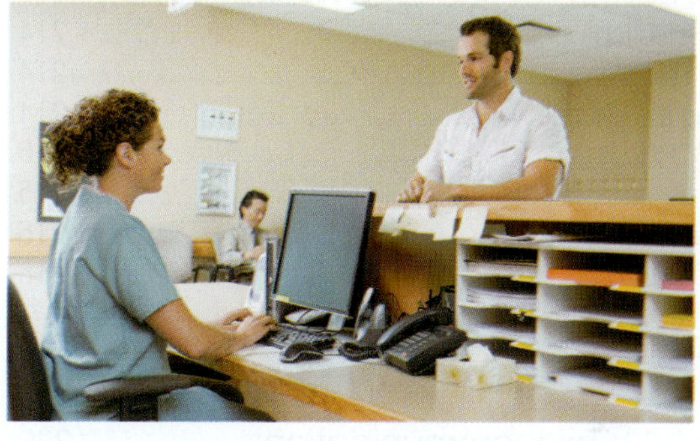

CHAPTER 10: Computers in the Medical Clinic 200

CHAPTER 11: Telecommunications 220

CHAPTER 12: Patient Scheduling 252

CHAPTER 13: Medical Records Management 276

LIST OF PROCEDURES

PREFACE

The world of health care continues to change rapidly, and, as medical assistants, you will be called on to do more and respond to an increasing number of responsibilities. Now is the time to equip yourself with the skills you will need to excel in the field to maximize your potential, expand your base of knowledge, and dedicate yourself to becoming the best multifaceted, multiskilled medical assistant that you can be.

The new edition of *Administrative Medical Assisting* will guide you on this journey. This text is part of a dynamic learning system that includes software, a study guide, and online materials. Together, this learning package includes coverage of the most current entry-level competencies identified by the Accrediting Bureau of Health Education Schools (ABHES) and the Commission on Accreditation of Allied Health Education Programs (CAAHEP). It will also help you prepare for certification examinations from the American Association of Medical Assistants (AAMA), the American Medical Technologists (AMT), and the National Healthcareer Association (NHA).

You will find this edition continues to provide you with opportunities to use your critical thinking skills through case studies, critical thinking boxes, patient education boxes, and scenarios. You will also see that the text addresses topics that will make you workplace-ready, including electronic health records (EHR), Practice Management (PM) software, ICD-10, professionalism, and confidentiality and privacy issues.

Some of the special new features and updates to this edition include:

- Increased emphasis on EHR and PM software, including many visual examples of EHR and PM systems, and sample electronic documentation
- Expanded coverage of ICD-10-CM and ICD-10-PCS, and their implementation
- Refreshed learning outcomes that map to the most current ABHES and CAAHEP competencies
- A refreshed *Attributes of Professionalism* feature in each unit opener that emphasizes behavioral skills
- A new *Quick Reference Guide* feature that highlights critical information in each chapter through a combination of photos, graphics, illustrations, and narrative text
- Dozens of new photos and illustrations portraying a greater number of procedures and showing the latest equipment
- Updated procedures that include language emphasizing professionalism skills
- Updated end of chapter content, including an expanded *Certification Review* section with multiple-choice questions that mimic the medical assisting certification examinations
- Updated certification and examination information for AAMA, AMT, and NHA
- Additional *Critical Thinking* boxes throughout the text

HOW THE TEXT IS ORGANIZED

Section I, "General Procedures" (Chapters 1 through 8), provides the groundwork for understanding the role and responsibilities of the medical assistant. Topics include the medical assisting profession, the health care team, communication skills, legal and ethical issues, and emergency and first aid procedures.

New material in this section includes:

- Quick Reference Guides
- Updated Attributes of Professionalism feature
- Expansion of factors causing stress in the work environment
- Patient coaching and navigation
- Americans with Disabilities Act
- Definition of expressed consent
- New Chapter 4 procedure that covers patient coaching
- New Chapter 6 procedures covering locating a state's legal scope of practice for medical assistants, and performing compliance-based reporting on public health statutes

- New Chapter 7 procedure that covers developing a plan for separating personal and professional ethics
- New Chapter 8 procedures covering performing first aid procedures for insulin shock, seizures, shock, and syncope
- New topics in Section I: patient-centered medical homes; accountable care organizations (ACO); influence of technology on communication; communication in end-of-life care; Affordable Care Act and Patients' Bill of Rights and Responsibilities

Section II, "Administrative Procedures" (Chapters 9 through 20), provides up-to-date information on all administrative competencies required of medical assistants. Topics include the facility environment, using computers and technology, clinic communications, scheduling, creating and managing medical records, insurance and coding, and financial practices.

New material in this section includes:

- Quick Reference Guides
- Expanded coverage of electronic health records (EHR) and related figures
- Expanded coverage of ICD-10-CM and ICD-10-PCS
- Expanded information on community resources
- New Chapter 11 procedures covering developing a list of community resources, and facilitating referrals to community resources
- New topics in Section II: patient portal systems; telemedicine; online scheduling; do-it-yourself appointments; traditional indemnity insurance

Section III, "Professional Procedures" (Chapters 21 through 24), examines the role of the medical assistant as clinic manager and human resources manager and provides tools and techniques to use when preparing for student practicums, medical assistant credentialing, and finding employment opportunities.

New material in this section includes:

- Quick Reference Guides
- Updated certification and examination information
- Revised section on using social media in the job search
- New Chapter 24 procedures covering how to write a résumé, and how to follow up on a job interview effectively
- New topics in Section III: generational expectations of employment; evaluating employees; online profiles

THE COMPLETE LEARNING PACKAGE: STUDENT SUPPLEMENTS

Study Guide (ISBN 978-1-3059-6485-3)

Explore the text content through Vocabulary Builder, Learning Review, Certification Review, and Application Activities for each chapter. The Study Guide has been fully revised to align with the content in the sixth edition.

Student Companion Website

(www.cengagebrain.com)

This student website is designed to provide students with the resources they will need to complete the text procedures. Editable Competency Checklists and Procedure Forms can be downloaded from the Student Companion Website.

Competency Checklists have been streamlined for ease of use and evaluation, and provide instructions on the specific scenario information needed to complete the procedure, as well as any forms to be used.

Procedure Forms are provided for the relevant checklists. The forms can be completed electronically and saved, or printed and completed manually.

Detailed instructions for accessing the Student Companion Website can be found on the Instructor Companion Website.

Critical Thinking Challenge 3.0

(ISBN 978-1-1339-3330-4 or 978-1-1339-3324-3)

The Critical Thinking Challenge 3.0 software simulates a 3-month practicum in a medical clinic. You will be confronted with a series of situations in which you must use your critical thinking skills to choose the most appropriate action in response to the situation. Your decisions will be evaluated in three categories: how your decisions affect the practice, the patient, and your career. The 3.0 version includes 12 all-new video-based scenarios with more branching options. After successfully completing the program, a Certification of Completion may be printed.

Learning Lab

(ISBN 978-1-1336-0956-8 or 978-1-1336-0953-7)

Learning Lab maps to learning objectives and includes interactive activities and case scenarios to build students' critical thinking skills and help retain the more difficult concepts. This simulated, immersive environment engages users with its real-life approach. Each Learning Lab has a pre-assessment quiz, three to five learning activities, and post-assessment quiz. The post-assessment scores can be posted to the instructor grade book in any learning management system.

MindTap for Comprehensive Medical Assisting: Administrative and Clinical Competencies, Sixth Edition

MindTap is a fully online, interactive learning experience built upon authoritative Cengage Learning content. By combining readings, multimedia, activities, and assessments into a singular learning path, MindTap elevates learning by providing real-world application to better engage students. Instructors customize the learning path by selecting Cengage Learning resources and adding their own content via apps that integrate into the MindTap framework seamlessly with many learning management systems.

The guided learning path demonstrates the importance of the medical assistant through engagement activities and interactive exercises. Learners can apply their understanding of the material through interactive activities taken from Critical Thinking Challenge 3.0 and the Medical Assisting Learning Lab, in addition to certification style quizzing and case studies. These simulations elevate the study of medical assisting by challenging students to apply concepts to practice.

To learn more, visit www.cengage.com/mintdtap

THE COMPLETE LEARNING PACKAGE: INSTRUCTOR SUPPLEMENTS

Instructor Companion Site

(ISBN 978-1-3059-6483-9)

(Access at www.cengage.com/login)

Spend less time planning and more time teaching with Cengage Learning's Instructor Resources. Log on to the Instructor Companion Site to gain access to the Instructor's Manual, Cognero Test Bank, and PowerPoint slides. Access at www.cengage.com/login with your Cengage instructor account. If you are a first-time user, click Create a New Faculty Account and follow the prompts.

Instructor's Manual The Instructor's Manual provides mapping to the most current ABHES and CAAHEP curriculum, lesson outlines, suggestions for classroom activities, and answer keys for the text and Study Guide.

Online Cognero Test Bank An electronic test bank makes and generates tests and quizzes in an instant. With a variety of question types, including multiple choice and matching exercises, creating challenging exams will be no barrier in your classroom. This test bank includes a rich bank of over 1,000 questions that test students on retention and application of what they have learned in the course. Answers are provided for all questions so instructors can focus on teaching, not grading. Each question also contains a reference to the text page number and ABHES and CAAHEP curriculum standard.

Instructor PowerPoint Slides A comprehensive offering of more than 900 instructor support slides created in Microsoft PowerPoint outlines concepts and objectives to assist instructors with lectures.

ABOUT THE AUTHORS

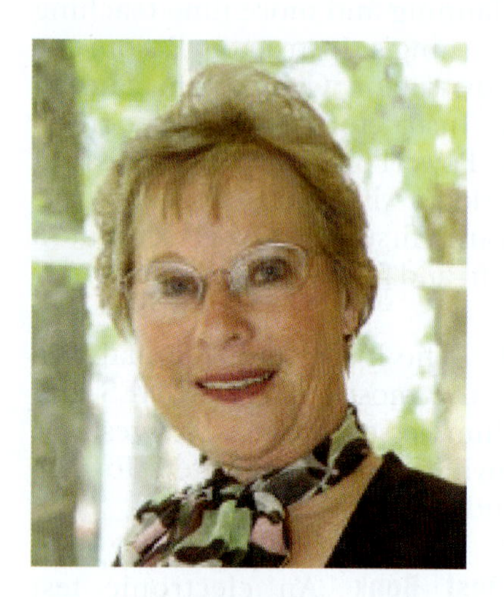

Wilburta (Billie) Q. Lindh, CMA, (AAMA), is Professor Emerita at Highline College in Des Moines, Washington, where she served as Program Director and consultant to the Medical Assistant Program. She received the Outstanding Faculty Member of the Year award for her efforts in revamping the program. An active member of SeaTac Chapter of the American Association of Medical Assistants (AAMA), and the National American Association of Medical Assistants, Ms. Lindh conducted workshops and lectured across the country. She is the co-author of several textbooks on medical assisting.

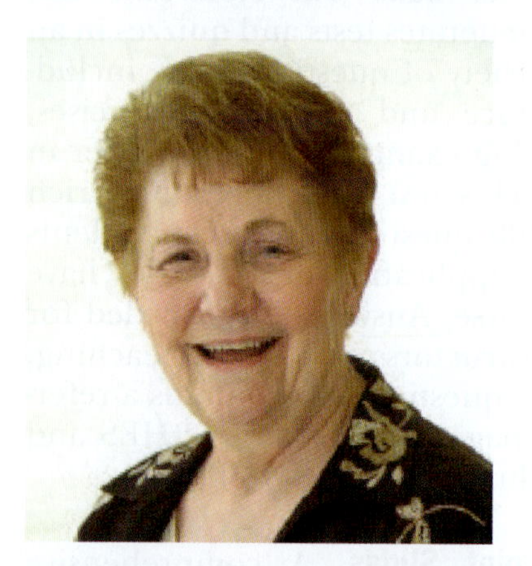

Carol D. Tamparo, CMA (AAMA), PhD, is the former Dean of Business and Allied Health at the Lake Washington Institute of Technology in Kirkland, Washington, and founder of the Medical Assistant program at Highline Community College. Author and Co-author of four texts for allied health professionals, she is also a member of the SeaTac American Association of Medical Assistants and the National American Association of Medical Assistants.

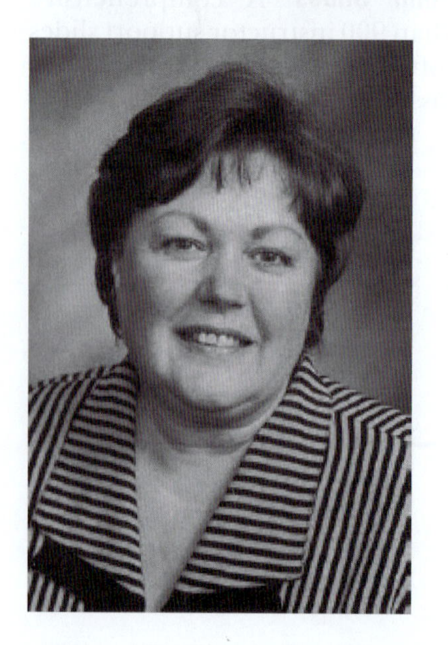

Barbara M. Dahl, served as a tenured faculty member and coordinator of the Medical Assisting Program at Whatcom Community College in Bellingham, Washington, for over 20 years. She was a very active member of several professional organizations, including the Whatcom County Chapter of Medical Assistants, the Washington State Society of Medical Assistants, the American Association of Medical Assistants (AAMA), and the Washington State Medical Assisting Educators and the American Academy of Professional Coders (AAPC). Ms. Dahl is currently involved in medical management and personnel consulting, curriculum development, and program accreditation advising, as well as advocating for medical assistants to enjoy the right to practice in Washington.

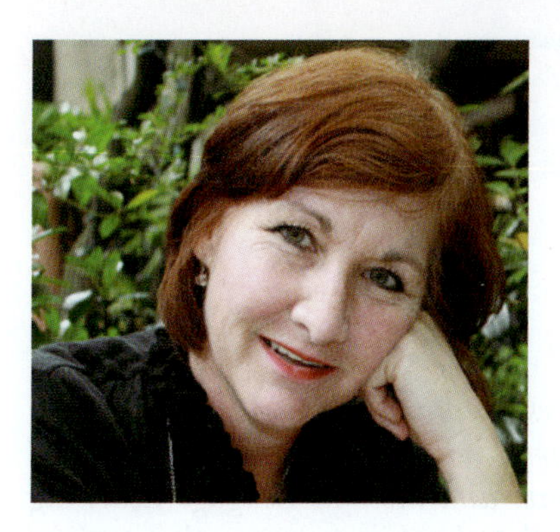

Julie A. Morris, RN, BSN, CBCS, CCMA, CMAA, decided to become a nurse at the age of 16. Ms. Morris has been involved in health care for more than four decades. She graduated from the Lurleen B. Wallace School of Nursing at Jacksonville State University with a Bachelor of Science degree in nursing. Her career has included directorship positions in case management, home infusion care, clinical education and clinic management. She has spent the last ten years pursuing her dream of educating adults in the allied healthcare field; holding positions as Instructor, Program Director, Externship Coordinator, and Director of Career Services. Currently, Ms. Morris is involved in integrating active learning in the classroom, curriculum development, and strategies to engage students and assist them in successful completion of educational programs. She is an active member of the Cobb Chapter of the American Association of Medical Assistants in Georgia.

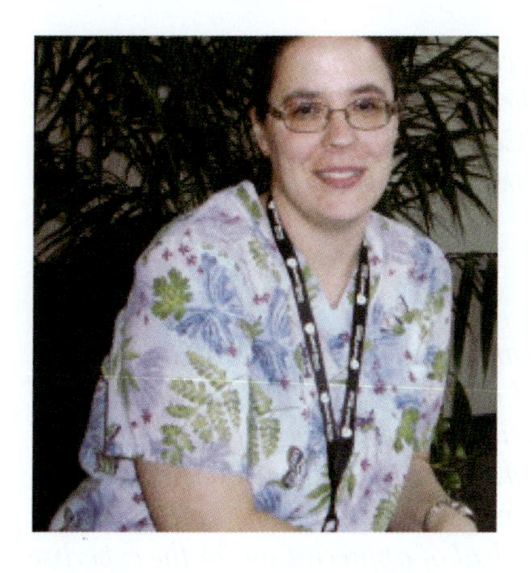

Cindy Correa, AHI (AMT), is the former Allied Health Educational Coordinator at City University of New York at Queens College. Cindy was responsible for the initial creation and curricula development of at least seven certificate programs of the Allied Health Program, including the Medical Assistant program at Queens College. She has extended her expertise to satellite courses in adult education programs. Her experience working in the private practice and administrative hospital environments includes oncology, cardiovascular surgery, pulmonology, and thoracic surgery. Cindy is actively involved in technical writing, software development projects, and serves on advisory boards of technical colleges in her home state of Colorado.

ACKNOWLEDGMENTS

A special thank you to my husband, DeVere, who continually supports, encourages, and assists me in so many ways. Thank you to my family and friends, who understood when I was not available for activities, but continually accepted and encouraged my commitment to excellence. Collaborating with the author team and those at Cengage Learning encouraged forward thinking and a 6th edition that is progressive and current with technology to ensure that medical assisting students are well prepared for tomorrow's challenges.

—Billie Q. Lindh

Many thanks are expressed to my husband, Tom, who assumed many household chores and took us out to dinner at just the right times. Writing a textbook, even the revision of a textbook, requires the input and dedication of many individuals, especially in the field of health care where changes occur almost daily. Collaborating with the other authors on this edition has ensured that the most recent information is included in this text. Thank you Stephen Smith and Lauren Whalen for your vision and guidance.

—Carol D. Tamparo

First I would like to thank my husband, Ed, for his continued support and encouragement during this 6th edition revision. It has been an exciting experience—making sure our textbook is the best and most current representation of what today's medical assistant student needs to know to enter the profession; covering the cognitive, psychomotor, and affective domains; as well as using the most current technology and new clinical diagnostics and equipment. I appreciate the opportunity to continue working with my diversely talented team members, Billie and Carol, and I welcome the fresh perspective of our new team members, Julie and Cindy. I also have a great deal of appreciation for the expertise and patience of Lauren Whalen, Stephen Smith, as well as the rest of our Cengage Learning team and Aravinda Doss with Lumina Datamatics in updating this nationally respected resource.

—Barbara M. Dahl

Of the things that I revere and find valuable in the profession of medical assisting, expanding knowledge and the delivery of quality patient care rank at the top. It is my hope that this text provides a guide to attain essential knowledge and the tools to apply that knowledge to the care of every patient. Each minute that was spent on the revision of this text will result in hours, days, months, and years of teaching and learning. That thought makes it all worth it! Dear future medical assistant, I wish you success and satisfaction in this career that you have chosen.

Thank you, co-authors and the team at Cengage. The sixth edition is a result of amazing collaboration. Specifically, Lauren Whalen and Stephen Smith, thank you for the kindness and support you have shown me during this and other Cengage projects.

Special thanks and appreciation to my family. Phillip Rutledge; Bryan, Casey, and Arleigh Mountjoy; and Sam Huckaby, you fill my heart with gratitude and love. Thank you for caring for me, supporting me, and always being around for a diversion when one is desperately needed.

—Julie A. Morris

Many thanks to Lauren Whalen for her guidance and support, and always having a sharp eye, valuable suggestions, and a helping hand. I appreciate the patience from the entire team during some challenging personal experiences during this project. I especially owe a tremendous debt to Audrey Theisen for her generous assistance and expertise—thank you! Billie, Carol, Barbara, and Julie, it was a pleasure working with such a professional team of authors. I am grateful to Stephen Smith and everyone at Cengage Learning for the opportunities extended and allowing me to be part of your ongoing projects. To my family and friends, who have propped me up and have made it possible for me to focus on my work by taking care of all the other details when needed, it would never have gotten done without you.

—Cindy Correa

CONTRIBUTOR

The authors and publisher would like to acknowledge the following professional for contributing to the content of this book:

Audrey Theisen, BS, RHIA, MSCIS, PhD
HIM Professor
Contributing author for Chapter 17

REVIEWERS

Deneen Dotson, CCMA (NHA)
Clinical Medical Assistant Program Director
Brookline College
Tucson, AZ

Alicia C. Dumas-Pace, MA, PA, AHI
College Administrator & Consultant/Instructor
Masters Vocational College
Riverside, CA

Amy Eady, MT(ASCP), MS, RMA (AMT)
Dean of Health Occupation
Montcalm Community College
Sidney, MI

Lisa Graese, CHDS
Intructor, Medical Office Careers
Spokane Community College
Spokane, WA

Karon Green-Walton, CMA (AAMA), BS
Program Director
Augusta Technical College
Augusta, GA

Kim Hashem-Dugal, MBA, NCMA (NCCT)
Medical Assisting Training Program Developer, Consultant
Great Bay Community College
Portsmouth, NH

Susan Holler, MSEd, CPC, CMRS
Medical Administrative Assistant, Medical Reimbursement & Coding
Bryant & Stratton College
Orchard Park, NY

Judith Hurtt, M.Ed.
Instructor
East Central Community College
Decatur, MS

Madeline Y. Jones, BSN, MBA, RN
Regional Director, Health Science Programs for VA, WV, and TN
American National University
Roanoke, VA

Michelle McCranie, A.A.S., CPhT, CMA (AAMA)
Medical Assisting Instructor
Ogeechee Technical College
Statesboro, GA

Nancy Measell, BS, AAS, CMA (AAMA)
Assistant Professor
Ivy Tech Community College
South Bend, IN

Janet Melton, MBA
VP of Education
Brookline College
Phoenix, AZ

Sandra Metcalf, M.Ed.
Professor and Program Director of Office & Computer Technology
Grayson College
Denison, TX

Karen Minchella, Ph.D., CMA (AAMA)
Educational Consultant
Consulting Management Associates, LCC
Warren, MI

Pamela Neu, CMA (AAMA), MBA
Medical Assisting Program Chair
Ivy Tech Community College
Fort Wayne, IN

Margaret Noirjean, BSN, RN
Medical Assistant Program Instructor
Dakota County Technical College
Rosemount, MN

Linda Pace, BS, CMA (AAMA)
Director of Medical Assisting and Phlebotomy
Red Rocks Community College
Arvada, CO

Cathy Salazar, MS, MA, EdS
Director
ITT Technical Institute
Pensacola, FL

Patricia Seydlitz, RHIT
Professor
Clark College
Vancouver, WA

Loreane Sheets, CMA (AAMA), BSH, BLS-I
Assistant Professor, Program Chair Medical Assisting
Belmont College
St. Clairsville, OH 43950

Deanna Stephens, AABA, RMA (AMT), CMOA
Instructor
Virginia College
Baton Rouge, LA

Gayla Taylor, MSM
Director of Education
PCI Health Training Center
Dallas, TX

Kathleen Tettam, CMA (AAMA), PBT (ASCP)
Medical Assistant Instructor
Dakota County Technical College
Rosemount, MN

Holly Tumbarello, RN, BSN
Certified Allied Health Instructor, MA Coordinator
Clatsop Community College
Astoria, OR

Marilyn Turner, RN, CMA (AAMA)
Medical Assisting Program Director
Ogeechee Technical College
Statesboro, GA

Jeanne Von Ohlsen, CMA (AAMA)
Program Chair, Medical Assisting
Hodges University
Naples, FL

Barb Westrick, AAS, CMA (AAMA), CPC
Program Chair, Medical Assisting and Medical Billing
Ross Education, LLC
Brighton, MI

Micheline B. Wheeler, ADN, RN, RMA (AMT)
Medical Assisting Program Manager
Central Carolina Technical College
Sumter, SC

Aprilan F. Woolworth, RHIT, CPC, CRC
Education Manager
Os2 Healthcare Solutions
Killeen, TX

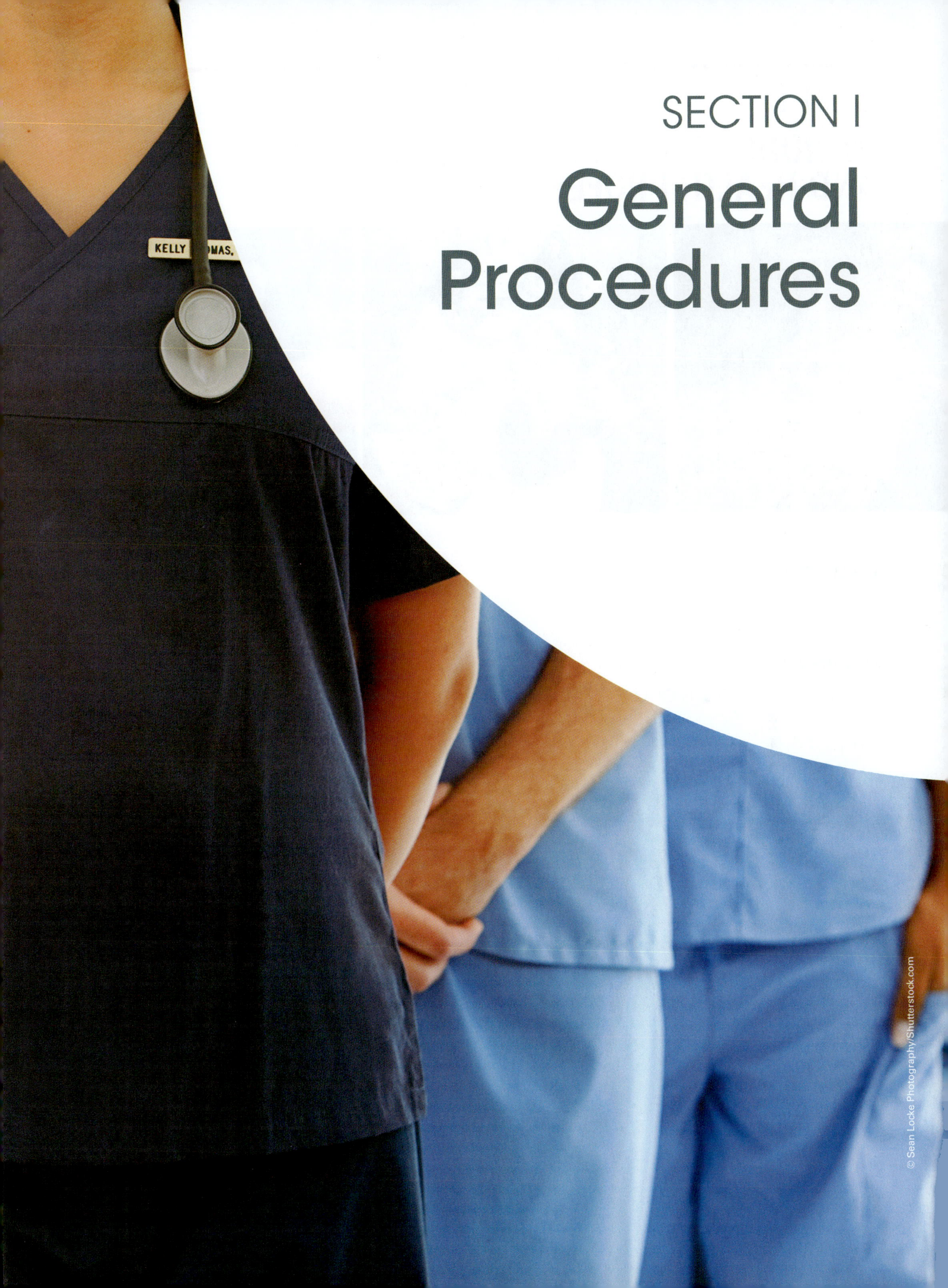
SECTION I
General Procedures

UNIT I

INTRODUCTION TO MEDICAL ASSISTING AND HEALTH PROFESSIONS

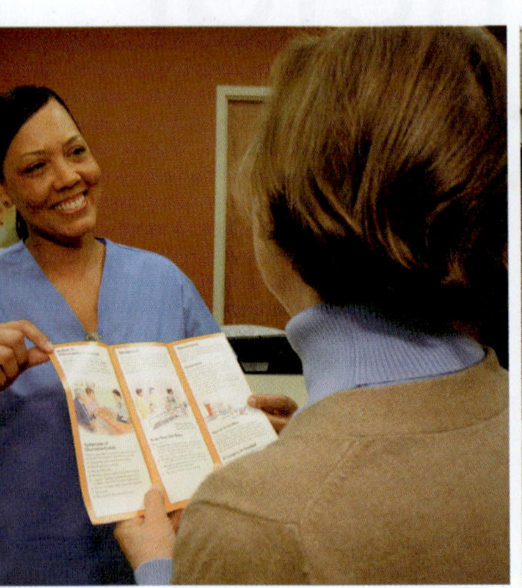

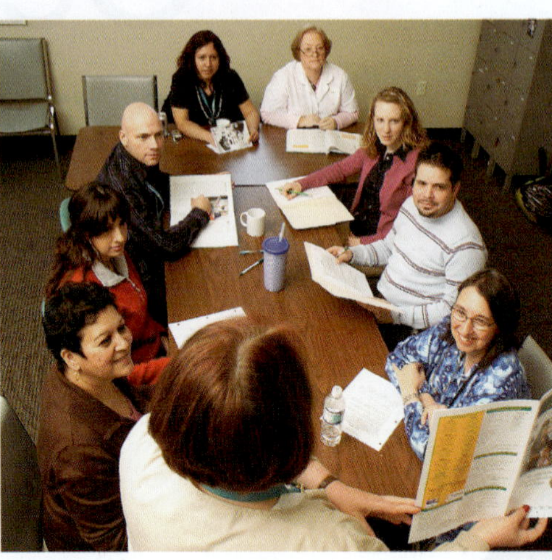

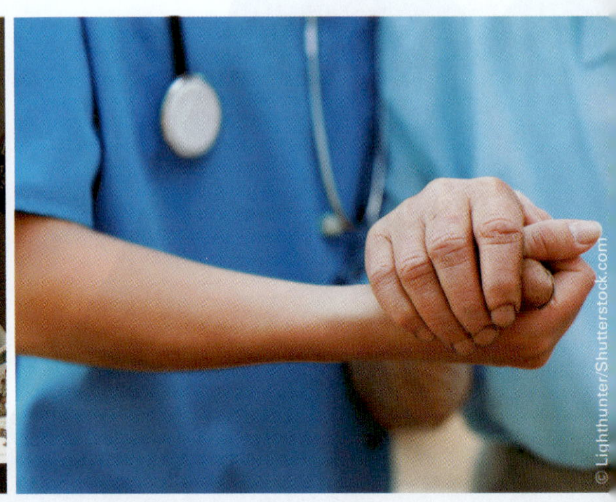

ATTRIBUTES OF PROFESSIONALISM

An essential attribute of a professional medical assistant is respect. Every person that enters your presence must be treated with respectful reverence. Patients, peers, and co-workers must all be held in high regard. Your willingness to show appreciation and consideration will facilitate a positive experience for all involved, and foster a true team atmosphere. On occasion, difficult patients will test the tolerance of even the most experienced medical assistant, because they seldom seem content with the care or services received. However, patients should never be treated with disinterest or in an unfriendly manner. You must always be pleasant and courteous. Seeking health care is a very personal experience. As a medical assistant, that means you must always respect the patient's information, resulting care, and documentation of that care, regardless of the circumstances.

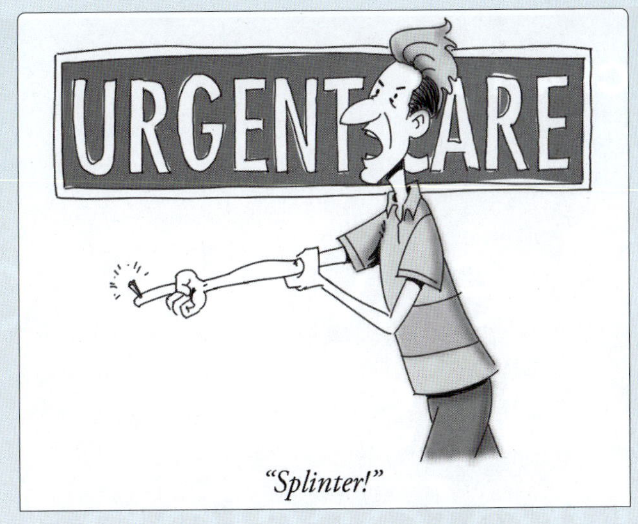

"Splinter!"

Listed below are a series of questions for you to ask yourself, to serve as a professionalism checklist. As you interact with patients and colleagues, these questions will help to guide you in the professional behavior that is expected every day from medical assistants.

Ask Yourself

COMMUNICATION

- ☐ Do I apply active listening skills?
- ☐ Do I display professionalism through written and verbal communication?
- ☐ Do I demonstrate appropriate nonverbal communication?
- ☐ Do I display appropriate body language?
- ☐ Does my knowledge allow me to speak easily with all members of the health care team?

PRESENTATION

- ☐ Am I dressed and groomed appropriately?
- ☐ Do I display a positive attitude?
- ☐ Do I display a calm, professional, and caring manner?

COMPETENCY

- ☐ Do I pay attention to detail?
- ☐ Do I ask questions if I am out of my comfort zone or do not have the experience to carry out tasks?
- ☐ Do I display sound judgment?
- ☐ Am I knowledgeable and accountable?

INITIATIVE

- ☐ Do I show initiative?
- ☐ Do I seek out opportunities to expand my knowledge base?
- ☐ Am I flexible and dependable?
- ☐ Do I implement time management principles to maintain effective office function?
- ☐ Do I assist co-workers when appropriate?

INTEGRITY

- ☐ Do I work within my scope of practice?
- ☐ Do I demonstrate respect for individual diversity?
- ☐ Do I immediately report any error I made?
- ☐ Do I do the "right thing" even when no one is observing?

CHAPTER 1

The Medical Assisting Profession

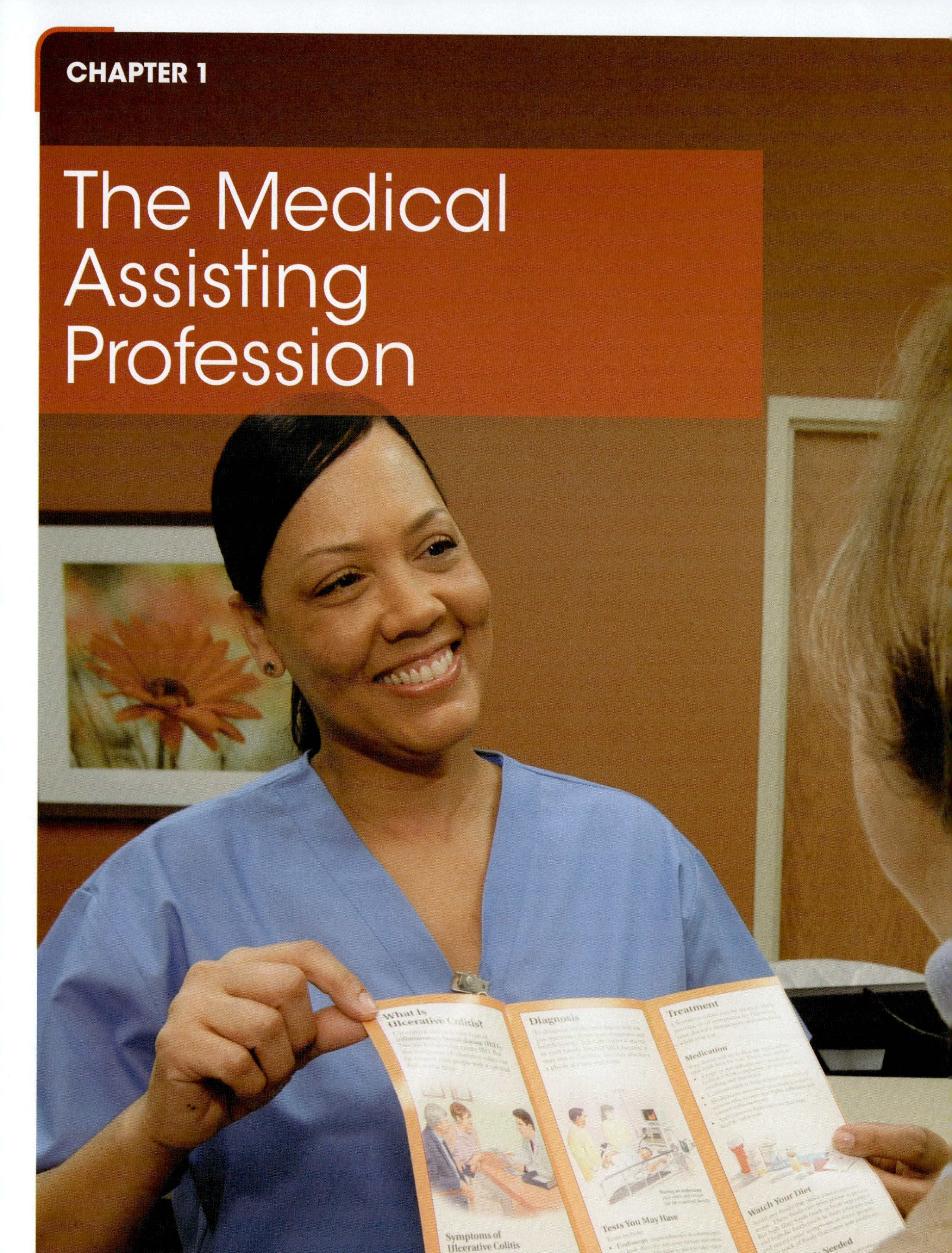

LEARNING OUTCOMES

1. Define and spell the key terms as presented in the glossary.
2. Discuss the history of medical assisting.
3. Describe the practicum experience.
4. Recall two criteria for the selection of practicum sites.
5. Identify three benefits of the practicum to the student and the site.
6. Describe the profession of medical assisting and analyze its career opportunities in relationship to your interests.
7. Identify and discuss five attributes that are essential to a professional medical assistant's career.
8. Describe the American Association of Medical Assistants and discuss its major functions.
9. Discuss the role of the American Medical Technologists in the credentialing of medical assistants.
10. Explain the purpose of the National Healthcareer Association.
11. Explain accreditation, certification, and continuing education as they pertain to the professional medical assistant.
12. Differentiate the requirements for certification and recertification for each of the credentialing bodies.
13. Identify the importance of the accreditation process to an educational institution.
14. Recall at least two methods available to obtain recertification.
15. Compare the five means of obtaining continuing education units.
16. Differentiate among certification, licensure, and registration.
17. Identify the importance of understanding the scope of practice for the medical assistant.

KEY TERMS

accreditation
Affordable Care Act (ACA)
ambulatory care setting
associate's degree
attributes
bachelor's degree
certification
Certified Clinical Medical Assistant (CCMA [NHA])
Certified Medical Administrative Assistant (CMAA [NHA])
Certified Medical Assistants (CMAs [AAMA])
competency
compliance
credentialed
dexterity
diploma
disposition
empathy
externship
facilitate
improvise
internship
license
licensure
practicum
professionalism
proprietary
Registered Medical Assistant (RMA [AMT])
scope of practice

SCENARIO

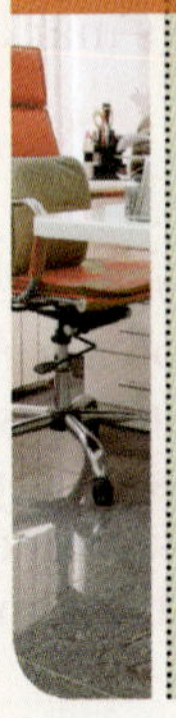

A group of high school freshmen have come to tour a medical assisting class and laboratory areas. The Program Director of Medical Assisting is showing the students around the department. The Program Director then takes them into the medical assisting laboratory, where senior medical assistant students are practicing their clinical skills. Each senior student pairs up with a high school freshman, and each pair talks about medical assisting, with the medical assistant students answering questions the others may have. The medical assistant students are in uniform as part of their preparation to go into various health care agencies to do their externship or practicum. The medical assistant students look professional, clean, fresh, and motivated. They tell the high school students about medical

continues

Scenario *continued*

assisting and describe the personal and physical attributes desirable for those who want to become medical assistants. They explain the importance of these attributes, as well as what duties a professional medical assistant performs and what education is needed to pursue a career in medical assisting.

Throughout the question and answer discussions, the senior medical assistant students and the program director stress the importance of ethics, empathy, attitude, dependability, and teamwork as necessary attributes. Individuals seeking a career in medical assisting must develop and maintain these characteristics.

Chapter Portal

There are many fascinating aspects of the medical assisting profession. When a person pursues formal education to enter the world of medicine as a professional medical assistant, he or she may take on a new role in his or her family and community. In this new role, the medical assisting student can have a major, positive influence on the community-wide knowledge of health and the process for seeking medical care. This influence is just the beginning of the many highly rewarding aspects of becoming a medical assistant.

The medical assistant is defined by the American Association of Medical Assistants (AAMA) Board of Trustees as "A multi-skilled member of the health care team who performs administrative and clinical procedures under the supervision of licensed healthcare providers." According to the 2015 statistics released by the Bureau of Labor Statistics, the majority of medical assistants are employed in provider offices, with outpatient care centers following as the next largest employer. The list of licensed health care providers that can supervise medical assistants has expanded to include nurse practitioners, physician's assistants, podiatrists, chiropractors, and optometrists.

Medical assistants come from a variety of backgrounds and educational experiences. Due to the sophistication of the health care consumer and the complexity of delivering health care, employers are seeking medical assistants who are educated and are credentialed for employment in their practices.

There is an entire body of knowledge—such as anatomy and physiology, medical terminology, and practical clinical skills—that must be acquired in your studies to become a professional medical assistant. An equally important aspect of a medical assistant's career is **professionalism**. Professionalism combines your acquired knowledge and skills with the types of behavior that demonstrate your moral, ethical, and respectful attributes when interacting with patients and colleagues.

HISTORICAL PERSPECTIVE OF THE PROFESSION

There is a rich history of medical assisting and the medical assistants who enjoy the profession. Historically, medicine has included the role of the handmaiden. This person served to assist the provider in his daily tasks caring for an ill population. This role was essential, but undefined. The first recognition of this important aspect of health care was nursing. As time progressed, another vital role emerged—that of the medical assistant.

The last 100 years have brought an acceleration of medical technology that has impacted both the diagnosis and treatment of many disease processes as well as the maintenance of wellness. With advancing technology, the provider has increased the demands on the staff of the practice. The American Association of Medical Assistants defines medical assistants as "multiskilled members of the health care team who perform administrative and clinical procedures under the supervision of licensed health care providers." As the availability of testing and treatment has moved from a more acute-care setting to the provider's clinic, there has been an expanding role for the medical assistant in the delivery of care. The medical assistant must possess a wide array of skills including excellent communication skills, clinical skills that relate to patient care, and administrative skills that are required to manage the facility and the practice's finances. These skills are all part of the requirements for a professional medical assistant in today's market.

CAREER OPPORTUNITIES

Medical assistants have been described as health care's most versatile, multifaceted professionals.

According to the Bureau of Labor Statistics, there are well over half a million medical assisting jobs in the United States, with the job outlook expected to increase by 23% from 2014 to 2024. This significant growth in available employment highlights the vital role that medical assistants currently play in the provision of health care. There are multiple factors recognized as the driving force for this expanding role. The aging baby-boom population requires health maintenance, preventive care, and outpatient management of chronic illness. With the implementation of the **Affordable Care Act (ACA)**, millions of people that previously had no insurance coverage are now seeking health care. There was a reported shortage of health care providers prior to the ACA, and with expanded patient demand due to the law's implementation, the shortage has grown. To help fill the gap, providers have hired medical assistants to perform routine administrative and clinical duties. This allows professional provision of care to a practice's increased patient population.

That medical assistants possess a broad scope of knowledge and skills makes them ideal professionals for any **ambulatory care setting**. Indeed, because of such versatility, medical assistants find employment in a variety of settings: clinics, medical laboratories, insurance companies, government agencies, pharmaceutical companies, educational institutions, surgical centers, urgent-care facilities, and electrocardiography (ECG or EKG) departments in hospitals. Other career opportunities are available to the medical assistant. Some medical assistants work as phlebotomists, coding specialists, medical laboratory assistants, and medical administrative specialists. The broad application of the skills of a medical assistant is relevant to many aspects of a medical practice. This ensures the continued growth of responsibilities and opportunities for medical assisting.

EDUCATION OF THE MEDICAL ASSISTANT

Prior to the 1950s, medical assistants were trained on the job. Organizing professionally brought about the need for a formalized education that incorporated a standardized curriculum. Today, education of medical assistants takes place in community and junior colleges, as well as in **proprietary** schools. In 1997, in coordination with the National Board of Medical Examiners, educators, and practicing **Certified Medical Assistants (CMAs [AAMA])**, the AAMA developed the Medical Assistant Role Delineation Chart, now known as the Occupational Analysis of the CMA (AAMA). This analysis can be found on the AAMA website at www.aamantl.org. Entry-level competencies must be mastered by students in academic programs.

Instruction takes place in a variety of settings. A future medical assistant will be educated in the classroom and in the laboratory, allowing both an understanding of foundational knowledge and processes, as well as an opportunity to practice the hands-on skills required to master the responsibilities of the profession. An important new mode of education is online education. Some schools offer medical assistant courses online, and if the school is accredited many students who cannot or desire not to take traditional classroom courses can work toward becoming certified or registered through this method. Upon graduation from a medical assisting program, the student will receive a **diploma** or certificate of completion. If a student decides to pursue general education courses, it could take another year to complete an **associate's degree** (a total of 2 years) or longer for a **bachelor's degree**.

Courses in a Medical Assisting Program

Some of the administrative, general, and clinical content taught in a medical assisting program is listed in Table 1-1.

Practicum

Practicum, **externship**, and **internship** are all terms used to define the transition period between the classroom and actual employment. A practicum

TABLE 1-1

SOME TYPICAL ADMINISTRATIVE, GENERAL, AND CLINICAL CONTENT TAUGHT IN AN ACCREDITED MEDICAL ASSISTING PROGRAM

Administrative Content	Electronic medical records (EMRs) and electronic health records (EHRs) Document management Appointments and scheduling Insurance claims/coding Billing, collections, and patients' accounts
General Content	Anatomy and physiology Medical terminology Pathophysiology Law and ethics Patient education
Clinical Content	Infection control Disease prevention Pharmacology Temperature, pulse, respirations, and blood pressure Assisting the provider with physical exams Assisting the provider with minor surgery Drawing blood samples Medication Administration Urine and blood testing in the laboratory CPR (provider-level certification), first aid

is planned and supervised by a coordinator from the medical assisting program and the health care facility that agrees to become a partner in the education and employability of the student. The benefit of this practical training is to allow the student a safe environment to implement their knowledge and, if needed, return to the educational setting for reinforcement of skills or knowledge.

Practicum Sites. Sites for practicums are chosen carefully to ensure that a variety of experiences are available for the student. The sites should provide the student with adequate administrative, clinical, and general experiences. The staff at the various sites must be willing to make a commitment to the medical assistant's education by spending appropriate time observing and instructing the student (see Chapter 21 for more information on supervising student practicums).

Benefits of Practicum. The practicum experience is mutually beneficial to the student and staff at the health care facility that is providing the educational experiences. Students are able to apply classroom knowledge and skill in a real-world medical setting, while using the practicum experience to build a résumé and begin to establish a network of support through colleagues. As students progress in their skills and abilities, they become oriented to the practice. The practicum may be considered an extended interview for possible job placement.

Associate's and Bachelor's Degrees

The expanding role and applicable job openings for medical assistants have allowed a new focus on degrees in medical assisting. Both proprietary schools and more traditional educational institutions have added both associate's and bachelor's degrees in medical assisting to their curriculum.

The primary benefit of these degrees is positioning in the job market. With an expanded curriculum, the medical assistant is prepared with college-level classes that include college math, English, and psychology as well as more in-depth classes related to medical assisting. Employers are eager to hire candidates with a demonstrated commitment to education and to their profession. Movement up the career ladder in health care is assisted by educational credentials as well as job experience.

With the increase of allied health education programs in the United States ranging from the certificate level to degree levels, a new opportunity has been created for tenured medical assistants: that of instructor. Required credentials for instructors in each medical assisting program are outlined by the credentialing bodies of each educational organization.

ACCREDITATION OF MEDICAL ASSISTING PROGRAMS

Educational institutions seeking **accreditation** for a medical assisting program must develop the curricula to meet the *Standards and Guidelines* set by the Commission on Accreditation for Allied Health Education Programs (CAAHEP), or the standards set by the Accrediting Bureau of Health Education Schools (ABHES) to ensure the highest quality medical assistant education and employment preparedness.

CAAHEP

The Commission on Accreditation for Allied Health Education Programs (CAAHEP) is an accrediting body for medical assisting programs in private and public postsecondary institutions and programs that prepare individuals for entry into the profession.

A medical assisting program that is accredited by CAAHEP meets the standards as outlined in the *Standards and Guidelines for an Accredited Education Program for the Medical Assistant*. Standards are the minimum standards of quality used in accrediting programs that prepare individuals to enter the medical assisting profession.

On-site review teams evaluate the program's **compliance** with, or adherence to, the standards. All aspects of programs seeking accreditation status undergo scrutiny to ascertain the program's quality and to ensure continued compliance with the standards.

For more information, see the CAAHEP Web site at www.caahep.org.

ABHES

The Accrediting Bureau of Health Education Schools (ABHES) is the agency that also grants accreditation to medical assisting programs. ABHES is recognized by the United States Department of Education (USDE) as an accrediting agency of public and private schools and colleges that primarily offer health education. This includes medical assisting, medical laboratory technology, and surgical technology programs. Besides being recognized by the USDE, recognition for ABHES comes from the AAMA, American Medical Technologists (AMT), National League for Nursing Accrediting (NLNA), and National Board of Surgical Technology and Surgical Assisting (NBSTSA).

More information about ABHES can be obtained through the ABHES Web site at www.abhes.org.

ATTRIBUTES OF A MEDICAL ASSISTANT PROFESSIONAL

Medical assistants should strive to cultivate certain characteristics or personal qualities. These are the **attributes** that identify a true professional; when caring for patients, these qualities should be sincere. They will enable the patient to trust you, the caregiver. Figure 1-1 lists some of the questions you must ask yourself as you work to develop your professional attributes. As you interact with patients and colleagues, the questions listed in the figure will serve as guidelines for the

COMMUNICATION

- ☐ Do I apply active listening skills?
- ☐ Do I display professionalism through written and verbal communication?
- ☐ Do I demonstrate appropriate nonverbal communication?
- ☐ Do I explain to patients the rationale for performance of a procedure?
- ☐ Do I speak at each patient's level of understanding?
- ☐ Do I display appropriate body language?
- ☐ Do I respond honestly and diplomatically to my patients' concerns?
- ☐ Do I refrain from sharing my personal experiences?
- ☐ Do I include the patient's support system as indicated?
- ☐ Do I reassure patients of the accuracy of test results?
- ☐ Do I show sensitivity when communicating with patients regarding third party requirements?
- ☐ Does my knowledge allow me to speak easily with all members of the health care team?
- ☐ Do I accurately and concisely update the provider on any aspect of a patient's care?
- ☐ Do I utilize tactful communication skills with medical providers to ensure accurate code selection?

PRESENTATION

- ☐ Am I dressed and groomed appropriately?
- ☐ Do my actions attend to both the psychological and the physiological aspects of a patient's illness or condition?
- ☐ Am I courteous, patient, and respectful to patients?
- ☐ Do I display a positive attitude?
- ☐ Do I display a calm, professional, and caring manner?
- ☐ Do I demonstrate empathy to the patient?
- ☐ Do I show awareness of patients' concerns related to the procedure being performed?
- ☐ Do I show awareness of patients' concerns regarding a dietary change?
- ☐ Do I display sensitivity when managing appointments?

COMPETENCY

- ☐ Do I pay attention to detail?
- ☐ Do I ask questions if I am out of my comfort zone or do not have the experience to carry out tasks?
- ☐ Do I display sound judgment?
- ☐ Am I knowledgeable and accountable?
- ☐ Do I incorporate critical thinking skills in performing patient assessment and care?
- ☐ Do I recognize the implications for failure to comply with CDC regulations in health care settings?
- ☐ Do I demonstrate professionalism when discussing the patient's billing record?
- ☐ Do I display sensitivity when requesting payment for services rendered?
- ☐ Do I interact professionally with third party representatives?
- ☐ Do I recognize the physical and emotional effects on persons involved in an emergency situation?
- ☐ Do I demonstrate self-awareness in responding to an emergency situation?

INITIATIVE

- ☐ Do I show initiative?
- ☐ Have I developed a strategic plan to achieve my goals? Is my plan realistic?
- ☐ Do I seek out opportunities to expand my knowledge base?
- ☐ Am I flexible and dependable?
- ☐ Do I direct the patient to other resources when necessary or helpful, with the approval of the provider?
- ☐ Do I implement time management principles to maintain effective office function?
- ☐ Do I assist co-workers when appropriate?
- ☐ Do I make adaptations for patients with special needs?

INTEGRITY

- ☐ Do I demonstrate the principles of self-boundaries?
- ☐ Do I work within my scope of practice?
- ☐ Do I demonstrate respect for individual diversity?
- ☐ Do I demonstrate sensitivity to patient rights?
- ☐ Do I protect the integrity of the medical record?
- ☐ Do I recognize the impact personal ethics and morals have on the delivery of health care?
- ☐ Do I protect and maintain confidentiality?
- ☐ Do I immediately report any error I made?
- ☐ Do I report situations which are harmful or illegal?
- ☐ Do I maintain moral and ethical standards?
- ☐ Do I do the "right thing" even when no one is observing?

FIGURE 1-1 Medical assistants should reflect on these questions to ensure that they are embodying the characteristics and qualities of a true medical professional.

type of professional behavior that is expected from medical assistants. It is difficult to list all of the requirements for presenting the demeanor of a competent professional. Many of the aspects of professionalism are those that cannot be measured. Communication and competency can be monitored and evaluated to improve performance, but other aspects—such as presentation, initiative, and integrity—are harder to quantify. Being a professional incorporates all of these attributes. You should continue to reflect on these important aspects of professionalism as you increase your knowledge of anatomy and physiology, medical terminology, procedures, and other concrete aspects of the profession.

Communication

Communication

It is important that medical assistants learn to develop the ability to communicate well both verbally and nonverbally with patients, staff, and other professionals (see Chapter 4). Written communications must be clear and concise and reflect on the practice's professional reputation. Letters and other professional communications must utilize correct grammar, punctuation, and medical terminology.

Compliance with the provider's treatment plan is important for a positive outcome of patients' illnesses (Figure 1-2). Also, patients will feel more comfortable and less threatened in a medical clinic or ambulatory center that encourages staff to keep them informed. Consistent kindness and concern help patients develop trust in you.

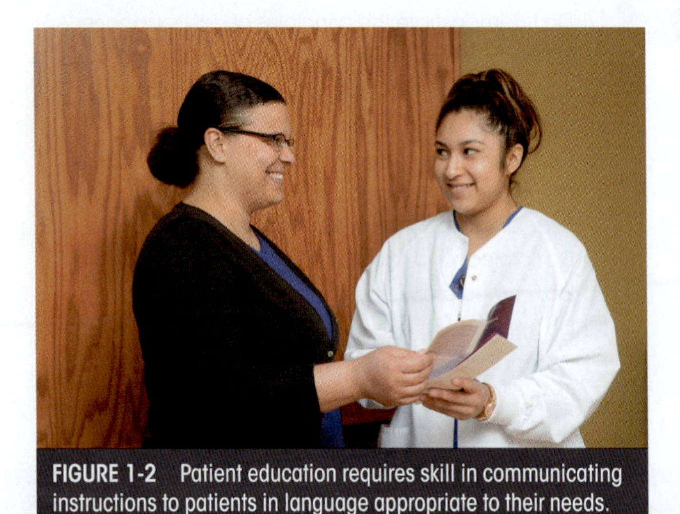

FIGURE 1-2 Patient education requires skill in communicating instructions to patients in language appropriate to their needs.

Presentation

Presentation

Presentation is the style or manner in which something is displayed. The professional medical assistant is required to present professionalism even when there is no conversation going on, no procedure being performed, and no documentation being recorded. Medical assistants should always be groomed and dressed appropriately in order to project a professional image. In addition to maintaining a professional appearance, medical assistants must also be able to communicate and interact with patients, family, and staff in an effective and constructive manner. Treating others with care and respect while displaying a positive attitude are equally important aspects of presenting a professional image.

Physical Attributes. Appearance is important in patients' perceptions of the delivery of their care. Imparting the look of a professional requires an appearance that is clean, fresh, and wholesome—in general, an appearance that reflects good health habits (Figure 1-3). Good personal hygiene practices (daily shower, deodorant), weight control, and healthy-looking skin, hair, teeth, and nails all contribute to a professional appearance. Rest, good

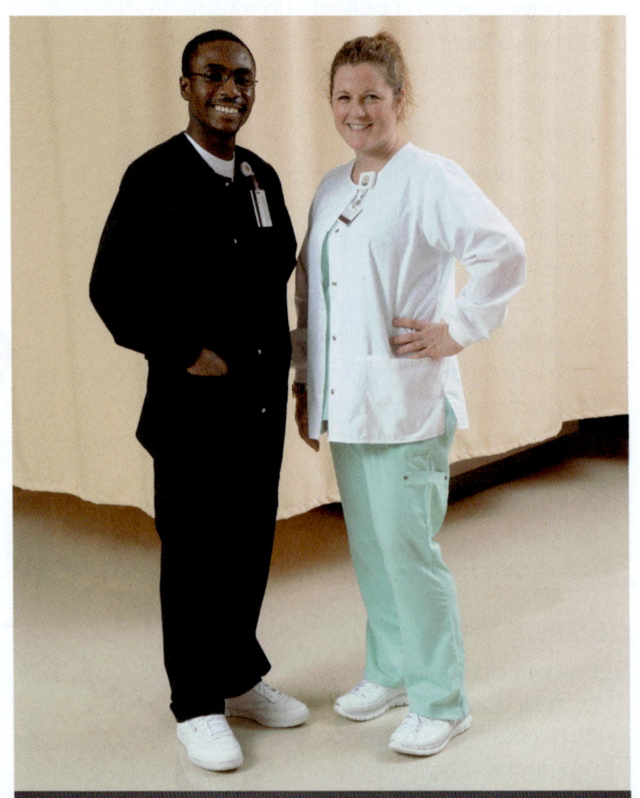

FIGURE 1-3 Medical assistants should always look very professional. Uniforms should always be crisp and clean.

nutrition, scheduled dental care, regular exercise, and recreation all promote good health. A smile can help alleviate some of the anxiety a patient may be experiencing. Your smile gives a pleasant and encouraging appearance to the patient.

Female medical assistants should wear only appropriate light daytime makeup. For the safety of both the professional and the patient, no necklaces or dangling earrings should be worn. The only jewelry worn should be single earposts or wedding rings. Hair should be neat. Fingernails should be short and manicured. Male medical assistants should be clean-shaven and have short hair. Colognes, perfumes, and aftershave should not be worn at work. Body piercings and tattoos should not be visible. There are a variety of cosmetic products manufactured specifically for the covering of visible tattoos. These cosmetics come in a variety of colors to match skin tone and are waterproof. Proper appearance instills confidence in your skills and abilities.

It is important to know and follow the appropriate dress code for your facility. The Centers for Disease Control and Prevention (CDC) recommends that artificial nails and nail extenders not be worn when caring for "high-risk" (intensive care, surgery, or dialysis) patients. Many ambulatory facilities have more stringent rules about artificial nails and extenders.

Patient care can place physical demands on medical assistants. Lifting and moving patients are often required, and the use of correct body mechanics will help minimize injuries to the back. Although every reasonable accommodation is made for medical assistants with physical challenges, it is important to be mobile without assistance because medical assistants move about throughout the day while performing tasks and procedures. It is frequently necessary to bend, stoop, kneel, and crouch, especially when filing and retrieving patients' records, as well as for other tasks. Most procedures require that medical assistants have the ability to hear and see well for the accurate completion of tasks (Figure 1-4). Listening to blood pressures, taking a medical history, observing patients, performing phlebotomy, and identifying microorganisms under a microscope are some of the routine tasks and procedures performed daily in a medical facility.

Manual **dexterity** is also needed for manipulating certain instruments, administering medications, and for entering data using a computer.

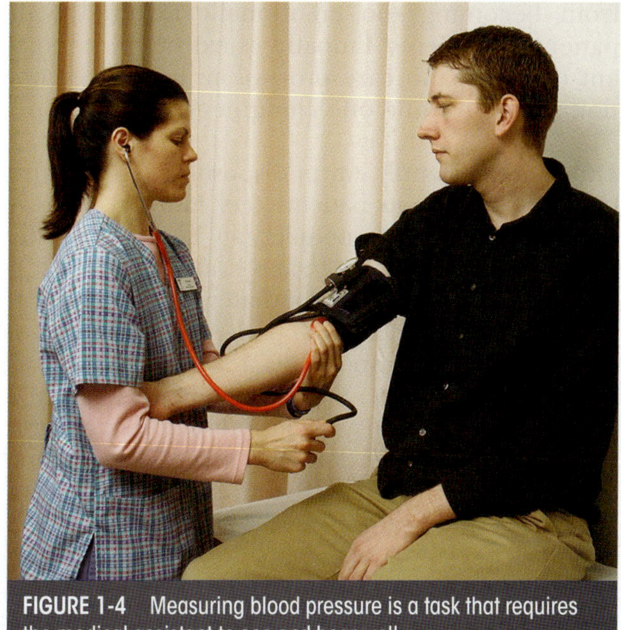

FIGURE 1-4 Measuring blood pressure is a task that requires the medical assistant to see and hear well.

Empathy. To have **empathy** means to consider the patient's welfare and to be kind. It means stepping into the patient's place, discovering what the patient is experiencing, and then recognizing and identifying with those feelings.

Medical assistants should treat patients as they themselves would want to be treated. A visit to the providers' clinic is often a time of fear and anxiety. Patients can feel vulnerable. Apprehension can be allayed tremendously when patients realize that their caregiver understands their feelings and desires to make their lives more pleasant and comfortable (Figure 1-5).

It is important to realize that patients' health problems can have a profound effect on you, the medical assistant. By maintaining a balanced outlook, medical assistants can safeguard themselves

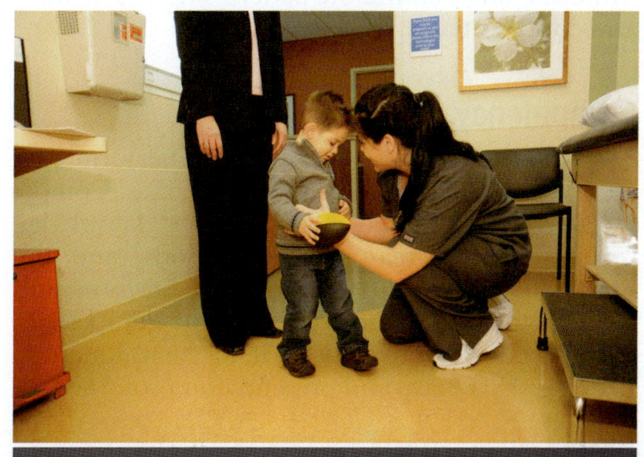

FIGURE 1-5 The medical assistant should have a friendly disposition and communicate empathy for the patient.

from becoming too emotionally involved with patients' problems. Empathy is extremely important in the health care profession; however, emotionalism can cloud one's judgment.

Attitude. A friendly, warm **disposition** and a sense of humor will help patients feel more at ease. A sincere affection for people can be conveyed by actions that **facilitate** open and honest communication. Your attitude should radiate genuine interest. Be sure that all contact with patients is positive.

An essential aspect of a good attitude is respect. Every person that enters the presence of a professional medical assistant must be treated with esteemed reverence. Patients, peers, co-workers, and other clients of the practice must be held in regard. A medical professional's willingness to show appreciation and consideration is an attitude that facilitates a positive experience for all involved. Seeking health care is a very personal experience. On the part of the medical assistant, it necessitates a respect for the patient's information, resulting care, and documentation of this care.

On occasion, difficult patients can test the tolerance level of the most experienced medical assistant because they seldom seem to be content with the care or services received. But no matter what the circumstances, patients should never be treated with disinterest or in an unfriendly manner. The medical assistant should always be pleasant and courteous.

Patients should be treated equally, with no reservations about their disease, race, religion, economic status, or sexual orientation. As a member of the health care delivery team, the medical assistant needs to be cooperative and supportive of all other members, working with the team in an honest, open manner while keeping in mind the patient's right to privacy and confidentiality.

Competency

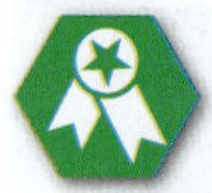

Competency is the ability to perform a set of skills on a reproducible basis. Competent medical assistants have knowledge of the reason, the methods, and the expected outcomes of the tasks they perform, and are able to execute them consistently. Competency is not just doing your job well. It is a commitment to keeping skills sharp and presentation professional.

Dependability. When providing for a patient's well-being, it is important to focus attention on activities in the office or clinic environment that will demonstrate that you are well organized, accurate, and responsive to patients' needs.

Being dependable means that the employer and coworkers rely on the medical assistant to be respectful of them, patients, and equipment and materials. Other members of the health care team will expect you to be accountable for the duties and responsibilities you undertake. A dependable person interacts with coworkers in a supportive manner, is punctual, and limits absences from work.

Flexibility. The ability to be adaptable is a trait that serves all professionals well. When caring for ill people, unexpected situations arise daily, and medical assistants must be able to respond to a variety of situations (many of them emergencies and unanticipated) without losing a sense of equilibrium. Finding solutions to problems and developing alternative action plans demonstrates flexibility. To **improvise**, or solve problems that arise either routinely or spontaneously, is a characteristic worth nurturing. Willingness to help with various aspects of the clinic offers opportunities to adjust to various situations. It shows your adaptability and willingness to respond to new circumstances.

Initiative

The willingness and ability to work independently shows initiative. A person with initiative is observant, notices work that needs to be done, and then takes action to complete those tasks without being told to do them. Employers and coworkers must be able to count on one another to anticipate patients' needs and be attentive to work that needs to be accomplished. The successful medical assistant will be ready to pitch in and recognize when others need assistance. Teamwork and a positive work ethic are valuable characteristics.

By asking appropriate questions and seeking information that will improve performance, medical assistants will demonstrate that they have the foresight and the "get up and go" needed to complete the numerous and varied tasks of the ambulatory care environment.

Desire to Learn. A willingness to continually learn and grow is the mark of a true professional. With the growing use of technology in medicine, there is an ongoing necessity for constant learning. Medical assistants must be dedicated to high standards of performance, which can be accomplished by showing a desire to acquire information and by constantly updating their knowledge and skills. Keeping abreast of the latest diseases, treatments, procedures, and techniques can be achieved in a variety of ways, such as college courses, seminars, workshops, reading, and simply by being observant. The sharper the power of observation, the more the medical assistant will learn from the provider and co-workers.

The gaining and maintaining of competency through participation in continuing education is the responsibility of every medical assistant. Active involvement and membership in the medical assistant professional organizations allows students and CMAs (AAMA) and RMAs (AMT) to participate in meetings and events that can increase professional skills. This benefits medical assistant skills as well as future careers. Students can attend medical assisting meetings (usually free of charge), enjoy student discounts, and network at the meetings.

Integrity

Integrity

Another crucial attribute of professionalism is integrity. Being honest is just one of the hallmarks of integrity. Adherence to moral and ethical principles also describes those who have integrity. The application of integrity is one of the professional characteristics that is in high demand in the profession of medical assisting. Integrity applies to every aspect of patient care, beginning with the first encounter with a patient and continuing through the end of the patient's episode of care. Integrity is not a learned trait, but rather a core personal attribute that can be nurtured and honed to become the cornerstone of one's reputation in the medical field.

Accountability. Accountability is the willingness to accept responsibility. If you reflect upon the numerous aspects of the role of an allied health care provider, you will discover that responsibility plays a key role. The medical assistant is responsible for collecting data, maintaining accurate documentation, interacting with the financial record, planning, and patient teaching, just to name a few tasks. Accountability is demonstrating the highest level of integrity when accepting the responsibility for a patient's care and management of his or her confidential information.

Ethical Behavior. No discussion about personal attributes is complete without the mention of ethics. Ethics is a system of values each individual has that determines perceptions of right and wrong. Our life experiences mold this set of values, which is considered a personal code of ethics.

Medical ethics govern medical conduct or that behavior practiced as health care providers. These ethics involve relationships with patients, their families, fellow professionals, and society in general. Ethical behavior will have a positive impact on the profession of medical assisting and on the medical community as well.

By adhering to the medical assistants' Code of Ethics, we endeavor to elevate the profession to a position of dignity and respect. Medical assistants interact on a daily basis with patients and are entrusted with information about their medical and personal histories. Such information must, by law, be kept confidential. (A more in-depth discussion of ethics and the Code of Ethics can be found in Chapter 7.)

The personal qualities of empathy, professional attitude, dependability, initiative, integrity, accountability, flexibility, the desire to learn, a wholesome physical presence, the ability to communicate well, and ethical behavior are some of the characteristics that most professionals have and that medical assistants should strive to develop. When entering into the profession of medical assisting, it is important to learn more about these and other qualities and to begin to use and refine them. Skills and knowledge alone do not guarantee success. There are personal characteristics that must go along with them.

Professional attitudes, attributes, and values are important for beginning medical assistant students to understand. Students' behaviors can impact the public's opinion of both the provider and the medical assistant profession.

The public has a right to expect that the medical assistant will be competent to practice medical assisting in accordance with the medical assistants' Code of Ethics (see Chapter 7) and with the standards and guidelines set by their professional organizations (such as AMT, AAMA, and NHA).

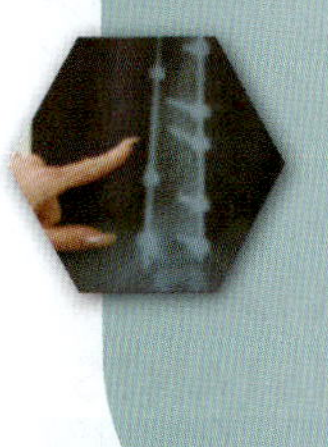

Critical Thinking

Of all the personal attributes that your text describes, which do you think is your most developed attribute? Give an example of that attribute that comes from your daily life.

AMERICAN ASSOCIATION OF MEDICAL ASSISTANTS (AAMA)

In the mid-1950s, there was a movement to form a national organization for medical assistants. The Kansas Medical Assistants Society met in Kansas City, Kansas, and accepted by vote the name American Association of Medical Assistants (AAMA) (see Figure 1-6). In 1956, this organization was supported by the American Medical Association by the passage of a resolution commending the objectives of the AAMA. By 1962, the AAMA had developed a sample certification exam, and in 1963, it offered the first certification. In order to continue to promote and gain recognition for this special set of medical assisting skills, with the collaboration of the American Medical Association, the AAMA began in 1966 to have influence over curriculum and accreditation of postsecondary levels of education. (See Chapter 23 for more information about credentialing for medical assisting.)

Certification

As the profession grew and developed, some states came to require special licensure or certification to perform certain tasks; in other states, other health professionals were challenged by the skill and broad spectrum of the medical assistant's abilities. To defend medical assistants whose right to practice clinical procedures was being challenged, the AAMA responded at their 1995 convention with the following policy:

> that any candidate for the AAMA Certification Examination be a graduate of a CAAHEP-accredited medical assisting program or a graduate of an ABHES-accredited program with one year of documented work experience. Anticipated benefits of the recommendation are to: (1) safeguard the quality of care to the consumer; (2) ensure the CMA's role in the rapidly evolving health care delivery system; and (3) continue to promote the identity and stature of the profession.

In order to sit for the CMA exam, a medical assistant must have not only completed an accredited program, they must also have a clean legal record. If a candidate for the exam has pled guilty to or been convicted of a felony, they generally are not permitted to take the CMA exam. There is a waiver that may be granted based on mitigating circumstances. A request must be submitted for waiver consideration.

Certified Medical Assistant. **Certification** is voluntary, not mandatory, for medical assistants to practice, although an increasing number of employers prefer (or even require) that their medical assistants be CMA (AAMA) certified. The examination measures professional knowledge at the job-entry level. Successful completion of the examination earns the individual the CMA (AAMA) credential (Figure 1-7). (For information on recertification, please see Chapter 23). The initials follow the individual's name. Conferring of the CMA (AAMA) status is referred to as being **credentialed**. The Certification Program of the Certifying Board of the American Association of Medical Assistants is accredited by the National Commission for Certifying Agencies (NCCA) as a result of demonstrating compliance with the *NCCA Standards for the Accreditation of Certification Programs.*

Continuing Education

The AAMA vigorously encourages continuing education for all medical assistants. This can be accomplished through various means such as educational meetings, seminars, workshops, conventions, and the AAMA's self-study publications, a series of study courses for continuing education credit.

Membership in the AAMA is trilevel: local, state, and national. Educational meetings are held regularly at local and state meetings and conventions. The annual AAMA national convention provides an

AMERICAN ASSOCIATION OF MEDICAL ASSISTANTS®

FIGURE 1-6 Logo of the AAMA, a professional organization founded in 1956.

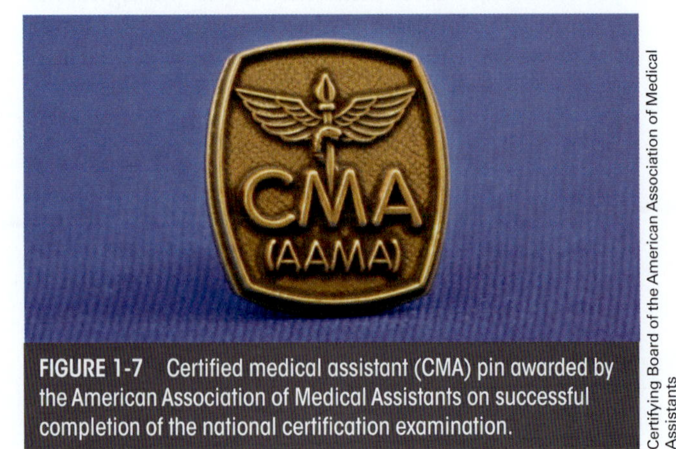

FIGURE 1-7 Certified medical assistant (CMA) pin awarded by the American Association of Medical Assistants on successful completion of the national certification examination.

excellent forum for attaining knowledge through its educational offerings and for networking with other medical assistants.

Continuing an education is a lifelong process and serves as testimony to a commitment to professionalism (see the AAMA Web site at www.aama-ntl.org).

AMERICAN MEDICAL TECHNOLOGISTS

Founded in 1939, the American Medical Technologists (AMT) is a national certification and professional membership association that represents 60,000 allied health care individuals. Its purpose is to certify and credential medical assistants, clinical laboratory personnel, allied health instructors, dental assistants, medical administrative specialists, and others. The AMT has its own bylaws, conventions, committees, state chapters, officers, and registration and certification examinations.

Registered Medical Assistant (RMA)

In 1972, the AMT established the certification examination for medical assistants. The designation of **Registered Medical Assistant (RMA [AMT])** is conferred on those individuals who successfully pass the examination (Figure 1-8).

AMT
American Medical Technologists
Certifying Excellence in Allied Health

Courtesy of the American Medical Technologists

FIGURE 1-8A AMT Logo.

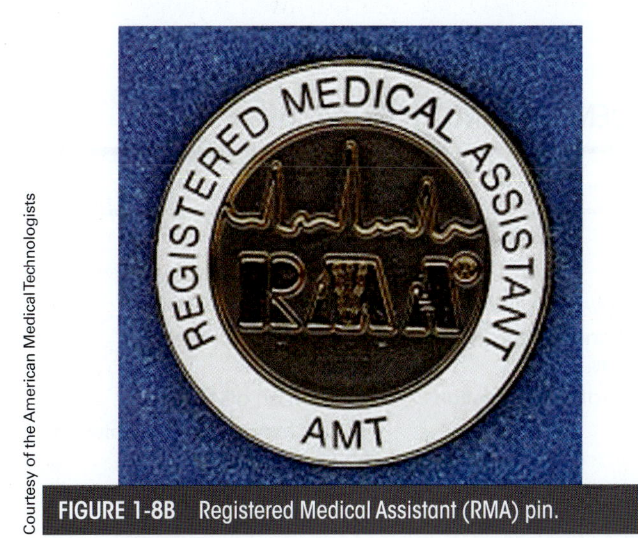

Courtesy of the American Medical Technologists

FIGURE 1-8B Registered Medical Assistant (RMA) pin.

The RMA certification examination includes general medical assisting topics, medical terminology, clinical medical assisting, medical law and ethics, human relations, administrative medical assisting, pharmacology, therapeutic modalities, laboratory procedures, electrocardiography, and first aid.

RMAs have been active in legislation to protect medical assistants, ensuring improvement in medical assistant education. American Medical Technologists advocate education and the evolution of professionalism in medical assisting.

Certified Medical Administrative Specialist (CMAS)

Another profession that the AMT certifies is the Medical Administrative Specialist (CMAS). Individuals who successfully pass the AMT certification examination are conferred with the credential of Certified Medical Administrative Specialist (CMAS). The CMAS exam is given in both computerized and paper and pencil formats.

The CMAS serves an important role in the hospital, clinic, or medical office. The CMAS is competent in a multitude of skills such as medical records management, coding and billing for insurance, practice finance management, information processing, and fundamental management practices. The CMAS also is familiar with the clinical and administrative concepts that are required to coordinate office functions in the health care setting.

Continuing Education

AMT encourages and promotes continuing education. The Certification Continuation Program (CCP) requires members to document activities that attest to their continued effort to carry the competencies needed to maintain certification. Proof of compliance is required every three years.

OTHER CERTIFICATION

National Healthcareer Association (NHA)

The National Healthcareer Association (NHA) is a certifying body for health care professionals (Figure 1-9). Its main goals are to certify and to offer continuing education course development, membership services for professionals, and a registry for certified professionals. The NHA offers

National Healthcareer Association®

National Healthcareer Association® (NHA®) is a division of Assessment Technologies Institute, L.L.C. (ATI) and use of its logo is prohibited without express written permission.

FIGURE 1-9 Logo of the National Healthcareer Association.

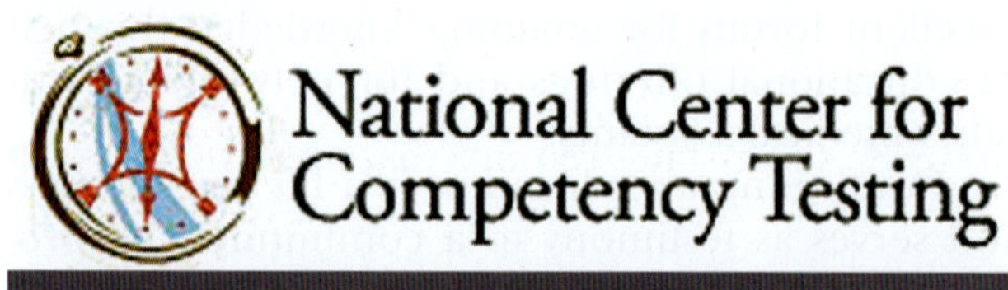

FIGURE 1-10 NCCT Logo.

Courtesy of the National Center for Competency Testing

certification for many allied health professions, including the **Certified Clinical Medical Assistant (CCMA [NHA])** and the **Certified Medical Administrative Assistant (CMAA [NHA])**.

National Center for Competency Testing (NCCT)

The National Center for Competency Testing (NCCT) (Figure 1-10) is an independent certifying body for many allied health professions, including Medical Assistant, Medical Office Assistant, and Phlebotomy Technician. There are two routes to qualify to sit for a certification exam with NCCT. These two routes are graduation from an approved educational program or qualifying work experience with the goal of validating competency.

National Certified Medical Assistant (NCMA). The NCMA certification exam is offered by the NCCT. It measures job knowledge, skills and abilities in the front and back office, general medical clinic management duties, medical procedures, and pharmacology. To assure proficiency, this exam also tests knowledge of anatomy and physiology as well as medical terminology.

REGULATION OF HEALTH CARE PROVIDERS

One way health care providers can be regulated is through the process of credentialing. Credentialing recognizes health care providers who are professionally and technically competent. Recognition comes from professional associations, certifying agencies, and the state or federal government. Regulation ensures:

- The competence of health care providers
- A minimum standard of knowledge, training, and skill
- The limiting of the performance of certain procedures to a specific occupation

Licensure, certification, and registration are three kinds of regulations/credentialing (Table 1-2).

TABLE 1-2

COMPARISON OF REQUIREMENTS FOR CERTIFICATION, LICENSURE, AND REGISTRATION

	CERTIFICATION	LICENSURE	REGISTRATION
Practice Requirement	Voluntary	Mandatory	Voluntary
Conferred by	Nongovernmental agency or professional association If qualified and meets requirements Must pass national examination	Legislated by each state If qualified and meets requirements Must pass state examination	Professional association If qualified and meets requirements Listed on an official roster Passing examination not always required
How restrictive	Used by most professionals	Most restrictive	Least restrictive

Scope of Practice

Medical assisting is not licensed as a profession; however, some states require that medical assistants be graduates of an accredited medical assisting program and be certified to work as medical assistants.

Two examples of licensed professions are medicine and nursing. A licensing body regulates the activities of these professions by enacting laws that specify educational requirements and by defining the **scope of practice**. A **license** is conferred on an individual who successfully completes specialized educational requirements and successfully passes an examination administered by the state in which the individual resides. The state grants a license to that individual to practice medicine or nursing. Licensure is mandatory and forbids anyone who is not licensed from performing activities that are designated by that particular license. For example, the law states that the medical license allows diagnosing and prescribing treatment. If someone were to diagnose or prescribe without a medical license, that individual would be committing an illegal act and would be practicing medicine without a license, which is considered a felony.

There are state laws that govern the practice of medicine and nursing (medical practice acts, nursing practice acts), and many states have acts that give providers the right to delegate certain clinical procedures to qualified allied health professionals. Because medical assistants are not required to be licensed, they can become certified voluntarily. They are allowed to perform clinical procedures only under the supervision of the provider or other licensed health care professional who is granted that right and who delegates the specific clinical procedures to the medical assistants.

In some states, including California, Washington, and others, unlicensed health care providers are required to have authorization from the state to perform allergy testing and venipuncture and to give injections. A registration fee and mandatory training are required. In such circumstances, medical assistants or other health care providers would be breaking the law if they performed these procedures without registration and training. In some states, authorization is required for unlicensed health care providers to expose patients to X-rays. It is essential that you research your state's scope of practice for medical assistants.

There has been an effort by the U.S. Senate to introduce legislation that would require additional education and credentialing for health care professionals that provide radiologic imaging and radiation therapy. Initially introduced in 2007, the Consistency, Accuracy, Responsibility and Excellence in Medical Imaging or Radiation Therapy (CARE) bill was sent to the Subcommittee on Health in April 2013. Since that time, there has been no further action on the bill.

The AAMA supports legislation that would require specific educational and certification standards for individuals performing medical imaging. Medical assistants do not perform procedures for which they have not been educated and in which they are not proficient. The AAMA's Occupational Analysis for the CMA (AAMA) (which can be accessed at www.aama-nlt.org) and the AMT's Medical Assisting Task List (which can be accessed at www.americanmedtech.org) are excellent reference sources that identify the clinical, administrative, and general procedures medical assistants are educated to perform. However, because of the variability of state statutes, the medical assistant would be wise to check with the AAMA or AMT if in doubt about the legality of certain clinical procedures.

The AMT and the AAMA (the two leading organizations that certify medical assistants) agreed on a model state law outlining the medical assistant's scope of practice. Both the AMT and AAMA took from existing state laws regarding medical assistants' right to practice the most important aspects of these and developed the model. Both organizations agreed to require a medical assistant to graduate from an accredited medical assistant program and to obtain certification from AMT, AAMA, or other approved agencies that certify. A nonexclusive list of functions that a supervised medical assistant may perform was developed. The purpose of the model state legislation is to protect the medical assistant's right to practice. A copy of the model legislation is available at state medical assistant societies.

As the scope of medical assisting practice expands and diversifies, there are many questions regarding state-by-state legislation. Resources to answer these questions are available at www.aama-ntl.org.

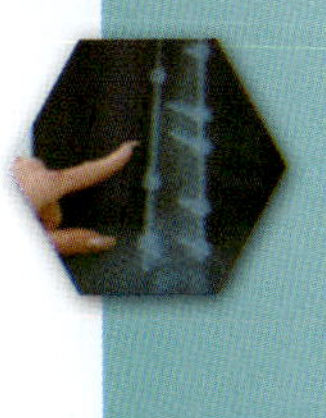

Critical Thinking

A medical assistant relates to a patient on the telephone that her symptoms are "probably the flu" and to "take over-the-counter cough syrup" for her cough. Is this an appropriate or inappropriate action for the medical assistant to take? Discuss your answer and explain why you came to your decision.

CASE STUDY 1-1

Refer to the scenario at the beginning of the chapter.

CASE STUDY REVIEW

1. If you were a freshman in high school and interested in medical assisting, would you like to have an opportunity to visit a program and tour the classroom and laboratories? Why or why not?
2. List three or four questions you might ask of the senior medical assistant students while you are touring the medical assisting department that would help to clarify what the profession is, the course requirements, etc.

Summary

- Progress has been made in the advancement of the profession of medical assisting since the first group of medical assistants gathered to become organized and formed the AAMA and the AMT.
- The total number of medical assistants in the work force is nearly 600,000, and employment opportunities continue to grow.
- The AAMA, AMT, and NHA continue to promote standards of excellence for their members, encouraging continuing education and awarding continuing education credits to members of AAMA, AMT, and NHA via various means.
- Becoming a professional is a gradual process and cannot be learned in its entirety from a textbook.
- The challenge of becoming a professional medical assistant will require open-mindedness and a desire for continued learning and education, certification and recertification of the professional credential, and professional involvement through organizational participation.
- As the scope of work done by medical assistants broadens and medical assistants seek and require formal education, the professional medical assistant will gain additional respect and be in even greater demand.
- Medical assistants must continuously pursue excellence, which is the hallmark of all professional behavior.

Study for Success

To reinforce your knowledge and skills of information presented in this chapter:

- Review the *Key Terms* and *Learning Outcomes*
- Consider the *Critical Thinking* features and *Case Studies* and discuss your conclusions
- Answer the questions in the *Certification Review*

CERTIFICATION REVIEW

1. Which of the following has resulted in an increase in employment opportunities for medical assistants?
   a. The volume of paperwork
   b. Managed care's emphasis on ambulatory care
   c. Baby boomers beginning to retire
   d. All of these
2. Which professional organization awards the CMAS designation?
   a. AAMA
   b. ABHES
   c. AMA
   d. AMT
   e. CAAHEP

3. Which of the following is the definition of ethics?
   a. A system of values each individual has that determines perceptions of right and wrong
   b. A code established by an agency that has nothing to do with the medical assistant's belief in right or wrong
   c. Making patients more comfortable
   d. Willingness to work as a team member
4. Which of the following describes accreditation?
   a. Meeting appropriate standards
   b. Obtaining the CMA (AAMA) or RMA (AMT) credential
   c. Being listed on an official roster
   d. Having a curriculum with courses that are unrestricted
   e. Sitting for an examination that proves mastery of a body of knowledge
5. Which of the following describes licensure?
   a. It is voluntary and up to the individual practitioner.
   b. It is unrestrictive in scope.
   c. It is conferred on an individual through a non-government agency.
   d. It is mandatory and legislated by states.
6. Medical assistants possess a skill set that is appropriate for which of the following settings?
   a. Provider's clinics
   b. Urgent care clinics
   c. Insurance companies
   d. Hospitals
   e. All of these
7. Benefits of a medical assistant practicum or externship include which of the following?
   a. Receiving a paycheck for experience gained
   b. Obtaining references for future employment
   c. Improving performance and knowledge
   d. Both b and c
8. Which of the following statements is true?
   a. Medical assisting is a licensed profession.
   b. Medical assistants must obtain an associate's degree.
   c. Medical assistants are governed by state laws.
   d. Medical assistants have mandatory certification.
   e. Medical assistants may perform any procedures that nurses can.
9. Which of the following is a true statement regarding the American Association of Medical Assistants (AAMA)?
   a. It provides certification for Registered Medical Assistant (RMA).
   b. It was the first national organization for medical assisting.
   c. It defined the occupation of medical assisting.
   d. Both b and c
10. Which of the following are attributes of the professional medical assistant?
   a. Communication skills
   b. Integrity
   c. Empathy
   d. Initiative
   e. All of these

CHAPTER 2

Health Care Settings and the Health Care Team

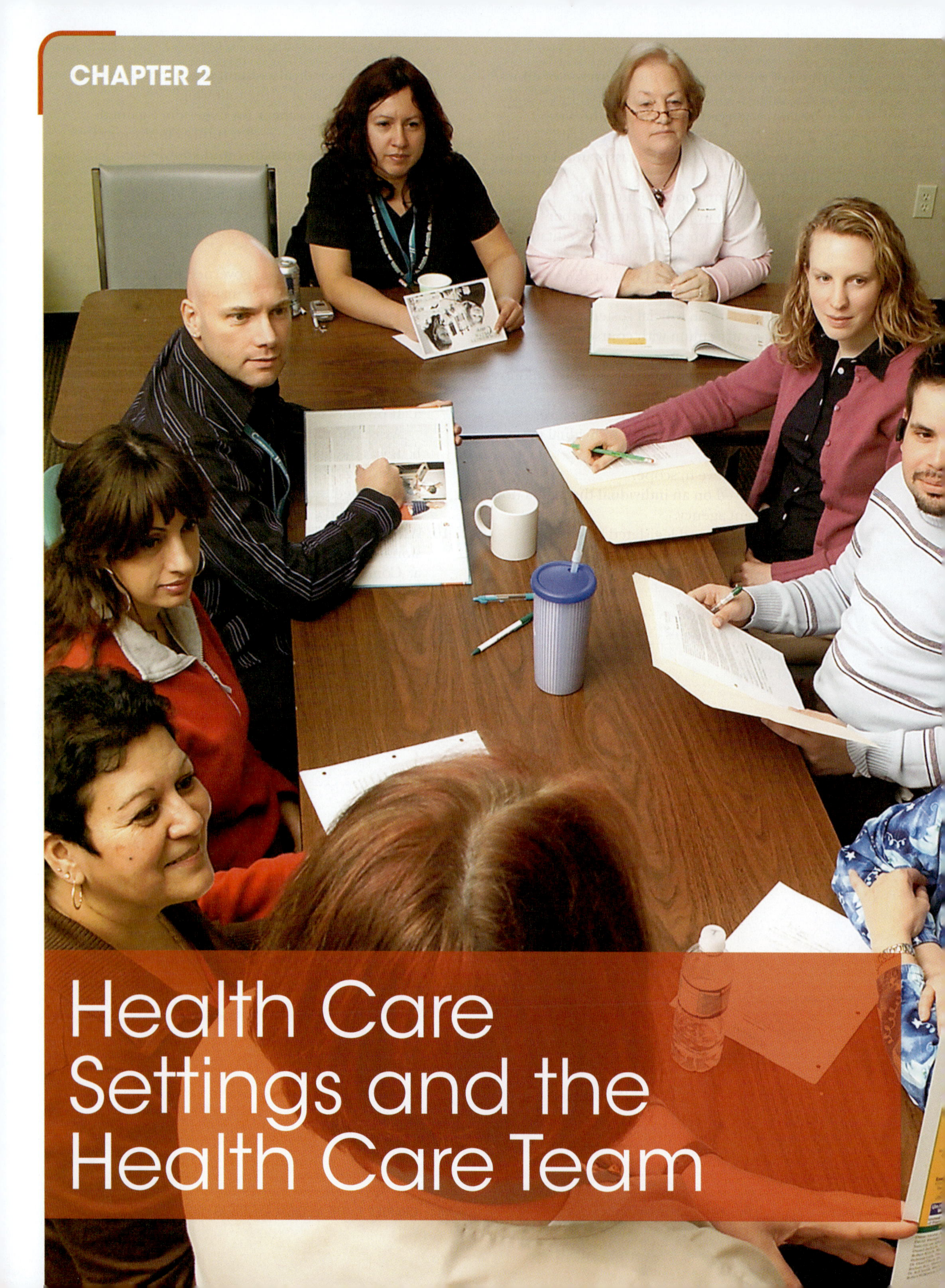

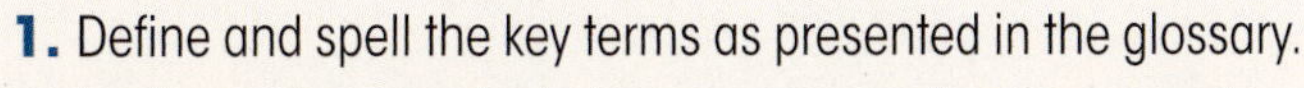

LEARNING OUTCOMES

1. Define and spell the key terms as presented in the glossary.
2. Critique the three primary medical management models.
3. Analyze the benefits and limitations of working in the different ambulatory health care settings.
4. Assess the role of managed care in the health care environment.
5. Compare the patient-centered medical home to accountable care organizations.
6. Describe the function of the health care team.
7. List and describe a minimum of 12 health care providers.
8. Research a minimum of three complementary health care specialists.
9. Compare a minimum of 12 allied health professionals.
10. Discuss the role of the medical assistant in ambulatory health care.
11. Critique complementary and alternative therapies and discuss their role in today's health care setting.
12. Comment on the value of the medical assistant to the health care team.

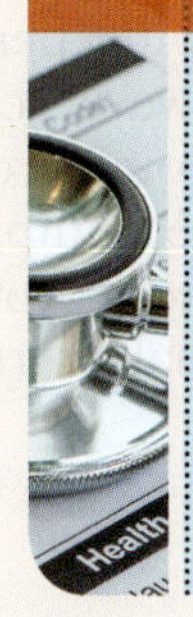

KEY TERMS

accountable care organization (ACO)
acupuncture
ambulatory care setting
complementary and alternative medicine (CAM)
health maintenance organization (HMO)
homeopathy
independent provider association (IPA)
integrative medicine
managed care operation
patient-centered medical home (PCMH)
preferred provider organization (PPO)

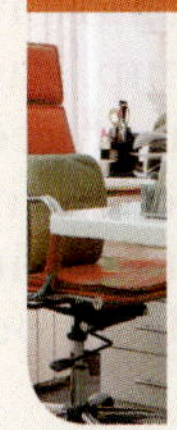

SCENARIO

You always had thought you wanted to be a medical assistant and work in a clinic where you would see a variety of patients. But after discussing this chapter in class, you are really intrigued with becoming a physical therapy assistant and want to investigate the profession further. What kind of research can you do to make certain you have chosen the right path? Consider working hours, rate of pay, patient contact, required schooling and attributes of professionalism, and job availability.

Chapter Portal

There are few professions in our society as rich and complex as the health care profession. Particularly in recent years, the health care environment has changed radically and continues to evolve as the profession seeks ways to provide quality care while containing costs. The Affordable Care Act that became law in March 2010 was created to address unsustainable health care spending, to enhance the "preventive" model of health care coverage, to reduce the high uninsured rate and health disparities across demographic lines, and to hopefully improve health outcomes for our nation's citizens.

Even before the Affordable Care Act was passed, the effort to curtail costs resulted in the rise of managed care, which, in turn, spawned a number of medical models such as **health maintenance organizations (HMOs)** and **preferred provider organizations (PPOs)**.

Many other types of networks and alliances are also being established as providers merge to give patients the best of care while controlling their costs. **Ambulatory care settings**, where services are

continues

Chapter Portal, continued

provided on an outpatient basis, are the focus of this text, but note that outpatient care is provided via many and varied avenues. Hospitals more frequently provide outpatient care as it has become more common for patients to appear at the emergency department (ED) for routine ailments when they have nowhere else to go. Large retail stores such as Walmart, Target, and CVS have also entered the field of outpatient care through their walk-in clinics. These retail sites, commonly staffed by nurse practitioners, provide routine medical services for a set fee.

Just as the medical setting continues to evolve to meet new societal needs, health care technology is ever changing. Health care is a dynamic, stimulating industry that requires the medical assistant and other professionals to constantly develop new skills if they are to contribute to the team effort. The range of skills within the health care team is astonishing and includes providers in more than 30 specialties, an increasing number of nontraditional complementary/integrative practitioners, and more than 20 kinds of allied health professionals.

AMBULATORY HEALTH CARE SETTINGS

Although medical assistants work in a number of different environments, including laboratories and hospitals, most are employed in an ambulatory care setting such as a medical clinic (either a solo provider or group practice), an urgent or primary care center, or a managed care organization where they give outpatient care.

Often, the medical assistant chooses to work in one setting rather than another based on interests, personality, and work preferences. For instance, the individual practice may provide medical assistants with the opportunity to use their full array of skills, whereas in larger group practices, the work of the medical assistant is often more specialized in nature.

It is helpful if medical assistants recognize the three major and basic forms of medical practice management and how they affect salary, benefits, and liability issues (Figure 2-1).

Medical assistants employed in ambulatory care settings or medical clinics are likely to see three major forms of medical practice management or a combination of three: sole proprietorships, partnerships, and corporations.

Sole Proprietorships

In the past, many providers preferred a solo practice. A solo practice entitles the sole proprietor to hold exclusive right to all aspects of the medical practice or sole proprietorship, including profits and debts. If the business fails, the sole proprietor's personal property may also be attached. As a self-employed sole proprietor, health and dental insurance is a deductible expense. A sole proprietorship may employ other providers to participate in the practice. Any employed providers are entitled to any employee fringe benefits such as health insurance and paid vacation, also.

The sole proprietor sees and treats all patients. Although this type of arrangement is limited in the number of people it can serve, many patients feel secure in this kind of health care setting because they come to know and trust their provider, and they feel their health care is being managed in a personal way. The sole proprietor practice, however, can be an expensive arrangement, because one provider must undertake the costs of clinic space, equipment, and personnel. Today, the majority of solo providers are found in many of the nontraditional alternative or complementary medical practices.

Partnerships

When two or more providers join together under a legal agreement to share in the total business operations of the practice, a partnership is formed. Several providers who share a facility and practice medicine are often referred to as a group. Partners share income, expenses, debt, equipment, records, and personnel according to a predetermined agreement. Partners are liable for only their own actions but may be liable for the whole amount of the partnership debts.

Professional Corporations

Providers may form a corporation, usually referred to as a professional service corporation. The shareholders are considered employees of the corporation. A corporation allows income and tax advantages to all employees. A variety of fringe benefits can be offered to the employees, which may include pension; profit-sharing plans; medical expense reimbursement; and life, health, and disability insurance. These benefits are separate from salary. Another advantage is that professional employees of a corporation are liable only for their own acts, and personal property cannot be attached in litigation. A sole proprietor may incorporate if the practice is large enough.

FORMS OF MEDICAL PRACTICE MANAGEMENT			
	Sole Proprietor	**Partnership**	**Professional Corporation**
Ease of Formation	Very Easy	Written agreement is helpful	Articles of Incorporation
Management	Owner	Often divided among partners	Board of Directors
Number of Owners	One	Unlimited	State law dictates
Owner Liability	Unlimited	Unlimited if general partner; investment is determined for limited partners	Limited to investment
Allocation of Income	100% to owner	Based on partnership agreement	Normally based on per share/per day rule
Retirement Plans	Any retirement plan	Any retirement plan; must be established by partnership; contributions are deductible by partner	Keogh plans not allowed; deductible at corporate level

FIGURE 2-1 Different forms of medical practice management.

Group Practices

Corporations or group practices are attractive arrangements where providers can share the costs of space, equipment, and personnel. The advantages of a group practice, however, are not solely economic; providers learn from and consult one another, and patients receive the benefit of this exchange of information and knowledge. Often, a group practice has more than one clinic, and some employees are asked to travel between sites to cut overhead. Group practices may be formed to offer specialized care, such as oncology or women's health care.

In many group practices, patients may request that they see the same provider for all appointments, although sometimes patients are assigned to the next available provider. For emergencies, group practices have the staff and flexibility to ensure that there is always a provider on call.

Many providers in small groups turn to large practice management firms, seeking to decrease the time spent managing the business side of their practice. These services often include coding, billing, collecting, or the complete financial management of a practice, and even human resource management. Such a plan is designed to allow providers and their medical assistants more time in patient care activities and less time in paper processing. The health maintenance organization (HMO) is one type of corporation in which providers often practice. Basically, providers are employees of the HMO and are paid by various methods; providers in the HMO usually serve as the primary care provider (PCP). In this situation, a referral from the PCP may be necessary before a patient can see a specialist or allied health professional.

Whatever form of management is chosen by providers, they are responsible for the employees that serve with them. (Refer to the discussion of *respondeat superior* in Chapter 6.) Employers and their medical assistants must have the kind of healthy working relationship where mutual trust and respect are apparent. The provider must understand the skill level of the medical assistant, and the medical assistant must feel secure enough to ask any necessary questions or admit any errors. Critical errors are often made when this trust does not exist between employer and employee. This causes a breakdown in the delivery of the best health care for patients.

Urgent Care Centers

Urgent care centers are usually private, for-profit centers that provide services for primary care, routine injuries and illnesses, and minor surgery. Sometimes laboratory services and a radiology department are located on the premises. The number of urgent care centers in the United States is estimated to be between 7,000 and 9,000, depending upon the inclusion of walk-in care clinics. Providers and other health care professionals in the center are often salaried employees, not owners who share in the profits, and some are associated with other medical facilities, sometimes even hospitals.

The pace in many urgent care centers is brisk, and typically a number of providers are working at one time. Patients are usually encouraged to make appointments, but drop-ins are accepted, so long as providers are available. Serious emergencies are still referred to the emergency department. As mentioned earlier, certain retail chain stores, including Walmart, Target, and CVS, have entered into this market. All over the country, there are walk-in urgent care chains such as Concentra and U.S. Healthworks providing patient care. According to the Urgent Care Association of America, an estimated 3 million patients visit these centers each week. About 25% of patients who patronize these locations have a primary care provider (PCP), but feel they can be seen quicker in this environment. It is also estimated that close to 25% of urgent care patients are uninsured and are required to pay cash for their services. Insurance may be accepted, but most of the centers do not accept Medicaid.

Because these centers often see a higher volume of patients during expanded hours (often 10 AM to 10 PM, 365 days of the year), usually for a lower cost than a hospital emergency department, urgent care centers have continued to grow in popularity. This increase in popularity is also partly due to patients who are used to doing their banking 24/7 seeking greater accessibility in their health care as well.

Managed Care Operations

Health maintenance organizations, or HMOs, are a common **managed care operation**. Originally, HMOs were designed to provide a full range of health care services under one roof. Today, the "HMO without walls" is more common and typically consists of a network of participating providers within a defined geographic area.

Originally, the HMO with walls was conceived to provide patients with comprehensive health care services at one facility. Today, as managed care and managed competition sweep through the health care industry, other arrangements include the preferred provider organization (PPO), where providers network to offer discounts to employers and other purchasers of health insurance, and the **independent provider association (IPA)**, the members of which agree to treat patients for an agreed-upon fee.

"Boutique" or "Concierge" Medical Practices

According to the American Academy of Family Physicians, there are now more than 12,000 "boutique" or "concierge" practices in the United States that are growing in popularity with both patients and providers. Providers who are discouraged by their shrinking insurance reimbursements and by managed care plans dictating what procedures and tests will be performed have turned to another avenue for providing health care. Patients who are disappointed in the quality of care received and frustrated by being bounced from one insurer to another as employers seek a cost reduction in their health care benefits are increasingly willing to pay the extra amount for the concierge care.

Concierge care generally offers patients the following services for a monthly or annual fee:

- Immediate access to their provider by phone 24 hours a day, 7 days a week
- Convenient and unhurried same-day appointments
- Unlimited email, fax, or phone consultation with the provider
- Home or work visits as needed
- Coordination of specialist referrals
- Friendly staff who understand each patient's unique health needs
- Free parking, luxury robes, shower facilities, and Internet access

There are two main types of concierge practices—retainer-based (concierge) and direct primary care (DPC). Neither of these have co-pays, deductibles, or co-insurance fees. About 80% of providers offering concierge service will accept insurance in their practice. DPCs do not accept insurance.

Patients who choose this type of service pay a set fee per year from $2,000 to $3,000 for one individual, and up to $5,000 to include a spouse or $6,000 to include children. Patients are expected

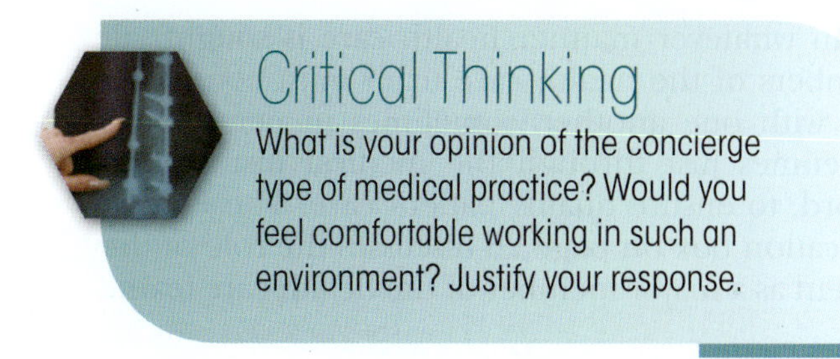

Critical Thinking

What is your opinion of the concierge type of medical practice? Would you feel comfortable working in such an environment? Justify your response.

to carry a major medical plan to cover referrals to specialists, hospitalization, and emergency care.

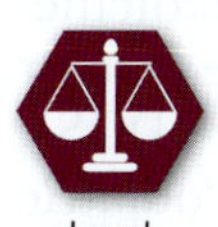
Legal

Ethical concerns have been raised regarding concierge services. Some say the "extra" services should be available to everyone; others believe the extra fees make the service very exclusive. There is concern that today's decreasing number of PCPs is only made worse when providers choose a concierge-type service over the traditional model of care, sometimes leaving as many as 2,000 patients to find a new PCP. There is speculation that concierge providers also hand-pick the healthiest patients for their service, leaving the sicker patients to be absorbed in traditional health care. Legal concerns surface also. For instance, those concierge providers who accept insurance run into issues with federal Medicare laws that prohibit charging recipients more than the allowable amount. They often turn to the DPC model of not accepting any type of insurance. Also, patients making a decision to embrace concierge medical care must realize that fees paid to these providers are not tax deductible as are fees paid to providers in the traditional model of health care.

Providers practicing in a concierge service report a greater satisfaction with their chosen profession, enjoy really getting to know their patients, and serve a few hundred patients rather than a few thousand as are seen in a traditional practice. Patients report satisfaction with receiving more time and personal care from a provider who determines the best options for maintaining their health.

Patient-Centered Medical Home (PCMH)

In the continuing effort to provide the best of medical care to the largest number of individuals, another model has surfaced. The **patient-centered medical home (PCMH)** is a model that listens to what patients want and seeks to provide better quality, experience, and cost. Presently more than 15% of PCP practices are recognized as PCMHs by the National Committee for Quality Assurance (NCQA). To be recognized by NCQA, practices must meet rigid standards for addressing patient needs. These include the following:

- After-hours and online access to providers
- Long-term relationships established in team-based care
- Patients seen as partners in health and health care decision making
- Higher quality and experience of care
- Reduced emergency department and hospital care, reducing costs

PCMH transformation is not without difficulty, however. A long-term commitment is required of each team member and a significant financial investment is involved. The goals of PCMHs are admirable. These goals include the best possible care being given to patients and coordination with better prevention methods to reduce emergency department and hospital care. PCPs give "whole" person care at the first contact, and every person in the practice is respectful and responsive to patients' individual needs. It is hoped that all this will bring greater satisfaction to providers, making their PCMH medical practice more successful.

In the future, the hope is for PCMHs to expand to include a medical neighborhood of specialists and hospitals, with practitioners of behavioral health, mental health, public health, and worksite/retail clinics and pharmacies. The Department of Defense is transforming its primary care practices into NCQA PCMHs. The Department of Health and Human Services is assisting community health centers in becoming recognized. Congress is looking toward legislation to move Medicare into support of PCMHs nationwide with new payment systems. Currently, 37 states have public and private PCMHs recognized by NCQA.

The road to success for the PCHM model, however, is a bumpy one. Many providers balk at the detailed assessment of practice capabilities and processes required for NCQA certification. Measuring patients' experiences, the original and ongoing cost of PCMH recognition, and on-site patient surveys are problematic. Providers, already bogged down in the paperwork required for insurance reimbursement and patient record-keeping, resist the addition of any program that requires more paperwork and valuable time. Other providers argue that the goals of PCMH practices are no different from what the goals of every medical facility ought to be right now, even without the NCQA recognition.

Accountable Care Organization (ACO)

Another model for health care is known as the **accountable care organization (ACO)**, which was launched in 2012. The ACO is much like the PCMH practices in its goals. An ACO is a network of providers and hospitals that agree to manage all the health care needs for a group of patients. For example, under the Affordable Care Act, an ACO would agree to provide health care for a minimum of 5,000 Medicare beneficiaries for at least three years. ACOs are intended to reduce health care costs by creating savings incentives, offering bonuses to providers who keep costs down or meet certain benchmarks, focusing on prevention of illness, and carefully managing patients with chronic illnesses. ACOs are similar to HMOs, except that patients in ACOs can and often do receive treatment outside the network.

ACOs have similar problems as the PCMH model. In addition, there is often concern about who is in charge—hospitals, providers, or insurers? In most cases, the answer to that question depends upon where and how the ACO was organized. There is also the concern that in a rural area, the ACO might grow so large that all the providers in the region are involved, often eliminating choice for patients.

THE HEALTH CARE TEAM

In every kind of health care setting, the team concept is critical to the quality of patient care. A PCP is most likely the main source of health care for patients. From time to time, however, a specialist is sought or recommended. A number of different allied health professionals, including the medical assistant, supply additional health care as ordered by the provider. Increasingly, patients are looking outside traditional medicine for portions of their health care. The Centers for Disease Control and Prevention's (CDC) National Health Interview Survey revealed that 38% of adults in the United States use some form of CAM care. The percentage is higher for those persons 50 years and older. The survey also indicated greater use of **complementary and alternative medicine (CAM)** among women and individuals with higher education. In 2012, the World Health Organization (WHO) estimated that between 65% and 80% of the world's population relied on alternative medicine as their primary health care source. Most medical schools in the United States now have courses in CAM. Although CAM care is not always covered by medical insurance, traditional and nontraditional health care practices are nonetheless blending in many areas. Today, many practitioners recognize the benefits of merging the traditional with some of the nontraditional therapies found in complementary medicine; this is recognized as integrative medical care.

In whatever manner health care is sought, all members of the health care team must communicate with one another, sometimes in person and sometimes just through the medical history and record, to ensure quality patient care. The Patient Education box on page 28 discusses the role of the patient as a major member of the health care team.

The Title *Doctor*

The public is often confused by the title *doctor.* The term implies an earned academic degree of the highest level in a particular area of study. Physicians have earned the MD, or Doctor of Medicine, degree. Other medical degrees include the Doctor of Osteopathy (DO), Doctor of Dentistry (DDS), Doctor of Optometry (OD), Doctor of Podiatric Medicine (DPM), Doctor of Chiropractic (DC), and Doctor of Naturopathy (ND). In the medical field, the abbreviation *Dr.* is used and the title *doctor* is used to address these individuals qualified by education, training, and licensure to practice medicine.

In nonmedical disciplines, persons who have achieved a doctorate conferred by a college or university include the Doctor of Education (EdD), the Doctor of Philosophy (PhD), and the Doctor of Psychology (PSYD). All three have several areas of specialty and are referred to as *doctor.*

Health Care Professionals and Their Roles

Doctor of Medicine. A doctorate degree in medicine and a license to practice allows a person to diagnose and treat medical conditions. The doctor of medicine candidate attends four years of medical school after receiving a bachelor's degree. Newly graduated MDs enter into a residency program that consists of three to seven years of additional training and education depending on the specialty chosen. This residency comes under the direct supervision of senior medical doctor educators. Family practice, internal medicine, and pediatrics each require a three-year residency; general surgery requires a five-year residency. Some refer to the first year of residency as an internship; however, the American Medical Association (AMA) no longer uses this term. At this point, many medical doctors choose to be board certified, which is optional and voluntary. Certification assures the public that the doctor's knowledge, experience, and skills in a particular specialty area have been tested and he or she has been deemed qualified to provide care in that specialty. Doctors of medicine can be certified through 24 specialty medical boards and in 88 subspecialty fields. Table 2-1 gives a partial listing of these fields.

TABLE 2-1

SELECTED MEDICAL AND SURGICAL SPECIALTIES

SPECIALTIES	TITLE OF DOCTOR	DESCRIPTION
Allergy and Immunology	Allergist and Immunologist	Evaluates diseases/disorders of the immune system and problems related to asthma and allergy
Anesthesiology	Anesthesiologist	Evaluates sleep and pain control
Cardiology	Cardiologist	Evaluates and treats medical conditions of the heart
Dermatology	Dermatologist	Evaluates disorders/diseases of skin, hair, nails, and related tissues
Emergency Medicine	Emergency Medical Doctor	Evaluates and treats medical conditions that result from trauma or sudden illness; manages the emergency department
Family Medicine	Family Practitioner	Treats the whole family from infancy to death
General Surgery	Surgeon	Operates to repair or remove diseased or injured parts of the body
Colon and Rectal Surgery	Colorectal Surgeon	Operates to remove or repair diseased colon and rectal areas of the body
Neurological Surgery	Neurosurgeon	Treats conditions of the nervous systems, often through surgery
Plastic Surgery	Plastic Surgeon	Repairs and reconstructs physical defects; provides cosmetic enhancements
Thoracic Surgery	Thoracic Surgeon	Performs surgery on the respiratory system, chest, heart, and cardiovascular system
Internal Medicine	Internist	Provides comprehensive care, practices preventive care, and treats long-term and chronic conditions
Medical Genetics and Genomics	Geneticist	Provides information in medical and genetic pathology
Nuclear Medicine	Doctor of Nuclear Medicine	Evaluates molecular and metabolic conditions using radiopharmaceuticals
Obstetrics and Gynecology	Obstetrician and Gynecologist	Provides care to pregnant women, delivers babies, and treats disorders/diseases of the female reproductive system
Ophthalmology	Ophthalmologist	Provides comprehensive care of the eye and its structures and offers vision services
Orthopedic Surgery	Orthopedist	Examines, diagnoses, and treats diseases and injuries of the musculoskeletal system
Otolaryngology	Otolaryngologist	Treats diseases/disorders of the ears, nose, and throat
Pathology	Pathologist	Evaluates body tissues
Pediatrics	Pediatrician	Treats diseases/disorders of children and adolescents; monitors growth and development of children
Physical Medicine and Rehabilitation	Doctor of Physical Medicine and Rehabilitation	Evaluates pain, orders rehabilitation, and practices sports medicine
Preventative Medicine	Doctor	Encourages healthy living

continues

Table 2-1 continued

SPECIALTIES	TITLE OF DOCTOR	DESCRIPTION
Psychiatry and Neurology	Psychiatrist and Neurologist	Diagnoses and treats patients with mental, emotional, or behavioral disorders as well as disorders of the brain and central nervous system
Radiology	Radiologist	Interprets diagnostic images, performs special procedures, and manages radiological services
Urology	Urologist	Treats diseases/disorders of the urinary tract

Medical doctors must still obtain a license to practice medicine from the state or jurisdiction of the United States in which they are planning to practice. They apply for the permanent license after completing a series of examinations and completing a minimum number of years of graduate medical education. Medical doctors must continue to receive a certain number of continuing medical education (CME) requirements each year to ensure that their knowledge and skills are current. CME requirements vary by state, professional organizations, and hospital staff organizations. Medical assistants are often required to maintain their employer's CME records for easier reporting at the time of license renewal.

Doctor of Osteopathy. Osteopaths are generally recognized as equal to medical doctors in all respects. The Doctor of Osteopathy, or DO, is a fully qualified provider licensed to perform surgery and prescribe medication. The training and education are quite similar to that of the MD. Osteopathic medicine was established in 1874 by Dr. Andrew Taylor Still, who was one of the first practitioners to study the attributes of good health to better understand the process of disease. He identified the musculoskeletal system as a key element of health and encouraged preventive medicine, eating properly, and keeping fit. The education of an osteopath includes a four-year undergraduate degree plus four years of medical school. After graduation from medical school, a DO can choose to practice in any of the 18 American Osteopathic Association specialty areas, requiring from two to six years of additional training. Approximately 65% of all osteopaths practice in primary care areas such as family practice, pediatrics, obstetrics/gynecology, and internal medicine. DOs must pass a state licensure examination and maintain currency in their education. Most patients find little difference between an MD and a DO. However, doctors of osteopathy can incorporate osteopathic manipulative treatment (OMT) in their treatment of patients as deemed helpful.

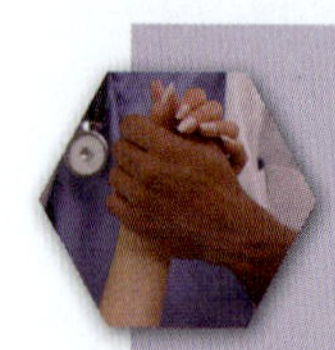

Patient Education

Continually remind your patients of the important role they play in their own health care. *Only your patients* know exactly what happens to their bodies and minds in any particular illness. *Only your patients* know if their pain is too much to bear. *Only your patients* know whether they will remain on any treatment regimen that has been established. *Only your patients* know if they are already embracing some alternative form of treatment. *Only your patients* know how much financial burden they can handle for health care. In initial interviews and preprovider preparations, ask your patients questions that encourage them to tell you what is happening, whether they are coping, and how their particular problem affects their daily lives. Listen to them carefully. Do not rush or second-guess their responses. Be mindful of the special needs of older adult patients and individuals for whom English is their second language. They are likely to be unfamiliar with taking a major role in their own health care. Always remember to be therapeutic and observe nonverbal cues. Empower your patients to be a member of their own health care team.

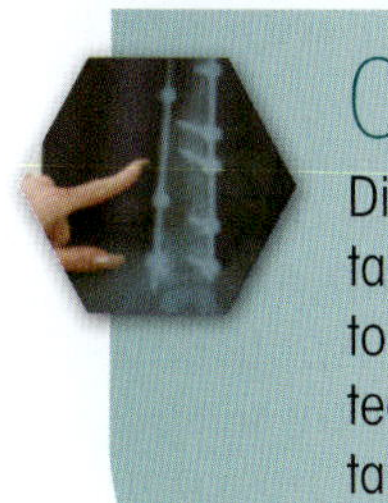

Critical Thinking

Discuss with a peer what action might be taken when patients refuse all opportunities to be a member of their own health care team. How might you encourage patients to take even a small part in their own health care? How would major decisions be made?

Integrative Medicine and Alternative Health Care Practitioners

Many **integrative medicine** and alternative health care practitioners also carry the title *doctor,* but they have a different training regimen than required for the MD or DO. The training is highly specialized and specific; when licensed, these professionals are allowed to diagnose and treat medical conditions.

As mentioned earlier, alternative therapies are increasingly being perceived as complements to traditional health care in a form of integrative medicine. In this text, three broad alternative therapy disciplines are identified: chiropractic, naturopathy, and Oriental medicine/acupuncture.

Doctor of Chiropractic. Chiropractic is a branch of the healing arts that gives special attention to the physiological and biochemical aspects of the body's structure and it includes procedures for the adjustment and manipulation of the bones, joints, and adjacent tissues of the human body, particularly of the spinal column. Chiropractic is a nonsurgical science that also does not include pharmaceuticals.

The roots of chiropractic care can be traced back to the beginning of recorded time. Text from China and Greece written in 2700 BCE and 1500 BCE, respectively, mention spinal manipulation and maneuvering of the lower extremities to ease lower back pain. Daniel David Palmer founded the chiropractic profession in the United States in 1895. Throughout the twentieth century, doctors of chiropractic (DC) gained legal recognition and licensure in all 50 states.

Doctors of chiropractic complete four to five years of study at an accredited chiropractic college. The curriculum includes a minimum of 4,200 hours of classroom, laboratory, and clinical experience. About 555 hours are devoted to adjustive techniques and spinal analysis. This specialized education must be preceded by a minimum of 90 hours of undergraduate courses focusing on science. On successful completion of their education and training, doctors of chiropractic must also pass the national board examination and all examinations or licensure requirements identified by the particular state in which the individual wishes to practice.

Doctors of chiropractic frequently treat patients with neuromusculoskeletal conditions such as headaches, joint pain, neck pain, lower back pain, and sciatica. Chiropractors also treat patients with osteoarthritis, spinal disk conditions, carpal tunnel syndrome, tendonitis, sprains, and strains. Chiropractors also may treat a variety of other conditions such as allergies, asthma, and digestive disorders. There are obstacles to chiropractors in some areas, however, because states vary in what they authorize chiropractors to practice and may limit their ability to practice **homeopathy** or **acupuncture** or to dispense or sell dietary supplements.

Doctor of Naturopathy. Naturopathy, often referred to as "natural medicine," is based on the belief that the cause of disease is violation of nature's laws. The goal of the naturopath is to remove the underlying causes of disease and to stimulate the body's natural healing processes. Naturopathic treatments may include fasting; adhering to natural food diets; taking vitamins and herbs; tissue minerals; counseling; homeopathic remedies; manipulation of the spine and extremities; massage; exercise; naturopathic hygienic remedies; acupuncture; and applications of water, heat, cold, air, sunlight, and electricity. Most of these treatment methods are used to detoxify the body and strengthen the immune system.

In the United States, a Doctor of Naturopathy (ND) or Doctor of Naturopathic Medicine (NMD) receives education, training, and credentials from a full-time naturopathy college. Full-time education includes two years of science courses and two years of clinical work. Naturopaths are currently licensed to practice in 16 states, the District of Columbia, four Canadian provinces, and Puerto Rico and the Virgin Islands. In many states, naturopaths practice independently and unlicensed, or they practice under the direction of a physician.

Oriental Medicine and Acupuncture. Oriental medicine is a comprehensive system of health care with a history of more than 3,000 years. Oriental medicine includes acupuncture, Chinese herbology and bodywork, dietary therapy, and exercise based on traditional Oriental medicine principles. This form of health care is used extensively in Asia and is rapidly growing in popularity in the West.

Oriental medicine is based on an energetic model rather than the biochemical model of Western medicine. The ancient Chinese recognized a vital energy behind all life-forms and processes called *qi* (pronounced "chee"). Oriental healing practitioners believe that energy flows along specific pathways called *meridians.* Each pathway is associated with a particular physiological system and internal organ. Disease is the result of deficiency or imbalance of energy in the meridians and their associated physiological systems. Acupuncture points are specific sites along the meridians. Each point has a predictable effect on the vital energy passing through it. Modern science has measured the electrical charge at these points, corroborating the locations of the meridians. Traditional Oriental medicine uses an intricate system of pulse and tongue diagnosis, palpation of points and meridians, medical history, and other signs and symptoms to create a composite diagnosis. A treatment plan then is formulated to induce the body to a balanced state of health.

The WHO recognizes acupuncture and traditional Oriental medicine's ability to treat many common disorders, including the following:

- *Gastrointestinal disorders.* Food allergies, peptic ulcer, chronic diarrhea, constipation, indigestion, anorexia, gastritis
- *Urogenital disorders.* Stress incontinence, urinary tract infections, sexual dysfunction
- *Gynecological disorders.* Irregular, heavy, or painful menstruation; premenstrual syndrome (PMS); infertility
- *Respiratory disorders.* Emphysema, sinusitis, asthma, allergies, bronchitis
- *Neuromusculoskeletal disorders.* Arthritis; migraine headaches; neuralgia; insomnia; dizziness; low back, neck, and shoulder pain
- *Circulatory disorders.* Hypertension, angina pectoris, arteriosclerosis, anemia
- *Eye, ear, nose, and throat disorders.* Otitis media, sinusitis, sore throats
- *Emotional and psychological disorders.* Depression; anxiety; addictions to alcohol, nicotine, and drugs
- *Pain.* Elimination or control of pain for chronic and painful debilitating disorders

In the hands of a comprehensively trained acupuncturist, patients do not find acupuncture painful. Sterile, very fine, flexible needles about the diameter of a human hair are used in treatment. Practitioners may also recommend herbs, dietary changes, and exercise, together with lifestyle changes.

Training for acupuncture and Oriental medicine can be obtained in schools and colleges accredited by the Accreditation Commission for Acupuncture and Oriental Medicine. Applicants must have a bachelor's degree. Most of these specialized programs are three years, and on completion graduates are conferred with a master's degree in Acupuncture and Oriental Medicine (MAOM) or a master's degree in Acupuncture (MA) degree. Nearly all states regulate the practice of acupuncture and Oriental medicine, either through licensure or a ruling by the Board of Medical Examiners. In most cases passing a national certification examination or other testing procedure is required before licensure. Many doctors (MDs, DOs, DCs, and NDs) have become qualified to perform acupuncture and to use Oriental medicine in their practices through additional education and training.

Future of Integrative Medicine

There was a time when osteopaths and chiropractors were not accepted by the medical establishment and had difficulty with licensure. Naturopaths, acupuncturists, and Oriental medicine practitioners face similar challenges, and states vary greatly in their regulations of any form of alternative medicine and the scope of practice for each.

The road may be bumpy for CAM practitioners, but their numbers continue to increase. Managed care health plans are offering increased access to CAM practitioners, mostly because of the ability to expand patient choices at a lower cost. It is expected, however, that states will continue to wrestle with licensure and scope of practice issues for the increased numbers of well-educated and trained CAM practitioners.

Neither the growth in the number of CAM practitioners nor the laws and insurance practices that facilitate their access by patients likely would have occurred without broad public acceptance of alternative and complementary medicine. Americans seem quite willing to pay out-of-pocket expenses for alternative forms of treatment, such as massage therapy, aromatherapy, biofeedback, guided imagery, hydrotherapy, hypnotherapy, and homeopathy. Furthermore, many patients are seeking the more integrated form of medicine that occurs when primary care providers are willing to refer to a CAM practitioner and vice versa. Table 2-2 gives a brief description of a few alternative modalities that integrate fairly easily with traditional medical practices.

TABLE 2-2

SELECTED ALTERNATIVE MEDICINE MODALITIES

Ayurveda	5,000-year-old system of natural healing from India; three "energies" shape mind/body characteristic. A person's ideal state is determined and diet, herbs, aromatherapy, massage, music, and medication are used to reestablish harmony when there is illness.
Biofeedback	Biofeedback machines gauge internal bodily functions and help patients tune in to these functions and identify the triggers that evoke symptoms. Relaxation can be taught to relieve the symptoms.
Guided Imagery	Uses images or symbols to train the mind to create a definitive physiological or psychological effect; relieves stress and anxiety and reduces pain.
Homeopathy	Healing that claims highly diluted doses of certain substances can leave an energy imprint in the body and bring about a cure. Homeopathic remedies are made from naturally occurring plant, animal, or mineral substances and are manufactured by pharmaceutical companies under strict guidelines.
Hydrotherapy	Hydrotherapy uses the buoyancy, warmth, and effects of water and its turbulence to speed recovery after surgery and to reduce pain and stress, spasm, and discomfort. It is especially beneficial for work- or sports-related injuries and arthritis.
Hypnotherapy	Hypnotherapy facilitates communication between the right and left sides of the brain with the patient in a state of focused relaxation when the subconscious mind is open to suggestions. It is currently used to help people lose weight; stop smoking; reduce stress; and relieve pain, anxiety, and phobias.
Massage	Massage reduces stress, manages chronic pain, promotes relaxation, and increases circulation of the blood and lymph. Hand stroking on the body helps patients become more familiar with their pain.
Movement Therapies	A group of therapies that include movement to establish balance, enhance relaxation, correct posture, elevate the spirit, and invigorate the mind. Pilates, Tai Chi, and Feldenkrais are examples.

ALLIED HEALTH PROFESSIONALS AND THEIR ROLES

In the health care team, allied health professionals bring specific educational backgrounds and a broad array of skills to the medical environment. Medical assistants are allied health professionals with a very specific set of skills for ambulatory care.

The Role of the Medical Assistant

In the ambulatory care setting, a critical and most beneficial allied health professional is the medical assistant. The medical assistant, performing both administrative and clinical tasks under the direction of the provider, is an important link between patient and provider (Figure 2-2). The medical assistant serves in many capacities—receptionist, secretary, office manager, bookkeeper, insurance coder and biller, sometimes transcriptionist, patient educator, and clinical assistant. The latter requires the medical assistant to be able to administer injections, perform venipuncture, prepare patients for examinations, assist with examinations and special procedures, and perform

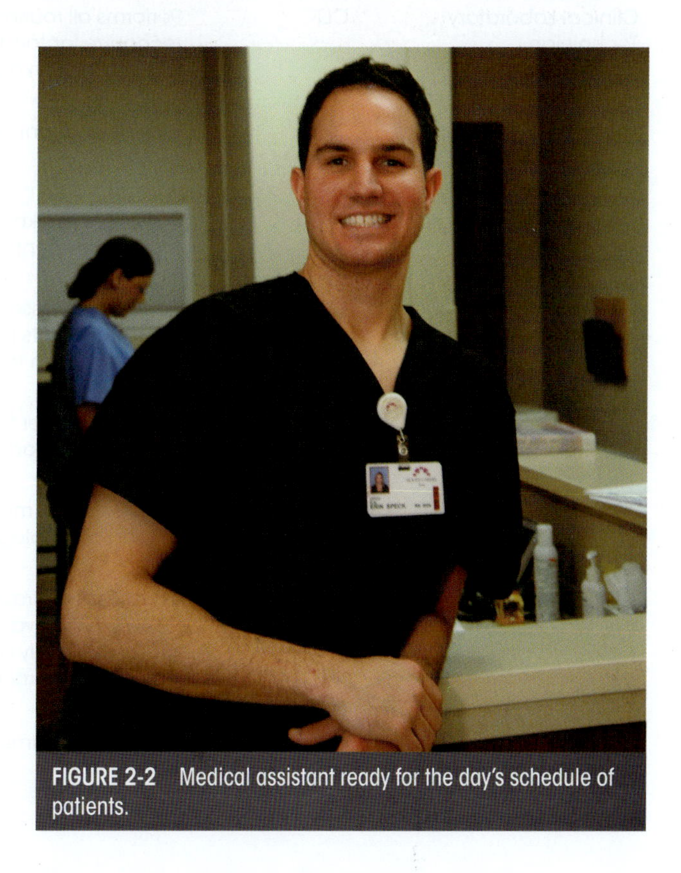

FIGURE 2-2 Medical assistant ready for the day's schedule of patients.

electrocardiography and various laboratory tests. Medical assistants screen and assess patient needs when scheduling appointments and tests. Although medical assistants have a broad range of responsibilities, it is critical that they perform only within the scope of their training, education, and personal capabilities and always function within ethical and legal boundaries and state statutes. To perform outside the scope of training is both illegal and unethical.

Because medical assistants are often the patient's first contact with the facility and its providers, a positive attitude is important (see Chapter 1). They must be excellent communicators, both verbally and nonverbally, and project a professional image of themselves and their employer. Medical assistants who believe in their work, who are proud of their career, and who convey compassion and caring provide a positive experience for patients who are ill or in a great deal of discomfort.

Table 2-3 lists some of the allied health professionals recognized by the Commission on Accreditation of Allied Health Education Programs (CAAHEP) and the Accrediting Bureau of Health Education Schools (ABHES).

As a medical assistant, you may not work directly with all the identified allied health care professionals, but you likely will have contact with many of

TABLE 2-3

SELECTED ALLIED HEALTH PROFESSIONS

OCCUPATION	ABBREVIATION	JOB DESCRIPTION
Anesthesiologist Assistant	AA	Performs preoperative tasks; performs airway management and drug administration for induction and maintenance of anesthesia during surgery under direction of a licensed and qualified anesthesiologist
Athletic Trainer	AT	Provides a variety of services, including injury prevention, recognition, immediate care, treatment, and rehabilitation after athletic trauma
Clinical Laboratory Technician *Associate Degree*	CLT	Performs all routine tests in a medical laboratory and is able to discriminate and recognize factors that directly affect procedures and results. Works under direction of pathologist, provider medical technologist, or scientist
Diagnostic Medical Sonographer	DMS	Provides patient services using medical ultrasound under the supervision of a provider
Electroencelphalographic Technologist	EEG-T	Possesses the knowledge, attributes, and skills to obtain interpretable recordings of a patient's nervous system functions
Emergency Medical Technician—Paramedic	EMT-P	Recognizes, assesses, and manages medical emergencies of acutely ill or injured patients in prehospital care settings, working under the direction of a provider (often through radio communication)
Medical Assistant	MA	Functions under the supervision of licensed medical professionals and is competent in both administrative/office and clinical/laboratory procedures
Medical Illustrator	MI	Creates visual material designed to facilitate the recording and dissemination of medical, biological, and related knowledge through communication media
Occupational Therapist	OT	Educates and trains individuals in the application of purposeful, goal-oriented activity in the evaluation, diagnosis, and treatment of loss of ability to cope with the tasks of daily living and impairment caused by physical injury, illness, or emotional disorder; congenital or developmental disability; or the aging process
Ophthalmic Medical Technician or Technologist	OMT	Assists ophthalmologists to perform diagnostic and therapeutic procedures

continues

Table 2-3 continued

OCCUPATION	ABBREVIATION	JOB DESCRIPTION
Personal Fitness Trainer	PFT	Develops an activity plan for each individual that integrates a complete approach to fitness and wellness through exercise, strength training, and proper diet
Radiographer	RT(R)	Provides patient services using imaging modalities, as directed by providers qualified to order and perform radiologic procedures
Registered Health Information Administrator	RHIA	Manages health information systems consistent with the medical, administrative, ethical, and legal requirements of the health care delivery system
Registered Health Information Technician	RHIT	Possesses the technical knowledge and skills necessary to process, maintain, compile, and report patient data
Respiratory Therapist	RRT	Applies scientific knowledge and theory to practical clinical problems of respiratory care
Surgical Technologist	ST	Works as an integral member of the surgical team, which includes surgeons, anesthesiologists, registered nurses, and other surgical personnel delivering patient care and assuming appropriate responsibilities before, during, and after surgery

them by telephone and written or electronic communication. Knowledge of the roles these health professionals play enables you to interact more intelligently with all members of the health care team.

In addition to the professionals listed in Table 2-3, you may encounter some or all of the following health care professionals in daily patient care.

Health Unit Coordinator

Health unit coordinators (HUCs) perform nonclinical patient care tasks for the nursing unit of a hospital. General secretarial and clerical duties allow HUCs to maintain patients' charts, schedule tests, order supplies, screen new patients, and give directions to visitors. This profession requires a self-motivated, mature individual who can handle the stress and hectic pace of coordinating personnel and their duties at the nurses' station. Also called unit secretary, administrative specialist, ward clerk, or ward secretary, a health unit coordinator receives on-the-job training or completes a six-month to one-year certificate program.

Medical Laboratory Technologist

Medical laboratory technologists (MLTs) physically and chemically analyze, as well as culture, urine, blood, and other body fluids and tissues

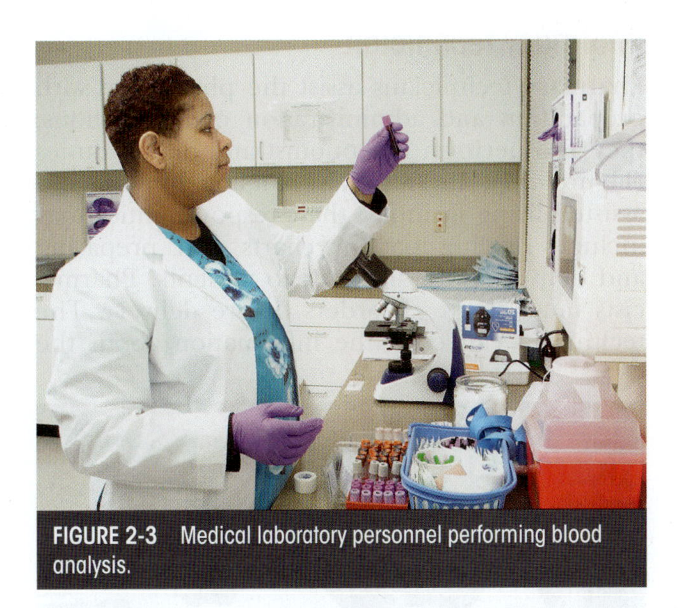

FIGURE 2-3 Medical laboratory personnel performing blood analysis.

(Figure 2-3). They work closely with specialists such as oncologists, pathologists, and hematologists. Knowledge of specimen collection, anatomy and physiology, biochemistry, laboratory equipment, asepsis, and quality control is essential. The American Society of Clinical Pathology (ASCP) is a professional organization that oversees credentialing and education in the medical laboratory professions.

Registered Dietitian

Registered dietitians (RDs) have specialized training in the nutritional care of groups and individuals and have successfully completed an examination conducted by the Commission on Dietetic Registration. Dietitians assist patients in regulating their diets. Although they are typically employed in hospitals and clinics, they can also be found working with the public in personal nutritional counseling. Education includes a bachelor's degree with a major in dietetics, food and nutrition, or food service systems management, in addition to completion of an approved internship.

Pharmacist

Pharmacists (RPh) are licensed by each state to prepare and dispense all types of medications as well as medical supplies related to medication administration. They can practice in hospitals, medical centers, and pharmacies. The minimum training for a pharmacist is a five-year bachelor's degree; some pharmacists pursue a Doctor of Pharmacy degree (PharmD), which is offered by major universities in the United States.

Pharmacy Technician

Pharmacy technicians assist the pharmacist with preparation and administration of medications; they also perform receptionist and billing duties (Figure 2-4). In hospitals, nursing homes, and assisted living facilities, their responsibilities may include reading patient charts and preparing and delivering medications to patients. Pharmacists must check all orders before delivery. The technician can copy the information about the prescribed medication onto the patient's profile. Professional certification of pharmacy technicians varies from state to state and is administered by state pharmacy associations.

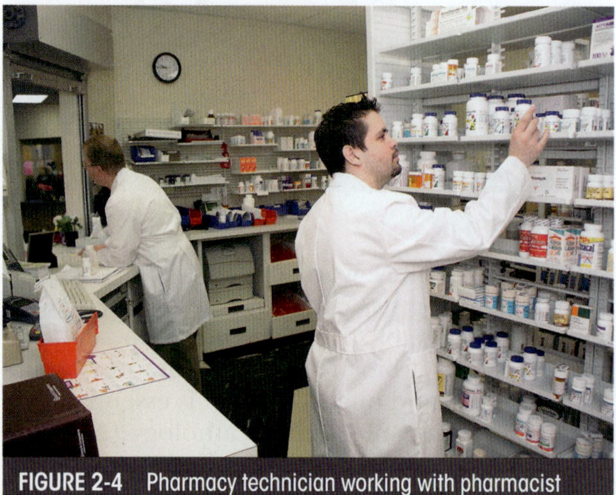

FIGURE 2-4 Pharmacy technician working with pharmacist preparing medications.

Phlebotomist

Phlebotomists are trained in the art of drawing blood for diagnostic laboratory testing. Phlebotomists are also referred to as laboratory liaison technicians. Phlebotomists may be nationally certified and are employed in medical clinics, hospitals, and laboratories. Training consists of one to two semesters in a community college program or on-the-job training.

Physical Therapist

Physical therapists (PTs) are licensed professionals who assist in the examination, testing, and treatment of physically disabled or challenged people. They also assist in physical rehabilitation of patients after an accident, injury, or serious illness, using special exercises, application of heat or cold, ultrasound therapy, and other techniques. Educational requirements for a PT are a minimum of a four-year bachelor's degree (bachelor of science) or a special certificate course after obtaining the bachelor of science in a related field. PTs must also successfully complete a state licensure examination.

Physical Therapy Assistant

Physical therapy assistants (PTAs) are trained to use and apply physical therapy procedures, such as exercise, and physical agents under the supervision of a physical therapist. The PTA has earned an associate of science degree from an accredited program and must pass a licensure or registry examination in selected states.

Nurse

Neither ABHES nor CAAHEP is responsible for nurse education or accreditation, but nurses are listed here as a major participant in health care. Nurses are licensed by the state in which they practice. Although nurses' education and training are oriented to bedside care, some may be employed in medical clinics as clinical assistants, especially in clinics where surgery is performed. Nurses play a number of roles on the health care team.

Registered Nurse. In the United States, registered nurses (RNs) are professionals who have completed, at a minimum, a two-year course of study at a state-approved school of nursing and have passed the National Council Licensure Examination (NCLEX-RN). Employment settings most often include hospitals, convalescent homes, clinics, and home health care.

Licensed Practical Nurse. A licensed practical nurse (LPN) is a professional trained in basic nursing techniques and direct patient care. LPNs practice under the direct supervision of an RN or provider and are employed in similar settings to RNs. Training includes completion of a state-approved program in practical nursing and successful completion of the National Council Licensure Examination (NCLEX-PN).

Nurse Practitioner. Sometimes referred to as an advanced registered nurse practitioner (ARNP), a nurse practitioner (NP) is an RN who, by advanced education (usually a master's degree) and clinical experience in a branch of nursing, has acquired expert knowledge in a specific medical specialty. Nurse practitioners are employed by providers in private practice or in clinics and sometimes practice independently, especially in rural areas. They have increased in numbers as the number of primary care providers continues to decrease. ARNPs may or may not be licensed to prescribe medications.

Physician Assistant

Physician assistants (PAs) receive formal education and training to provide diagnostic, therapeutic, and preventive health care services delegated by and under the supervision of providers and surgeons. PAs take medical histories, examine and treat patients, order and interpret laboratory tests and X-rays, and make diagnoses. They also treat minor injuries by suturing, splinting, and casting. PAs write progress notes, instruct and counsel patients, and order tests and therapy. In all 50 states, the District of Columbia, and Guam, PAs may prescribe certain medications. They can supervise technicians and medical assistants. PAs may be primary care providers in areas where the supervising physician is not present all the time but is always available for conferring as necessary and required by law. PAs, too, are growing in numbers.

Most PA programs are two years in length with the added requirement of at least two years of college and some health care experience. For licensure, all states require PAs to complete an accredited, formal education program and to pass the Physician Assistant National Certifying Examination administered by the National Commission on Certification of Physician Assistants (NCCPA). The examination is available only to graduates of an accredited PA education program. Upon successful completion of the examination, the credential "Physician Assistant–Certified" can be used.

THE VALUE OF THE MEDICAL ASSISTANT TO THE HEALTH CARE TEAM

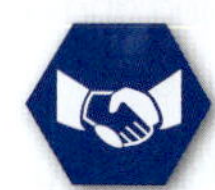
Professional

With their broad range of competencies in both administrative and clinical areas, medical assistants are the most valued ambulatory health care team member. Medical assistants are the great communicators, serving as liaisons between provider and hospital staff and between provider and any number of allied and other health professionals. Because they often are the first providers to see or speak with patients, they undertake responsibility for directing, informing, and guiding patient care while establishing a professional and caring tone for the entire health care team. The value of a competent, professional, compassionate medical assistant is immeasurable in today's fast-paced and challenging health care environment.

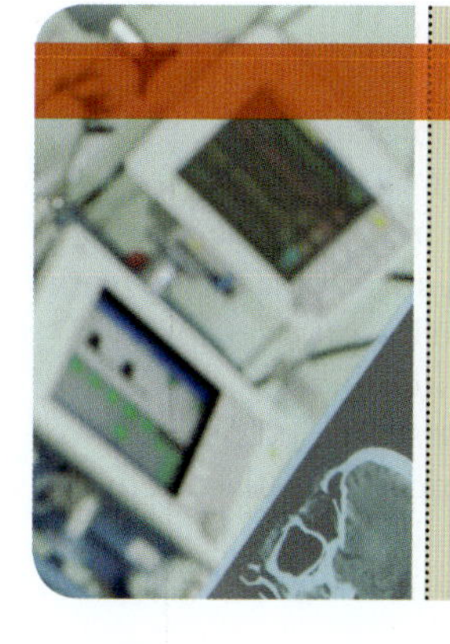

CASE STUDY 2-1

Refer to the scenario at the beginning of the chapter.

CASE STUDY REVIEW

1. Where will you research additional information on being a physical therapy assistant?
2. Compare the working hours, rate of pay, contact with patients, required schooling, and job availability to those of the medical assistant in your geographic location.
3. If other health professions discussed in the chapter are of special interest to you, answer the same questions. This review helps to clarify the position of the medical assistant for you.

CASE STUDY 2-2

You are the medical assistant for a family-practice provider, Dr. Bill Claredon, who is close to retirement. He is much adored by all his patients, but he thinks any complementary therapies are outright quackery. Marjorie Johns, a patient with debilitating back pain, tells you she is seeing an acupuncturist and is taking less and less of her prescribed medications. You quietly mention this to Dr. Claredon before he enters the examination room to see Marjorie. He glares at you with disgust at the information and is quite agitated when he enters the examination room.

CASE STUDY REVIEW

1. Describe the discussion that you think might occur between Dr. Claredon and Marjorie.
2. If Marjorie is unhappy when she is ready to leave the facility, what professionalism skills can you use to help her?
3. As the medical assistant, what attributes of professionalism can be utilized to ease Dr. Claredon's concern and help bridge this gap for Marjorie?

Summary

- The health care environment is a dynamic service that changes rapidly in response to new technology and societal needs.
- Some form of managed care likely will dominate the health care industry for years to come.
- A strong health care team is critical in the health care setting, as primary care providers, specialists of all disciplines, complementary care practitioners, and allied and other health professionals collaborate on the best way to provide integrative medicine and quality patient care.
- The medical assistant is a vital link in the team and is responsible for a range of responsibilities, both clinical and administrative.

Study for Success

To reinforce your knowledge and skills of information presented in this chapter:

- Review the *Key Terms* and *Learning Outcomes*
- Consider the *Critical Thinking* features and *Case Studies* and discuss your conclusions
- Answer the questions in the *Certification Review*

CERTIFICATION REVIEW

1. Where are the majority of medical assistants employed?
   a. Hospitals
   b. Nursing facilities
   c. Ambulatory care settings
   d. Insurance companies
2. Which term best describes a health maintenance organization?
   a. Managed care operation
   b. Individual practice
   c. Sole proprietorship
   d. Hospital
   e. PCMH
3. With its emphasis on controlling costs, what will managed care likely affect the most?
   a. Only hospitals
   b. All health care settings
   c. Only providers in private practice
   d. Only patients
4. How is the health care team best described?
   a. It should exclude the patient as part of the team.
   b. It is only important in the hospital setting.
   c. It consists of physicians and nurses.
   d. It includes physicians, nurses, allied health care professionals, patients, and integrative medicine practitioners.
   e. It refers to only the PCP and the patient.

5. Which of the following statements best identifies integrative health care approaches?
   a. It is increasingly accepted as complementary to traditional health care.
   b. It is always covered by insurance.
   c. It is seldom approved for licensure.
   d. It is not important to understand.
6. When a medical assistant permitted by law to draw blood for diagnostic laboratory testing performs such a procedure, it is similar to those performed by which of the following?
   a. A health unit coordinator
   b. A health information technician
   c. A phlebotomist
   d. A respiratory therapist
   e. A nurse
7. Which of the following best describes a "boutique" or "concierge" medical practice?
   a. It is another form of managed care.
   b. It allows patients special privileges in their health care.
   c. It is covered by all major insurance plans.
   d. It does not require special fees for services.
8. Providers just establishing their practice often seek to work with another provider in the same field. When expenses and profits are shared, what is the name given to this form of management?
   a. HMO
   b. Corporation
   c. Sole proprietor
   d. Group or partnership
   e. Community care organization
9. Which of the following will the medical assistant *not* do in health care?
   a. Code and bill insurance, bookkeeping
   b. Diagnose and treat ailments
   c. Screen when making appointments
   d. Assist provider, perform clinical and laboratory procedures
10. What is an alternative approach to medicine that treats patients using thin, flexible needles called?
   a. Acupuncture
   b. Naturopathy
   c. Chiropractic
   d. Homeopathy
   e. Ayurveda

UNIT II
THE THERAPEUTIC APPROACH

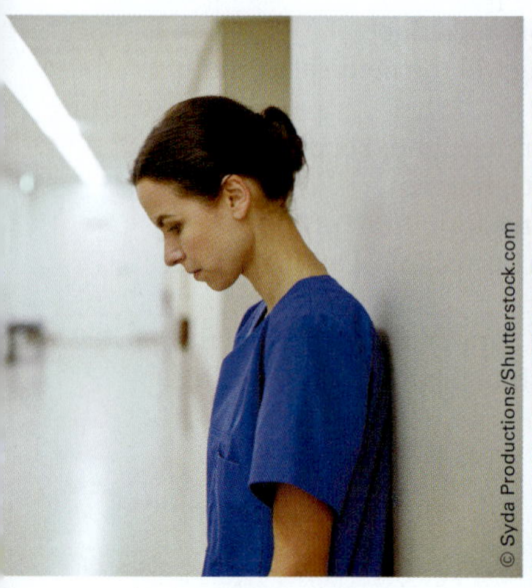

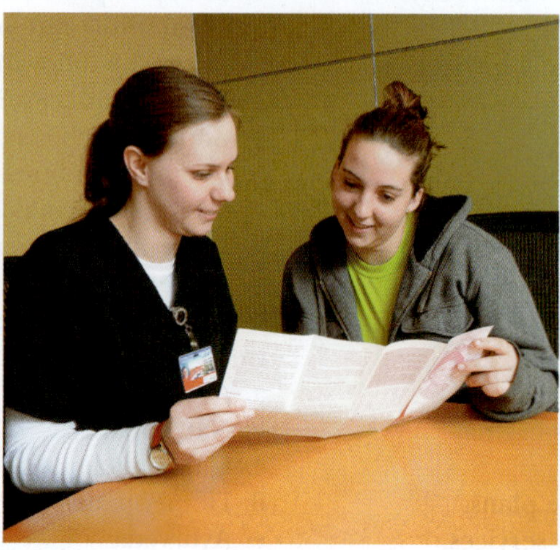

© Syda Productions/Shutterstock.com

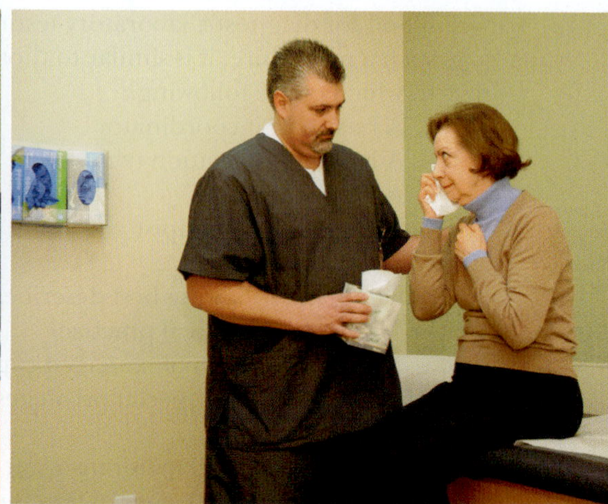

ATTRIBUTES OF PROFESSIONALISM

The professional medical assistant is very aware of the importance of communication skills and strives to be therapeutic in all situations. Therapeutic communication requires clear communication of technical information in a manner that is empathetic to the patient's emotional state. It requires adherence to accepted social behavior and political correctness. It is also important to remember that nonverbal communication or body language can be an even stronger communicator than words. Body language generally communicates our true feelings and often we are not even aware of the messages we are sending. Because nonverbal communication can easily be misinterpreted, the professional medical assistant will look for agreement between verbal and nonverbal communication in order to send and receive a clear message.

Listening is often identified as the passive aspect of communication. However, if it is done well, listening is very active. Good listeners focus on the speaker, are attentive, and are aware of the nonverbal messages as well as the verbal information being shared. The professional medical assistant should have three listening goals: (1) to improve listening skills so that patients are heard accurately; (2) to listen for what is not being said or for information transmitted only by hints; and (3) to verify that the information was heard accurately.

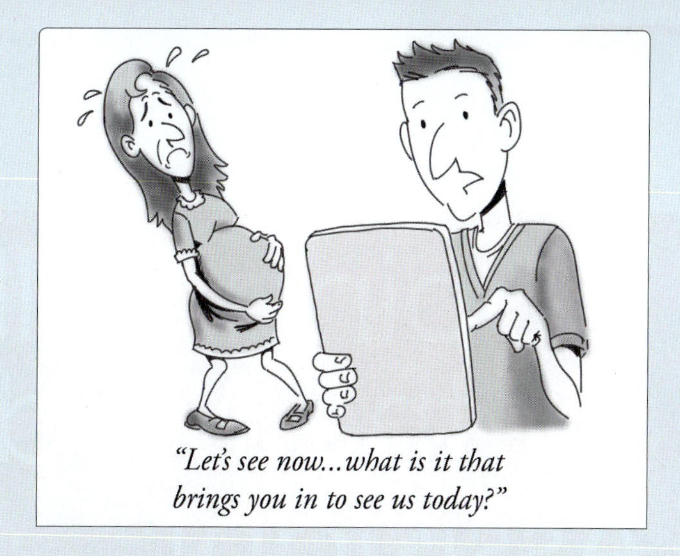

"Let's see now...what is it that brings you in to see us today?"

Listed below are a series of questions for you to ask yourself, to serve as a professionalism checklist. As you interact with patients and colleagues, these questions will help to guide you in the professional behavior and therapeutic communication that is expected every day from medical assistants.

Ask Yourself

COMMUNICATION

- ☐ Do I apply active listening skills?
- ☐ Do I display professionalism through written and verbal communication?
- ☐ Do I demonstrate appropriate nonverbal communication?
- ☐ Do I speak at each patient's level of understanding?
- ☐ Do I display appropriate body language?
- ☐ Do I respond honestly and diplomatically to my patients' concerns?
- ☐ Do I refrain from sharing my personal experiences?
- ☐ Do I include the patient's support system as indicated?
- ☐ Does my knowledge allow me to speak easily with all members of the health care team?
- ☐ Do I accurately and concisely update the provider on any aspect of a patient's care?

PRESENTATION

- ☐ Am I courteous, patient, and respectful to patients?
- ☐ Do I display a positive attitude?
- ☐ Do I display a calm, professional, and caring manner?
- ☐ Do I demonstrate empathy to the patient?

COMPETENCY

- ☐ Do I pay attention to detail?
- ☐ Do I ask questions if I am out of my comfort zone or do not have the experience to carry out tasks?
- ☐ Do I display sound judgment?

INITIATIVE

- ☐ Do I show initiative?
- ☐ Have I developed a strategic plan to achieve my goals? Is my plan realistic?
- ☐ Am I flexible and dependable?
- ☐ Do I direct the patient to other resources when necessary or helpful, with the approval of the provider?
- ☐ Do I assist co-workers when appropriate?
- ☐ Do I make adaptations for patients with special needs?

INTEGRITY

- ☐ Do I demonstrate the principles of self-boundaries?
- ☐ Do I demonstrate respect for individual diversity?
- ☐ Do I demonstrate sensitivity to patient rights?
- ☐ Do I recognize the impact personal ethics and morals have on the delivery of health care?

CHAPTER 3

Coping Skills for the Medical Assistant

LEARNING OUTCOMES

1. Define and spell the key terms as presented in the glossary.
2. Analyze the difference between stress and stressors.
3. Describe the three categories of stressors.
4. Discuss Hans Selye's General Adaptation Syndrome (GAS) theory.
5. Differentiate between short-duration and long-duration stress.
6. Analyze the body's response to stress as displayed by the sympathetic and parasympathetic nervous systems.
7. Summarize stress in the work environment and discuss ways to eliminate or cope with it.
8. Model ways a positive attitude may reduce the level and duration of stress.
9. Discuss physical illnesses and psychological symptoms of stress on the body.
10. Describe characteristics of prolonged stress.
11. Compare the four stages of burnout.
12. Identify persons most vulnerable to burnout.
13. Differentiate between long-range and short-range goals.

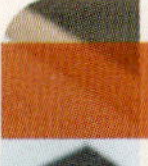

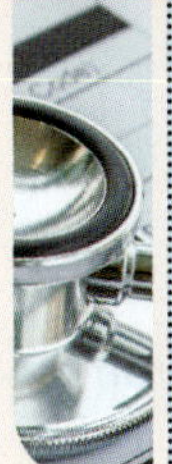

KEY TERMS

acute stress
burnout
chronic stress
episodic stress
goal
inner-directed people
long-range goals
outer-directed people
parasympathetic nervous system
self-actualization
short-range goals
stress
stressors
sympathetic nervous system

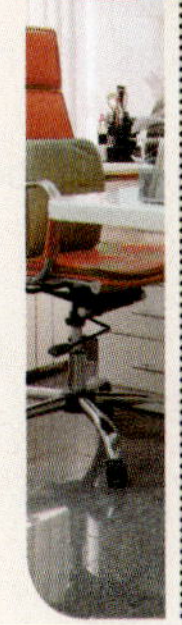

SCENARIO

At Inner City Health Care, there are four full-time medical assistants who collaborate to make the clinic run smoothly, both administratively and clinically. One day a month, though, clinic manager Marilyn Johnson, CMA (AAMA), is out of town, leaving Ellen Armstrong, CMAS (AMT), the administrative medical assistant, in charge of a busy reception area and an ever-ringing telephone.

On these days, Ellen pays close attention to details and is particularly careful to organize her work so that things run as they should. Implementation of time management principles helps ensure the clinic functions effectively. Although Ellen cannot anticipate every emergency, she does try to influence the situation rather than let events control her.

Chapter Portal

Even in the most well-managed ambulatory care setting, medical assistants and other health providers are likely to feel the effects of stress from time to time. They may be overworked on certain days, they may face difficult patient situations, and they may find that the administrative and paperwork load is getting ahead of them.

This chapter helps today's busy, multifaceted medical assistant pinpoint the symptoms of stress and provides ideas for coping with stress as it occurs. The better equipped the medical assistant is to confront and solve the sources of stress, the less likely stressors will become so overwhelming as to lead to burnout on the job. Goal setting, recognizing one's limitations and potentials, setting priorities, and keeping a balanced perspective can work together to reduce stress and enable the medical assistant to take pleasure in working with patients and colleagues.

WHAT IS STRESS?

The body's response to mental or emotional strain or tension is termed **stress**. Walter Cannon, a neurologist, is credited with first determining that both emotional and physical events act as **stressors** and that the body reacts in a similar way to either type of event. What constitutes stress is highly individual and depends to a great extent on personality type. Events that may be stressful to one person may be enjoyable to another. A delayed airplane flight may be very stressful to a person who worries about making another connection or missing a meeting. Another person will simply look for an alternative flight or notify the people that he was to meet and then take the time to enjoy a good book, experiencing little or no mental or physical change. The key is to learn how to manage stress so that it works for you rather than against you.

Adaptive behavior patterns we assume in response to real physical threats or emotional effects result in either eustress (positive feelings) or distress (negative feelings). Moving to a new city or receiving a promotion usually are perceived as positive events, whereas going through a divorce or losing a job are, conversely, perceived as negative events; however, each of these events can result in inducing stress in the body. These events are called stressors. Stressors can be divided into three categories:

1. *Frustrations.* Circumstances that prevent us from doing what we want to do
2. *Conflicts.* Incompatibility between two important things or objectives equally important to us
3. *Pressure.* Demands of schedule, workload, or expectations placed on us by ourselves or others

Complete the "How Stressed Are You????" exercise in Figure 3-1 to help assess your current stress level.

HOW STRESSED ARE YOU????

Answer each question with a 0, 1, 2, 3 or 4.

0 = never 1 = rarely 2 = sometimes 3 = often 4 = very often/always

Instructions for scoring follow the questions.

1. ____ My sleep is poor—delayed onset, wake early or not restful.
2. ____ I have headaches regularly (tension or migraine).
3. ____ I feel tense and anxious.
4. ____ I rarely have enough time to complete tasks.
5. ____ I experience frustration when trying to get things accomplished.
6. ____ I feel like escaping, I wish I were somewhere else.
7. ____ I feel like my schedule is controlled by outside factors or other people.
8. ____ I feel angry even for no reason.
9. ____ I feel overwhelmed by things that shouldn't be that hard.
10. ____ I eat more sugar and junk food than I want.
11. ____ I am not happy with the way I look.
12. ____ I have digestive difficulties (gas, cramping, irregularity).
13. ____ I feel like I want to cry, I am tearful more often than normal.
14. ____ I can't concentrate.
15. ____ I have constant colds/flu/infections.
16. ____ I feel isolated even when around others.
17. ____ I am forgetful, even important things slip my mind.
18. ____ I have pain in more than one place in my body.
19. ____ I feel irritable.
20. ____ I am unorganized and lose things.
21. ____ I have cold hands and/or feet.
22. ____ I am late for appointments or meetings.
23. ____ I have moist or sweaty hands.
24. ____ I talk rapidly.
25. ____ My heart pounds in my chest.

Scoring

Add all your points together. You can have a total of 100 points.

The higher the score, the greater your stress response.

Keep in mind that your symptoms may not be just stress related—it is important to see your doctor if you are not feeling well!

0–25: low
26–36: low-moderate
37–50: moderate-high
50–65: high
+ 65: VERY HIGH

John Jordy, The Stress Clinic, LLC

FIGURE 3-1 Determining how well you handle stress will help identify personal strengths and weaknesses and point you toward the skills needed to be a successful health care professional. Complete the stress self-test.

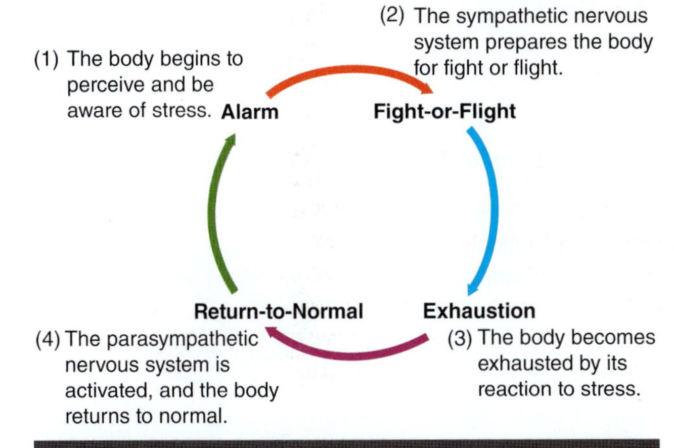

FIGURE 3-2 Hans Selye's General Adaptation Syndrome (GAS) theory proposes that four stages are involved in adapting to stress.

According to Hans Selye, who first conceived the theory of nonspecific reaction as stress, which is the body's response to any demand or stressor, the body does not differentiate between positively and negatively induced stress. It is only the level of the stress and its duration that affect the body. See Figure 3-2 illustrating Hans Selye's General Adaptation Syndrome cycle.

Types of Stress

Short-duration stress, sometimes termed **acute stress**, can be beneficial. Acute stress adds anticipation and a feeling of "being alive." For example, when we experience bungee jumping from a cliff, we experience acute stress. The short-lived adrenaline rush brings the world into sharper focus and enhances our lives. It helps us focus on details, achieve difficult goals, and perform at our best.

When we have a last-minute rush in the clinic or are hurrying to get an assignment finished for school, we are experiencing short-duration stress. Short-duration stress is experienced when the telephone rings, the examination rooms are full, and the provider is called to the hospital for an emergency. Immediately, the body's stress mode is activated and adrenaline is produced, enabling you to make quick judgments and decisions, to be organized and efficient, and to accomplish tasks within minimal time limits. Recovery from acute stress occurs when the stress has been dealt with.

Acute stress that is experienced frequently or lasts longer in duration is termed **episodic stress**. Examples of episodic stress include taking on too many projects and placing unrealistic demands on one's self, and then worrying needlessly. Individuals who are very competitive and demanding or referred to as "Type A" personalities may experience episodic stress. Episodic stress ceases from time to time or once the stress has been managed.

Chronic stress is an unhealthy form of stress. Often chronic stress is the result of events over which we have little control, such as long-term unemployment, dysfunctional relationships, or chronic illness. Long-duration stress that results from chronic stress can be life-threatening, leading the person to resort to violence, self-harm, or even suicide.

The Body's Response to Stress

The body's response to stress helps humans survive whatever fearful crisis they experience. The **sympathetic nervous system** prepares the body for "fight or flight" by signaling specific body systems.

Short term, these responses are not harmful, and the body's **parasympathetic nervous system** returns the body to normal after the stressor has been removed. Long-duration stress, over an extended period of time, can have harmful, even life-threatening results. For more information, see the "How Body Systems React to Stress" Quick Reference Guide.

Clinical responses to stress include emotional, physical, behavioral, and cognitive signs and symptoms, as described in Table 3-1. The more signs

TABLE 3-1

CLINICAL RESPONSES TO STRESS

CLINICAL RESPONSE	SIGNS AND SYMPTOMS
Emotional	Anxiety, worry, guilt, nervousness, anger, frustration, hostility, feeling overwhelmed, loneliness, isolation, mood swings, depression
Physical	Aches, pains, muscle spasms, dizziness, lightheadedness, feeling faint, nausea, diarrhea, constipation, difficulty breathing, chest pain, palpitations, rapid pulse, belching, flatulence
Behavioral	Increased or decreased appetite, sleep disorders (insomnia, nightmares), nervous habits (fidgeting, feet tapping, nail biting, pacing, procrastinating or neglecting responsibilities), lies or excuses to cover up poor work
Cognitive	Difficulty concentrating, racing thoughts, forgetfulness, disorganization, confusion, difficulty making decisions or making poor judgments, decreased interest in appearance and punctuality

QUICK REFERENCE GUIDE

HOW BODY SYSTEMS REACT TO STRESS

Body System	Fight-or-Flight Response	Response to Long-Duration Stress	Organ(s)
Nervous	Brain signals adrenal glands to release adrenaline and cortisol. This causes heart to beat faster, increasing blood pressure.	Depression, anxiety, stroke, degenerative neurological disorders such as Parkinson disease	Brain
Musculoskeletal	Large muscles and heart muscles dilate to increase blood flow.	Tension headaches, migraines, various musculoskeletal conditions	Muscles
Respiratory	Increased respiration rate supplies plenty of oxygen to the body.	Hyperventilation, panic attacks	Lungs
Cardiovascular	Increased heart rate and stronger contractions increase blood flow.	Inflammation in the coronary arteries, which may lead to heart attacks	Heart
Endocrine	Hypothalamus causes adrenal cortex to produce cortisol, and the adrenal medulla to produce epinephrine. The liver produces more glucose to provide increased energy.	Increased blood pressure and heart rate, increased glucose from glycogen in the liver, increased fatty acid in the blood, and decreased activity in the gastrointestinal (GI) tract	Glands
Gastrointestinal	Changes here increase glucose levels in the bloodstream.	Eating disorders, heartburn, acid reflux, butterflies, nausea or pain in stomach; diarrhea or constipation	Intestinal Tract

(continues)

Body System	Fight-or-Flight Response	Response to Long-Duration Stress	Organ(s)
Reproductive	Changes here may lead to reproductive dysfunction.	Males may experience impaired testosterone and sperm production, or impotence. Females may experience irregular menstrual cycles or painful periods, reduced sexual desire.	Male Female

and symptoms you notice, the closer you may be to stress overload. It is important to remember that many of these signs and symptoms can also be indicators of other psychological or medical problems.

FACTORS CAUSING STRESS IN THE WORK ENVIRONMENT

Stress in the work environment may come from many different sources, some of which you may control by making a few adjustments to resolve the stress. Conditions that cannot be changed may need to be accepted as a part of the job. Examples of work environment conditions that may cause stress include the following, but are not limited to these mentioned.

Overwhelming Situations

Initiative

Inability to control expectations, workload, and duties; feelings of frustration; and panic because of schedules can all result in feelings of powerlessness and not knowing where to start. Planning and prioritization can help to prevent panic and reduce stress when faced with the inevitable situation of too much work and too little time. A job that looks impossible can be broken down into elements that are manageable. Prioritization of the smaller elements and proceeding without wasting any time procrastinating usually results in getting the job finished in the allotted time, or at least with a minimum amount of stress. Requesting that you have a written job description can control powerlessness. You will then know your duties and responsibilities, and you will not experience sudden change when you least expect it. A job description will also help to avoid some of the instability resulting from a manager who is too sanguine (laid back) or manages from one crisis to another. If you know what your job entails, you can anticipate the events and take action to prevent a crisis.

Round Peg in Square Hole

Competency

Being a round peg in a square hole means not being emotionally suited or qualified for the position you hold. The only solution for this situation is changing jobs or obtaining training to become qualified for the requirements of the present job. Medical assistants can find themselves in emotional distress if a provider asks them to do tasks that they are not allowed to perform under the scope of their education and training. An example of this could be a medical assistant working for a provider who does outpatient surgery and expects the medical assistant to suture the incision after he or she has completed the major part of the procedure.

Traumatic Events on the Job

You may not be emotionally prepared for trauma involved in the job. Not every medical assistant can handle assisting with surgery or performing invasive procedures. A medical assistant finding himself or herself in this position could be proactive and seek a move from clinical to administrative duties or take steps to obtain another position having fewer traumatic events.

Physical Environment

Physical conditions such as noise, lighting, or some other types of stressors are frequently within the control of the worker. Additional lighting could be added or light shields could be used as suits the situation, and dressing in layers to accommodate temperature changes could mitigate the "too cold" stressor. The main point is not to sit back and become upset about situations over which you have some control. Take proactive steps to alleviate the stress-causing condition.

Management Style

Your manager's management style may cause uproar or instability in work demands. Talking to the manager might affect the situation, but it is highly unlikely. Obtaining a detailed job description; being able to say "no"; and utilizing goal-setting techniques, as discussed later in this chapter, are the best ways to reduce stress from this cause.

Difficult Coworkers

Integrity

Difficult people are all around us; in fact, you may be one to someone else. Maintaining a good interpersonal relationship with fellow employees is important to achieving a satisfying work experience and has a remarkable effect in reducing the problem of difficult people. Before a strong interpersonal relationship is established with others, a positive self-attitude is needed. The choices we make affect our positive attitude. Making positive decisions will affect the work environment, and hence the level and duration of stress experienced. Following are some choices we all make in our lives:

- To be respectful of others
- To be a diligent worker
- To be willing to learn
- To be honest
- To be willing to assume responsibility for one's actions
- To express appropriate humor
- To have an attitude of humility
- To be goal directed
- To understand Maslow's hierarchy of needs (see Chapter 4 for information related to Maslow's hierarchy of needs)

If you do all these things and still have difficult people in your work environment, develop a plan and take steps to have the least contact possible with those people. Taking proactive steps will in itself reduce stress.

Failure to Meet Needs

Certain job conditions do not permit achievement of Maslow's needs. Failure to meet our needs results in frustration, lack of job satisfaction, and ultimately burnout. Failure to meet needs can result from low salary, little opportunity for career growth, and discrimination in opportunities available and perceived distribution of assignments.

Job Instability

Job instability is an example of a stressor capable of causing worry. Worry is excessive concern about situations over which we have no direct control. Ensuring job stability is not directly within the medical assistant's control, but the medical assistant can be proactive in developing an employment plan and working toward its implementation. Taking these proactive steps to alleviate a potentially difficult situation over which you have no direct control will reduce worry and stress.

Technological Changes

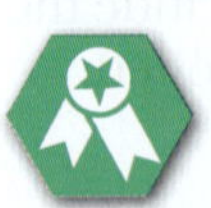
Competency

Change, even good change, can cause stress. Implementation of a practice management (PM) system (see Chapter 10) into a medical facility is an excellent example of an event that will result in stress for almost all employees; they are divorcing themselves from the familiar and being asked to embrace the unknown. The resulting level and duration of stress would be dependent on the comfort level of each individual with computer technology. For some older employees it may create stress until they retire. The best way to avoid stress from technological change is to remain current with the tools of your profession through continued education programs.

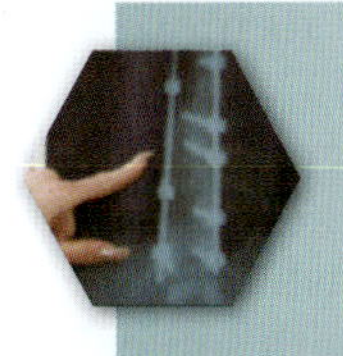

Critical Thinking

Practice in Time Management Analysis

List all of the tasks you do in a typical day. Beside each task write down how many minutes/hours you spend on each task. At the conclusion of the exercise, draw a histogram showing the percentage of each day spent on each task. This will quickly show where you spend most of your time. How could you save time? Develop a plan to reduce time spent in nonproductive, inessential activities.

Organization Size

Working in a large organization may lead to less understanding of the total job picture by the worker, resulting in less predictability and less control of the job to which the employee is assigned. This frequently results in feeling overwhelmed and frustrated. As the formalization and centralization of an organization increase, the stress experienced by an employee also increases. Downward delegation by management is the best approach to minimizing this problem.

Overspecialization

Overspecialization represents a limited practice exposure that isolates the employee from seeing the big picture and patient outcomes. This results in the employee receiving little or no satisfaction from his or her work, causing boredom, dissatisfaction and frustration.

WAYS TO REDUCE STRESS

Internal factors that influence your ability to handle stress include your nutritional status, overall health and fitness, and emotional well-being. There are numerous methods of reducing stress. A beginning place might be to review your diet and eating habits. Nutritious meals and snacks can boost the immune system, making it easier to cope with stress. Reducing the amount of caffeine and sugar in your diet has many health benefits. Alcohol, smoking, and drugs should be avoided.

Start an exercise regime. Exercising on a regular basis helps reduce the production of stress hormones and associated neurochemicals. Studies have found that exercise is a potent antidepressant, combats anxiety, and serves as a sleeping aid for many people. The amount of sleep and rest you get can determine your body's ability to respond to, and deal with, external stress-inducing factors. Sleep relaxes and refreshes the body and promotes clear thinking. Relaxation techniques such as meditation, yoga, deep breathing, aromatherapy and music are great stress relievers as well.

Goal Setting as a Stress Reliever

Do you direct your life, or do you allow others to influence and make decisions for you? **Outer-directed people** let events, other people, or environmental factors dictate their behavior. By contrast, **inner-directed people** decide for themselves what they want to do with their lives.

Studies prove that goal-oriented employees are more effective and assertive than are colleagues with no goals or future objectives. Recognizing the value of goal planning, many employers arrange planning sessions or seminars to encourage goal setting as a practical application for coping with stress and burnout and to develop career objectives. If your employer does not offer these outlets, seek your own seminars for goal setting. Such an activity not only "centers" you in your current employment, but also helps you clearly picture your future plans and hopes.

What is a **goal**? According to *Merriam-Webster's Collegiate Dictionary*, a goal is "the result or achievement toward which effort is directed." To reach a desired goal, a person must implement planning supported by a sincere desire to work hard. Skill in goal setting allows the medical assistant to clarify what must be accomplished and to develop a strategic plan to successfully achieve that goal.

A goal must be specific, challenging, realistic, attainable, and measurable. Specific goals are focused and have precise boundaries. A goal that is challenging creates enthusiasm and interest in achievement. Realistic goals are practical and beneficial both for the present and for future **self-actualization**, or fulfilling one's ultimate potential. An attainable goal refers to the fact that the goal is possible to fulfill. Measurable goals achieve some form of progress or success. By reflecting on the process, one is encouraged to establish additional goals.

Long-range goals are achievements that may take three to five years to accomplish. Long-range goals give direction and definition to our lives and serve to keep us "on track," so to speak. Much discipline, perseverance, determination, and hard work will be expended in accomplishing long-range goals. Some adjustment and readjustment to your goals may be necessary, however. The rewards of goal achievement include satisfaction, pride, a sense of accomplishment, and a job well done.

Short-range goals take apart long-range goals and reassemble the required activities into smaller, more manageable time segments. The time segments may be daily, weekly, monthly, quarterly, or yearly periods. Successfully completing a short-range goal encourages you to go on to the next goal and promotes a sense of achievement.

As a graduate and new employee, one of your long-range goals might be to become the clinic manager in the ambulatory care setting in which you are currently employed. You may wish to attain this goal within the next three to five years; by breaking it into three longer range goals and a series of short-range goals, you will be able to measure progress and feel a sense of accomplishment. Examples of long- and short-range goals might include:

Long-range goal 1:

- To become proficient in all clinical skills during the first year of employment.

Short-range goals necessary to achieve this:

- Practice accuracy and proficiency when performing tasks and skills.
- Practice efficiency by planning ahead for the equipment and supplies needed for each task performed.
- Evaluate your progress on a regular basis, and identify areas that need improvement.

Long-range goal 2:

- To add administrative tasks and skills to your routine during the second year of employment.

Short-range goals necessary to achieve this:

- Practice accuracy and proficiency when performing all administrative tasks and skills.
- Practice efficiency by planning ahead for the equipment and supplies needed for each task performed.
- Evaluate your progress on a regular basis, and identify areas that need improvement.

Long-range goal 3:

- To begin to focus on clinic management during the third year of employment.

Short-range goals necessary to achieve this:

- Develop a procedure manual for all clinical and administrative tasks and skills.
- Enroll in clinic management classes.
- Focus on team-building skills.

By the fourth year, you will be ready to move into the clinic manager position.

Long- and short-range goals work together to help make changes in our lives. Goals keep life interesting and give us something for which to strive. We can all reach goals successfully with some planning, hard work, discipline, and dedication.

EFFECT OF PROLONGED STRESS—BURNOUT

Burnout is a psychological term for the experience of long-term emotional, mental, and physical exhaustion accompanied by a diminished interest and motivation that affects job performance, health-related outcomes, and mental health issues. Burnout has four stages:

- *Honeymoon.* Love your job and have unrealistic expectations placed on you either by your manager or by yourself if you are a perfectionist; take work home and look for all the work you can get; cannot say "no" to accepting additional work.
- *Reality.* Begin to have doubts you can meet expectations; feel frustrated with your progress and work harder to meet expectations; begin to feel pulled in many directions; may not have a role model to follow and guidelines may not be established or defined.
- *Dissatisfaction.* Loss of enthusiasm; try to escape frustrations by binges of one sort or another: drinking, partying, shopping, or excessive eating or sexual activity; fatigue and exhaustion develop.
- *Sad state.* Depression, work seems pointless, lethargic with little energy, consider quitting, and look on yourself as a failure; represents full-blown burnout.

All of these stages are part of the process leading to burnout. The honeymoon stage might seem desirable, and it is pleasant; however, the seeds of the illness are present in the unrealistic expectations and the workaholic attitude of the employee. Unless these causes are eliminated, the progression to full burnout is ensured.

Burnout results in physical illnesses such as headaches, insomnia, allergies, cancer, acute indigestion, stomach ulcers, hypertension, blood clots, stroke, and immune system disorders. Psychologically, the body also is influenced by long-duration stress. Onsets of depression and anxiety, as well as eating problems resulting in weight loss or gain, are associated with the body's psychological response to stress. Anorexia and bulimia are common eating disorders attributed to long-duration stressful events. Long-duration stress can also affect our ability to think clearly, and objectivity may be impaired. Animal studies strongly suggest that maternal stress can also affect a fetus in later life. Physical symptoms of these emotional effects include alcohol abuse, drug abuse, cigarette smoking, obesity, depression, and lack of interest in or excessive sexual activity. A person in danger of burnout may also experience loss of energy and make poor exercise and nutritional choices, leading to a further cycle of medical problems and a more serious burnout condition.

Persons Most Vulnerable to Burnout

People with inadequate social support networks who are poorly nourished, sleep deprived, or physically ill have a reduced capacity to handle the pressures and stressors of everyday life and consequently are at greater risk of burnout. Some stressors are particularly associated with certain age groups or life stages. Persons facing life transitions such as children, adolescents, working parents, and older adults are vulnerable simply because of the increased stress associated with these transitional changes.

Personality type can have a role in susceptibility to burnout. When individuals with a high need to achieve do not reach their goals, they are apt to feel angry and frustrated and become negative toward their job. Failing to recognize these signs as symptoms of burnout, they may throw themselves even more fully into work-related goals. Unless there is some type of revitalization outside of the workplace, burnout occurs. Perfectionists try to do everything equally well without setting priorities; thus fatigue and exhaustion associated with burnout begin to set in after time.

Tips to Avoid Burnout

If you are stressed, or recognize that you are in one of the stages of burnout, you have reached a turning point. It is imperative that you make some changes in your relationship with your job. The following changes are appropriate and helpful in stress management or once you have entered the burnout stage:

- Make a concerted effort to say "no" when asked to assume additional work. Job scope creep is a leading factor in burnout.
- If you have more work than you can realistically accomplish, either prioritize it with the approval of your superior or delegate it within the limits of your authority.
- Change your work-related environment by creating variations. Modify your work routine slightly, rearrange your workstation to make it more personal, or change the computer desktop picture or screensaver to something you find pleasant that generates positive emotions.
- Evaluate the negative feelings you have regarding your job and attempt to replace them with more positive thoughts (i.e., instead of thinking the glass is half empty, think of the glass as half full).
- Try to look on work as a "fun" experience and an adventure.
- Establish some long- and short-term realistic goals and write them down along with a plan to make them happen.
- Develop strong social support networks by promoting friendships with coworkers; with family; or in outside religious, fraternal, or professional organizations. Occasionally going to lunch together with coworkers to laugh a little will promote a strong clinic support network and may help with that difficult person in your clinic life. Embark on a program of relaxation and meditation to reduce stress. Relaxation reduces muscle tension resulting from stress and can be achieved in a few minutes. Meditation requires about 20 minutes each day. Meditation affects body processes such as heart rate, blood pressure, metabolic rate, and brain activity and helps to obtain a feeling of "well-being."

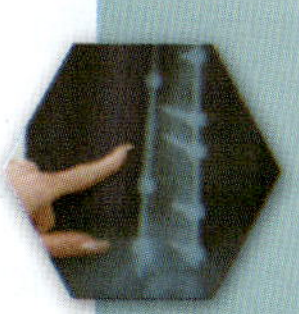

Critical Thinking

Self-Evaluation

- List several situations in your life that are stressful. Select the one that is most stressful.
- List as many things as possible about the situation that make it stressful to you.
- How would you change each of the things you have listed to make them less stressful?
- List the things you "could do" to effect the changes you listed.
- Rank the items in your "could do" list in terms of achievability.
- Select one or two of the items that are achievable and discuss them with a classmate. Now attempt to put them into practice for a week. Report back to your classmate on how effective these items were in reducing stress in your life.

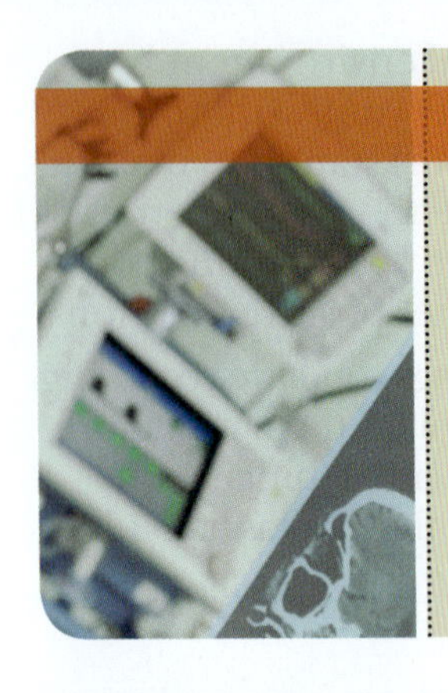

CASE STUDY 3-1

Refer to the scenario at the beginning of the chapter.

CASE STUDY REVIEW

1. What work can Ellen Armstrong, CMAS (AMT), organize the night before the clinic manager is out of town, leaving Ellen in charge of the reception area and the ever-ringing telephone the next day?
2. What professional skills should Ellen implement in this scenario?
3. How might Ellen relieve stress as the hectic day progresses?

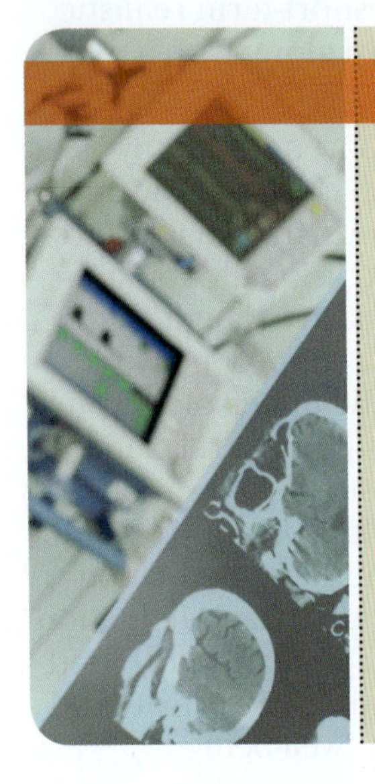

CASE STUDY 3-2

Ellen Armstrong, CMAS (AMT), has been employed for five years as an administrative medical assistant with Inner City Health Care. Ellen is a perfectionist and has pushed herself to achieve many of her short-and long-term goals. The clinic staff has become aware that Ellen does not have a sense of humor lately. She seems frustrated and irritable, and she is becoming critical of herself and others. Ellen has felt physically and emotionally exhausted, yet she continues to focus on her high standard of job performance; however, work is becoming a chore. At the end of the day, if everything has not been completed to her satisfaction, she feels like a failure.

CASE STUDY REVIEW

1. Do you think Ellen is stressed or experiencing burnout? On what do you base your conclusions?
2. What might Ellen do to differentiate these two conditions?
3. What changes might Ellen implement to resolve this problem?

Summary

- Stress is the body's response to mental and emotional strain or tension.
- Stressors are mental and emotional events that create stress and may be divided into three categories: frustrations, conflicts, and pressure.
- The four stages involved in adapting to stress according to the General Adaptation Syndrome cycle include alarm, fight-or-flight, exhaustion, and return-to-normal.
- Different kinds of stress include acute, episodic, and chronic stress.
- The sympathetic nervous system prepares the body for fight-or-flight. The parasympathetic nervous system returns the body to normal function. Long-duration stress can lead to harmful effects on the body, even life-threatening conditions.
- Clinical responses to stress include emotional, physical, behavioral, and cognitive signs and symptoms. The more signs and symptoms you notice, the closer you may be to stress overload. It is important to remember that many of these signs and symptoms can also be indicators of other psychological or medical problems.
- Stress in the work environment comes from many contributing factors, such as the physical environment, management style, difficult workers, failure to meet needs, job instability, technological changes, organization size, and overspecialization.
- Ways to reduce stress include reviewing your diet and eating habits. Nutritious meals and snacks boost the immune system, making it easier to cope with stress. Reduce caffeine and sugar, and avoid alcohol, smoking, and drugs. Exercise on a regular basis to strengthen the body and build core muscles. Sleep relaxes and refreshes the body and

continues

Summary continued

promotes clear thinking. Relaxation techniques such as meditation, yoga, deep breathing, aromatherapy, and music are great stress relievers.

- The benefits of goal setting are satisfaction, pride, a sense of accomplishment, and a job well done. Successfully completing short-range goals encourages you to go on to the next goal and promotes a sense of achievement. Long- and short-range goals work together to help make changes in our lives. Goals keep life interesting and give us purpose and something for which to strive.
- The four stages of burnout are honeymoon, reality, dissatisfaction, and sad state.
- Tips to reduce burnout include making a concerted effort to say "no" when asked to assume additional work; evaluating the negative feelings you have regarding your job and attempting to replace them with more positive thoughts; trying to look on work as a "fun" experience and an adventure; establishing some long- and short-term realistic goals and writing them down along with a plan to make them happen; developing strong social support networks by promoting friendships with co-workers, family, or in outside religious, fraternal, or professional organizations; and embarking on a program of relaxation and meditation to reduce stress.

Study for Success

To reinforce your knowledge and skills of information presented in this chapter:

- Review the *Key Terms* and *Learning Outcomes*
- Consider the *Critical Thinking* features and *Case Studies* and discuss your conclusions
- Answer the questions in the *Certification Review*

CERTIFICATION REVIEW

1. Which answer is *not* true about stress?
   a. It does not occur suddenly.
   b. It has physical and emotional effects on the body.
   c. It may be positive or negative in its effects on the body.
   d. It is the body's response to change.
2. How many stages occur in Hans Selye's General Adaptation Syndrome theory?
   a. 2 stages
   b. 3 stages
   c. 4 stages
   d. 5 stages
   e. 6 stages
3. Which is *not* a stage in the General Adaptation Syndrome?
   a. Fight-or-flight
   b. Exhaustion
   c. Burnout
   d. Alarm
4. Which of the following signs and symptoms is *not* associated with burnout?
   a. Physical illnesses such as headaches and insomnia
   b. Psychological influences such as anxiety and depression
   c. Feelings of accomplishment and pride in work
   d. Ability to think clearly and objectively
   e. Loss of energy; poor exercise and nutritional choices
5. The four stages of prolonged stress–burnout include which of the following?
   a. Honeymoon, reality, dissatisfaction, sad state
   b. Honeymoon, frustrations, conflicts, pressures
   c. Honeymoon, reality, conflicts, pressures
   d. Honeymoon, dissatisfactions, frustrations, pressures
6. Which response is *not* true of long-range goals?
   a. They may take 3 to 5 years to accomplish.
   b. They are divided into a series of short-range goals.
   c. They don't involve too much hard work.
   d. They may need to be adjusted and readjusted.
   e. They give direction and keep us on track.
7. The GAS theory proposes which order for its stages?
   a. Fight-or-flight, alarm, exhaustion, return-to-normal
   b. Exhaustion, alarm, fight-or-flight, return-to-normal
   c. Exhaustion, fight-or-flight, alarm, return-to-normal
   d. Alarm, fight-or-flight, exhaustion, return-to-normal

8. Stressors can be divided into which three categories?
   a. Frustrations, conflicts, pressure
   b. Pressure, anxiety, depression
   c. Conflicts, resolution, burnout
   d. Frustrations, conflicts, burnout
   e. Depression, burnout, suicide
9. Which of the following is *not* considered a sign and symptom of burnout?
   a. Anger
   b. Frustration
   c. Negativity
   d. Self-actualization
10. Which of the following is *not* true of the sympathetic nervous system?
    a. Returns the body to normal after the stressor has been removed
    b. Prepares the body for fight-or-flight
    c. Signals adrenal glands to produce adrenalin and cortisol
    d. Releases hormones into the bloodstream
    e. Causes stronger contractions of the heart muscle

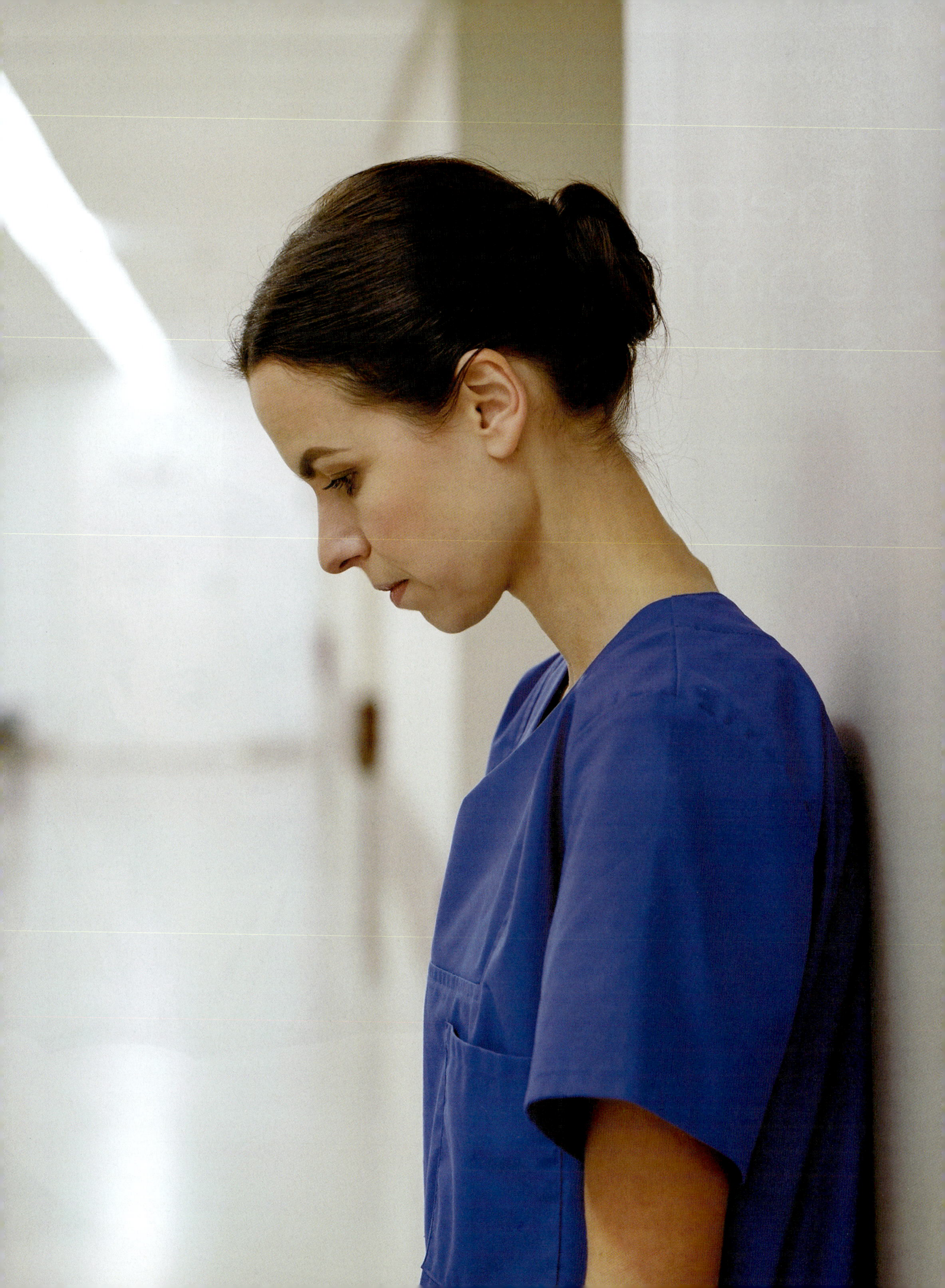

CHAPTER 4

Therapeutic Communication Skills

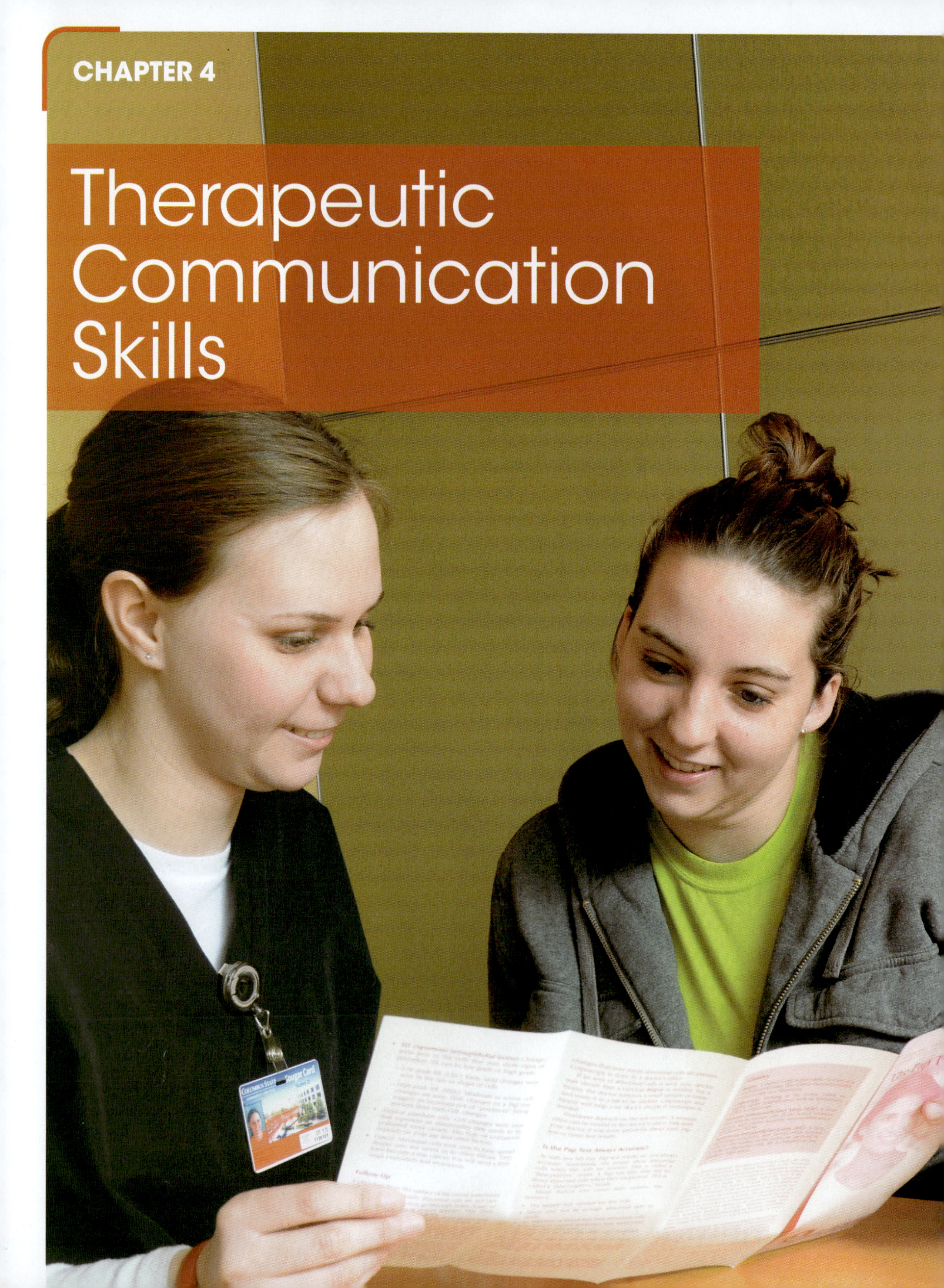

LEARNING OUTCOMES

1. Define and spell the key terms as presented in the glossary.
2. Identify the importance of communication.
3. Describe the four basic elements of the communication cycle.
4. Explain the five modes or channels of communication most pertinent in our everyday exchanges.
5. Model the importance of active listening in therapeutic communication.
6. Recognize differences between the terms *verbal* and *nonverbal communication.*
7. Discuss the five Cs of communication and describe their effectiveness in the communication cycle.
8. Analyze the following body language or nonverbal communication behaviors: facial expressions, personal space, position, posture, gestures/mannerisms, and touch.
9. Explain congruency in communication.
10. Differentiate between low-context and high-context communication styles.
11. Discuss generalizations of cultural/religious effects on health care.
12. Summarize the use of Maslow's Hierarchy of Needs in therapeutic communication.
13. Recall at least three steps to building trust with culturally diverse patients.
14. Recognize eight significant roadblocks or barriers to therapeutic communication.
15. Analyze common defense mechanisms.
16. Contrast closed questions, open-ended questions, and indirect statements.
17. Differentiate between coaching and navigation in health care.

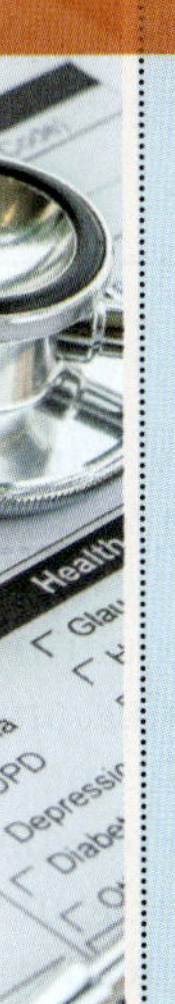

KEY TERMS

active listening
bias
body language
closed questions
clustering
coach
compensation
congruency
culture
decode
defense mechanisms
denial
displacement
encoding
Hierarchy of Needs
high-context communication
indirect statements
kinesics
low-context communication
masking
navigator
open-ended questions
prejudice
projection
rationalization
regression
repression
roadblocks
sublimation
suppression
therapeutic communication
time focus
undoing

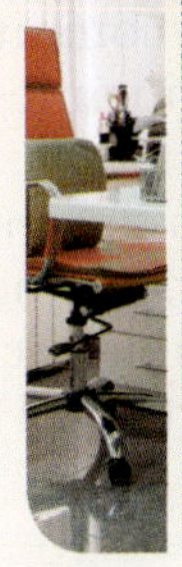

SCENARIO

At Inner City Health Care, four medical assistants constantly interact with patients, allaying their concerns, scheduling their appointments, instructing them on medications, and helping them understand their insurance coverage. On this busy day, clinic manager Marilyn Johnson, CMA (AAMA), is arranging for a patient whom it has just been discovered needs an interpreter, wants to personally greet new patients Anna and Joseph Ortiz, but is also concerned about Ellen Armstrong, the administrative assistant who informed her this morning her brother is gravely

continues

Scenario *continued*

ill in a neighboring state and she must take time off to be with him. Marilyn's warm manner and calm demeanor put everyone at ease.

Ellen is able to greet Martin Gordon, who has prostate cancer, and seems depressed and anxious. Setting aside their personal concerns, both Marilyn and Ellen try to create an environment where patients feel free to share their concerns and anxieties.

Ellen demonstrates therapeutic communication by acknowledging each patient as they arrive for appointments and puts them at ease by providing instructions. Medical assistants who project a warm and courteous presence while maintaining composure, even during difficult situations, and who ask the right questions in a nonthreatening manner will achieve therapeutic communication.

This scenario would be quite different if Marilyn were upset and angry that prior warning was not given of the need for an interpreter, she never has time to greet new patients to the practice, and Ellen is so upset by her brother's sudden illness that she accidently drops a call on hold and scowls at Martin Gordon and tells him to just take a seat.

Chapter Portal

Of all the tasks and skills required of the medical assistant in the ambulatory care setting, none is quite so important as communication. Communication is the foundation for every action taken by health care professionals in the care of their patients. Because medical assistants are often the liaison between patient and provider, it is critical to be aware of all the complexities of the communication process.

Every day, Marilyn, Ellen, and the two clinical medical assistants at Inner City Health Care face many communication challenges. This chapter describes effective communication principles, applies those principles to face-to-face communication, and describes the basic roadblocks to communication. The key word to all communication in the medical setting is therapeutic. In all conversations with patients, the more *therapeutic* the conversation, the more satisfied the patient will be with the care provided.

THERAPEUTIC COMMUNICATION DEFINED

Therapeutic communication differs from normal communication in that it introduces an element of empathy into what can be a traumatic or difficult experience for the patient. It imparts a feeling of comfort in the face of even the most frightening news about the patient's prognosis. The patient is made to feel validated and respected. Therapeutic communication uses specific and well-defined professional skills.

Therapeutic communication in the health care setting is the foundation of all patient care and is of the utmost importance. Communication must be in nontechnical language the patient can understand, delivered with feeling for the patient's emotional situation and state of mind, and yet it still must be technically accurate. The medical staff must be alert to the patient's state of stress and whether **defense mechanisms** have taken over to the extent that the patient has "tuned out" and is no longer communicating with the staff.

Patients seeking an ambulatory care service look for medical professionals with technical skills and a competent clinical staff capable of communicating with them. Questions frequently asked by individuals seeking a new provider and clinic include "Will the doctor talk with me so that I understand?" "Will the doctor listen to what I have to say?" and "Can I talk to the doctor honestly and openly?" The answer to all of these questions needs to be "yes."

THE COMMUNICATION CYCLE

All communication, whether social or therapeutic, involves two or more individuals participating in an exchange of information. The communication cycle involves sending and receiving messages even when not consciously aware of them.

Five basic elements are included in the communication cycle. They are (1) the sender, (2) the message, (3) the channel or mode of communication, (4) the receiver, and (5) feedback (Figure 4-1).

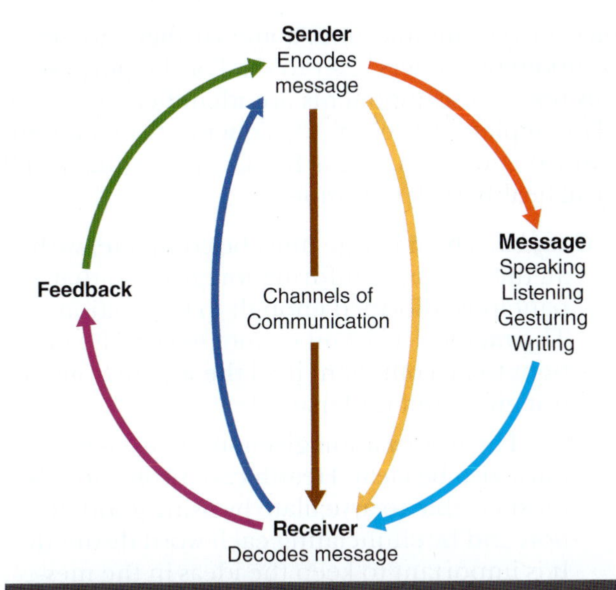

FIGURE 4-1 The communication cycle and modes or channels of communication.

The Sender

The sender begins the communication cycle by **encoding** or creating the message to be sent. Before creating the message, the sender must observe the receiver to determine as much as possible the complexity of the words to be used within the message, the receiver's ability to interpret the message, and the best channel by which to send the message. Encoding is an important step, and much care should be taken in formulating the message.

The Message

The message is the content being communicated. The message must be understood clearly by the receiver. Various levels of complexity in communication are used depending on the ability of the receiver to recognize and understand the words contained within the message. Children do not have the vocabulary base or the cognitive skills to communicate and understand at the same level as adults. Individuals with special needs will require special attention as well. The health of the receiver also must be considered. A patient who is distressed or is in pain may find it difficult to concentrate on the message. If the patient is of a different nationality or culture from the sender, verbal communication may require special skill. When visual or hearing acuity is impaired, this challenge must be surmounted.

The Channel or Mode of Communication

The three channels of communication, also called modes of communication, most pertinent in our everyday exchange are (1) speaking and listening, (2) gestures or body language, and (3) writing. These channels or modes are affected by our physical and mental development, our culture, our education and life experiences, our impressions from models and mentors, and how we feel about and accept ourselves as individuals. Each channel or mode of communication has its appropriate usage and must be considered when formulating the message.

The Receiver

The receiver is the recipient of the sender's message. The receiver must **decode**, or interpret, the meaning of the message. The primary sensory skill used in verbal communication is listening. It is hard work to concentrate and listen. When decoding the message, the receiver must be aware that not only the spoken word but the tone and pitch of the voice and the speed at which the words are spoken carry meaning and must be evaluated. Body language and how it is interpreted is a critical piece in face-to-face communication. The written word as a mode of communication (see Chapter 14) adds a dimension not realized in verbal communication—the ability to review the information or message being sent.

Feedback

Feedback takes place after the receiver has decoded the message sent by the sender. Feedback is the receiver's way of ensuring that the message that is understood is the same as the message that was sent. Feedback also provides an opportunity for the receiver to clarify any misunderstanding regarding the original message and to ask for additional information.

Listening Skills

A vital part of feedback in the communication cycle is listening. A good listener is alert to all aspects of the communication cycle—the verbal and nonverbal message, as well as verification of the message through appropriate feedback.

Active listening is one method used in therapeutic communication. In this technique, the received message is sent back to the sender, worded a little differently, for verification from the sender.

Sender:	How can I possibly pay this fee when I have no insurance?
Receiver:	You're worried about paying your bill?

The preceding example illustrates how the receiver is able to validate the sender's concerns at the same time the message is checked for accuracy. The door is then left open for a therapeutic response, such as:

Sender: Our bookkeeper will be glad to work out a payment plan with you that will fit your resources.

Active listening involves listening with a "third ear," that is, being aware of what the patient is *not* saying or picking up on hints to the real message by observing body language. The health care professional should have three listening goals:

- To improve listening skills sufficiently so that patients are heard accurately
- To listen either for what is *not* being said or for information transmitted only by hints
- To determine how accurately the message has been received

So many health professionals try to "fix" everything with a recommendation, a prescription, or even advice. Sometimes, none of those things is necessary. The patient simply needs someone to listen, to acknowledge the difficulty, and to remember that the patient is not helpless in finding a solution to the problem.

Skill in communication takes years of practice and frequent review. It will never become perfect; we can only hope that we will become better at it with each passing day.

VERBAL AND NONVERBAL COMMUNICATION

Communication

We communicate not only by what we say, but also by our tone of voice, body movements, and facial expressions. The following paragraphs present important aspects of verbal communication, the importance of listening skills, and nonverbal communication. The importance of maintaining consistency between verbal and nonverbal messages also is stressed.

Verbal Communication

Verbal communication takes place when the message is spoken. To be effective, it involves both speaking and listening. It is a two-way process. The purpose of verbal communication is to relay a message to one or more recipients. The majority of communication taking place in the health care community is verbal and has many purposes.

The Five Cs of Communication. Numerous authors, in and out of health care, have identified important pieces to communication. Some say there are seven components; others refer to six. For the purpose of this text, five components are identified. They are (1) complete, (2) clear, (3) concise, (4) coherent, and (5) courteous. These five Cs apply equally well in all health care professions.

Complete. The message must be complete, with all the necessary information given so that a patient is informed enough to take action. The medical assistant cannot expect the patient to be compliant if all the instructions are not given and understood.

Clear. The information given in the message must also be clear. Health care professionals must be able to articulate by using good diction and by enunciating each word distinctly. It is important to keep the ideas in the message to a minimum. The patient must be allowed time to process the message and verify its meaning. They should not have to read between the lines or make assumptions about the message.

Concise. A concise message is one that does not include any unnecessary information. It should be brief and to the point. Patients must not be overloaded with technical terms that may not be understood or that tend to distract them by diverting their attention away from the balance of the message.

Coherent. A coherent message is organized and logical in its progression. The coherent message does not ramble and does not jump from one subject to another. The patient should be able to follow the message easily. The medical assistant should always allow time to summarize detailed messages and use responding skills to verify that the patient fully understands the message.

Courteous. Courtesy is important in all aspects of communication. It takes only a moment to acknowledge a patient with a smile or by name. Be friendly, open, and respectful. There should be no hidden tones of disinterest. Remember to be courteous to colleagues in the clinic, also. Good working relationships and professionalism are always enhanced by simple courtesy.

When communicating within health care professions and to patients, keep in mind the following:

1. Good communication skills and following the five Cs are necessary in establishing rapport with co-workers and patients.

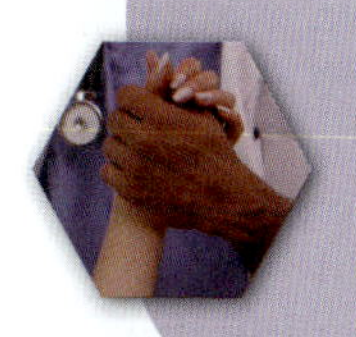

Patient Education

Sensitive medical assistants will encourage patients to verbalize their concerns. The ability to ask questions in a nonprobing way to elicit patient responses is an important function in any ambulatory care setting, because it is critical to know a patient's history, current medications, and other relevant data.

2. Patients feel respected and validated when called by their full name, such as Mary O'Keefe or Mrs. O'Keefe.
3. Patients should be encouraged to verbalize their concerns and to ask questions.
4. Patients should be given technical information (verbally and written) in a manner that they can understand.
5. Patients should have the opportunity to suggest and discuss any personal applications to their health care.

Nonverbal Communication

Verbal communication alone is not always adequate in conveying the message being sent. In most instances, more than one mode or channel of communication is used. Nonverbal communication, often referred to as **body language**, includes the unconscious body movements, gestures, and facial expressions that accompany speech. The study of body language is known as **kinesics**. Experts tell us that 70% of communication is nonverbal. The tone of voice communicates 23% of the message—only 7% of the message is actually communicated by the spoken word.

Nonverbal communication is the language we learn first. It is learned seemingly automatically when infants learn to return a smile or respond to touches on the cheek. Much of our body language is a learned behavior and is greatly influenced by the primary caregivers and the culture in which we are raised.

Feelings and emotions are communicated most often through nonverbal means. The body expresses its true repressed feelings using body language. Expressions and appearances communicate volumes of information. For instance, their appearance, attitude, and behavior sends messages about what health care professionals are thinking and feeling. Similarly, patients often convey their discomfort nonverbally before they verbalize a concern. Most of the negative messages we communicate are also expressed nonverbally and usually are unintentional (Figure 4-2).

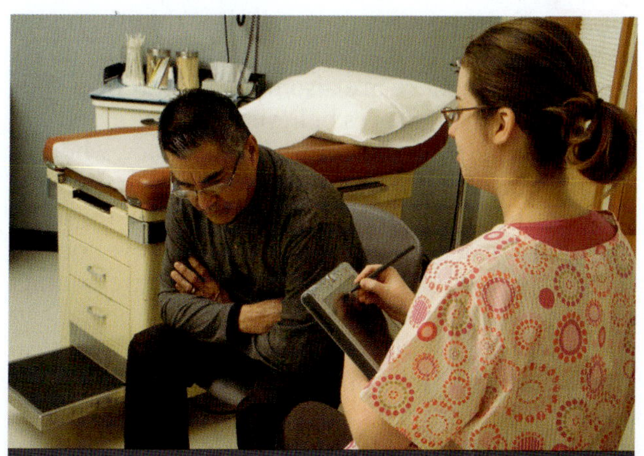

FIGURE 4-2 Body language can communicate more than spoken words.

Facial Expression. Facial expression is considered one of the most important observed nonverbal communicators. Each facet or aspect of the anatomy of the face sends a nonverbal message, most commonly through a smile or a frown.

Often expressions of joy and happiness or sorrow and grief are reflected through the eyes. The anatomy of the eyes does not change, but the movements of the structures surrounding the eyes enhance or magnify the message being communicated. Very brief or broken eye contact may express nervousness, shyness, or mistrust.

Children are told it is not polite to stare at people. It is acceptable to stare at animals in the zoo or art objects in the museum, but not at humans. Staring is dehumanizing and is often interpreted as an invasion of privacy.

The medical assistant must learn not to stare when patients present with ailments that make them "look" different. Patients such as these are individuals who have needs, who feel pain and discomfort, and who have decreased self-esteem and value. These feelings will only be amplified if the medical assistant and other health professionals are unable to "see" them as humans. A lack of eye contact may also be viewed as avoidance or disinterest in being involved.

The movements of the eyebrows indicate many nonverbal cues as well. Surprise, puzzlement, worry, amusement, and questioning are often nonverbal messages reflected by the position of the eyebrow. It may be difficult to "read" a patient's body language when they have lost their hair, even their eyebrows, during chemotherapy treatments. Wrinkling of the forehead sends similar messages.

Diversity

Cultural influences affect customs and different forms of facial expressions. It is important to remember that there are many cross-cultural similarities in body language, but there are also many differences. For example, some cultures believe that prolonged eye contact is rude and an invasion of privacy, whereas others consider it a sign of intimacy. Some people stare at the floor when concentrating or thinking through a process. Other cultures avoid eye contact to display modesty, whereas others feel eye contact expresses hostility or aggression. It is important to understand the cultures of the patients treated in the facility in which you are employed.

Personal Space. Personal space is the distance at which we feel comfortable with others while communicating. In the classroom, for example, students claim their personal space the first day of class. The area is well defined by using books and papers, or by placing the arm, hand, or chair on boundary lines. When another invades the personal space, a shift in body position or the use of eye contact sends the message, "This is my area." Individuals may feel threatened when others invade their personal space without permission. Some examples of comfortable personal space for U.S. culture are as follows:

- Intimate: touching to 1½ feet
- Personal: 1½ to 4 feet
- Social: 4 to 12 feet (most often observed)
- Public: 12 to 15 feet

Diversity

As with facial expressions, personal space is handled differently by various cultures. For example, there is no word for privacy in the Japanese language. Population numbers require crowding together publicly, as well as privately. Public crowding is often viewed as a sign of warmth and pleasant intimacy in Japan. In the private home, several generations may live together; however, each considers this space to be their own and resents intrusion into it.

Arabs like to touch their companions, to feel and to smell them. To deny a friend your breath is to be ashamed. When two Arabs talk to each other, they look each other in the eyes with great intensity. U.S. businessmen often end a business arrangement with a handshake; however, Native Americans view a handshake as an act of aggression or an offensive behavior. Each culture has its own distinct nonverbal communication cues.

It is beneficial to explain procedures that invade their space to patients before beginning the procedure so that it will not be perceived as threatening. This helps to empower the patient by involving the patient in the decision-making process and builds a sense of trust in the medical assistant.

Posture. Like personal space, posture is important to health care professionals. Posture relates to the position of the body or parts of the body. It is the manner in which we carry ourselves, or pose in situations. We tend to tighten up in threatening or unknown situations and to relax in nonthreatening environments. Those who study kinesics believe that a posture involves at least half the body, and that the position can last for nearly five minutes.

When the patient is seated with the arms and legs crossed, the message of closure or being opinionated may be relayed. In contrast, sitting in a chair relaxed with the hands clasped behind the head indicates an attitude of being open to suggestions. Slumped shoulders may signal depression, discouragement, or, in some cases, even pain.

Position. Position, the physical stance of two individuals while communicating, is a key factor to consider while communicating with the patient. Most provider–patient relationships use the face-to-face communication arrangement. When speaking with a patient, the provider or medical assistant will want to maintain a close but comfortable position, enabling observation of all cues being sent, both verbal and nonverbal (Figure 4-3).

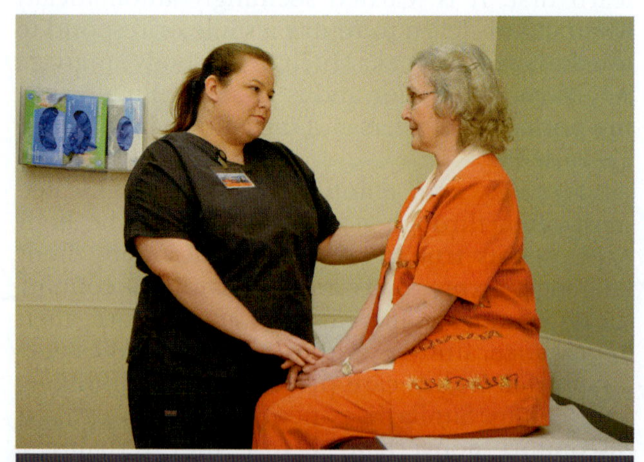

FIGURE 4-3 Positive posture and position encourage therapeutic communication.

Standing over a patient can convey a message of superiority, and too much distance between the two parties may be interpreted as avoidance or exclusivity. Generally, leaning toward the patient expresses warmth, caring, interest, acceptance, and trust. Moving away from the patient may be interpreted as dislike, disinterest, boredom, indifference, suspicion, or impatience.

Whenever possible, it is best to have a chair in the examination room and to have the patient seated comfortably in the chair to begin the communication cycle. The medical assistant or provider can sit on a stool that can be moved easily toward the patient. This arrangement aids the patient in feeling valued, listened to, and cared for as a fellow human being.

Gestures and Mannerisms. Various cultures denote different meanings to various gestures. If your patient is from another culture, never assume that gestures used hold the same meaning for the patient as they do for you. Most of us use gestures and mannerisms when we "talk" with our hands. This form of body language may be useful in enhancing the spoken word by emphasizing ideas, thus creating and holding the attention of others. Some common gestures and their possible meanings are as follows:

Finger-tapping	Impatience, nervousness
Shrugged shoulders	Indifference, discouragement
Rubbing the nose	Puzzlement
Whitened knuckles and clenched fists	Anger
Fidgeting	Nervousness

Touch. The medical assistant may perform many invasive tasks during the course of a clinic visit. Examples include taking vital signs or giving injections, both of which require touching the patient. Touch is a powerful tool that communicates what cannot be expressed in words. Its appropriateness in the patient–health professional relationship has well-defined boundaries and requires the use of good judgment on the part of the professional. Infants who are not touched, cuddled, and loved do not grow and develop as do those who receive these reassuring gestures. Touch is personal and is linked closely to personal space.

Diversity

Understanding touch as it relates to various cultures must also be considered. For example, Vietnamese, Cambodian, Hmong, and Thai families traditionally consider the head to be the site of the soul. During conversation and patient assessment, avoid touching the patient's head unless it is necessary for the examination. Southeast Asian patients may fear bodily intrusion; therefore, physical examination and treatment procedures should be explained carefully and completely before they are performed. The touch that communicates caring, sincerity, understanding, and reassurance is usually welcomed and considered to be a therapeutic response. Most patients will understand and accept the touching behavior as it relates to the medical setting; however, we must remember that not all patients are comfortable with touch. Whenever the patient is not comfortable with touch, explain the procedure fully, ask permission, and create as safe and reassuring an environment as possible.

Congruency in Communication

There must be **congruency** between the verbal and nonverbal communication. For example, shaking your head "no" while saying "yes" verbally sends a mixed message. In most cases, the nonverbal messages will be accepted as the intended message.

It is also important to remember that most nonverbal messages are sent in groups of various forms of body language. The grouping of nonverbal messages into statements or conclusions is known as **clustering**. **Masking** involves an attempt to conceal or repress the true feeling or message. The perceptive professional will be aware of all these messages. Perception as it relates to communication is the conscious awareness of one's own feelings and the feelings of others. To be most useful and therapeutic as health professionals, we must first explore our own feelings and appreciate and accept ourselves.

Learning to use perception involves the ability to sense another's attitudes, moods, and feelings. It takes practice and experience to develop and use this skill effectively. Being attentive to other professionals and observing their use of perception will yield insight into its usefulness and provide an example to emulate. A word of caution—the use of perception may easily be misinterpreted, especially when going with your feeling or assessment of what is happening regarding the patient. Always follow perceived assessments with verbal validation before assuming your perception of the circumstance is correct.

Nonverbal communication is easily misinterpreted. Careful observation for congruency between verbal and nonverbal communication, and clustering nonverbal cues being sent into nonverbal statements will strengthen your ability to interpret the message accurately.

INFLUENCE OF TECHNOLOGY ON COMMUNICATION

There will always be face-to-face and telephone conversations in the medical clinic, but clinics are also establishing secure portals to permit their patients access to their medical records. This approach permits the patient to schedule and review appointments, view laboratory reports, renew prescriptions, and communicate with medical personnel.

Social media has also created a niche in health care. Currently, it is being used for education, networking, goal setting, and receiving support (for example, weight loss, diabetes monitoring, and tracking personal progress). Health care providers use Facebook, Twitter, and YouTube to connect with patients and share information related to health issues through blogging. The Internet can be used to search for information related to health issues and treatment options. The CDC uses the number of searches on medical conditions, such as the flu and communicable diseases, as an indicator for epidemic warnings.

In some cases, satellite video and teleconferencing are being used to share information, receive education and training, or conduct meetings that include participants from various locations. Robots make rounds in the hospital setting and electronically communicate information regarding a patient's health. The patient can also see the provider on the robot's monitor and voice their concerns. (See Chapter 10 for more information related to the virtual medical clinic.) The major downside to using technology to communicate in the medical setting is security issues. Another disadvantage of technology is minimized interpersonal interaction. Chapter 10 discusses ways to ensure security at various levels and also presents ways to help the patient feel valued and included during interpersonal interactions via electronic means.

FACTORS AFFECTING THERAPEUTIC COMMUNICATION

Anything that interferes with the patient's ability to focus has a negative impact on therapeutic communication. The following paragraphs discuss significant barriers. The medical assistant must recognize that until these barriers are dealt with or minimized, therapeutic communication will be significantly affected.

Age Barriers

Professional medical assistants must understand human growth and development and be able to adapt their communications appropriately to any age group. Many scientists and researchers have studied human growth and development and have proposed guidelines for communication with patients during each stage. Erik Erikson (1902–1994) taught that each stage or phase is part of a continuum throughout the life cycle. The "Stages of Human Growth and Development" Quick Reference Guide lists Erikson's stages of human growth and development and identifies communication problems and suggested actions to be taken during each stage.

Economic Barriers

The influence of economics may reveal discomfort if the clinic staff and patients have a different perception about how billing is managed and when and how payment is expected. A discussion of billing and payment procedures at the first clinic visit or before a major procedure will be beneficial to all concerned parties.

Educational and Life Experience Barriers

Educational and life experiences will, in part, determine how patients react to their care. Patients with family members being treated for a chronic illness will have more knowledge and understanding of that illness in their own lives. Individuals who have already suffered a great deal of loss and grief in their lives may handle the information of a life-threatening illness more calmly than someone who has experienced little grief.

Bias and Prejudice Barriers

Personal preferences, biases, and prejudices will enter into many provider–patient relationships. Such biases affect the types of communication possible.

For therapeutic communication to take place, biases must be examined, a person's comfort level with each bias should be determined, and measures need to be taken to ensure that a hostile attitude is not present. **Bias** is defined as a slant toward a particular belief. **Prejudice** is defined as an opinion or judgment that is formed before all the facts are known; prejudice is a preconceived and unfavorable concept of some other person or group.

QUICK REFERENCE GUIDE

STAGES OF HUMAN GROWTH AND DEVELOPMENT

	Age Group	Communication Problem	Action Taken
	Infant 0–1 years Trust versus Mistrust	Total dependence on others for life support	• Respond to social smiles • Provide warm, friendly atmosphere • Consider safety issues • Wear colorful uniform
	Toddler 2–3 years Initiative versus Guilt	Limited vocabulary, fear of encounter with medical staff, separation anxiety if separated from caregiver	• Use child's own vocabulary and rephrase • Encourage and praise • Use simple commands • Allow child some control by permitting ambulation • Establish consistent clinic visit routine • Display a cordial relationship with parent to promote trust by child
	Preschooler 3–6 years Initiative versus Guilt	Unable to comprehend abstract ideas, cannot tolerate direct eye contact, creative imagination, short attention span, seeks control	• All of the above as appropriate • Physical contact at child's eye level if possible • Role play therapy (for example, give pretend injection to stuffed toy) • Allow control by permitting child to make as many choices as possible (for example, say, "Would you like to be measured to see how tall you are or weighed first?")
	School Age 6–11 years Industry versus Inferiority	Developing ability to comprehend, taking some ownership of health care, concern for privacy	• Include child in explanation of treatment and protocols using child's vocabulary • Encourage and praise • Make health care a teaching opportunity • Respect privacy of child
	Adolescent 12–18 years Identity versus Role Confusion	Increased comprehension, capable of abstract thought, may be fiercely independent, may use colloquial language, sexually maturing, concerned about confidentiality	• Actively listen, using patient's own language idioms as much as possible • Use abstract thought, but be alert to lack of understanding • Reassure that confidentiality will be protected, but state limits • Recognize peer pressure • Be aware of body image impacts

(continues)

	Age Group	Communication Problem	Action Taken
	Early Adulthood 19–40 years Intimacy versus Isolation	Greater comprehension and abstract thought capability, usually more in touch with reality than adolescents	• All of the items listed for adolescent • Provide health care options • Describe benefits and expectations of good health care
	Middle Adulthood 40–65 years Generativity versus Stagnation	Established socioeconomically, thinks of charities, concerns for succeeding generation	• Listen • Validate • Provide health care choices when appropriate
	Late Adulthood 65 years to death Integrity versus Despair	Anxious and stressed, hearing or vision impaired, slow to respond to inquiries, prone to omitting facts, overemphasis on somatic concerns, fear or embarrassed by loss of physical control, fear of being alone at death	• Be in proximity to patient and gently touch as appropriate • Speak slowly and clearly • Pace the encounter to match patient's tolerance • Be gentle and truthful

Common biases and prejudices in today's society include:

1. A preference for Western-style medicine
2. Choosing providers according to gender
3. Prejudice related to a person's sexual preference
4. Discrimination based on race or religion
5. Hostile attitudes toward people with different value systems than one's own
6. A belief that people who cannot afford health care should receive less care than someone who can pay for full services

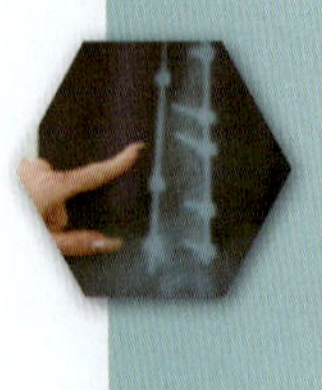

Critical Thinking

Define in your own words the terms *bias* and *prejudice*. Now identify one bias and one prejudice that you have. How will these impact your ability to respond therapeutically in the medical setting? What steps can you take to become more accepting of the uniqueness of others, thereby improving therapeutic communication?

Medical assistants must recognize such biases and prejudices so that their own culture with its biases does not prevent them from responding therapeutically in communications with all patients. Such recognition requires being aware of the differences among human beings and willingly accepting the uniqueness of each person.

ROADBLOCKS TO THERAPEUTIC COMMUNICATION

Being sensitive to patients' unique personalities and needs will enable the health care professional to avoid **roadblocks** to communication (see Table 4-1).

It must be the concern of each health care professional to facilitate communication by encouraging and enabling patients to express themselves honestly without fear. Roadblocks close therapeutic communication and prevent quality care of the total person.

Well-intentioned attempts to make the patient feel more comfortable can sometimes have negative effects on therapeutic communication. The following are some examples:

- Attempting to dispel the patient's anxiety by implying that there is not sufficient reason for it to exist is to completely devaluate the

TABLE 4-1

ROADBLOCKS TO COMMUNICATION

ROADBLOCK	EXAMPLE
Reassuring clichés	"Don't worry about not having a job, Mr. McKay; you'll find another one really soon."
Moralizing/lecturing	"If you were smart, Mrs. Johnson, you'd lose 50 pounds and you wouldn't have such a problem with your diabetes and hypertension."
Requiring explanations	"Why would you not want to have chemotherapy, Mr. Gordon? Seeing your wife die of cancer should surely make you want to seek treatment."
Ridiculing/shaming	"Ha, ha, Mr. Gordon! It's not *prostrate* cancer—it's *prostate* cancer."
Defending/ contradicting	"Mr. Marshal, I assure you the physician is *very busy*. He will not see you until he has finished with his other patients."
Shifting subjects	"Yes, Mrs. Jover, your work is very interesting, but I must ask you to sign this permission form to test for HIV."
Criticizing	"Mrs. O'Keefe, why in the world would you stay with an abusive husband?"
Threatening	"There is no way you will get rid of this cough if you do not stop smoking, Mr. Fowler."
Giving advice/ approval	Often occurs when health care professional is doing more talking than listening or feels the need to control the patient's thoughts or actions. "If I were you…" or "You should…"
Stereotyping	A preconceived notion that all people are the same. Anytime you group races or individuals together and make a judgment about them without knowing them, you are stereotyping. Remarks about racial groups, sexual orientation, and gender are the most common stereotyping subjects.

patient's own feelings. Developing a sincere interpersonal relationship more readily helps the patient. The health care professional should remain neutral in regard to the patient's condition. He or she should remain empathetic, but nonjudgmental.

- Rejecting the patient's ideas or comments causes therapeutic interaction to cease and thwarts the patient's expression.
- Indicating accord with the patient by using statements such as "That's right" or "I agree" can result in the health care professional speaking for the patient and can sometimes unintentionally put the health care professional's conclusions in the patient's mind.

Defense Mechanisms as Barriers

Therapeutic communication becomes difficult if a patient is in a highly emotional state. A patient who is frightened, ashamed, guilty, or threatened often will resort to defense mechanisms as a means of avoiding injury to the ego. We all use defense mechanisms to some limited extent, but they become harmful when they result in a breakdown in therapeutic communication. Failure by the patient to face problems often results in inability to provide satisfactory treatment on the part of the health care professional. Recognizing common defense mechanisms enables the medical staff to minimize the triggering event and to communicate more effectively.

Defense mechanisms are defined as behaviors that are used to protect the ego from guilt, anxiety, or loss of esteem. Use of defense mechanisms is most often subconscious to the person using them. It is the body's way of seeking relief from uncomfortable or painful reality. A mentally healthy person uses defense mechanisms to put a problem on hold until sufficient time has passed to permit him or her to address it without unacceptable emotional pain. Excessive use of defense mechanisms or failure to address a problem even after sufficient time has elapsed may be a sign of mental health issues.

Defense mechanisms are usually readily apparent to the disaffected observer; however, they are difficult to analyze without knowledge of the motive behind the behavior. Study each defense mechanism presented in the "Defense Mechanisms" Quick Reference Guide.

QUICK REFERENCE GUIDE

DEFENSE MECHANISMS

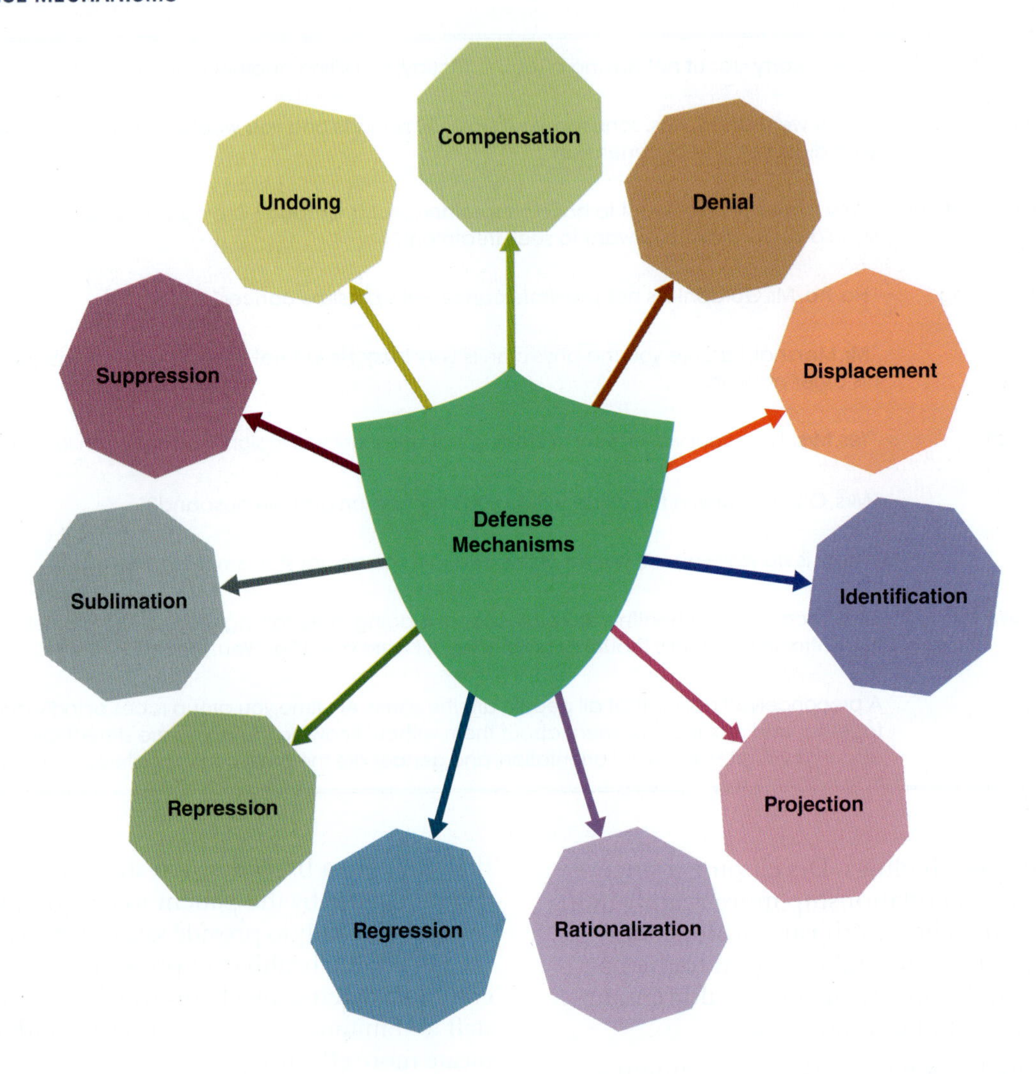

COMPENSATION

A conscious or subconscious overemphasizing of a characteristic to offset a real or imagined deficiency.

Example: A young boy whose physical stature keeps him from being a football star, so he compensates by achieving an academic award.

DENIAL

The refusal to accept painful information that is readily apparent to others. Careful attention to what the person is saying will reveal that he or she does not accept his or her situation and is not mentally conscious that it is happening.

Example: Often occurs when a person is diagnosed with a disease such as cancer or experiences the death of a close family member or associate.

(continues)

DISPLACEMENT

The subconscious transfer of unacceptable emotions, thoughts, or feelings from one's self to a more acceptable external substitute.

Example: A patient who is angry with the provider for some reason slams the door as he or she leaves the clinic.

IDENTIFICATION

An unconscioous defense mechanism in which a person assimilates or copies the identifying characteristics, traits, or actions of other persons or groups. Overuse of this defense mechanism denies the person the benefits and self-actualization of their own accomplishments.

PROJECTION

Attributing unacceptable desires, impulses, and thoughts falsely to others to avoid acknowledging they are actually the person's own experiences.

Example: A mother who abuses her child might accuse the medical assistant of being rough with the child while performing patient assessment to conceal her own feelings of wanting to throttle the child.

RATIONALIZATION

The mind's way of making unacceptable behavior or events acceptable by devising a rational reason in order to avoid embarrassment or guilt.

Example: A patient who tells the provider that he or she did not take his or her blood pressure medication because he or she did not have enough time before leaving for work.

REGRESSION

An attempt to withdraw from an unpleasant circumstance by retreating to an earlier, more secure stage of life. Usually occurs when a person feels powerless or desperate.

Examples: A toddler soiling himself after the arrival of a new baby sibling; An adult or child using a security blanket.

REPRESSION

The mind's way of defending itself from mental trauma by forgetting or wiping things out of the conscious memory.

Example: A child subconsciously forgetting to tell parents that he or she got into trouble at school.

SUBLIMATION

The channeling of a socially unacceptable behavior into a socially acceptable behavior.

Example: An overly aggressive person directed to play football to relieve aggression.

SUPPRESSION

The conscious or unconscious attempt to keep threatening material out of consciousness.

Example: The failure to remember a significant childhood event, such as the death of a grandmother.

UNDOING

Acting in ways designed to make amends or to cancel out inappropriate behavior.

Example: An abuser showering the abused person with gifts to compensate for unacceptable actions that took place in the past.

BARRIERS CAUSED BY CULTURAL AND RELIGIOUS DIVERSITY

Diversity

True therapeutic communication cannot take place without taking into consideration the cultural and religious background of the patient. **Culture** is a pattern of many concepts, beliefs, values, habits, skills, instruments, and art of a given group of people in a given period. Culture and religion influence the patient's communication context, caregiving expectations, time focus, and attitude toward Western medicine practiced in the United States. Table 4-2 presents characteristics that are typical of different cultural and religious groups.

TABLE 4-2

GENERALIZATION OF CULTURAL/RELIGIOUS EFFECTS ON HEALTH CARE

CULTURE OR RELIGION	MEDICAL CARE BACKGROUND	CAREGIVING STRUCTURE	COMMUNICATION TRAITS	TIME FOCUS*
Caucasian, Western Culture	**Western medicine,** rely on prescription medications, practice preventive medicine, may rely on folk medicine in some rural areas.	**Individual,** immediate family, close friends.	**Low context,** direct, eye contact expected, not adverse to therapeutic touching, may challenge medical opinions, basic English, speaks loudly.	**Future**
African American, Western Culture	**Western medicine,** rely on prescription medications, practice preventive medicine, may rely on folk medicine in some rural areas.	**Extended family,** relatives, close friends, neighbors, church family.	**Low context,** direct, eye contact expected, not adverse to therapeutic touching, may challenge medical opinions and can distrust medical personnel, basic English sometimes mixed with street language (Ebonics).	**Present/Future**
Black, African, or Caribbean Culture	**Mixture** of Western combined with spiritualism.	**Extended family,** relatives, close friends, neighbors, church family, tribal affiliation.	**Low context,** eye contact expected, highly emotional, basic English strongly mixed with local dialect.	**Present**
Asian Culture Asian, Indian, Chinese, Filipino, Japanese, Korean, Thai, Laotian, Vietnamese	**Mixture** of Western combined with Confucian principals, i.e., mind control of the body and maintaining a balance between natural forces and energy in the body, eating foods designated as having hot and cold properties to cure illness is common, mental illness is considered shameful and is denied.	**Immediate family,** opinions of family and particularly elders are important.	**High context,** indirect, avoid eye contact, show little emotion, avoid therapeutic touching, youth speak basic English, elders may speak little English, may agree with what is said even when they do not understand in order to avoid conflict or to avoid losing face, speak softly.	**Present/Past**
Native American, South Sea Island Cultures	**Mixture** of Western and folk medicine combined with importance of a balance between the forces of nature.	**Extended family,** relatives, close friends, neighbors, tribal affiliation.	**High context,** avoid eye contact, speak softly and slowly, basic English mixed with tribal dialects.	**Present**
Hispanic and Latino Cultures	**Mixture** of Western combined with a strong belief in intervention by God, eating foods designated as having hot and cold properties to cure illness is common.	**Extended family,** relatives, church family, collective community.	**High context,** be respectful and make direct eye contact, speak softly, some basic English, most speak Spanish.	**Present/Past**
Judaism	**Western medicine,** religion does not allow eating pork and requires kosher food.	Culturally dependent.	Culturally dependent.	**Future/Present**
Hinduism/ Buddhism	**Western medicine,** religions do not allow eating meat, modest regarding their body.	Culturally dependent.	Culturally dependent.	**Future/Present**
Islam	**Mixture** of Western combined with a strong belief in intervention by Allah, match gender of care-giver and patient, women may not be permitted to be examined by male medical professional, mental illness denied, do not ingest alcohol, believe complete rest is proper for all illnesses, do not eat pork.	**Immediate family,** opinions of family and particularly male head of household are important.	**High context,** touching between men and women is prohibited for strict believers, do not discuss sexual dysfunction, females do not make direct eye contact, will not discuss many taboo subjects (mental illness, birth defects, contraception, hospice), those from Middle East speak loudly to indicate the importance of what they are saying.	**Future/Present**
Christian Science	Most are unfamiliar with Western medicine, preferring to rely on prayer and spiritual intervention; accept clinical diagnosis, but attribute the causation to an underlying spiritual condition, healed by prayer; do not believe in drug therapy and may reject vaccination; each has freedom to seek modern medical treatment.	**Immediate family** and the use of Christian Science practitioners and nurses committed to a ministry of healing, but none have medical training or knowledge.	Christian Scientists could have any cultural background and hence communicate in the context of that culture; because of their lack of medical knowledge, the provider should clearly explain any procedures.	**Present/Future**

*The bold term represents the predominant focus.

Communication Context. Communication context can be one of two styles: low-context or high-context. **Low-context communication** uses few environmental idioms to convey an idea. It relies on explicit and highly detailed language. **High-context communication** relies on body language, reference to environmental objects, and culturally relevant phraseology to communicate an idea. Neither communication style is superior to the other. It is important, however, that both the speaker and the listener be cognizant of the style being used in the conversation. In the medical clinic, the medical assistant should be aware of communication content and attempt to utilize the style used by the patient to the extent that it is practical.

Persons having different communication styles can easily develop an incorrect impression of the other person. Low-context communication is direct and in your face, whereas high-context communication is indirect and seems to take forever to reach a conclusion. The high-context speaker is often thought of as mentally slow or uneducated, and the low-context speaker is thought of as being rude or arrogant. Conclusions based on communication style usually are preconceived misconceptions and should be considered at all times when health care professionals are working with patients.

Caregiving Expectations. Caregiving expectations refer to the arrangements for taking responsibility for medical requirements. Most persons from Western cultures are individualistic and take personal responsibility for their medical care, though children and older adults generally must rely on family or medical professionals for caregiving. However, many other cultures and religions do not share this individualistic philosophy, focusing more on the immediate or extended family for support. This can result in problems related to privacy requirements and patient compliance if a medical power of attorney has not been established.

Time Focus. The cultural background as well as the socioeconomic environment of the patient have considerable impact on time focus. **Time focus** relates to whether the patient's attitude toward life is focused on the future, present, or past. Time focus is usually related to culture and religion and is not necessarily related to current circumstances, though children, regardless of culture or religion, are present focused and older adults are more likely to be past focused.

Future time focus is found in persons whose physical needs have been met and who can sacrifice immediate gratification to achieve perceived greater future returns. Future-oriented persons are time conscious and plan out their daily lives in considerable detail. Persons from affluent Western cultures usually are future oriented.

Present time focus is found in persons who are less assured of being able to meet their physical needs. It is difficult to plan for the future when basic items in the hierarchy of needs have not been met. Punctuality usually is not important to present-focused persons, as they are immersed in the present and oblivious to time.

Past time focus is associated with persons from cultures having long-standing traditions. Tradition and past life experience become the central focus of their life.

Human Needs as Barriers

Human needs, such as those discussed in Maslow's Hierarchy of Needs, are barriers to effective therapeutic communication if they are not met. A patient who does not know where he or she will find food or shelter or who feels rejected and unloved will frequently make these needs first and of primary concern in their mind. It is nearly impossible to focus on communication regarding other concerns until these basic needs have been met. This section discusses human needs and how they can be addressed by the medical assistant or by referrals provided by health care professionals.

Maslow's Hierarchy of Needs. Abraham Maslow is considered the founder of humanistic psychology and is most well known for his **Hierarchy of Needs** (Figure 4-4). *Webster's Dictionary* defines *hierarchy* as "a group of persons or things arranged in order of rank, grade, class, etc." According to Maslow's theory, human needs are grouped into five levels. He

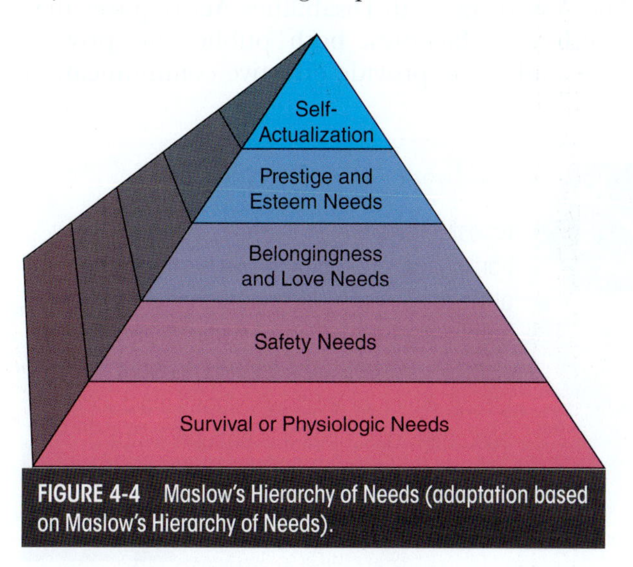

FIGURE 4-4 Maslow's Hierarchy of Needs (adaptation based on Maslow's Hierarchy of Needs).

also theorized that each level of need must be satisfied before one can move on to the next level.

The needs in the first level include physiologic or survival needs. These needs include food, water, and air to breathe—homeostasis for the body. The second level includes needs of safety and security, that is, the need for security, stability, and protection. Everyone has the desire to be free from fear and anxiety. Safety needs also include the need for structure, law and order, and limits.

The third level involves belonging and love needs. This level of need involves both giving and receiving affection. Additional words that express our connectedness are *roots, origins, peers, friends, family, neighborhood, territory, clan, class,* and *gang.* We have a basic animal tendency to herd, flock, join, and belong.

The fourth level, prestige and esteem needs, comes from a basic need for a stable, healthy self-respect for ourselves and others. There is the desire for achievement, strength, and confidence. Also, there is the need for recognition, prestige, reputation, status, and even fame. Satisfaction of these needs leads to feelings of self-confidence and worth. The final level is self-actualization. In this stage, we are at our peak, doing what truly fits us. It is an achievement of potential.

Individuals may move back and forth from one need to another depending on circumstances. Understanding this hierarchy helps to assess a patient's needs. If the most basic of needs are not met, it is highly unlikely that a patient can be successful with any treatment protocol. Keeping this hierarchy in mind will help to facilitate therapeutic communication.

Patients with Special Needs

The Americans with Disabilities Act requires that health care facilities, both public and private, large and small, provide effective communication alternatives to patients with language and hearing loss or speech impairment. The provider can choose the communication method or device as long as it results in effective communication. The expense for this accommodation must be charged against the overhead of the clinic and may not be billed to the patient.

A language deficiency can be overcome by using an interpreter, employing a human translator, using a telephone or service translator, or using online translation systems with software applications such as Google Translate, Speak and Translate, FaceTime, or Skype. These applications can translate in real time with text or with voice recognition software. Current technology has the capability to translate some 100 languages. The main disadvantage of voice systems is that they require speaking slowly and have difficulty translating technical terminology. When a person-to-person interpreter has been considered to be the translation mode used in the clinic, a resource list of interpreters should be compiled. The Registry of Interpreters for Deaf, Inc. is an excellent resource (www.rid.org). Your local city or state registry of interpreters may also be useful. It is also important to document the mode of preferred communication within the patient's medical record.

Patients who are visually challenged may be able to understand the spoken language; however, their vocabulary may be limited because of their disability. Utilize large-print materials and assure adequate lighting in all patient areas. Always speak in a normal voice to the patient as you enter the examination room or before you touch them. Extra caution must be exercised to ensure that patients who are visually impaired understand the message you are attempting to transmit.

Challenges with mental cognition will be a deterrent to communication. Dementia or other types of mental impairment, or even a serious illness, may make communication difficult if not impossible. Communication should include the patient's legal guardian or caregiver. Even so, every attempt should be made to have the patient involved in the conversation so he or she is not frustrated and feeling powerless and overwhelmed by the situation.

Critical Thinking

An established patient arrives 20 minutes early for his appointment. He is in obvious pain and discomfort and tells the administrative medical assistant, "I can't sleep, I can't eat, and I can't go to work today." Which of Maslow's stages most accurately describes this patient? What actions should the medical assistant take to assist this patient?

Environmental Factors

Environmental factors such as noise or any visual commotion that causes a distraction for either the patient or the health care professional will be an extreme barrier to communication of any type. Your conversation with the patient should be stopped until you can either move to a more suitable environment or the distraction has stopped. Physical barriers such as a computer screen or a desk between the patient and health care professional should be avoided. The medical professional should attempt to take a position close to the patient and at eye level, taking care not to invade his or her personal space. Always be vigilant to ensure there are no privacy issues violated.

Time Factors

Therapeutic communication requires time. Rushing a conversation with a patient and expecting effective conveyance of a message is unrealistic. The patient will listen but not retain your message if he or she is being rushed. The emotional state of the health care professional will be conveyed by body language in such circumstances.

ESTABLISHING MULTICULTURAL COMMUNICATION

Multicultural communication is the ability to communicate effectively with individuals of other cultures while recognizing one's own personal cultural biases and prejudices and putting them aside.

Approximately one third of the population of the United States comes from a culture other than Caucasian, English-speaking, Judeo-Christian. Figure 4-5 illustrates the percentage of various cultures living in the United States.

Medical professionals working within a specific cultural community should seek further information relating to that particular culture. In many instances, health care professionals can develop rapport with their ethnically diverse patients by simply demonstrating an interest in their culture and background.

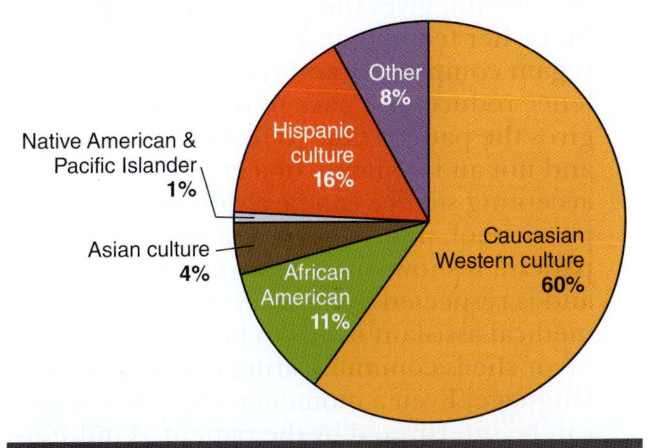

FIGURE 4-5 United States demographic make-up (2010 Census).

Before multicultural or any therapeutic communication can begin, the patient must first be willing to discuss his or her health care issues, listen to the professional's questions, and give honest answers to those questions. The patient must trust the professional. Several steps to building trust include:

- *Risk/trust.* It is essential for the helping professional to build an atmosphere of trust, making it easier for the patient to risk expressing feelings and attitudes about the problem. Trust has to be earned. Remember to promise no more than you can deliver, be honest, and carefully and thoroughly explain procedures and policies. Answer all questions truthfully and honestly.
- *Empathy.* Empathy is the ability to accept another's private world as if it were your own. Empathy communicates identification with and understanding of another's situation. It states, "I'm available to walk this road with you."
- *Respect.* Respect values another person and considers him or her as a special individual. It is important to respect the patient's personal space, to provide privacy, and to use his or her full name and title when appropriate.
- *Genuineness.* This means being real and honest with others. The health care professional must be able to communicate honestly with others, while being careful not to blame or condemn.
- *Active listening.* Active listening involves verbal and nonverbal clues that send the message you are completely involved in the communication. Sit facing the patient with no barriers, such as a desk, between you. Lean toward the patient slightly to convey genuine concern and interest. Establish and maintain appropriate eye contact to elicit interest and concern. Maintain an open, relaxed posture to establish a nonthreatening environment for the patient. Listen carefully to the words the patient uses to describe problems, and use those terms rather than medical terminology when discussing symptoms.

THERAPEUTIC COMMUNICATION IN ACTION

The following section identifies the proper communication techniques medical assistants should use as part of the most important communication function they perform: patient interview techniques.

Interview Techniques

All health professionals must be adept at interview techniques—knowing how to encourage the best communication between themselves and the patient. It is important to remember that an unequal relationship exists between the health professional and the patient. The health professional, whether it be the provider or the medical assistant, is in the power position and has a great deal of control over the patient. Therefore, it is important to equalize the relationship as much as possible.

Early in the interview, the patient must feel comfortable enough to risk being honest with the health professional. The health professional must build an atmosphere of trust by showing concern for the patient. A gentle touch and a warm, caring facial expression may be all that is necessary. Always be honest and genuine in your responses to patients. Be sympathetic and empathic and use responding skills such as sharing observations, validation and acknowledging, and paraphrasing to create an environment that is free of hypocrisy.

When the medical assistant is interviewing the patient for the presenting problem or chief complaint, it is important to listen with a "third" ear. Listen to what the patient is not saying but is apt to exhibit through nonverbal communication.

You might choose to share your observation of the nonverbal message with the patient, thus encouraging the patient to verbalize more freely. When concerns are shared, validate and acknowledge those concerns through statements such as "I can understand why you would be concerned." You can verify the communication by reflecting or paraphrasing what the patient has said. Reflecting focuses on the patient's emotional expression as well as observation of her body language. "You feel …" will often be used at the beginning of or within your response to the patient. Paraphrasing restates in the health professional's own words what the patient has said. The patient has opportunity to verify the accuracy of his message and that the professional understood the message as intended. Using words such as "You feel … because …" connects the two skills. For example, "You feel the back exercises are not working because you are still experiencing pain and discomfort."

When the health care professional is not sure of the meaning of the message communicated, clarifying skills are useful. Statements such as "I'm not sure I understand what you mean" or "Do you mean ...?" are examples of asking for clarification.

Knowing how to ask questions that help the patient express concerns takes practice and skill. The answers to these questions are vital to patient care and for accuracy of the medical record. Three basic types of questions are used to elicit information.

Closed questions are useful when collecting information for the patient history. They can be answered with a simple yes or no and usually begin with *do, is,* or *are.* Examples include:

"Are you still taking your medication?"

"Do you have pain in your back now?"

You will also use **open-ended questions** with the patient. These questions encourage therapeutic communication because they encourage the patient to express more detail. Open-ended questions usually begin with *how, what,* or *could.* Examples include:

"What kind of help will you have at home during your recovery?"

"How are you coming along on this diet?"

Indirect statements will also prove helpful in facilitating therapeutic communication. An indirect statement will elicit a response from a patient without the patient feeling questioned. Such statements encourage verbalization and express interest in the patient from the health care professional. Examples include:

"Tell me what you've been doing since you retired."

"I'd like to know more about your exercise program."

Additional helpful approaches to establishing therapeutic communication include:

- *Silence.* Utilizing the absence of verbal communication gives the patient time to put his or her feelings and thoughts into words, regain composure, and continue talking. Silence reduces the pace of the encounter and gives the patient time to feel like a human and not an inanimate object. A positive and accepting silence can be a valuable therapeutic tool, particularly for a shy and quiet patient; it shows that he or she has worth and is respected by another person. The medical assistant needs to be alert to what he or she is communicating through body language. Even a momentary loss of interest can be interpreted by the patient as indifference. In long periods of silence, the medical assistant must not become bored or allow his

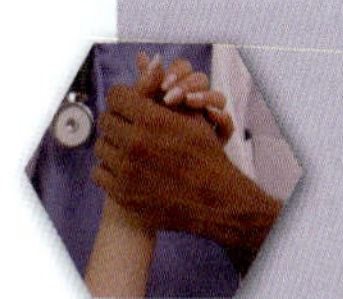

Patient Education

Education of a patient or caregiver should consist of the following fundamentals regardless of the subject:

- Do not attempt to educate the patient while he or she is emotionally upset or distressed. Under these conditions the individual will not be communicative; that is, he or she is listening but not hearing what is said. Make every effort to calm the patient. If necessary, reschedule another time for the educational session.
- Use multiple teaching methods, such as visual (including multimedia), verbal, and action, to convey the message. This approach ensures that your communication style will be versatile and meet the needs of the patient. Convey information in a clear, concise manner using context that is relevant to the patient.
- Limit the amount of material covered. If necessary, schedule additional sessions so that the patient is not overwhelmed.
- Communicate in simple words, avoiding medical terminology that may not be understood by the patient.

or her attention to wander from the patient. The medical assistant should give a broad opening such as "Where would you like to begin" and avoid small talk. Let the use of silence encourage patients to express themselves.

- *Feedback.* Nodding "yes," saying "I understand" if you do, or just "uh hmm" are forms of feedback. Offer general leads and give encouragement to the patient to continue by using statements such as "Go on," "And then?" or "Tell me about it." Acknowledge the patient's right to his or her opinion, to make decisions, and to think for himself or herself. Seeking to make clear that which is not meaningful or that which is vague provides useful feedback. Attempt to verbalize what the patient has hinted at or suggested. Search for mutual understanding and for accord in the meaning of words.
- *Giving recognition.* Give recognition and acknowledge his or her presence through greeting the patient by name. When the patient makes an effort or accomplishes something, the medical assistant should acknowledge it and give encouragement.
- *Offering comfort.* Help the patient to be comfortable during the medical encounter by showing empathy with the patient's situation. Introduce yourself and explain what is about to happen or to be done to the patient. Make available the facts the patient needs to feel at ease and to make the encounter less stressful.

PATIENT COACHING AND NAVIGATION

Primary care providers struggle to adequately cover every agenda item a patient may have within the 15-minute clinic visit. This is especially true for patients with chronic conditions. As a result, a paradigm shift away from a provider diagnosing and prescribing a treatment plan toward a collaborative approach where the patient and provider discuss options for health care has developed, utilizing both coaching and navigation. The primary objective of the **coach** is to educate patients regarding self-health management and to encourage patients to take a more active role in staying healthy. Each member of the health care team can integrate elements of coaching into their interactions with patients; however, at least one team member should be designated as a coach. It is the responsibility of the coach to help patients gain the knowledge, skills, tools, and confidence to become active participants in the management of their health care.

Health coaches may act as advocates or intermediaries in the patient–provider relationship by sharing relevant information with the provider and by motivating and encouraging the patient to follow provider protocols. The coach may also instruct the patient about diagnostic and therapeutic modalities and guide the patient in making informed choices about when, how, and where to use community health care resources. (See Chapter 11 for community resource information.)

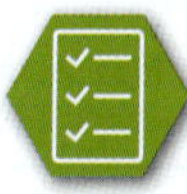
Procedure

A **navigator** works in conjunction with the medical home health care team and assists with answering questions about care and medications, keeping the family informed and engaged in patient care, providing one-on-one education aimed at improving health, helping schedule appointments, and arranging community resources as needed. These resources may include home health care, skilled nursing facilities, and rehabilitation centers. The navigator can also help with transition care, including specialist to specialist, hospital to home, and hospital to skilled nursing or rehabilitation centers. Procedure 4-1 provides the steps to coach or navigate a patient regarding a collaborative approach to health care.

Qualifications for the role of coach or navigator include being an excellent listener; having good communication skills; and utilizing planning, organization, and follow-up techniques. Medical assistants are prime candidates for this role due to their multifaceted professional education. They are ideally suited to provide linguistic and cultural coaching as well. Since scope of practice varies from state to state, you will want to check your state's regulations as they relate to coaching and navigation. Generally, medical assistants are not permitted to make medical assessments.

PROCEDURE 4-1

Coach or Navigate a Patient Regarding a Collaborative Approach to Health Care

PURPOSE:

To educate patients regarding self-health management, to encourage patients to take a more active role in staying healthy, and to assist them in navigating the medical home health care team.

EQUIPMENT/SUPPLIES:

- Paper and pen
- Computer
- Information ordered by provider for coaching/navigation session

PROCEDURE STEPS:

1. Check your state's scope of practice regulations. RATIONALE: You must always ensure you are working within your scope of practice.
2. Develop a written plan (approved and included in the clinic's procedure manual) on who the coach/navigator will be and what information will be disseminated by the coach/navigator. RATIONALE: Communication skills and barriers, developmental life stages, and cultural and religious diversity issues should all be considered in the patient approach in order to foster a positive patient/provider relationship.
3. Introduce yourself by name and title, and identify the patient.
4. Provide a written copy of all instructions to the patient and review them verbally with the patient. RATIONALE: Ensures that all instructions are discussed.
5. Ask the patient to repeat instructions and answer any questions or concerns he or she may have regarding the instructions. Provide the office telephone number in case the patient has any additional questions. RATIONALE: Ensures clarification for all parties.
6. ***Demonstrate empathy, active listening, and respect for individual diversity*** throughout the session.
7. Document in the patient's medical record what information and instructions were given.

DOCUMENTATION:

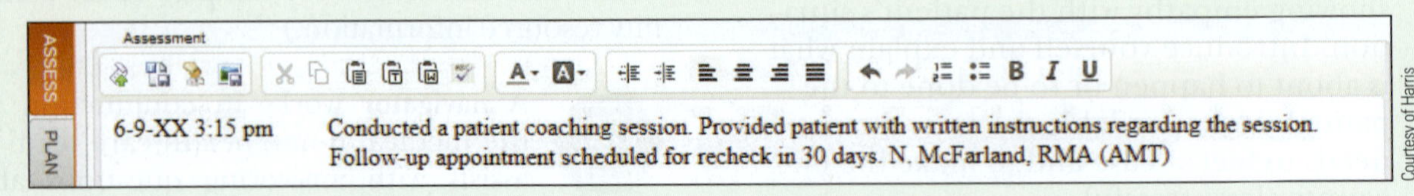

Courtesy of Harris CareTracker PM and EMR

When using a coach or a navigator, the benefits to the patient and the practice include:

- Helping patients navigate an increasingly complex health care system
- Reviewing progress since the last visit with the patient and the medical team
- Answering questions regarding medical instructions and processes
- Confirming that information is correct in the medical record
- Following up with the patient after a visit to the practice
- Strengthening patient satisfaction
- Motivating the patient to change behavior and to self-manage his or her health toward mutually agreed-on goals

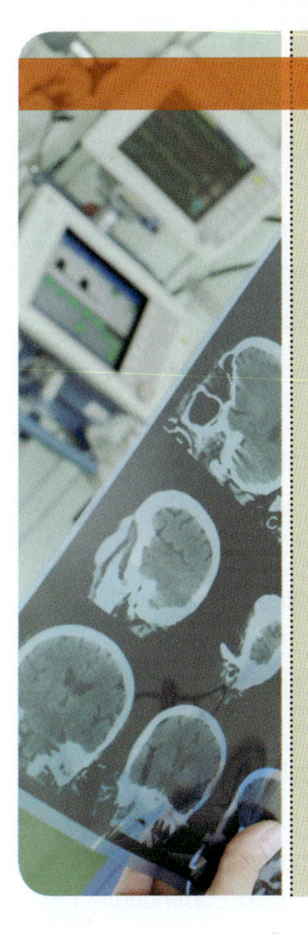

CASE STUDY 4-1

It is a very busy day at Inner City Health Care. Despite the three emergencies in the early afternoon and the full schedule of patients, everything is running smoothly with Dr. Lewis, and the entire staff, responding quickly but thoroughly to patient concerns.

At 4:00 PM another emergency patient arrives; at the same time, Jim Marshal, an architect in a downtown firm, comes in early for a routine appointment and demands to be seen immediately. Jim, a regular patient, has a history of being difficult and impatient; being a bit arrogant, he tends to put his needs first. However, Dr. Lewis is occupied with another patient. It is critical to treat the patient with the emergency as soon as possible, and Jim is half an hour early.

Ellen Armstrong, CMAS (AMT), the clinic's administrative medical assistant, calmly asks Mr. Marshal to please wait until his scheduled appointment time. When he threatens to leave, Ellen explains to Mr. Marshal that there are two patients ahead of him, but that the provider will see him at his scheduled appointment time.

CASE STUDY REVIEW

1. What communication roadblocks did medical assistant Ellen Armstrong avoid as she reacted to Jim Marshal's demands to see the provider?
2. With another student, role-play the scenario, with one student taking the role of patient and one student the role of the medical assistant. Identify roadblocks to communication imposed by the patient. How is the medical assistant using the five Cs of communication to deal with the situation?
3. Do you think the medical assistant reacted appropriately? What else could she have done? What should she *not* do in this situation?

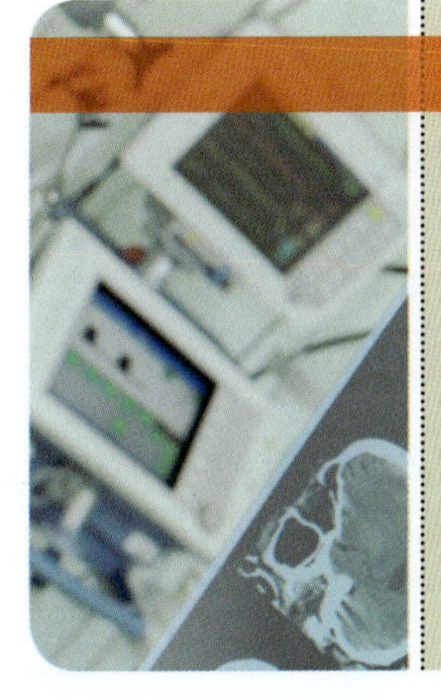

CASE STUDY 4-2

You have learned in this chapter that communication has not been successful until the communication cycle is complete. Consider the following scenario.

An 82-year-old woman with moderate dementia and a hearing impairment is brought to the surgeon's clinic for a follow-up appointment after hip replacement surgery. The woman's daughter, who is the patient's medical power of attorney, accompanies her. The goal of the appointment is to make certain the hip is healing nicely and to discuss precautions before the patient returns to her assisted-living apartment. Almost immediately, the conversation is directed toward the daughter because it is so much easier to explain to her what should be done.

continues

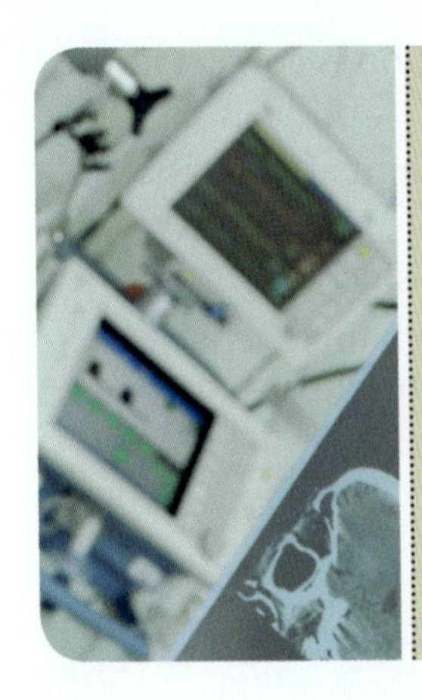

CASE STUDY 4-2 *continued*

CASE STUDY REVIEW

1. What might the staff do to help the patient understand the following?
   - Use the walker consistently.
   - Wear shoes that are leather, tennis-shoe type, or uniform style; consider Velcro closure as opposed to laces that have to be tied.
   - Do not walk your dog on a leash.
2. Should the patient be left out of the conversation? Should the daughter be included?
3. In cases such as these, is something other than verbal communication indicated?

Summary

- Therapeutic communication uses specific and well-defined professional skills. It is understandable to the patient, delivered with empathy, and technically accurate.
- Communication involves two or more individuals participating in an exchange of information. The communication cycle includes the sender, the message, the channel or mode of transmission, the receiver, and the feedback.
- Verbal communication involves speaking and listening while using the five Cs of communication.
- Nonverbal communication or body language includes the unconscious body movements, gestures, and facial expressions that accompany speech.
- To avoid miscommunication there must be congruency between the verbal and nonverbal communication.
- There will always be face-to-face and telephone conversations in the medical clinic; however, technology is rapidly breaking ground for the virtual medical clinic.
- The medical assistant must recognize that until the barriers affecting therapeutic communication are dealt with or at least minimized, therapeutic communication will be significantly impacted.
- Culture and religion influence the patient's communication context, caregiving expectations, time focus, and attitude toward Western medicine practiced in the United States.
- According to Maslow's Hierarchy of Needs, human needs are grouped into five levels and must be satisfied before one can move on to the next level.
- The Americans with Disabilities Act requires that all health care facilities provide effective communication alternatives to patients with language and hearing loss or speech impairment. Any expense incurred with the accommodation must be charged against the overhead of the clinic and may not be billed to the patient.
- Approximately one third of the population of the United States comes from a culture other than Caucasian, English-speaking, Judeo-Christian. Multicultural communication requires recognizing one's own personal cultural biases and prejudices and putting them aside to promote therapeutic communication.
- All health care professionals must be adept at interview techniques that build an atmosphere of trust by showing concern for the patient, being sympathetic and empathic, using appropriate responding skills, and asking questions in a nonthreatening manner.
- The primary objective of the coach is to educate patients regarding self-health management and to encourage patients to take a more active role in staying healthy. A navigator works in conjunction with the medical home health care team.
- Throughout this text you are reminded of the importance of effective communication techniques. Good communication takes practice. Use the techniques identified in this chapter with your family and with your peers. Watch for roadblocks, be aware of defense mechanisms, and remember the five Cs of communication.

Study for Success

To reinforce your knowledge and skills of information presented in this chapter:

- Review the *Key Terms* and *Learning Outcomes*
- Consider the *Critical Thinking* features and *Case Studies* and discuss your conclusions
- Answer the questions in the *Certification Review*

Procedure

- Perform the *Procedure* using the *Competency Assessment Checklist* on the *Student Companion Website*

CERTIFICATION REVIEW

1. Which of the following factors affect therapeutic communication?
   a. Gestures and mannerisms
   b. Posture
   c. Personal space
   d. Education and life experience
2. What does encoding mean in the cycle of communication?
   a. Deciphering a message
   b. Creating the message to be sent
   c. Sending the message
   d. Receiving the message
   e. Interpreting the message
3. What is true of body language?
   a. It is used to express feelings and emotions.
   b. It is not as important as verbal communication.
   c. It only makes up 7% of the message.
   d. It is only used in Eastern cultures.
4. What is a comfortable social space?
   a. Touching to 1½ feet
   b. 1½ feet to 4 feet
   c. 12 to 15 feet
   d. 5 to 16 feet
   e. 4 to 12 feet
5. Which of the following accurately describes a reassuring cliché?
   a. It is a way of calming down a patient.
   b. It is a means of rationalizing a decision.
   c. It is a roadblock to communication.
   d. It is always useful in daily communications.
6. Redirecting a socially unacceptable impulse into one that is socially acceptable is an example of which of these defense mechanisms?
   a. Sublimation
   b. Rationalization
   c. Projection
   d. Displacement
   e. Repression
7. Which of the following is true of open-ended questions?
   a. They usually require just a "yes" or "no" answer.
   b. They usually begin with *do, is,* or *are.*
   c. They elicit a response from a patient without the patient feeling questioned.
   d. They usually begin with *how, what,* or *could.*
8. Which statement is true of kinesics?
   a. It is the study of body language.
   b. It is the study of personal space.
   c. It is the study of touch.
   d. It is the study of congruency.
   e. It is the study of defense mechanisms.
9. High-context communication relies on which of the following?
   a. Body language
   b. Reference to environmental objects
   c. Explicit and highly detailed language
   d. Culturally relevant phraseology
10. Which of the following describes defense mechanisms?
    a. They are a refusal to accept painful information that is readily available to others.
    b. They are the conscious or subconscious overemphasis of a characteristic to offset a real or imagined deficiency.
    c. They are behaviors used to protect the ego from guilt, anxiety, or loss of esteem.
    d. They are the mind's way of making unacceptable behavior or events acceptable by devising a rational reason.

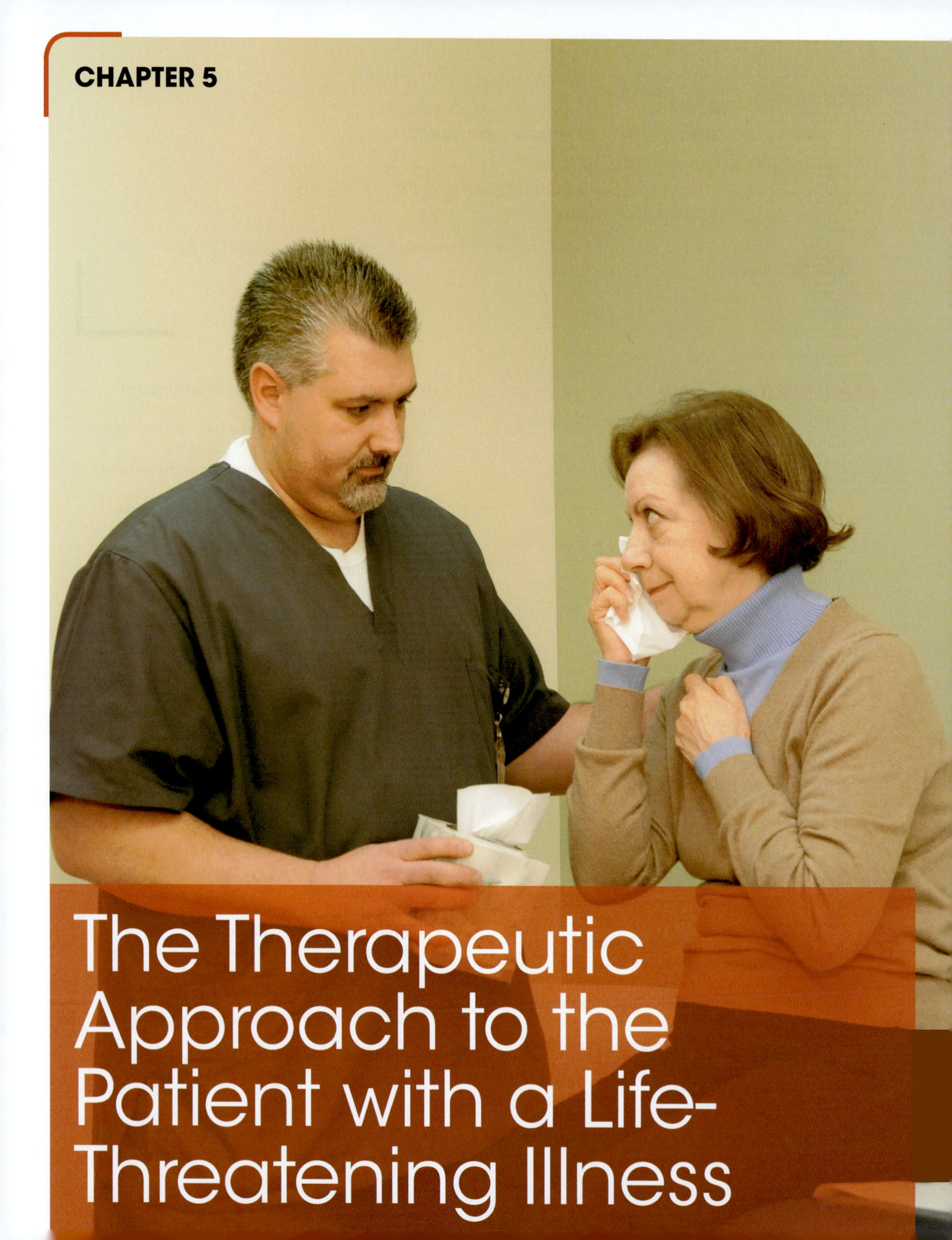

CHAPTER 5

The Therapeutic Approach to the Patient with a Life-Threatening Illness

LEARNING OUTCOMES

1. Define and spell the key terms as presented in the glossary.
2. Recognize possible patient perspectives when facing a life-threatening illness.
3. Define "life-threatening" illness.
4. Critique the cultural manifestations of life-threatening illness.
5. Identify the strongest cultural influence in the life of a patient.
6. List at least four choices to be made when facing a life-threatening illness.
7. Analyze the different forms of health care directives.
8. Explain how a durable power of attorney for health care is used.
9. Discuss the range of psychological suffering that accompanies life-threatening illnesses.
10. Summarize additional concerns/fears when the life-threatening illness is cancer, AIDS, or end-stage renal disease.
11. Demonstrate the therapeutic response to persons with a life-threatening illness.
12. Summarize four questions to help patients verbalize their feelings in end-of-life communication.
13. Explain the five stages of grief and the meaning of the acronym TEAR.
14. Recall a number of challenges faced by the medical assistant when caring for people with life-threatening illnesses.

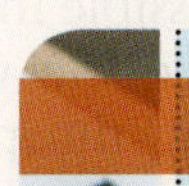

KEY TERMS

durable power of attorney for health care

health care directive

palliative

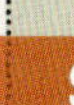

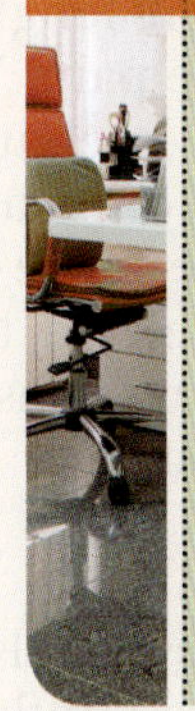

SCENARIO

You have seen the medical reports and agonize with your employer who must tell long-time patient Suzanne Markis when she comes in today that she has inoperable pancreatic cancer. When she arrives, you treat her as you normally would, making certain she suspects nothing from you. When she emerges from the provider's room, you make certain to meet her, take her arm, and ask if you can call someone for her. You do not present her with a bill or make another appointment at this time. You recognize that anything you say probably will not be remembered, so you focus entirely on this patient and her immediate needs. In a day or two, as instructed by your employer, you will telephone to make an appointment for Suzanne and anyone she might want present at her next visit with the provider so any questions can be answered.

Chapter Portal

Everything you learned in Chapter 4 regarding therapeutic communication is heightened and considered more challenging when the patient has a life-threatening illness. If you were told today that your life will probably be shortened because of a serious illness, your perspective likely would change. What was important yesterday may mean little or nothing now. Something that meant nothing to you yesterday suddenly takes on great importance to you now. It is essential for the medical assistant to remember this difference in perspective and remember what is likely to be important to patients with a life-threatening illness.

continues

Chapter Portal, *continued*

It also must be remembered that no two individuals respond to a life-threatening illness in the same way. Some respond with denial and act as if the information had never been shared with them. Others alter their lives radically and drastically change their priorities. Still others quietly continue their lives, changing little outwardly, but recognizing that their choices may now be limited (Figure 5-1).

LIFE-THREATENING ILLNESS

A life-threatening illness is not easily defined. Some use the word *terminal;* others refuse to use that word because they believe it removes any hope from the situation. Still others believe even the term *life-threatening* is too hopeless and prefer to use the term *life-altering;* however, a life-altering illness can quickly become life-threatening. Also, what one individual considers life-threatening may not be the same for another. For our purposes, life-threatening is used to imply a life that in all probability will be shortened because of a serious or debilitating illness or disease. It may be defined as death that is imminent; it may be defined in terms of a serious illness that a person will battle for many years but one that will ultimately shorten his or her life.

Cultural Perspective on Life-Threatening Illness

Diversity

Strong cultural manifestations will be seen during the treatment of a life-threatening illness and in anyone facing death. Culture is defined as how we live our lives, how we think, how we speak, and how we behave. Cultures can be accepting, denying, or even defying of death. Death can be considered either as the end of existence or as a transition to another state of being or consciousness. Death can be considered as profane or sacred. In some cultures, a life-threatening illness may be viewed or referred to as a "slow-motion" death because of degenerative diseases that often exhaust the resources and emotions of patients and their families.

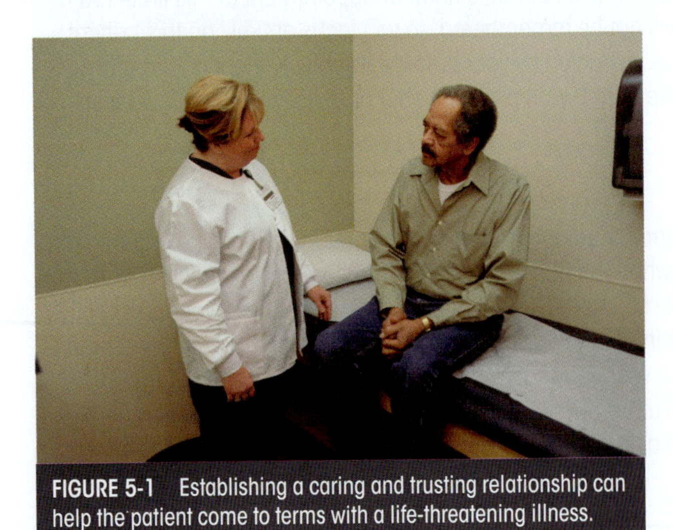
FIGURE 5-1 Establishing a caring and trusting relationship can help the patient come to terms with a life-threatening illness.

Some cultures prefer that the life-threatening illness not be shared with the patient in the beginning, but with the family who helps to prepare the patient for the inevitable. A few cultures generally do not seek care for an illness until it is quite advanced; this practice can make pain management and treatment more difficult or impossible in some cases. Some cultures surround the person who is ill with great attention, never leaving the person alone. Other cultures view the illness as something that must be removed from the body, perhaps even believing that the individual has been given this illness because of some past sin or transgression.

Pain is viewed in the same manner. Some cultures believe it is to be endured quietly without complaint; others believe there is to be no pain, and family members will go to great lengths to have health care providers relieve the pain. When questioning a patient about the pain level, it must be within a cultural perspective. For example, cultures with an Asian influence are more likely to describe pain in general terms related to the imbalance of the body rather than in terms such as "piercing, intermittent, or throbbing" or "on a scale from 1 to 10."

Integrity

Skilled health care professionals will remember that the strongest influence in managing any life-threatening illness in the life of the patient is *not* the health care team; it is the family and those closest to the patient. Therefore, great care must be taken to determine and understand the patient's cultural perspective as much as possible, and the patient must be given great respect. Often, the cultural influence may contradict the standard of care preferred by the health care provider. It is better to understand the culture and work within that parameter than to deny it and continually work

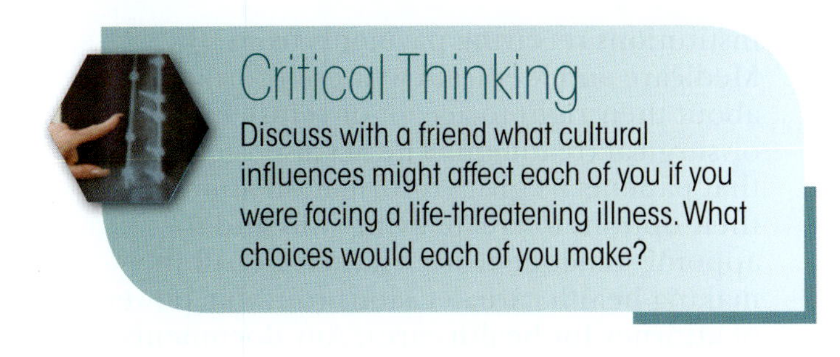

Critical Thinking

Discuss with a friend what cultural influences might affect each of you if you were facing a life-threatening illness. What choices would each of you make?

against the patient's belief system and the influence of family.

CHOICES IN LIFE-THREATENING ILLNESS

Many choices are available to a patient with a life-threatening illness, but there are also many decisions to be made. The urgency of the decisions will depend, in part, on possible life expectancy. Patients often want an answer to the question, "How long do I have?" Providers are unable to give a definitive answer; however, estimates may be given in terms of weeks, months, or even years. Patients may choose to make decisions that seem contrary to recommended medical intervention. Often, too, these decisions are clouded by a provider's desire and need to heal even in light of overwhelming odds.

Early in the process, it is a good idea for the provider to ask patients how they might like to be involved in the decision-making process. The question might be "How much do you want to know?" There is a fine line between overwhelming patients with information and providing them the information they need or want to make appropriate choices and necessary decisions.

Patients generally have the right to choose or to refuse treatment. Some rush into a treatment protocol only to discover later that their choices have brought them pain, disability, and expense far beyond what originally was assumed. Although it is the health care professional's goal to heal, if healing is not likely or possible, patients ought not to be "urged" into treatment protocols that are likely to be contrary to their personal wishes for the sake of treatment only.

Legal

In fact, those facing a life-threatening illness may make many different choices, and there are several schools of thought regarding those choices:

1. As stated earlier, patients may choose to forgo any treatment, including medications, transfusions, artificial hydration and feeding, respirators, surgery, chemotherapy, radiation, and dialysis.
2. The choice might be **palliative** care that focuses on quality of life while relieving symptoms of pain and suffering alongside of or instead of disease-focused treatment.
3. There is a growing group of individuals who consciously choose not to eat or drink anything by refusing all food and fluids for a more natural death. This choice is referred to as VSED (voluntarily stop eating and drinking) in medical circles.
4. Total sedation may be sought and is used when dying patients experience unbearable suffering and their bodies do not respond to other treatments. The medication causes unconsciousness and eventually death.
5. In an increasing number of states there is the option to seek aid in dying, usually through self-administration of medication prescribed by a physician.

Although health care professionals are generally less comfortable with some of these choices and death than they are with saving life, there are issues appropriate to consider with patients especially when facing life-threatening illness. Those issues include the following:

1. *Alternative methods of treatment should be discussed, as well as the outcome if no treatment is sought.* At some point, many patients will want to know *all* the treatment protocols that are feasible. This is a logical time to discuss any alternative or integrative medicine therapies that have shown success. Explanations should be made in language that the patient can understand. Illustrations and diagrams can be beneficial. Referrals might be made to integrative medicine practitioners, and patients are to be encouraged to discuss any chosen alternative therapies with their primary care provider. Sometimes treatment alternatives the patient may consider are not within the realm of recognized medical acceptability, but it is better to have that discussion than to ignore the possibility. Patients may also ask what happens if no treatment is chosen. This question can be difficult for health care providers who are anxious to provide some form of treatment for patients, but patients may have a number of reasons not to seek treatment. Remember the earlier statement indicating that family members and friends bring more influence to bear than does the health care professional.

2. *Discussion of pain management and treatment is essential.* The major fears patients have in facing life-threatening illness are pain, loss of self-image, and loss of independence. A frank discussion of pain control and how that can be accomplished can alleviate a fair amount of concern. Loss of self-image is devastating to many. To experience serious gain or loss of weight, loss of mobility, and the inability to perform daily tasks is seen by some as a fate worse than death. Providers will want to be ready to discuss loss of independence related to any life-threatening illness or to make a referral to someone who can be helpful. Patients have concerns such as wanting to know how long before the disease takes its toll, how long can they drive, what kind of care or assistance will be necessary, whether they can remain in their own home, and how long before they must have someone make decisions for them.
3. Legal *Health care directives such as a durable power of attorney for health care or health care proxy allows an individual to make decisions related to health care when the patient is no longer able to do so.* Such documents are increasingly important when a life-threatening illness is being faced. In the best of circumstances, these documents attempt to carry out the decisions the patient has already made regarding terminal conditions and whether to prolong life. Advances in medicine allow patients' lives to be sustained even when they are unlikely to recover from a persistent and vegetative state. The **health care directive** and the **durable power of attorney for health care** allow patients to make decisions before becoming incapacitated on whether life-prolonging medical or surgical procedures are to be continued, withheld, or withdrawn, as well as if or when artificial feeding and fluids are to be used or withheld. These documents can help providers and patients talk about dying and open the door to a positive, caring approach to death. The health care directive and the durable power of attorney for health care documents are legal in all 50 states. Although states may vary somewhat in the wording of these documents, they provide the same overall benefit to patients (see Chapter 6 for more information.) The federal government passed the Patient Self-Determination Act in 1990, which gives all patients receiving care in institutions receiving payments from Medicare and Medicaid written information about their right to accept or refuse medical or surgical treatment. The act also requires that patients be given information about their options to create living wills and to appoint someone to act on their behalf in making health care decisions (durable power of attorney for health care). Any documents of this nature that the patient has should be copied in the medical chart that goes with the patient when admitted to the hospital. Whenever the patient makes a change in such a document, the old document is to be replaced with the new one.
4. *Finances are to be considered.* If there is medical insurance, what will be covered? Who makes the decisions in a managed care environment? What family resources can or will be used? Finances are no one's favorite subject, especially for providers. However, such a discussion is important. Often, patients fear not being able to meet their financial obligations and leaving large debts to surviving family members almost as much as the life-threatening illness itself. As a medical assistant, you can help patients understand the parameters of their health insurance and any restrictions there might be on particular illnesses or treatments. Can medical insurance be canceled if the patient's employer pays a portion of the health insurance and the patient is no longer able to work? If there is a life insurance policy, help patients determine if any portion of the policy can be used for end-of-life expenses. Any services you can provide to the patient or family members in relieving the financial stress can bring great relief to everyone involved.
5. *Emotional needs of the patient and their family members are important.* Emotional support is vital when dealing with a life-threatening illness. Health care professionals will want to determine the source of that support for the patient. Can a support system be suggested for the patient and family members? For some patients and families, an individual giving spiritual guidance is seen as a member of the family and as a member of the health care team. For others, no spiritual influence is recognized or sought. For some life-threatening illnesses, there are support systems specifically related to the particular illness, for example, cancer support groups that offer coping strategies and management of personal struggles.

It is not the responsibility of health care professionals treating the individual with life-threatening illness to provide all these services, but a health care professional who suggests that patients and families address these issues is more closely in tune with a patient's power in the illness.

Life-threatening illnesses are *family* illnesses. There are primary (the person suffering from the illness) and secondary (family and friends) patients. Stress on a spouse or partner is enormous as they think about taking over the other person's role and as they try to deal with their own feelings. The stress on parents faced with the possible death of a child is especially devastating. Patients and their families and friends often feel angry. The situation is especially tragic if it might have been avoided (for example, a long-time smoker dying of lung cancer or a family member paralyzed in a crash caused by a drunk driver). There needs to be time for everyone to grieve. Depression is common among patients with life-threatening illnesses and their families. Warning signs should be reported to the provider. Remember that how patients live their last days are just as important as the numbers on the laboratory reports.

THE RANGE OF PSYCHOLOGICAL SUFFERING

The range of suffering associated with a life-threatening illness is extensive. Patients feel extreme distress. Anxiety and depression are common. At the time of diagnosis, patients' responses may include denial, numbness, and an inability to face the facts. Sadness, hopelessness, helplessness, and withdrawal often are exhibited.

The range of psychological suffering often leads to physical symptoms, such as tension, tachycardia, agitation, insomnia, anorexia, and panic attacks. The provider may be so intent on treating the physical ramifications of the illness that the psychological suffering is mostly ignored.

Relationships of individuals with a life-threatening illness often change. Close friends may feel uncomfortable with someone who is dying. Some fear touching or caressing the dying patient and become aloof and distant. However, new friendships can often be made if patients meet others with the same or similar life-threatening issues and help maintain each other's self-esteem. Relationships are important because they provide support and encouragement beyond any other source. Patients experience a loss of self-esteem when they are ill, are in pain, and have a body that is failing them. When self-image is lost, patients feel useless, see themselves as burdens, and have difficulty accepting help from anyone. The psychological effect of this "loss of self" can even hasten death.

It is often helpful to encourage patients to set goals for themselves. These can be small goals such as walking around the block, eating all their dinner, or connecting with a friend. The goals may also be much larger, such as staying alive until a son graduates from college, or putting all financial matters in order for surviving family members. Personal goals give the patient something other than the illness to plan for and work toward.

Communication

Carefully listening to patients and seeking clues for what *may not* be said is essential for the medical assistant and support staff caring for patients. Putting yourself in their shoes and asking what would be helpful is often beneficial. Be ready with a list of community resources that may benefit patients at this time.

It is not the intention of this chapter to specifically identify the many life-threatening illnesses and their particular needs, but some of the more common life-threatening diseases include coronary artery disease (CAD), chronic obstructive pulmonary disease (COPD), Alzheimer disease, and diabetes. Three of the most common life-threatening illnesses are identified in the following sections along with some specific information.

PATIENTS WITH CANCER

The first reaction patients with cancer usually have is the fear of loss of life. More than any other disease, patients think, "Cancer equals death. I am going to die." Following this reaction, issues begin to differ for each person. A few may choose no treatment and allow life to take its course. Most, however, will wonder about what treatment to choose, how to make that choice, and how effective it will be. Many patients are empowered by taking a major role in the decision making related to their cancer. Research can be helpful in studying the many options that may be available in treatment. The facts are that many patients diagnosed with cancer will die, whereas others diagnosed will live many years after diagnosis and treatment.

The three most widely known treatments of cancer are surgery, radiation, and chemotherapy. Often, treatment is a combination of the three. Patients can experience serious side effects from both radiation and chemotherapy. In today's world, there are other treatment options as well. They include hormone therapy, stem cell or bone

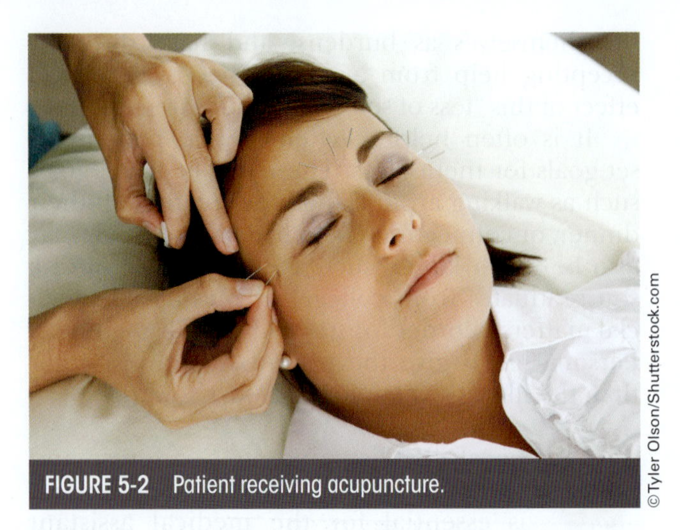

FIGURE 5-2 Patient receiving acupuncture.

©Tyler Olson/Shutterstock.com

marrow transplant, targeted therapy, and immunotherapy. Practitioners of complementary and integrative medicine have shown that many of their modalities can either enhance traditional treatment or ease their side effects. For instance, complementary practices that enhance the immune system give the body a stronger chance to overcome cancer cell growth. Meditation or acupuncture (Figure 5-2) can help ease the side effects for some patients. Loss of hair, nausea, vomiting, and pain are quite disconcerting to patients trying to cope, and they are relieved to find something that may be helpful. The American Cancer Society (http://www.cancer.org) has a number of resources for patients.

The most common signs and symptoms of advanced cancer are weakness, loss of appetite and weight, pain, nausea, constipation/diarrhea, sleepiness or confusion, and shortness of breath. Make certain patients understand your provider's willingness to relieve and treat these symptoms. Even when there is "nothing more to do" related to the cancer, there is still "much to do" to maintain comfort and to give patients the chance to do the things that are meaningful to them and their families.

PATIENTS WITH HIV/AIDS

Patients testing positive for human immunodeficiency virus (HIV) and those with acquired immune deficiency syndrome (AIDS) feel great stress from the infection, the disease, and the fear of other life-threatening illnesses. Some persons with HIV infection may have only a short time before the onset of AIDS; others may have a much longer period. AIDS is a disease that can have many periods of fairly good health and many periods of serious near-death illnesses. Recent developments in the treatment of HIV infection and AIDS help patients to live much longer, but there is no cure and their lives are greatly compromised because of their suppressed immune system.

Complex criteria determine whether a patient's illness is identified as AIDS rather than HIV infection. Some providers prefer not to use the term *AIDS;* rather, they discuss the illness as early or later stage HIV infection. Many providers in the United States and around the world use the term *AIDS* when patients' CD4 counts (healthy T4 lymphocytes) decline to less than 200. (The average healthy individual will have D4 lymphocyte counts of 800 to 1,500.) Many developing countries in the world, however, are unable to measure CD4 counts. AIDS is then diagnosed by the symptoms and any immunodeficient illnesses the patients have. Using only a CD4 count for diagnosis can be quite discouraging for patients who monitor those counts quite closely. Also, a patient's CD4 count can decrease dramatically into the "AIDS zone" one time, and then increase in sufficient numbers to move the patient back into HIV infection another time. Other criteria that may identify an illness as AIDS are a particular type of opportunistic infection or tumor, an AIDS-related brain or lung illness, and severe body wasting. Allied health professionals will need to take the lead from their employers.

In the three decades since HIV was first diagnosed, the stigma attached to the illness has lessened only a little. In some cases, guilt develops over past behavior and lifestyles or the possibility of having transmitted the disease to others. Individuals with HIV infection may feel added strain if this is the first knowledge their families have of any high-risk behaviors they have that are associated with the transmission of the disease. When the disease is contracted by individuals who feel they are protected or safe from the disease, anger is paramount. HIV affects mostly individuals who are relatively young. Thus, they are not as likely to have substantial financial resources or permanent housing. Treating HIV is expensive, and many patients have little or no insurance coverage.

Patients with HIV may experience central nervous system involvement. Forgetfulness and poor concentration may be followed by psychomotor retardation, or the slowing of physical and mental responses, decreased alertness, apathy, withdrawal, and diminished interest in work. Some patients later experience confusion and progressive impairment of intellectual function or dementia. When HIV-infected patients contract other opportunistic diseases, those symptoms are experienced as well.

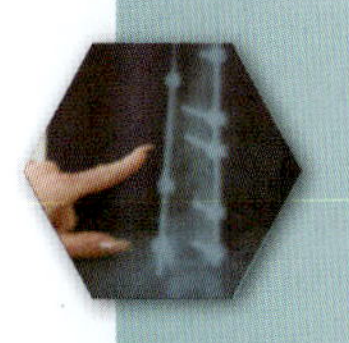

Critical Thinking

Many individuals in the end stages of both AIDS and cancer have lost their image of themselves. Their bodies have been diminished; they may have lost a great deal of weight from the disease or gained much weight from the medications taken. They may have no hair. They may have lost their ability to speak or to control bodily functions. What can you do or say to help them feel like a human being?

PATIENTS WITH END-STAGE RENAL DISEASE

Loss of kidney (renal) function leads to a serious illness known as end-stage renal disease (ESRD). When the kidneys fail completely, patients cannot live for long unless they receive dialysis or a kidney transplant. A successful kidney transplant relieves the person of kidney failure. However, there are not enough transplants for every person who needs one, and not all transplants are appropriate or successful. Dialysis is the process of artificially replacing the main functions of the kidneys—filtering blood to remove wastes (Figure 5-3). Choosing dialysis as a treatment plan can sustain life for years and is covered by Medicare, but it does have complications that burden patients and their caregivers.

Depending on age, a patient's general health, and other circumstances, some patients will opt not to have dialysis and to let death come from kidney failure. The by-products of the body's chemistry accumulate in renal failure and cause an array of symptoms. Mild confusion and disorientation are common. Upsetting hallucinations or agitation can occur. Certain minerals concentrated in the blood can cause muscle twitching, tremors, and shakes. Some patients experience mild or severe itching. Appetite decreases early, and breathing can be rapid and shallow. Many patients with kidney failure pass little or no urine. Fluid overload results in edema, or swelling of the body, particularly of the legs and abdomen. Patients with some urine output may live for months even after stopping dialysis. People with no urine output are likely to die within a week or two. Patients will lose energy and become sleepy and lethargic. Typically, patients slip into a deeper sleep and gradually lose consciousness. Kidney failure has a reputation for being a gentle death.

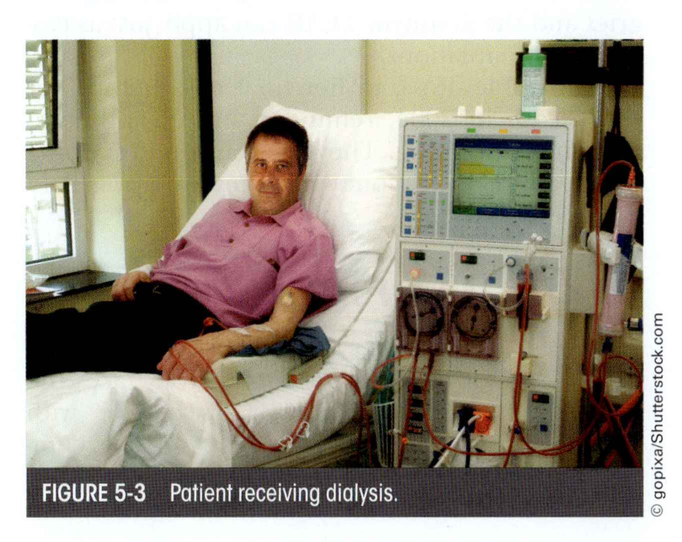

FIGURE 5-3 Patient receiving dialysis.

© gopixa/Shutterstock.com

THE THERAPEUTIC RESPONSE TO PATIENTS WITH LIFE-THREATENING ILLNESSES

Health care professionals will want to remember that when individuals face a danger such as a life-threatening illness, the brain's response of "flight or fight" kicks in before cognitive processes do. This means that patients often report hearing "nothing" after hearing the words "cancer" or some other feared diagnosis. Health care professionals who mostly focus on the cognitive data often miss a patient's reaction of surprise, shock, fear, and anger.

Presentation

Communication

For this reason, therapeutic health care professionals must carefully observe their patients' reactions. This is accomplished by being aware of the patient's displayed emotion and responding to it. Such a process is called empathy—putting yourself in the other person's shoes to imagine what her life is like under these circumstances. The therapeutic response then is to let your patients know you understand: "This has to be really difficult news to hear. I'm trying to imagine what this must be like for you." Then you assure patients that they have your support: "My team and I will help you every way we can through this process." Carrying out such a promise creates an openness in communication that is beneficial through the treatment of a life-threatening illness.

A word of caution here is to remind yourself that the tendency when caring for someone with a life-threatening illness is to care only for the patient's clinical needs, thus ignoring their very real needs as a human being whose life has been threatened to the core. Your compassion and empathy will go a long way in making life more meaningful and comfortable.

COMMUNICATION IN END-OF-LIFE CARE

Communication

There comes a time in a patient's life-threatening illness experience when a transition is made to end-of-life care. This may be when there are no further anticancer care options, and all treatment ceases. It may be when the antiviral medications so beneficial in the treatment of HIV are no longer effective. For patients with heart failure, it may be when the heart simply no longer functions properly. Either providers or their patients and family members may raise the issue of end-of-life care, but it can be an uncomfortable conversation either way. There is some research, however, that indicates that the majority of patients choose to have some control over the process.

Questions to help patients better verbalize their feelings might include the following:

- What is most important to you now that we have reached this stage?
- What are you hoping for?
- What plans, if any, have you made for this transition in your life?
- How can my team and I be of help?

The last question will help patients verbalize their wishes. Perhaps it is a discussion about comfort and lack of pain, not wanting to die on a machine in a vegetative state, or even donating organs after death. This stage is difficult at best for all involved, but following these guidelines fosters an atmosphere in which health care professionals will be remembered for their respectfulness, their attention to care and treatment, and their empathy.

THE STAGES OF GRIEF

Living with a life-threatening illness or making a transition to end-of-life care causes grief for both patients and family members. There are a number of different philosophies on grief and the stages patients are apt to experience when they know their lives are about to end, but none is so widely known as that of Dr. Elisabeth Kübler-Ross, who was one of the first to conduct research and determine possible stages of grief: denial, anger, bargaining, depression, and acceptance. These stages are discussed in greater detail in the "Stages of Grief" Quick Reference Guide.

Dr. Kübler-Ross reminds health care professionals that while not all patients go through all five stages, some patients go through all five stages over and over again, each time with a little less stress. When moving through these stages multiple times, the grief and pain is most pronounced in the beginning, but gradually diminishes as grief is resolved. Others get stuck in one stage, usually denial. Grief and dying are very personal. No two patients will follow the same pattern. Family members also suffer grief and are often in different stages; therefore, it is often difficult for them to communicate and help each other.

Remember that grief work is exhausting. So much energy is spent in the grief process that it is often difficult to carry on day-to-day tasks. Any help that can be made available is appreciated.

The acronym TEAR is fairly popular and is often used to describe the grieving process. It has similarities to the five stages of grief:

T: To accept the reality of the loss

E: Experience the pain of the loss

A: Adjust to what was lost

R: Reinvest in a new reality

Although the five stages of grief and the TEAR stages discussed in this chapter are directed toward patients with life-threatening illnesses, remember that the family members and loved ones of patients also will experience grief. Both of these principles can be applied to any kind of serious loss that occurs in one's life—loss of a job, divorce, disaster, war, famine, loss of a limb or important body function, Alzheimer disease, loss of a friend, or even the death of a beloved pet. The stages of grief and the acronym TEAR can apply just as easily to these situations.

Dr. Kübler-Ross, in her final days before her own death in 2004, reminded her co-author to "Listen to the dying. They will tell you everything you need to know about when they are dying. And it is easy to miss."

THE CHALLENGE FOR THE MEDICAL ASSISTANT

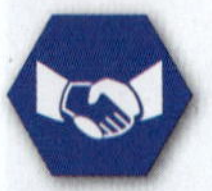
Professional

As a medical assistant, you face the challenge of caring for people with life-threatening illnesses; you can comfort those who face great suffering and death. You will become a source of information

QUICK REFERENCE GUIDE

Stages of Grief

DENIAL

This is the stage where patients cannot believe that this is happening. They are likely to experience shock and dismay. If the grief is for the loss of a loved one, it is difficult for them to believe that the loved one is dead. If the grief is for themselves and some incident in their lives, they have a hard time accepting the reality of the loss. Words such as "I can't believe it is true" and "There must be some mistake" are common.

It is difficult to help someone in denial. You may be able to reaffirm the reality of the circumstances, but there is little you can do to move someone from the stage of denial.

ANGER

Patients express anger, sometimes openly and assertively. Other times, the anger is turned inward and is difficult to accurately express. Patients ask the question "Why?" and often need explanations of what is occurring. Anger is often expressed to others who have no idea what is happening in patients' lives.

When possible, this type of anger should be realized for what it is and never taken personally. Patients are angry at the event, not at you. Patients can be helped to express the anger in a realistic and nonhurtful manner.

BARGAINING

In this stage, patients bargain with God or a higher being and even their providers and express their desire to make a certain milestone in their lives. "If you can just get me through this current crisis so I can make it to my 40th wedding anniversary, I can accept what is happening." Goals can be very helpful to patients, and they can be encouraged to continue to set realistic goals during their grieving.

DEPRESSION

Patients who reach this stage are sad and sometimes quiet and withdrawn. There is a feeling that they have given up. They often prefer not to be around anyone. The depression can be and often is treated so that patients' grief is eased somewhat. This is true especially when patients remain in this stage for a very long time.

ACCEPTANCE

This is the time that patients accept the loss. If it is death that is being faced, they often feel they are ready. Everything is in place, and peace has been made with the prognosis. If a loss is being suffered, it is the time when patients begin to move on and make other plans for their lives and their future.

for patients and their support members. Be sensitive and respectful toward individuals who may be shunned by society. Examine your own beliefs, lifestyle, and biases so that you can be comfortable treating all patients, no matter what the illness is or how it was contracted.

As well as assisting your employer in providing the best possible medical care, you may be required to provide many nonmedical forms of assistance for patients suffering from life-threatening illnesses. You may need to make referrals to community-based agencies or service groups. Health departments, social workers, trained hospice volunteers, and AIDS and cancer volunteers may also be helpful to you, your patients, and their families.

The best therapeutic response to the patient with a life-threatening illness will build on the person's own culture and coping abilities, capitalize on strengths, maintain hope, and show continued care and concern. Patients may want up-to-date information on their disease; its causes, modes of transmission, and treatments available; and sources of care and social support. Honor their wishes. Be prepared to recommend support systems where patients can further discuss their feelings and express their concerns. Treat patients with concern and compassion and assure them everything will be done to provide continuity of care and relief from distress. Patients also may be encouraged to call on a spiritual advisor.

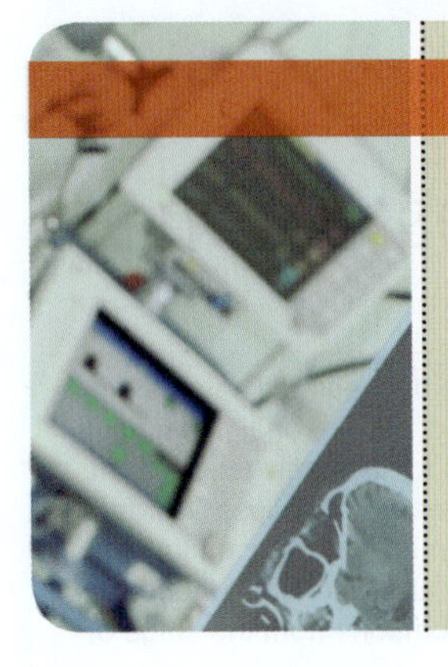

CASE STUDY 5-1

Refer to the scenario at the beginning of the chapter. As you prepare for the second visit of Suzanne Markis, you make a mental note of what kind of information you will have available.

CASE STUDY REVIEW

1. What paperwork might be necessary?
2. What questions might you have for Suzanne?
3. What might family members who may accompany Suzanne want to know?
4. As the medical assistant, how does your role differ from that of your employer?

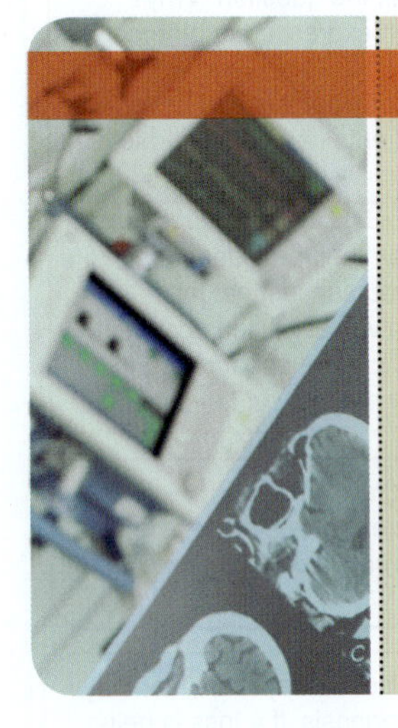

CASE STUDY 5-2

The extended family of Wong Lee is concerned about his illness and his care. Chronic obstructive pulmonary disease (COPD) has ravaged his body. He is on oxygen all the time now. He wants to remain at home to die; his family wants that, too. The family has been with him and has been involved in his care plan all along. However, you are uncertain of how much information to give to members of his extended family when they call.

CASE STUDY REVIEW

1. Are the questions that the extended family members raise intended to harm or help Mr. Lee?
2. Is there a durable power of attorney for health care in place?
3. Which, if any, of the family's desires are related to the culture?
4. What can you and your employer suggest to be of help to everyone involved?

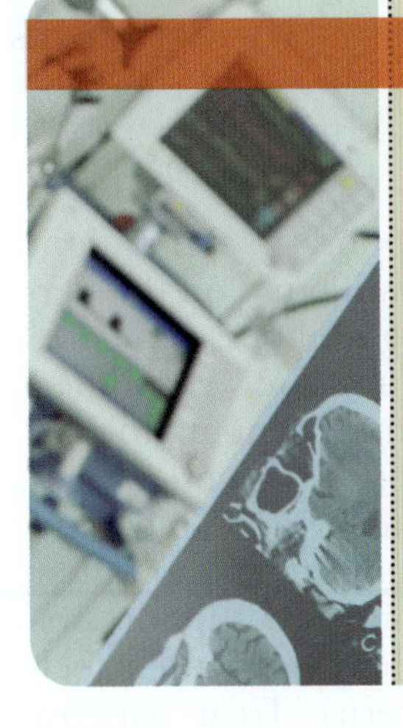

CASE STUDY 5-3

Jeff and Amy live in rural Tennessee. They are expecting their first baby and are excited beyond belief because they had so much trouble getting pregnant. You are the medical assistant for their family practice provider. Test results from their recent ultrasound have been returned to your clinic, and the news is not good. There appears to be some difficulty and one or more apparent birth defects in the developing fetus. You and your employer discuss possible resources.

CASE STUDY REVIEW

1. As the medical assistant, what is your first responsibility to these expectant parents?
2. Where might you look for possible resources?
3. Identify three to five possible resources.
4. If referral to a specialist is to be made, what role might you play in that referral?

Summary

- Note the differing expressions for "life-threatening" and recall the influence of cultural diversity on how an individual faces a serious or debilitating illness.
- Life-threatening illnesses create challenging and numerous options for decision making, such as type of treatment, if any; pain management; health care directives; financial concerns; and emotional needs of self and family.
- Grief and end-of-life decisions often result in anxiety, depression, sadness, helplessness, and withdrawal.
- Patients with ESRD, cancer, and AIDS will require special attention, understanding, and compassion.
- The best therapeutic response builds on a person's culture, coping abilities, and strengths. Recommend support systems and assure patients that everything will be done to provide continuity of care and relief from distress.
- Medical assistants will want to remember that when caring for patients with a life-threatening illness, having even the slightest fear of death can undermine the ability to respond professionally, with empathy and support.
- If you feel yourself losing the ability to be helpful, it is time to briefly step aside. This does not mean withdrawal from your position or refusal to care for your patients. It means that you do whatever is necessary so that your perspective is not lost.
- Take time to "fill up your psyche" and to give yourself a rest. If the ambulatory care setting has an abundance of patients with life-threatening illnesses, it may require that you spend some time in a support group of your own so that you are better able to cope.
- Never be afraid to feel sad or weep with your patients. It is better to sense their pain and, at times, feel the pain with them, than it is to be so clinically objective that you miss their true needs.

Study for Success

To reinforce your knowledge and skills of information presented in this chapter:

- Review the *Key Terms* and *Learning Outcomes*
- Consider the *Critical Thinking* features and *Case Studies* and discuss your conclusions
- Answer the questions in the *Certification Review*

CERTIFICATION REVIEW

1. When a practice treats patients with HIV/AIDS, cancer, or ESRD, what is it important for medical assistants to do?
   a. Warn other patients about the dangers of transmission
   b. Segregate these patient reception areas from other patient areas
   c. Be supportive and free of prejudice
   d. Deny any information to patients regarding the seriousness of the illness
2. What is characteristic of the Patient Self-Determination Act?
   a. It allows a patient to have a choice of providers.
   b. It ensures a patient's right to request a referral to another provider.
   c. It gives patients the right to formulate advance directives.
   d. It ensures that Medicare and/or Medicaid can help pay for treatment.
   e. It allows patients to choose their hospital care plan.
3. Who or what is the strongest influence on a patient with a life-threatening illness?
   a. The provider
   b. The hospital
   c. The patient
   d. The family
4. How is life-threatening illness best defined?
   a. A life shortened because of illness or disease
   b. An illness that is harmful but not dangerous
   c. An illness serious enough to require hospitalization
   d. An illness that makes palliative care improbable
   e. An illness that begins in childhood

5. How might a patient's culture affect his or her view of a life-threatening illness?
   a. It will have no impact on a patient's decisions.
   b. It can cause a patient to be accepting, denying, or even defiant of death.
   c. It will determine the type of care or pain medication used.
   d. It will dictate care outside the United States for treatment.
6. Which of the following statements is true regarding therapeutic communication with a patient with a life-threatening illness?
   a. It is no different than communicating with any patient.
   b. It comes naturally and requires no special skill.
   c. It is heightened and considered more challenging.
   d. It is left to nonmedical support staff.
   e. It often is unappreciated.
7. What is an appropriate therapeutic response to a patient with a life-threatening illness?
   a. I hope you'll feel better soon.
   b. You can conquer this; don't let it get you down.
   c. Everything will be fine once treatment begins.
   d. I'm having a hard time imagining how I might feel in your shoes.
8. What does a durable power of attorney for health care accomplish?
   a. It enables someone other than the patient to make only health care decisions.
   b. It enables someone other than the patient to make any decisions for the patient.
   c. It makes certain that patients' financial responsibilities are met.
   d. It makes certain an attorney's wishes are followed.
   e. It prevents hospitals from using experimental treatment.
9. Which stage of grief attempts to negotiate an event or experience?
   a. Acceptance
   b. Depression
   c. Denial
   d. Bargaining
10. What might effective pain management depend upon?
   a. The patient's wishes and needs
   b. The patient's loss of self-image
   c. Professional nursing criteria
   d. The patient's range of psychological suffering
   e. Insurance allowance for pain control

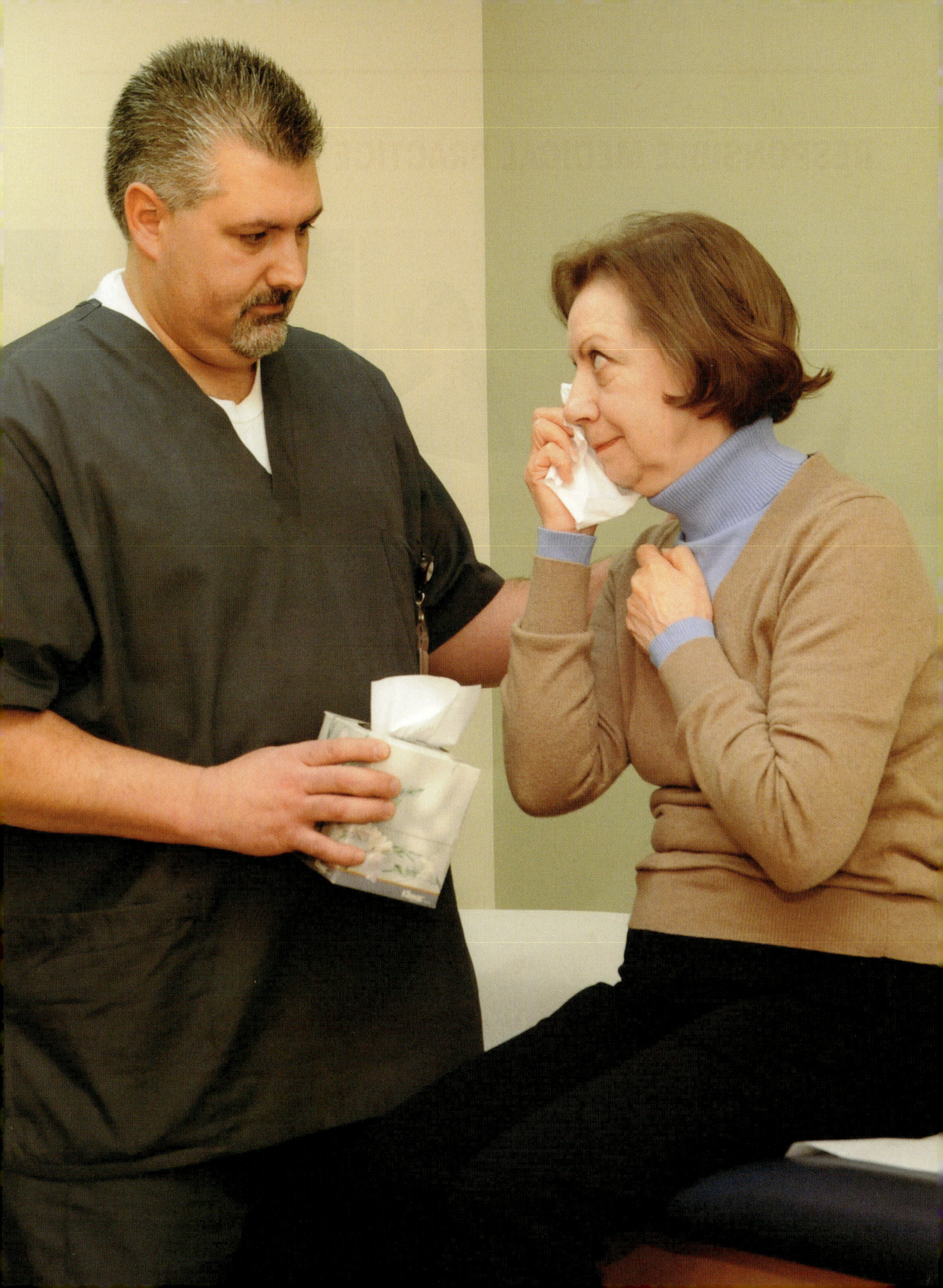

UNIT III

RESPONSIBLE MEDICAL PRACTICE

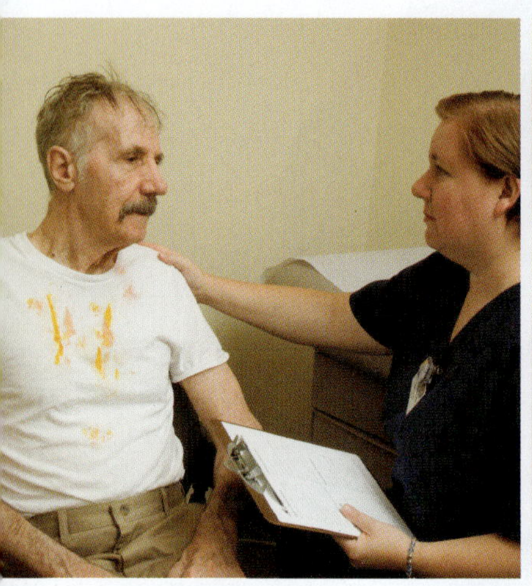
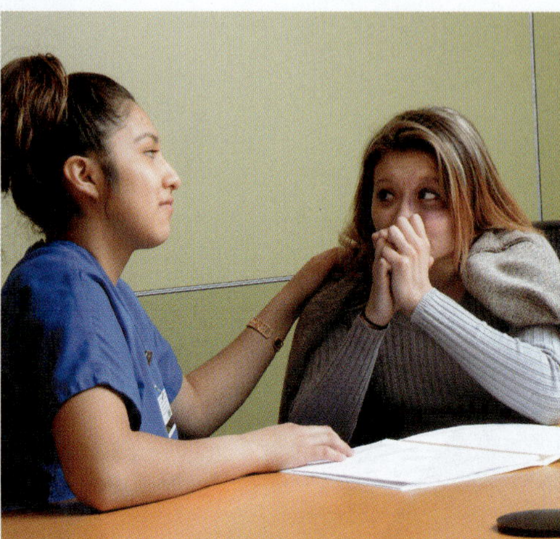
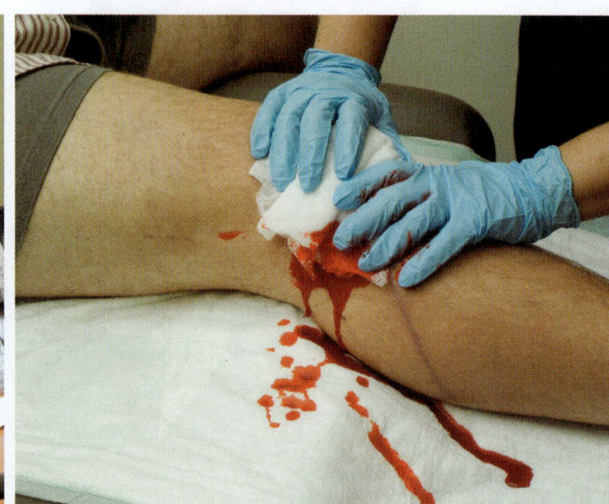

ATTRIBUTES OF PROFESSIONALISM

The professional medical assistant will understand the absolute necessity for abiding by all laws pertinent to outpatient care, and serving with the utmost moral integrity and absolute ethical behavior. Prior to entering into the profession, professional medical assistants must examine their prejudices and biases and realize that even when there is a difference of beliefs and personal ethics between the patient and the professional, bias can never enter into the care of that patient.

It is also imperative that the professional medical assistant maintain current first aid certification and understand how and when to give first aid both within the facility and when in public. You must never attempt to perform any procedure outside your scope of training, knowledge, and experience.

As a true professional medical assistant, you will maintain your personal integrity and practice within your personal ethical boundaries, always treating patients with compassion and understanding. In emergency circumstances, you will act appropriately, keeping in mind the patient's immediate safety and comfort, and understanding when additional assistance is needed.

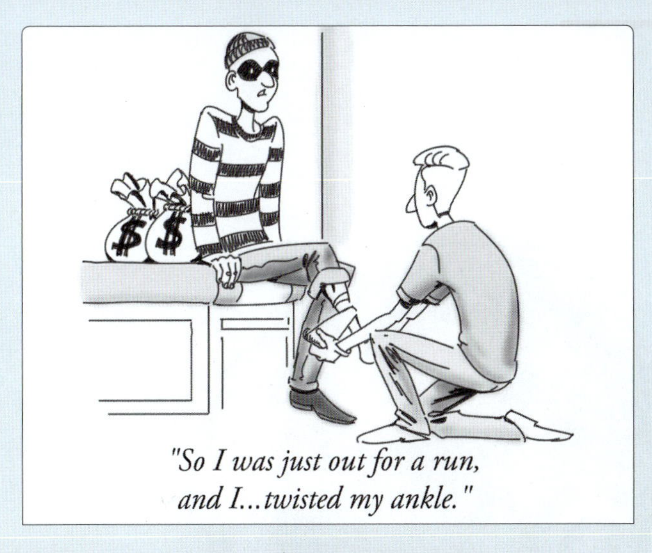

"So I was just out for a run, and I...twisted my ankle."

Listed below are a series of questions to ask yourself and to serve as your professionalism checklist. As you interact with patients and colleagues, these questions will help to guide you in the professional behavior that is expected every day from medical assistants.

Ask Yourself

COMMUNICATION

- ☐ Do I apply active listening skills?
- ☐ Do I display professionalism through written and verbal communication?
- ☐ Do I demonstrate appropriate nonverbal communication?
- ☐ Do I display appropriate body language?
- ☐ Does my knowledge allow me to speak easily with all members of the health care team?

PRESENTATION

- ☐ Am I dressed and groomed appropriately?
- ☐ Do I display a positive attitude?
- ☐ Do I display a calm, professional, and caring manner?
- ☐ Do I demonstrate empathy to the patient?

COMPETENCY

- ☐ Do I pay attention to detail?
- ☐ Do I ask questions if I am out of my comfort zone or do not have the experience to carry out tasks?
- ☐ Do I display sound judgment?
- ☐ Am I knowledgeable and accountable?
- ☐ Do I recognize the physical and emotional effects on persons involved in an emergency situation?
- ☐ Do I demonstrate self-awareness in responding to an emergency situation?

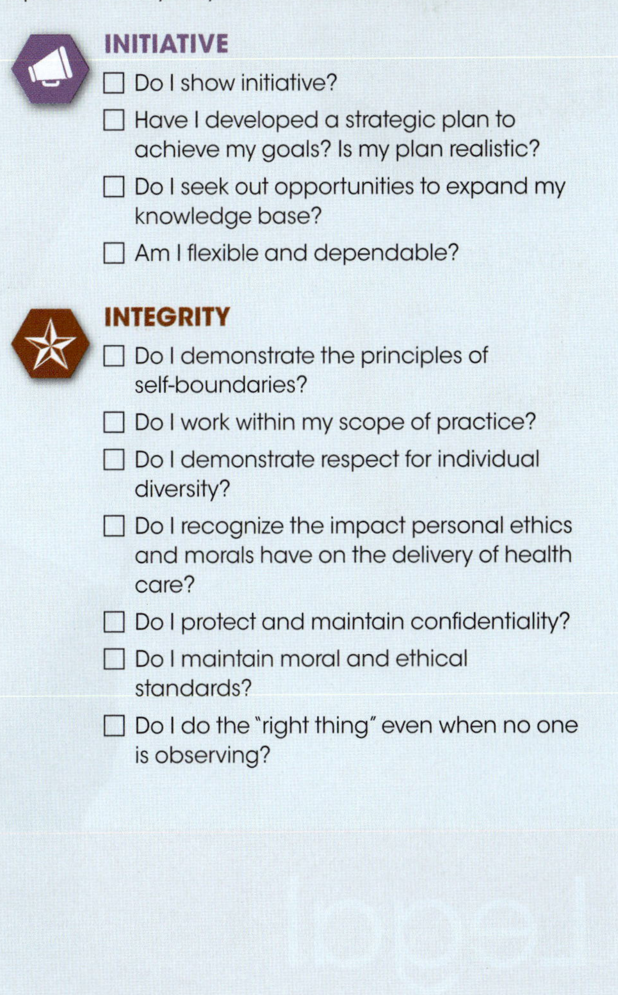

INITIATIVE

- ☐ Do I show initiative?
- ☐ Have I developed a strategic plan to achieve my goals? Is my plan realistic?
- ☐ Do I seek out opportunities to expand my knowledge base?
- ☐ Am I flexible and dependable?

INTEGRITY

- ☐ Do I demonstrate the principles of self-boundaries?
- ☐ Do I work within my scope of practice?
- ☐ Do I demonstrate respect for individual diversity?
- ☐ Do I recognize the impact personal ethics and morals have on the delivery of health care?
- ☐ Do I protect and maintain confidentiality?
- ☐ Do I maintain moral and ethical standards?
- ☐ Do I do the "right thing" even when no one is observing?

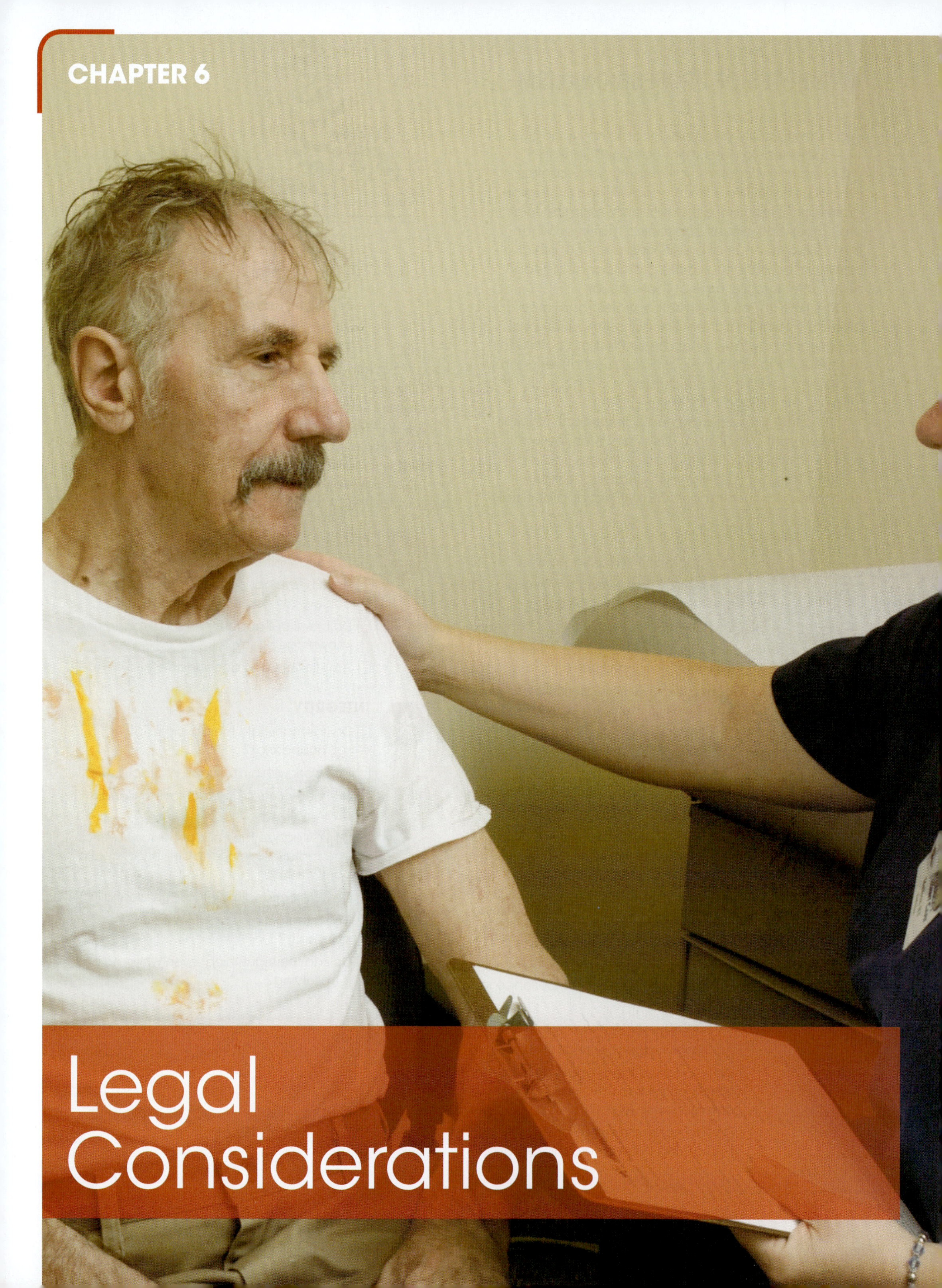

CHAPTER 6

Legal Considerations

LEARNING OUTCOMES

1. Define and spell the key terms as presented in the glossary.
2. Briefly describe the five sources of law, differentiating between civil and criminal law.
3. Recall at least seven of the nine administrative law acts important to the medical profession.
4. Outline the implications of HIPAA for the medical assistant.
5. Paraphrase administering, prescribing, and dispensing of controlled substances.
6. Describe the measures to take for disposal of controlled substances.
7. Discuss licensure renewal and revocation for physicians.
8. Follow established policies when initiating or terminating medical treatment.
9. List and characterize the four Ds of negligence.
10. Distinguish provider and medical assistant roles in terms of standard of care.
11. Identify three common torts that can occur in the outpatient care setting and what constitutes each one.
12. Discuss informed consent and classify types of minors.
13. Evaluate at least 10 practices to help in risk management.
14. Outline the necessary steps in civil litigation, including how and when subpoenas are used.
15. Recall special considerations for patients related to issues of confidentiality, the statute of limitations, and public duties.
16. Describe procedures to follow in reporting abuse.
17. Discuss Good Samaritan laws.
18. Recall maintenance of advance directives in the ambulatory care setting.

KEY TERMS

administer
administrative law
agents
alternative dispute resolution (ADR)
arbitration
civil law
common law
constitutional law
contract law
criminal law
defendant
deposition
discovery
dispense
durable power of attorney for health care
emancipated minors
expert witness
expressed consent
expressed contract
felony
Health Insurance Portability and Accountability Act (HIPAA)
implied consent
implied contract
incompetence
informed consent
interrogatory
intimate partner violence (IPV)
libel
litigation
malfeasance
malpractice
mature minors
mediation
medically indigent
minor
misdemeanor
misfeasance
negligence
noncompliant
nonfeasance
Patient Self-Determination Act (PSDA)
plaintiff
precedents
prescribe
risk management
slander
statutory law
subpoena
tort
tort law

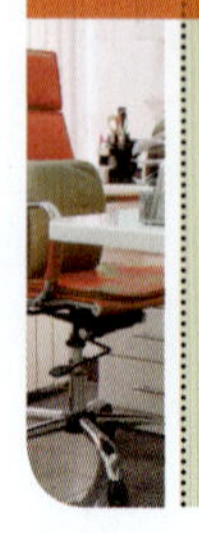

SCENARIO

Marilyn, the clinic manager at Inner City Health Care, is reviewing some concerns in a staff meeting. Even though each employee is well aware of privacy, confidentiality, and the many ways their actions are legally binding, Marilyn notices occasional carelessness creeping into their busy activities. Marilyn has heard voices of staff from the hallway discussing confidential matters and notices the staff carrying on personal conversations in the presence of patients. As well as reviewing HIPAA compliance, Marilyn spends some time discussing the importance of focusing all attention on patients.

Chapter Portal

The law as it relates to health care has grown increasingly complex in the last decade. The agendas of federal and state governments include an investigation of quality health care, a desire to control health care costs (while hoping to ensure equitable access to health care), and an interest in protecting the patient. The Patient Protection and Affordable Care Act of 2010 further added to this complexity. Today's medical assistant must have knowledge of federal, state, and local laws related to health care. A full discussion of health law requires several volumes; therefore, the aim of this chapter is awareness of the law and its implications and establishment of sound practices and procedures to both safeguard patient rights and protect the health care professional.

SOURCES OF LAW

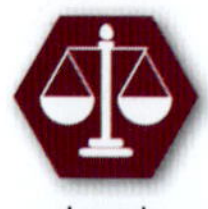

Law is a binding custom or ruling for conduct that is enforceable by an agency assigned that authority. Laws come from state statutes, common law, both civil and criminal laws, administrative law agencies, and contract and tort law. The highest authority in the United States is the U.S. Constitution. Adopted in 1787, this document provides the framework for the U.S. government. The Constitution includes 27 amendments, 10 of which are known as the Bill of Rights. This authority is sometimes referred to as **constitutional law**. The U.S. Constitution calls for three branches of the federal government:

- *Executive branch.* The president and vice president (elected by U.S. citizens), cabinet officers, and various other departments of the federal government.
- *Legislative branch.* Members of the U.S. Senate and the House of Representatives (elected by U.S. citizens) and the staffs of individual legislators and legislative committees.
- *Judicial branch.* The courts, including the U.S. Supreme Court, courts of appeals for the nine judicial regions, and district courts.

Laws enacted at the federal level are often referred to as acts or laws, or by a specific title. An example is Title XIX of Public Law, the Social Security Act, established in 1967 to provide health care for the **medically indigent**. This program is known as Medicaid. Federal law is the supreme law of the land.

Statutory Law

The body of laws made by states is known as **statutory law**. Constitutions in the 50 states identify the rights and responsibilities of their citizens and identify how their state is organized. States have a governor as the head and state legislatures (both elected by the state's citizens), as well as their own court systems with a number of levels. All powers that are not conferred specifically on the federal government are retained by the state, yet states vary widely in their interpretation of that power. State law cannot override the power of any laws defined in the U.S. Constitution or its amendments, although states often attempt to do so. State statutes commonly include practice acts for doctors and nurses. Some identify licensure or certification requirements for medical assistants, also. These practice acts broadly define the scope of practice for the profession as well as licensure and/or certification requirements.

Common Law

Common law is not so easily defined but is essential to understanding law in the United States. Common law was developed by judges in England and France over many centuries and was brought to the United States with the early settlers. Common law is often called judge-made law. The law consists of rulings made by judges who base their decisions on a combination of a number of factors: (1) individual decisions of a court, (2) interpretation of the U.S. Constitution or a particular state constitution, and (3) statutory law. These decisions become known as **precedents** and often lay down the foundation for subsequent legal rulings.

Criminal Law

Criminal law addresses wrongs committed against the welfare and safety of society as a whole. Criminal law affects relationships between individuals and between individuals and the government. Another term that might be used to describe a criminal act is *malfeasance*. **Malfeasance** is conduct that is illegal or contrary to an official's obligation. Criminal offenses generally are classified into the basic categories of a **felony** or a **misdemeanor** that are specifically defined in statutes.

Felonies are more serious crimes and include murder, larceny or thefts of large amounts of money, assault, and rape. Punishment for a felony is more serious than for a misdemeanor. A convicted felon cannot vote, hold public office, or own any weapons. Felonies often are divided into groups such as first degree (most serious), second degree, and third degree. Sentences are generally for longer than one year and are served in a penitentiary. Misdemeanors are considered lesser offenses and vary from state to state. Punishment may include probation or a time of service to the community, a fine, or a jail sentence in a city or county facility. Misdemeanors also can be divided into groups or classifications, such as A, B, or C class misdemeanors, denoting the seriousness of the crime (Class A is the most serious).

For a person to be found guilty of a crime, a judge or jury must prove the evidence against the individual "beyond a reasonable doubt." In a criminal case, charges are brought against an individual by the state with the intent of preventing any further harm to society. For example, a physician practicing medicine without a proper license may be subject to criminal action by the courts for endangering a patient's life.

Civil Law

Civil law affects relationships between individuals, corporations, government bodies, and other organizations. Terms that may be used in civil law are **misfeasance**, referring to a lawful act that is improperly or unlawfully executed, and **nonfeasance**, referring to the failure to perform an act, official duty, or legal requirement. The punishment for a civil wrong is usually monetary in nature. When a charge is brought against a **defendant** in a civil case, the goal is to reimburse the **plaintiff** or the person bringing charges with a monetary amount for suffering, pain, and any loss of wages. Another goal might be to make certain the defendant is prevented from engaging in similar behavior again. In civil law, cases need to show that a "preponderance of the evidence" is more than likely true against the defendant. The most common forms of civil law that directly affect the medical profession are administrative law, contract law, and **tort law**.

ADMINISTRATIVE LAW

Legal

Administrative law establishes agencies that are given power to specialize and enact regulations that have the force of law. The Internal Revenue Service is an example of an administrative agency that enacts tax laws and regulations. Health care professionals are bound by federal administrative law through the Medicare and Medicaid program rules administered by the Social Security Administration.

There are a number of other regulations in administrative law governing health professionals and their employees. It is important that medical assistants be informed of legislation and any federal or state regulations that are critical to patients and the medical profession. Identified here with a brief description are a number of administrative acts, some of which also are referred to in other chapters in this textbook.

Affordable Care Act and Patients' Bill of Rights

Congress passed the Affordable Care Act (ACA) and President Obama signed the act into law on March 23, 2010. In June 2012, the U.S. Supreme Court upheld the law as constitutional. Commonly referred to as Obamacare, the law has 10 titles or sections and includes the following provisions: (1) ending preexisting condition exclusions for children, (2) keeping young adults covered under parents' health care plans until age 26, (3) preventing insurers from cancelling coverage due to honest errors, (4) guaranteeing the right to appeal, (5) ending lifetime coverage limits, (6) reviewing premium increases, (7) maximizing services for premium dollars, (8) covering recommended preventive health care services, (9) allowing choice of primary care provider from a plan's network, and (10) removing insurance barriers to emergency services.

The ACA also provides for the Patients' Bill of Rights to make certain that patients receive all the benefits of the law. Today, health care providers, clinics, and hospitals provide a document outlining these benefits to their patients. Providers can vary in their approach, but must cover all the aspects of the 2010 law. Many of the documents also include a statement on the patient's responsibilities. See Chapter 7 for further discussion, and do a Web search for sample documentation.

The Civil Rights Act

Title VII of the Civil Rights Act of 1964 protects employees from discrimination. The act states that an employer with 15 or more employees must not discriminate in matters of employment related to age, sex, race, creed, marital status, national origin, color, or disabilities. (Some states are more restrictive in their laws and identify employers with 8 or more employees.)

Through the years, many additions have been made. They include such topics as voting rights, fair housing, and unlawful harassment in the workplace. The Genetic Information Nondiscrimination Act (GINA) was passed in 2008 and prohibits the use of genetic information in employment and health insurance decisions. This amendment was added in order to protect individuals from the misuse of genetic information brought about by the ever-increasing expansion and advances in the use of genetics in medicine.

The Equal Employment Opportunity Commission (EEOC) enforces Title VII and provides oversight of equal employment regulation and policies. The Departments of Labor, Health and Human Services, and the Treasury have responsibility for issuing regulations addressing the use of genetic information in health insurance. Although some health care settings have fewer than 15 or even 8 employees, it is best to follow state and federal guidelines on all matters of employment.

Currently, 22 states have laws banning employment discrimination because of sexual orientation. Those states are California, Colorado, Connecticut, Delaware, Hawaii, Illinois, Iowa, Maine, Maryland, Massachusetts, Minnesota, Nevada, New Hampshire, New Jersey, New Mexico, New York, Oregon, Rhode Island, Utah, Vermont, Washington, and Wisconsin. The District of Columbia, Guam, and Puerto Rico have passed similar legislation.

Harassment. Included in Title VII is an employee's protection from sexual harassment and a hostile work environment.

Harassment occurs when sexual favors are implied or requested by a supervisor in return for job advancement or special treatment on the job. Another form of harassment and a more common problem that may exist in the workplace is referred to as a hostile work environment. A hostile work environment exists when pervasive or severe sexual comments, jokes, or inappropriate touching create a workplace so negative that it interferes with an employee's work performance.

A written policy on sexual harassment detailing inappropriate behavior and stating specific steps to be taken to correct an inappropriate situation should be established. The policy will include (1) a statement that harassment is not tolerated, (2) a statement that an employee who feels harassed needs to bring the matter to the immediate attention of a person designated in the policy, (3) a statement about the confidentiality of any incidents and specific disciplinary action against the harasser, and (4) the procedure to follow when harassment occurs.

It is illegal for a supervisor or employer to ignore an employee's complaint. An employer or supervisor who does not take corrective action is liable. The EEOC guidelines make the employer strictly liable for the acts of supervisory employees, as well as for some acts of harassment by coworkers and clients (see Chapter 22).

Equal Pay Act of 1963

Ambulatory health care clinics may not have as much of an issue with this act as some other places of employment, but it is important to note. The Equal Pay Act (EPA) of 1963 protects men and women in the same place of business who perform substantially the same work with substantially equal skill, effort, and responsibility from sex-based wage discrimination. In other words, the starting salary for two medical assistants of the opposite sex is to be the same when they are performing essentially the same job with equal skill and experience under similar working conditions.

Federal Age Discrimination Act

The Federal Age Discrimination in Employment Act of 1967 protects certain individuals 40 years and older from discrimination based on their age in matters of employment, promotion, discharge, compensation, or privileges of employment. This act has become increasingly important as individuals are working longer and seeking employment in their later years. Age restriction may be applied *only* when required by law. For instance, servers of alcohol must be 21 years of age. Valid reasons to decline applicants for employment include (1) health issues that may interfere with the safe and efficient performance of the job, (2) unavailability for the work schedule of the particular job, (3) insufficient training or experience to perform the duties of the particular job, and (4) someone else is better qualified.

Americans with Disabilities Act

The Americans with Disabilities Act (ADA) of 1990 prohibits discrimination that prevents individuals who have physical or mental disabilities from accessing public services and accommodations, employment, and telecommunications. A disability implies that a physical or mental impairment substantially limits one or more of an individual's major life activities. ADA is identified in five titles. Title I, enforced by the EEOC, prohibits discrimination in employment (see Chapter 22 for further details). Essentially, Title I requires a potential employer to identify and prove that certain disabilities cannot be accommodated in performing the job requirements. Employers only have to provide reasonable accommodations rather than anything an employee demands or something that is extraordinarily expensive. Individuals who formerly abused drugs and alcohol and those who are undergoing rehabilitation also are covered by the ADA and cannot be denied employment because of their history of substance abuse.

Titles II, III, and IV mandate access to public services, public accommodations, and telecommunications for individuals with disabilities. The ADA protects persons with HIV infection or AIDS, making certain they cannot be refused treatment by health care professionals because of their health status. Generally speaking, health care professionals with HIV infection or AIDS cannot be kept from providing treatment either, unless that treatment could be found to be a significant risk to others. Title V covers a number of miscellaneous issues such as exclusions from the definition of *disability*, retaliation, insurance, and other issues. Again, the ADA applies to businesses with at least 15 employees, but some states have more stringent laws.

Of note is the 2008 amendment to the ADA, known as the Americans with Disabilities Act Amendments Act (ADAAA). In this act, Congress made it easier for individuals seeking protection under the ADA to establish their disability by broadening the scope of the term *disability*. Disability is now defined as a physical or mental impairment that substantially limits one or more major life activities. For example, individuals formerly denied protection from impairments caused by cancer, diabetes, and epilepsy can now be covered. For greater detail on the ADAAA, go to https://www.eeoc.gov and search for "ADAAA Fact Sheet."

Family and Medical Leave Act

The Family and Medical Leave Act (FMLA) of 1993 is important for large ambulatory care centers and hospitals. FMLA requires all public employers and any private employer of 50 or more employees to provide up to 12 weeks of job-protected, unpaid leave each year for the following reasons: (1) birth and care of the employee's child, or placement for adoption or foster care of a child; (2) care of an immediate family member who has a serious health condition; and (3) care of the employee's own serious health issue. Employees must have been employed for at least 12 months and have worked at least 1,250 hours in the 12 months preceding the beginning of the FMLA leave. Effective March 2015, the definition of spouse under FLMA covers employees in legal same-sex marriages, regardless of where they live.

Health Insurance Portability and Accountability Act

The **Health Insurance Portability and Accountability Act (HIPAA)** of 1996 required the Department of Health and Human Services to adopt national standards for electronic health care transactions. The law also required the adoption of privacy and security standards to protect an individual's identifiable health information. This mandate required greater protection of a patient's protected health information (PHI). The privacy of telephone conversations, all verbal exchanges, and all written data regarding a patient must be assured. The goal of HIPAA was also to assist in making health insurance more affordable and accessible to individuals by protecting health insurance coverage for workers and their families when they change or lose their jobs.

HIPAA law is identified in seven titles. They are summarized briefly as follows:

I. *Health insurance access, portability, and renewal.* Increases the portability of health insurance, allows continuance and transfer of insurance even with preexisting conditions, and prohibits discrimination based on health status.

II. *Preventing health care fraud and abuse.* Establishes a fraud and abuse system and spells out penalty if either event is documented; improves the Medicare program through establishing standards; establishes standards for electronic transmission of health information.

III. *Tax-related provisions.* Promotes the use of medical savings accounts (MSAs) to be used for medical expenses only. Deposits are tax-deductible for self-employed individuals who are able to draw on the accounts for medical expenses.

IV. *Group health plan requirements.* Identifies how group health care plans must provide for portability, access, and transferability of health insurance for their members.

V. *Revenue offsets.* Details how HIPAA changed the Internal Revenue Code to generate more revenue for HIPAA expenses.

VI. *General provisions.* Explains how coordination with Medicare-type plans must be carried out to prevent duplication of coverage.

VII. *Assuring portability.* Ensures employee coverage from one plan to another; written specifically for health insurance plans to ensure portability of coverage.

As of April 21, 2006, all covered health care entities were required to be in compliance of HIPAA's privacy regulations. Government and industry allocated billions of dollars to electronic medical records software and the transfer of the paper medical record to the digitized format through the Health Information Technology for Economic and Clinical Health (HITECH) Act. (See IV above.) Federal stimulus money approved in 2009 helped underwrite the cost to clinics or hospitals that serve Medicare and Medicaid patients when their electronic medical records software meets the required standards for sharing information between proprietary networks.

Occupational Safety and Health Act

The Occupational Safety and Health (OSH) Act of 1967 is a division of the U.S. Department of Labor. Its mission is to ensure that a workplace is safe and has a healthy environment. Penalties assessed by OSHA can be quite high for repeated and willful violations. (OSH Act refers to the actual law, while OSHA refers to the administration or group of individuals who oversee and govern the law.) Among these guidelines are those that make certain all employees know what chemicals they are handling, know how to reduce any health risks from hazardous chemicals that are labeled 1 to 4 for severity, and have Safety Data Sheets (SDSs) listing every ingredient in the product. Other sections of this law protecting medical assistants and patients are detailed in additional chapters. They include the Clinical Lab Improvement Amendments of 1988 (CLIA), the Bloodborne Pathogens Standard of July 1992, and the Needlestick Prevention Amendment of 2001.

Controlled Substances Act

The Controlled Substances Act of 1970 became effective in 1971. The act is administered by the Drug Enforcement Administration (DEA) under the auspices of the U.S. Department of Justice. The Controlled Substances Act lists controlled drugs in five schedules (I, II, III, IV, and V) according to their potential for abuse and dependence, with Schedule I having the greatest abuse potential and no accepted medical use in the United States. In the most recent years, there has been a move to either declassify or reclassify marijuana from its Schedule I listing—the highest potential for abuse. The Drug Policy Alliance of New York stresses scientific research that confirms marijuana's medical benefits and its wide margin of safety. Yet, the DEA and the National Institute on Drug Abuse (NIDA) continue to block any attempt to allow marijuana to be marked as a prescription medication. This issue is further complicated by the number of states that have legalized marijuana, against federal regulations.

The Controlled Substances Act and the U.S. Code of Federal Regulations regulate individuals who **administer**, **prescribe**, or **dispense** any drug listed in the five schedules. Any individual who administers, prescribes, or dispenses any controlled substance must be registered with the DEA. The DEA supplies a form for registration and mandates that renewal occur every 3 years.

A provider who prescribes only Schedules II, III, IV, and V controlled substances in the lawful course of professional practice is not required to keep separate records of those transactions. The majority of providers fall within this category. Providers who regularly administer controlled substances in Schedules II, III, IV, and V or who dispense controlled substances are required to keep specific records of each transaction.

For those providers who dispense or administer controlled substances, an inventory must be taken every 2 years of all stocks of any controlled substances on hand. The inventory must include (1) a list of the name, address, and DEA registration number of the provider; (2) the date and time of the inventory; and (3) the signatures of the individuals taking the inventory. This inventory must be kept at the location identified on the registration certificate for at least 2 years. All Schedule II drug records must be maintained separate from all other controlled substance records. These records must be made available for inspection and copying by duly authorized officials of the DEA. Some state requirements are even more restrictive than the federal requirements.

Any necessary disposal of controlled substances, usually occurring when they become outdated or when a medical practice is closed, requires specific action. The provider's DEA number and registration certificate should be returned to the DEA. Specific guidelines for destruction of the controlled substances will need to be obtained from the nearest divisional office for the DEA. Using the Internet, search using "Controlled Substances Act of 1970" for a listing of sites providing more information. You will find a listing of drugs in each of the five schedules. The listing changes from time to time as new drugs come on the market and are classified.

Uniform Anatomical Gift Act

The Uniform Anatomical Gift Act of 1968 allows persons 18 years and older who are of sound mind to make a gift of all or any part of their body (1) to any hospital, surgeon, or physician; (2) to any accredited medical or dental school, college, or university; (3) to any organ bank or storage facility; and (4) to any specified individual for education, research, advancement of medical/dental science, therapy, or transplantation. The gift may be noted in a will or by signing, in the presence of two witnesses, a donor's card. Some states allow these statements on the driver's license. There is no cost to donors or their families for gifts of all or part of the body, and there is a great need for organ donors in this country.

Critical Thinking

Research the DEA Web site to determine the steps required to dispose of contaminated or outdated Schedule II drugs.

Regulation Z of the Consumer Protection Act

Regulation Z of the Consumer Protection Act of 1967, referred to as the Truth in Lending Act, requires that an agreement by providers and their patients for payment of medical bills in more than four installments must be in writing and must provide information on any finance charge (see Chapter 19). This act is enforced by the Federal Trade Commission. These guidelines are often seen in fee-for-service plans in prearrangements for surgery or prenatal care and delivery, because patients may not be able to pay the entire fee in one payment.

Medical Practice Acts

Each state has medical practice acts that regulate the practice of medicine with the intent of protecting its citizens from harm. These statutes govern licensure, standards of care, professional liability and negligence, confidentiality, and torts. Table 6-1 summarizes licensure, renewal, and revocation rules for medical doctors. Medical assistants sometimes are asked to maintain their employer's records of continuing education for license renewal and to process the renewal at the proper time. In some states, the renewal may be done online if the license is active and in good standing.

TABLE 6-1

LICENSURE, RENEWAL, AND REVOCATION FOR MEDICAL DOCTORS

LICENSURE	RENEWAL	REVOCATION
Completion of medical education	Payment of a fee	Conviction of a crime
Completion of internship	Documentation of continuing medical education (CME)	Unprofessional conduct
Passing the U.S. Medical Licensing Examination (USMLE)	CMEs might include appropriate medical reading, teaching health professionals, and attending conferences and workshops	Personal or professional incapacity

PROCEDURE 6-1

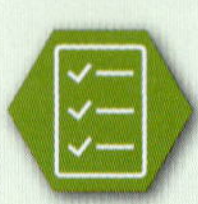
Procedure

Identifying a State's Legal Scope of Practice for Medical Assistants

PURPOSE:

To determine a medical assistant's scope of practice in the state where employment will take place.

EQUIPMENT/SUPPLIES:

Computer and Internet access

PROCEDURE STEPS:

1. Research the scope of practice for medical assistants in the state assigned to you by your instructor (sources to consider include local AAMA, AMA, and state statutes). RATIONALE: Allows students to learn about various states' rules and regulations regarding scope of practice for medical assistants.
2. Report your findings for your particular state in a summary that can be shared with the class. RATIONALE: Informs students of as many states' regulations as possible.
3. From your assigned state's report, identify any skills learned in your education that you will not legally be able to perform. RATIONALE: Demonstrates any limitations placed on medical assistants by state.

States also may regulate personnel who are employed in the outpatient care setting. Generally, medical assistants perform their duties and responsibilities under the direct supervision of the physician or doctor, and therefore are governed by medical practice acts or the state board of medical examiners. Medical assistants employed and supervised by independent nurse practitioners are governed by the nurse practice acts and the state board of nursing. Other health professionals, such as chiropractors and naturopaths, may have separate practice acts as well. Medical assistants employed by these practitioners will need to be knowledgeable of those laws. Some states require that medical assistants be licensed or certified to perform any invasive procedures. Other states require additional education and training in radiology for the medical assistant to be able to take radiographs. Furthermore, there are still a few states so strict in their regulations that medical assistants mostly perform clerical functions and noninvasive clinical duties.

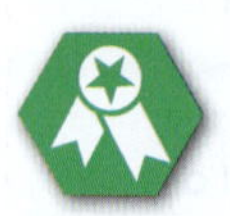
Competency

Integrity

Procedure

Certainly, medical assistants desiring to use their skills must be aware of state regulations and always perform only within the scope of those regulations as well as their education and professional preparation. Medical assistants will want to be as diligent as any other health professional about maintaining their certification, registration, and licensure and should monitor any legislation that pertains to licensure or certification (see Procedure 6-1).

CONTRACT LAW

The contractual nature of the provider–patient relationship necessitates a discussion of contracts, which are an important part of any medical practice. A contract is a binding agreement between two or more persons. A provider has a legal obligation, or duty, to care for a patient under the principles of **contract law**. The agreement must be between competent persons to do or not to do something lawful in exchange for a payment.

A contract exists when the patient arrives for treatment and the provider accepts the patient by providing treatment. An example of a valid contract occurs when a patient calls the office or clinic to make an appointment for an annual physical examination. Assuming both provider and patient are competent, and that the provider performs the lawful act of the physical examination and the patient pays a fee, all aspects of the contract exist.

There are two types of contracts: expressed and implied. An **expressed contract** can be written or verbal and specifically describes what each party in the contract will do. A written contract requires that all necessary aspects of the agreement be in writing. Examples of a written contract in the medical environment include a third party's agreement to pay a patient's bill, or the contract between a patient and the provider indicating a bill can be paid in four or more installments. An **implied contract** is indicated by actions, even silence, rather than by words. The majority of provider–patient contracts are implied contracts. It is not required that the contract be written to be enforceable as long as all points of the contract exist. An implied contract can exist either by the circumstances of the situation or by the law. When a patient reports a sore throat and the provider takes a swab for a throat culture to diagnose and treat the ailment, an implied contract exists by the circumstances. An implied contract by law exists when a patient goes into anaphylactic shock and the provider administers epinephrine to counteract shock symptoms. The law says that the provider did what the patient would have requested had there been an expressed contract.

For a contract to be valid and binding, the parties who enter into it must be competent; therefore, people who are mentally incompetent or legally insane, individuals under heavy drug or alcohol influences, infants, and some minors cannot enter into a binding contract.

Medical assistants are considered **agents** of the employers they serve, and as such must be cautious that their actions and words may become a binding contract for their employers. For example, to say that the provider can cure the patient may cause serious legal problems when, in fact, a cure may not be possible.

Termination of Contracts

A broken contract or breach of contract occurs when one of the parties does not meet contractual obligations. A provider is legally bound to treat a patient until:

- The patient discharges the provider
- The provider formally withdraws from patient care
- The patient no longer needs treatment and is formally discharged by the provider

Patient Discharges Provider. When the patient discharges the provider, a letter should be sent to the patient to confirm and document the termination of the contract. The notice is sent by certified mail with return receipt requested. Keep a copy of the letter in the patient's record (Figure 6-1).

Provider Formally Withdraws from the Case. To avoid any charges of abandonment, the provider should formally withdraw from the case when, for example, the patient becomes **noncompliant** or the provider feels the patient can no longer be served. Again, notice should be sent to the patient by certified mail with return receipt requested, and a copy of the notice should be filed in the patient's record (Figures 6-2 and 6-3).

The Patient No Longer Needs Treatment. Unless a formal discharge or withdrawal has occurred, a provider is obligated to care for a patient until the patient's condition no longer requires treatment.

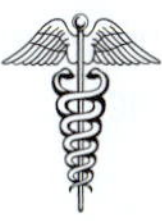

Inner City Health Care
8600 Main Street, Suite 200
River City, XY 01234

January 6, 20XX

CERTIFIED MAIL

Jim Marshal
76 Georgia Avenue
Millerton, XY 43912

Dear Mr. Marshal:

This will confirm our telephone conversation today in which you discharged me as your attending physician in your present illness. In my opinion your condition requires continued medical supervision by a physician. If you have not already done so, I suggest that you employ another physician without delay.

You may be assured that after receiving a written request from you, I will furnish the physician of your choice with information regarding the diagnosis and treatment which you have received from me.

Very truly yours,

Winston Lewis

Winston Lewis, DO
WL:ea

FIGURE 6-1 Letter confirming a physician's discharge by the patient.

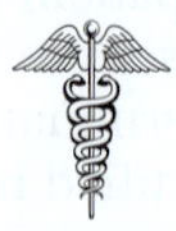

Inner City Health Care
8600 Main Street, Suite 200
River City, XY 01234

May 9, 20XX

CERTIFIED MAIL

Lenny Taylor
260 Second Street
River City, XY 01234

Dear Mr. Taylor:

You will recall that we discussed our professional relationship in my office on May 6, 20XX.

Your son, George Taylor, and Bruce Goldman, my medical assistant, were also present. As you know, the primary difficulty has been your failure to cooperate with the medical plan for your care.

While it is unfortunate that our relationship has reached this stage, I will no longer be able to serve as your physician. I will be available to you on an emergency basis only until June 10, 20XX. Meanwhile, you should immediately call or write the Medical Society, 123 Omega Drive, Carlton, MI 11666, Tel. 123-456-7899 and obtain a list of providers. Any delay could jeopardize your health, so please act quickly.

Your physical (and/or mental) problems include hypertensive heart disease, decreased kidney function, and arteriosclerosis. You could have additional medical problems that may also require professional care. Once you have found a new provider have him or her call my office. I will be happy to discuss your case with the provider assuming your care and will transfer a written summary of your case upon the receipt of a written request from you to do so.

Thank you for your anticipated cooperation and courtesy.

Very truly yours,

Winston Lewis

Winston Lewis, DO
WL:ea

FIGURE 6-2 Letter reiterating "for the record" the osteopath's decision to withdraw from the case discussed during a previous meeting with patient.

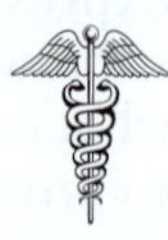

Inner City Health Care
8600 Main Street, Suite 200
River City, XY 01234

December 5, 20XX

CERTIFIED MAIL

Rhoda Au
41 Academy Road
River City, XY 01234

Dear Ms. Au:

I find it necessary to inform you that I am withdrawing further professional medical service to you because of your persistent refusal to follow my medical advice and treatment.

Because your condition requires medical attention, I suggest that you place yourself under the care of another provider without delay. If you so desire, I shall be available to attend you for a reasonable time after you have received this letter, but in no event later than January 7, 20XX. This should give you sufficient time to select someone from the many competent practitioners in this area.

You may be assured that, upon receiving your written request, I will make available to the provider of your choice your case history and information regarding the diagnosis and treatment that you have received from me.

Very truly yours,

Mark King

Mark King, MD
MK:ea

FIGURE 6-3 Letter notifying patient of provider's withdrawal from the case.

TORT LAW

A **tort** is a wrongful act, other than a breach of contract, resulting in injury to one person by another.

Standard of Care and Scope of Practice

To better understand torts, we must consider the standard of care and the four Ds of negligence. All health care providers have the responsibility and duty to perform within their scope of training and to always do what any reasonable and prudent health care professional in the same specialty or general field of practice would do. That is what is expected of every provider when a contact is made by a patient. Failure to do what any reasonable and prudent health care professional would do in the same set of circumstances can be seen as a breach of the standard of care.

Negligence is defined as the failure to exercise the standard of care that a reasonable person would exercise in similar circumstances. Negligence occurs when someone experiences injury because of another's failure to live up to a required duty of care. This is a primary cause of malpractice suits. **Malpractice** is professional negligence or the failure of a medical professional to perform the duty required of the position, causing injury to another.

Four Ds of Negligence. The four elements of negligence, sometimes called the four Ds, are:

1. *Duty.* Duty of care
2. *Derelict.* Breach of the duty of care
3. *Direct cause.* A legally recognizable injury occurs as a result of the breach of duty of care
4. *Damage.* Wrongful activity must have caused the injury or harm that occurred

If an individual has knowledge, skill, or intelligence superior to that of a layperson, that individual's conduct must be consistent with that status. For instance, medical assistants are held to a high standard of care by virtue of their skills, knowledge, and intelligence. As professionals, medical assistants are required to have a standard minimum level of special knowledge and ability. This is what is known as duty of care.

The Medical Assistant's Role in Negligence. Throughout this text, you will be reminded again and again of the critical role played by the medical assistant in patient care. Always remember to treat *all* patients with dignity and respect. Medical assistants must be certain to recall the four Ds of negligence and the standard of care required of their profession at all times. The first rule is to remember to *always* practice within the scope of one's instruction and education. The second rule is to remember that each state is likely different in what is included in the medical assistants' scope of practice. Understanding and performing within that scope of practice is essential.

Medical assistants may commit a tort that can result in **litigation**. When it can be proven that the injury resulted from the medical assistant (or other health care professional) not meeting the standard of care governing their respective professions, then litigation is a possibility. If, however, the medical assistant (or other health care professional) commits a wrongful act but the patient experiences no injury or harm, then no tort exists. For example, if the medical assistant changes a wound dressing and breaks sterile technique, and the patient suffers a severely infected wound, the medical assistant has committed a tort and can be held liable to any legal action taken. In contrast, if the medical assistant changes a wound dressing and breaks sterile technique, and the patient's wound does not become infected, no harm has occurred, and a tort does not exist. If a medical assistant fails to report to the provider an abnormal result on a blood test that prevents the provider from making an early diagnosis of a disease, the assistant's omission of an act has caused a breach in the standard of care.

Classification of Torts

There are two major classifications of torts: *intentional* and *negligent.* Intentional torts are deliberate acts of violation of another's rights. Negligent torts are not deliberate and are the result of omission and commission of an act. Malpractice is the unintentional tort of professional negligence; that is, a professional either failed to act in a reasonable and prudent manner and caused harm to the patient, or did what a reasonable and prudent person would not have done and in so doing caused harm to a patient.

There are two Latin terms that can be used to describe aspects of negligence. These are known as doctrines. *Res ipsa loquitur,* or "the thing speaks for itself," is the term used in cases that involve situations such as a nick made in the bladder when the surgeon is performing a hysterectomy. The negligence is obvious. The other doctrine, *respondeat superior,* or "let the master answer," expresses that providers are responsible for their employees' actions. If a medical assistant violates the standard of care, therein lies the basis for a suit of medical malpractice. For example, the medical assistant used the incorrect solution to clean the patient's wound and the patient sustained injuries to the wound. The provider-employer can be sued under the doctrine of *respondeat superior* because the provider-employer is responsible for the acts employees commit in the scope of their employment. The medical assistant also can be sued because individuals are responsible for their own actions.

Common Torts

Some common areas of negligence may result in torts when adherence to the standard of care has not been fulfilled. Specific examples of common torts that can occur in the office or clinic are *battery, defamation of character,* and *invasion of privacy.*

Battery. The basis of the tort of battery is unprivileged touching of one person by another. A patient must consent to being touched. When a procedure is to be performed on a patient, the patient must give consent in full knowledge of all the facts. It does not matter whether the procedure that constitutes the battery improves the patient's health. Patients have the right to withdraw consent at any time.

One example of battery is when a medical assistant insists on giving the patient an injection that was ordered for the patient even though the patient refuses the injection. Another example can be seen when a surgeon performs additional surgery beyond the original procedure (the surgeon performed a hysterectomy, for which consent was given, but is liable for battery for removing a suspicious looking abdominal nevus from the patient's abdomen without consent). It does not matter that the surgeon does not charge for the additional procedure. It also does not matter if the patient would have given consent if asked in advance.

Defamation of Character. The tort of defamation of character consists of injury to another person's reputation, name, or character through spoken or written words for which damages can be recovered. Two kinds of defamation are libel and slander. **Libel** is false and malicious writing about another, such as in published materials, pictures, and media. An example can be seen when the medical assistant writes in the patient's record, "Mr. O'Keefe's wife and her negative attitude appear to be the cause of his ulcer." A copy of Mr. O'Keefe's records were later sent to a new provider, who reviewed the record and read the remarks quoted by the medical assistant.

Slander is false and malicious spoken words. Slander can be seen in the following comment directed by a patient to the provider, "Dr. Woo is incompetent. He should have his license revoked." The statement is overheard by the clinic administrative medical assistant and other patients waiting in the reception area.

For a tort of defamation of character (either libel or slander) to exist, a third party must see or hear the words and understand their meaning.

Invasion of Privacy. Invasion of privacy is another kind of tort. It includes unauthorized publicity of patient information, medical records being released without the patient's knowledge and permission, and patients receiving unwanted publicity and exposure to public view. For example, if a minor unmarried girl has been examined for possible pregnancy, and the medical assistant telephones the girl's home and inadvertently gives the laboratory results to someone other than the patient, her privacy has been invaded. A second situation exists when persons other than those providing care and performing examinations and procedures (essential or nonessential personnel) are allowed to be present without the patient's consent. Yet another example of the patient's right to privacy being violated is when the patient is asked to walk from the examination room across the hall to a treatment room while wearing only a patient gown in full view of other patients and personnel.

Medical assistants and other health care professionals should:

- Close a door, pull a curtain, or provide a screen when looking at, handling, or examining the patient
- Expose only body parts necessary for treatment (drape the patient, exposing only the part that is being treated)
- Discuss the patient with no one except those individuals involved in the patient's care, and then discuss only those aspects of care that relate to the needs of the patient

It is not an invasion of privacy to disclose information required by a court order, subpoena, or statute to protect the public health and welfare, as in the reporting of violent crime.

INFORMED CONSENT

Documentation of **informed consent** becomes an important part of the patient care process. Every patient has a right to know and understand any procedure to be performed. The patient is to be told in language easily understood:

- The nature of any procedure and how it is to be performed
- Any possible risks involved, as well as expected outcomes of the procedure
- Any other methods of treatment and the risks they involve
- Risks if no treatment is given

It is the responsibility of the health care provider to make certain the patient understands. If an interpreter is necessary, the provider must procure one.

Often, consent forms will be signed if there is to be a surgical or invasive procedure performed. For specific samples of consent forms for medical treatment go to http://www.who.int and search "informed consent form templates." The medical assistant may be asked to witness the patient's signature and may be expected to follow through on any of the provider's instructions or explanations, but is not expected to explain the procedure to the patient. The signed consent form is kept with the medical record, and a copy also is given to the patient.

Increasingly, providers who perform invasive procedures on a regular basis (i.e., surgeons, dermatologists, etc.) use video to further explain the procedure(s) to be performed. Some formal consent forms ask patients to explain in their own words the procedure to be performed. The explanation given serves as a measure of the patient's understanding of the process.

Expressed Consent

When patients indicate to their providers they understand the process to take place, or when they are asked to sign an informed consent document, they are making an **expressed consent**. Expressed consent indicates that patients have directly communicated their consent to the provider either by a verbal "Yes, I consent," or by signing a consent form.

Implied Consent

Two circumstances related to consent are worth mentioning at this point. **Implied consent** occurs when there is a life-threatening emergency, or when the patient is unconscious or unable to respond. The provider, by law, is allowed to give treatment within his or her scope of practice without a signed consent. Implied consent also occurs in more subtle ways. For example, the patient who rolls up a shirtsleeve for the medical assistant to take a blood pressure reading is implying consent to the procedure by the action taken. Implied consent is generally understood from the facts and circumstances surrounding the treatment.

Consent and Legal Incompetence

Consent for treatment is not valid if the patient is legally incompetent to give consent. Legal **incompetence** means that a patient is found by a court to be insane, inadequate, or to not be an adult. In such instances, consent must be obtained from a parent, a legal guardian, or the court on behalf of the patient. Consent for treatment can be given only by the natural parent or legal guardian as determined by the court for a minor child. A **minor** is a person who has not reached the age of majority (18–21 years old), depending on the laws of each state. Generally, a minor is considered unable to give effective consent for medical treatment; therefore, without proper consent from parents or guardians, medical professionals can be held liable for battery if medical treatment is given. Exceptions to this rule are in cases of emergency and for mature and emancipated minors. **Emancipated minors** are minors younger than 18 years who are free of parental care and are financially responsible, married, become parents, or join the armed forces. **Mature minors** are persons, usually younger than 18 years, who are able to understand and appreciate the nature and consequences of treatment despite their young age. Nearly every state allows minors to give consent for treatment for pregnancy, drug or alcohol addiction, and sexually transmitted disease. Some states have passed legislation that names minors as statutory adults at 14 years old for the purpose of receiving medical care. In these states, minors may consent and be protected by confidentiality and privacy even though their parents or legal guardians may still be financially responsible for their medical bills.

Questions related to the ability of minors and emancipated minors to give consent often must be determined on a case-by-case basis because state statutes vary. Placing a telephone call to the state attorney general's office can help clarify issues, questions, and concerns that involve consent and treatment of minors.

RISK MANAGEMENT

Practicing good **risk management** makes the medical assistant and the provider-employer less vulnerable to litigation.

Following are some ways to avoid incidents that may lead to litigation:

- Perform only within the scope of your training and education.
- Comply with all state and federal regulations and statutes.
- Keep the clinic safe and equipment in readiness.
- Never leave a patient unattended; if you must leave, pass the responsibility for the patient's care on to another individual.
- Keep all patient information confidential.
- Follow all policies and procedures established for the clinic.
- Document fully only facts; formally document withdrawing from a case and discharging patients.

Critical Thinking

Identify the suggestions in the previous risk management list that are most likely not performed when the staff in the ambulatory care setting find themselves overworked, overwhelmed, and behind. What might be done to prevent carelessness brought on by such circumstances?

- Log telephone calls and return calls to patients within a reasonable time frame.
- Follow up on missed or canceled appointments.
- Never guarantee a cure or diagnosis, and never advise treatment without a provider's order.
- Secure informed consent as necessary.
- Do not criticize other practitioners.
- Explain any appointment delays.
- Be particularly watchful with patients who have special needs, such as the elderly, pediatric patients, and those with physical and emotional disabilities.
- Report any error that may have occurred to your employer.

Professional Liability Coverage

The vast number of legal concerns providers must attend to in the care of patients as well as all the many things that can go wrong demand that providers carry professional liability or malpractice insurance. Therefore, providers commonly carry professional liability insurance coverage in order to cover the costs of any litigation that may occur. In today's health care climate, there is a great deal of discussion regarding the cost of such insurance and the dollar amounts of awards being made to plaintiffs. While not recommended, some providers are doing without professional liability coverage and notifying their patients of such action. Others have chosen to limit their practice to procedures that are not high risk. For instance, a family practice provider may choose not to deliver babies because of the high cost of professional liability coverage for deliveries. Obstetrics, gynecology, and surgery professional liability coverage are among the highest.

Health care employees need their own professional liability coverage. While litigation activities may seek out the "highest-paid" individual to sue, employees can be and are sued quite regularly. Medical assistants can purchase professional liability coverage from the American Association of Medical Assistants (AAMA). Such insurance is designed to help protect personal assets from being taken in order to cover any judgment awarded the plaintiff.

CIVIL LITIGATION PROCESS

Legal

Despite all the best efforts of health care professionals and their employees, litigation can occur. Litigation is the process of taking a lawsuit or a criminal case through the courts. It is helpful to understand the steps taken for civil litigation to occur. The greatest amount of any litigation seen in the ambulatory care setting occurs when relationships between individuals break down for one reason or another. When this happens, the party, or plaintiff, bringing the action, usually a patient, seeks an attorney who agrees to bring the complaint to the courts. The provider, or defendant, is summoned to court. This summons or subpoena notifies the provider of the plaintiff's suit and allows the defendant to file an answer with the court.

Subpoenas

The **subpoena** is an order from the court naming the specific date, time, and reason to appear. A portion of a medical record or the entire medical record may be subpoenaed, the health care provider may be subpoenaed to testify in court, or both the medical record and the provider may be subpoenaed (*subpoena duces tecum*). The staff in the ambulatory care setting usually will have ample time to make certain the record is current and complete before its inclusion in court. Out of courtesy, a provider will notify patients whose records have been subpoenaed. If, for any reason, the patient does not want the record released, the provider must call for legal advice on how to respond to the subpoena.

Certain records, because of their sensitive nature, may require more than a subpoena to be released. These include records related to sexually transmitted diseases, including AIDS and HIV testing; mental health records; substance abuse records; and sexual assault records. For the courts to have access to these records, a *court order* is required in many states.

HIPAA law requires clinics to identify in written policies and procedures what information they will release regarding patients. Before patient information is released, the following must be identified: (1) the purpose or need for the information, (2) the nature or extent of the information to be released, (3) the date of the authorization, and (4) the signature(s) of the person(s) authorized to give consent. Release only what the subpoena or court order specifically requests rather than releasing the entire medical record. Many practitioners keep a patient's consent information in a specific section of the medical record for quick referral and to demonstrate HIPAA compliance.

The care taken with subpoenas and court orders for certain information is to ensure patients of confidentiality. The information in the medical record, including the information a patient shared with the provider and medical assistant, is private.

No patient information can be given to another person or entity (provider, patient's attorney, insurance carrier, or federal or state agency) without the expressed written consent of the patient. Care must be exercised at all times to ensure that the patient's right to confidentiality is not breached. For example, information given to unauthorized personnel associated with the provider's or clinic's practice in regard to the patient's condition, or financial status regarding payment of bills, violates the patient's right to confidentiality. Likewise, when discussing issues over the telephone that can be overheard by others, such as the patient's account being turned over to a collection agency, the patient's right to confidentiality has been violated.

Certain disclosures of information about a patient's conditions and suspected illnesses are required by law. Legally required disclosures are necessary when the public needs to know certain information for its safety and welfare. The disclosures supersede the patient's right to privacy and confidentiality (see the Reportable Diseases/Injuries discussion in the Public Duties section).

Discovery

In the litigation process, the period of **discovery** follows the subpoenas. This is the time in which both parties are allowed access to all the information and evidence related to the case. Rules of discovery vary from state to state but may include the following:

1. An **interrogatory** is a written set of questions that can come from either the plaintiff or the defendant and that must be answered, under oath, and within a specific time period.
2. A **deposition** is oral testimony taken with a court reporter present in a location agreed on by both parties. Both attorneys are usually present when depositions are taken.

Medical assistants may be asked to respond to an interrogatory or may be deposed by the plaintiff's attorney. The defendant's attorney will provide specific instructions in both situations. Because both are done under oath, honesty is an absolute. The medical assistant may be asked to refer to certain documents, recall specific information, or identify documentation in a medical record.

Expert Witnesses. Providers and members of their staff may be called to testify in court to the standard of care. In such a case, they are usually considered expert witnesses. An **expert witness** is one who has enough knowledge and experience in a field to be able to testify to what is the reasonable and expected standard of care. Expert witnesses are expected to tell what they know to be fact and are best counseled to use lay terms rather than complicated medical language. The goal is for jurors and judges to understand the nature of any medical information shared. Visual aids, charts, and computer simulations often are used to illustrate or clarify testimony given by expert witnesses.

Pretrial Conference

A pretrial conference is generally held close to the trial date to decide if there is just cause for the suit, to make certain that both parties are ready, and to determine if there might be an out-of-court settlement. If a trial seems imminent, **alternative dispute resolution (ADR)** may be suggested. ADR saves money, time, and adverse publicity that can come from a trial.

Mediation allows a neutral facilitator to help the two parties settle their differences and come to an acceptable solution. If no settlement is reached, the case can still look to the court for satisfaction. **Arbitration** allows the neutral party to settle the dispute. This arbitration can be binding or nonbinding. In binding arbitration, both parties agree at the outset to accept the neutral party's decision as final. In nonbinding arbitration, the case can look to the court for settlement.

Trial

A trial can be held before a judge or before a judge and a jury. When the trial begins, opening statements outlining the details of the case are made by both sides. The plaintiff's attorney calls witnesses

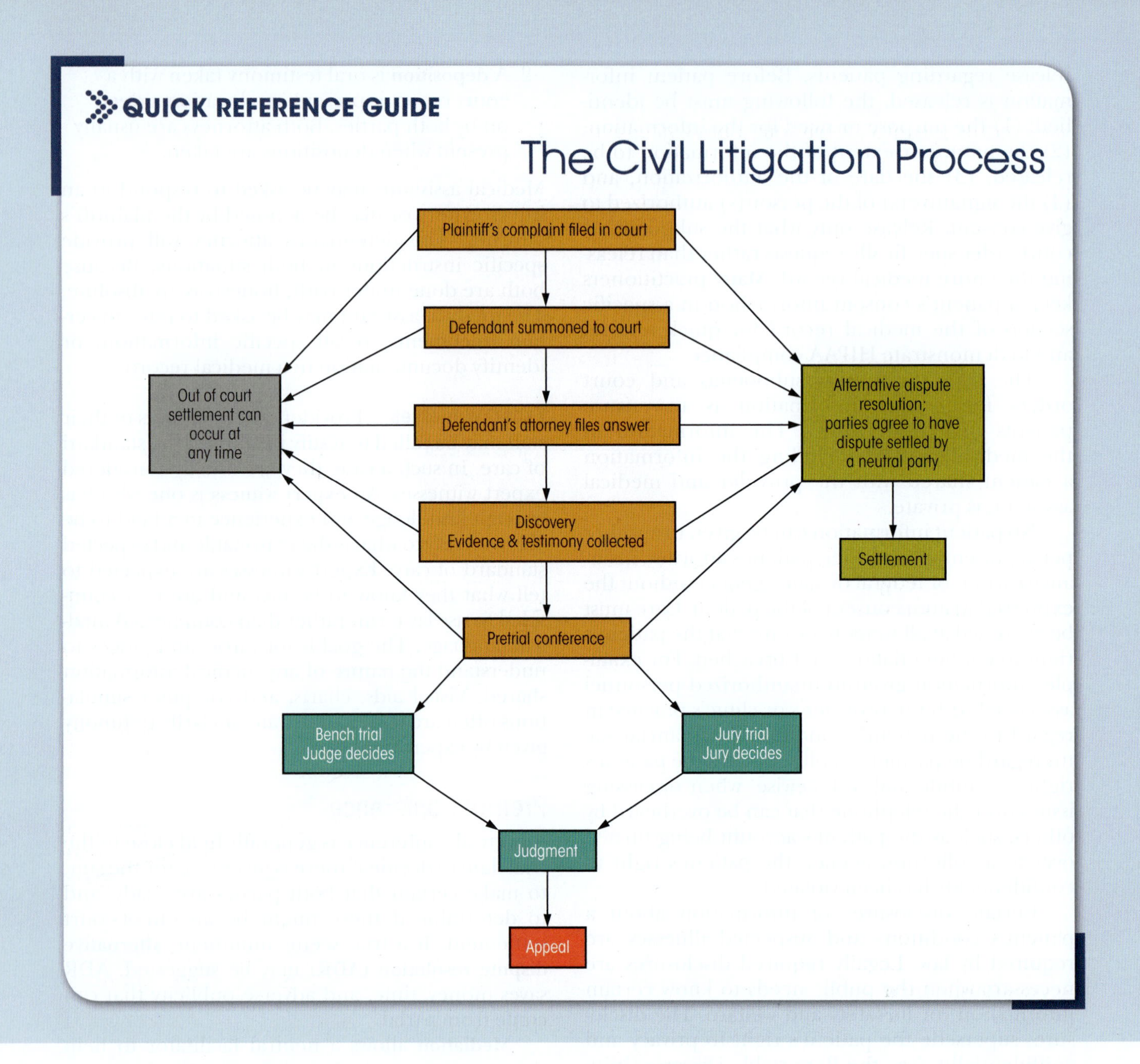

to produce evidence first. This is known as direct examination. In cross-examination, the defendant's attorney questions the witness. When the plaintiff's case is finished, the defendant presents the case in the same manner. When all the information has been presented, the case is turned over for judgment.

If the plaintiff's case is successful, the judge or jury may award a specific amount of money or damages. The judge will instruct the jury regarding the kinds of damages that can be considered in that state. A number of states have placed limits on monetary awards in malpractice cases, making it impossible to go above the maximum award allowed even when juries determine that the monetary award should be higher than allowed by the state. If the defendant's case is successful, the case is dismissed. After a court decision, the party that has lost the case can begin an appeal process. The appeal requests an opinion from higher courts that review cases usually on the basis of a faulty legal process or action.

See the "Civil Litigation Process" Quick Reference Guide for an outline of the civil case process.

STATUTE OF LIMITATIONS

No discussion of negligence, malpractice, or medical records is complete without a brief statement regarding the statute of limitations that will, in part, determine timelines for any litigation and how long medical records are kept. Statutes of limitations most commonly begin at the time a negligent act was committed, when the act was discovered, or when the care of the patient and the provider–patient relationship ended. Therefore, generally all records should be retained until after the statute has run out, usually 3 to 6 years. It is easy to understand why many providers choose to keep their records indefinitely, a plan made much easier with electronic files.

State and federal statutes set maximum time periods during which certain actions can be brought or rights enforced; there is a time limit for individuals to initiate legal action. The statute of limitations varies from one jurisdiction to another, and a lawsuit may not be brought after the statute of limitations has run. For example, in the Commonwealth of Massachusetts, the statute of limitations for an act of medical malpractice committed on an adult is 3 years. If harm to a patient resulted from a medical assistant administering the wrong dose of medication to a patient in Massachusetts, a lawsuit must be brought within 3 years from the time the medication error was made, with the 3 years commencing at the time the negligent act was committed.

PUBLIC DUTIES

Providers and their employees must comply with all federal, state, and local health care laws and regulations. When a good working relationship exists between providers and their employees, compliance to these regulations is less likely to be compromised. There are a number of public duties to be considered.

Reportable Diseases/Injuries

All medical providers have a duty to the public to report diseases and injuries that jeopardize public health and welfare. Transmittable or contagious diseases and/or injuries resulting from a knife or gunshot are examples; these must be reported to the appropriate authorities. This can be done without the patient's consent because it is required by law. When reporting, it is important to do so properly and according to the laws of the state in which one is employed. Knowledge of which illnesses, injuries, and conditions to report, to whom to report, and the appropriate forms to submit is essential. Copies of all information must be kept for the clinic.

MedlinePlus, a Web site sponsored by the U.S. National Library of Medicine and the National Institutes of Health, has an excellent site connected to the Medline Encyclopedia titled "Reportable Diseases" that identifies guidelines for reportable diseases. Local, state, and national agencies such as the Centers for Disease Control and Prevention (CDC) require such diseases to be reported when diagnosed by providers or laboratories. States may vary in the diseases that require reporting, but their lists are likely to include the list of "Nationally Notifiable Infectious Diseases" that can be found on the CDC's Web site (go to www.cdc.gov and search for "Nationally Notifiable Conditions"). Some diseases require written reports. Others require reporting electronically or by telephone; they include rubeola (measles) and pertussis (whooping cough). Still others ask for only the number of cases to be reported. Such reporting is beneficial to society and all health care managers in tracking and preventing illness. The list changes as new diseases occur and are diagnosed.

Other generally required facts to report include births; deaths; childhood immunizations; rape; and abuse toward a child, elder, or intimate partner.

Some states have laws specific to the release of information relative to mental or psychological treatment, HIV testing, AIDS diagnosis and treatment, sexually transmitted diseases, and chemical substance abuse.

Local or state health departments can provide lists of diseases and injuries to report and will also provide the appropriate forms (see Procedure 6-2).

Abuse

Child abuse, **intimate partner violence (IPV)**, and elder abuse are becoming more commonly known in today's society. As a result, patients experiencing such abuse may be seen in the ambulatory care setting. In all cases of abuse, medical records hold valuable information if a court procedure ensues. Careful documentation is critical. State laws are fairly specific and consistent in mandates to report child abuse, but laws related to elder abuse and domestic violence or intimate partner violence are not as detailed. In any case, the rights of the abused must be protected. (See Table 7-1 for a summary.)

PROCEDURE 6-2

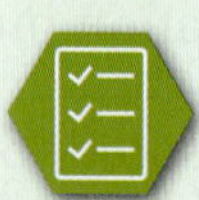
Procedure

Perform Compliance Reporting Based on Public Health Statutes

PURPOSE:

To report a communicable disease.

EQUIPMENT/SUPPLIES:

- Patient's medical record
- Local, state, and national guidelines for reporting communicable disease
- Computer and Internet access, telephone, and fax machine

PROCEDURE STEPS:

1. From the patient's medical record and/or provider's instructions, determine the disease to be reported. RATIONALE: Helps determine if local, state, or national reporting is necessary or all three are required.
2. Access the Medline Encyclopedia "Reportable Diseases" and the CDC's Web site to determine how the disease is to be reported. RATIONALE: Regulations may change; ensures the most recent guidelines.
3. Follow the instructions from the above sites to prepare the confidential report via telephone, fax, or written notice. RATIONALE: Makes certain proper protocol is followed.
4. Place a copy of the report in the patient's medical record. RATIONALE: Indicates completion of the reporting process.

Child Abuse. All 50 states and the District of Columbia mandate, or require, that health care professionals, teachers, social workers, and certain others who suspect child abuse report the incident to the proper authorities. Confidentiality in the provider–patient relationship does not exist when children are abused. If a person has a reason to suspect abuse and reports the abuse to the police and, in the case of child abuse, to the child protective agency, this individual is protected against liability as a result of making the report. Failure to report could result in criminal or civil penalties. Usually, the child protective unit of the state department of social services is called to investigate suspected cases of child abuse. Some injuries that are commonly seen in child abuse are bruises, welts, burns, fractures, and head injuries. Evidence of neglect, intimidation, or sexual abuse also may be seen.

If a suspicion of abuse exists, the provider should do the following:

- Treat the child's injuries.
- Send the child to the hospital for further treatment when necessary.
- Inform parents of the diagnosis and that it will be reported to the police and social services agency.
- Notify the child protective agency (keep phone number posted).
- Document all information.
- Provide court testimony if requested.

Elder Abuse. Elder abuse may consist of neglect, physical abuse, punishment, physical restraint, and/or abandonment. Examples are seen when elders are overmedicated or undermedicated, physically restrained, intimidated by shouting or profanity, sexually abused, neglected or abandoned, or in any other way have their rights and dignity violated. The person reporting the abuse is generally a health care professional who observes or suspects the abuse, and the reporting agency is most likely one of a social service or welfare nature. The majority of states have laws protecting vulnerable adults and the elderly from abuse.

Intimate Partner Violence (IPV). The term *domestic violence* has been changed to be more encompassing of an escalating problem. *Intimate partner violence (IPV)* is now used and refers to violence or abuse between a spouse or former spouse; boyfriend, girlfriend, or former boyfriend/girlfriend; and same-sex or heterosexual intimate partner or former same-sex or heterosexual intimate partner. The abuse may include physical or sexual violence, threats of the same, and psychological or emotional violence. Physical violence is a criminal act, and failure to report it is considered a misdemeanor in some states. Victims of IPV should be treated as soon as possible after the assault so that evidence can be preserved for legal purposes. Some forms of IPV are considered acceptable behavior in many cultures, even in the United States. Some cultures believe the woman is chattel, or property, of her spouse; that she has no rights or authority; and that she must submit to her husband's, brother's, or father's demands.

An individual who manages to come to the ambulatory care setting with signs of IPV is courageous and probably is extremely frightened as well, because reporting the violence may increase the risk for continued violence and even death in some instances.

Make certain that community resources are readily available for survivors of IPV, even if they choose to stay in the abusive situation. In many cases, the abused patient's options are so few that leaving is more frightening than staying in the abusive relationship. Do not pass judgment on these survivors; they desperately need understanding and compassion.

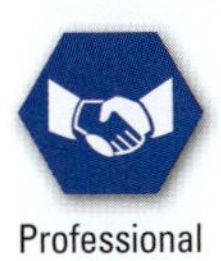

Your understanding and compassion are perhaps the only door through which they might feel comfortable enough to leave the abusive relationship.

Good Samaritan Laws

All 50 states have laws regarding the rendering of first aid by health care professionals at the scene of an accident or sudden injury. Good Samaritan laws, although not always clearly written, encourage health care professionals to provide medical care within the scope of their training without fear of being sued for negligence. In an emergency situation, medical assistants cannot be held liable should an injury result from some form of first aid rendered or from first aid they omitted to render as long as they acted in a reasonable way within the scope of their knowledge. Medical assistants and other health care professionals with skills in cardiopulmonary resuscitation (CPR) who are present when CPR is needed must perform the procedure on the victim or otherwise could be declared negligent. Emergencies that arise in the ambulatory care setting generally are not covered by Good Samaritan laws.

FRAUD

Unfortunately, illegal activities can and do take place in the health care environment. As a result, it is important to discuss how fraud may occur. Following is a list of the most common violations committed:

1. Billing for services not provided
2. Billing a noncovered service as if it is covered
3. Misrepresenting dates, locations, and providers of service
4. Incorrect reporting of diagnoses or procedures
5. Taking kickbacks and bribery
6. False or unnecessary issuance of prescription drugs, especially opioids

This list may seem obvious, but without appropriate checks and balances, an illegal act is often committed due to carelessness rather than malicious intent. Consider the following examples:

- The PCP is on maternity leave and the team's nurse practitioner fills in, but all charges are made at the PCP level of service.
- The PCP indicates a higher level of service during the appointment and/or indicates procedures the medical assistant observes to be inaccurate.
- The PCP misrepresents dates of services on a labor and industry case in order to assure payment of the claim.
- The PCP continues to issue opioid prescriptions without following proper procedures.

In a very large medical clinic or a hospital clinic, there likely is a quality assurance protocol in place. However, illegal matters should be reported to proper authorities. Billing fraud can be reported to the appropriate agency (e.g., Medicare/Medicaid or to the clinic's accountant). Providers who create these acts can be reported to the local branch of the American Medical Association and to the police. Employees must recall that not reporting illegal activities makes them an accessory to the crime.

ADVANCE DIRECTIVES

Medical assistants in the ambulatory care setting will be asked to attach advance directives or living wills to patients' medical records These directives are legal documents in which patients indicate their wishes in the case of a life-threatening illness or serious injury.

Health care providers in many states and cities have adopted the Physician Orders for Life-Sustaining Treatment (POLST) form. This form is to be completed by a health care provider based on the patient's preferences regarding the type of life-sustaining treatment wanted and medical indications. POLST is most often brightly colored (neon pink or green). To be valid, the form must be signed by the proper authority. Some states may use another name than POLST, but the intent is quite similar. POLST is appropriate for seriously ill individuals with life-threatening or terminal illnesses. Some providers believe that even with an advance directive in place, it is advisable to complete a POLST form. This form goes with the patient when he or she is moved between care settings. For those living at home, it is recommended that the form be posted on the refrigerator where emergency responders can locate it easily. For a current listing of states' development of POLST, go to www.polst.org and click on the "Programs in Your State" link. Such documents should always accompany patients to the hospital for any treatment or care. They may be updated from time to time, and patients can ask to rescind such a document at any time. Medical assistants must remember that these documents reflect the choices of their patients and are to be respected as such.

Living Wills/Advance Directives

Patients who desire to make known in advance their choices related to health care, especially when death is near, are likely to have living wills, advance directives, a health care proxy, or a POLST order. The title of such a document is largely determined by the state in which the document is made. These documents are necessary because advances in medicine allow medical professionals to sustain life even if the individual will not recover from a persistent vegetative state. Persons who prefer not to remain in that state can use the living will or advance directive to make decisions about life support and to direct others to implement their wishes in that regard. Such a document allows individuals to indicate to family and health care professionals whether life-prolonging medical or surgical procedures are to be continued, withheld, or withdrawn, and whether artificial feeding and fluids are to be used or withheld. The document allows individuals to make this decision before incapacitation.

To be valid, the proper and particular form, which is different in each state, must be used, and it must be lawfully executed. States vary in the number of witnesses required and whether a notary public is required for those signatures. The form goes into effect when provided to a patient's health care provider *and* when the patient is no longer capable of making health care decisions. Examples of incapacity include permanent unconsciousness, life-threatening illness in the latter stages, and inability to communicate. The U.S. Legal Forms Web site (http://USlegalforms.com) has samples of living wills for all 50 states and the District of Columbia under the heading "Living Will." A sample from each state is available without a fee.

Durable Power of Attorney for Health Care

Another document seen in the ambulatory care setting is the **durable power of attorney for health care** or designation of health care surrogate or health care proxy. This document allows a patient to name another person as the official spokesperson for that patient should he or she be unable to

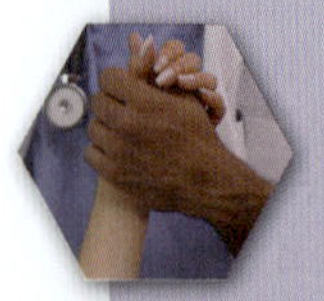

Patient Education

Legal

Because of the increased awareness of confidentiality as a result of HIPAA, medical assistants can be helpful by suggesting that any family member(s) who might be involved and need to know about the patient's care be indicated in the patient's medical record with a signed release from the patient. There have been examples recently of adult children of elder adults who were either not informed when their ailing parent was taken to emergency services in another state or were unable to get any information about their parent from a hospital or provider even though a durable power of attorney for health care was in place. If that directive does not go with the patient, no information can be given. For that reason, it is suggested that patients may want to keep a wallet card containing a notice of the advance directive, any appointed agent named, and any family member(s) who is allowed information.

make health care decisions. A basic durable power of attorney document allows another person to manage finances and personal matters; however, it takes a durable power of attorney for health care for that person to make medical decisions.

Every state has a slightly different version of their living will, advance directive, durable power of attorney for health care, or POLST. Most forms and specific information can be found on the Internet by keying in a particular state and the title of the document wanted. Also, the Web site for Compassion and Choices (http://www.compassionandchoices.org), located in Portland, Oregon, is quite helpful.

Patient Self-Determination Act

In 1991, the federal government passed the **Patient Self-Determination Act (PSDA)**, which applies to all health care institutions receiving payments from Medicare and Medicaid. PSDA requires that all adults receiving health care from these institutions be given the opportunity to provide information about their wishes in an advance directive.

Copies of advance directives are to be given to patients' providers so the documents can be transferred to a hospital or nursing facility as necessary. Any named agent should have a copy, and family members also may have a copy.

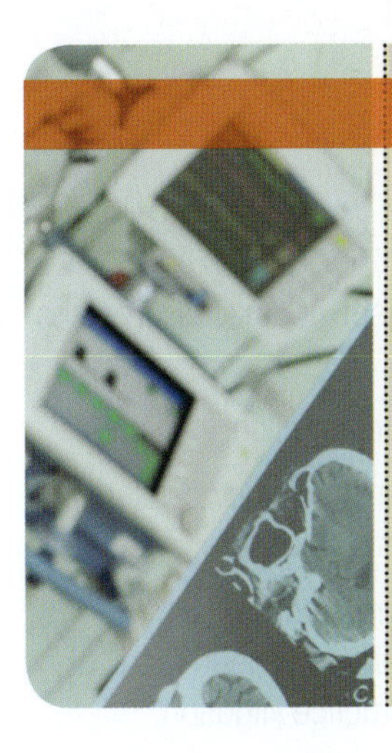

CASE STUDY 6-1

Refer to the scenario at the beginning of the chapter. You realize that any breach of confidentiality is a serious matter, whether intentional or accidental, and that the lack of professionalism can lead to such errors in judgment.

CASE STUDY REVIEW

1. What corrective measures can you suggest to decrease voices heard in the hallway or from examination rooms?
2. How can private patient information be kept private even among staff?
3. What suggestions do you make to keep personal conversations and interactions out of view and/or sound of patients?

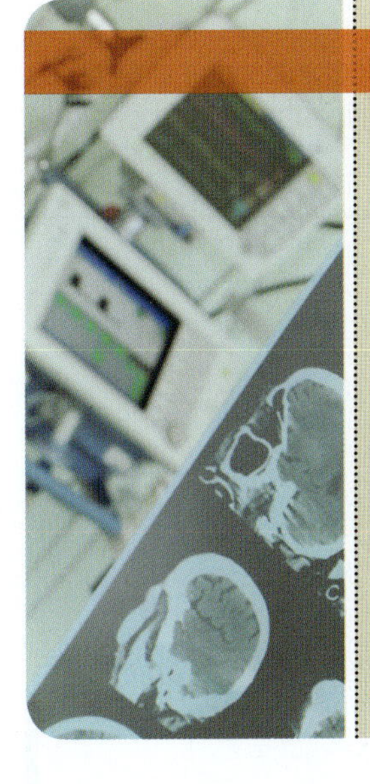

CASE STUDY 6-2

Three weeks ago, Dr. King treated a new patient, Boris Bolski, for lower back pain, which the patient believed was the result of consistent heavy lifting at his job. Medical assistant Joe Guerrero, CMA (AAMA), assisted Dr. King during the examination. Today, both Joe and Dr. King were served with subpoenas by Mr. Bolski's attorney. Mr. Bolski is alleging that unsafe conditions at his workplace caused severe strain on his back, and he is suing his employer for damages. Dr. King and Joe Guerrero were called as expert witnesses to a civil hearing; Joe, especially, is a bit nervous about this, because he has never been on the witness stand in court and is not sure what is expected of him.

CASE STUDY REVIEW

1. How will Mr. Bolski's medical record help Joe answer questions at the hearing?
2. What information should Joe gather so that he is prepared to testify?
3. As an expert witness, what might Joe be expected to communicate to the judge in this case?

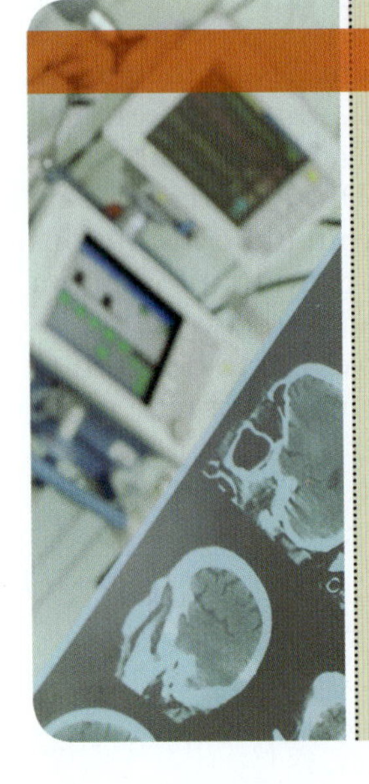

CASE STUDY 6-3

Wanda Hanson, RMA (AMT), is working on a part-time basis in Hudson, Florida, as an administrative medical assistant on the phone desk in the emergency department at Hudson Community Hospital when a frantic long-distance call is received. The caller is Larry Nelson from Cheyenne, Wyoming. He received a call from the nursing home where his 95-year-old mother is living informing him that she was taken by ambulance to your hospital. Larry wants to know if Muriel Nelson has arrived and what her condition is. Wanda is aware of a patient's right to privacy, confidentiality, and the HIPAA regulations. Wanda observed Mrs. Nelson arrive at the emergency department quite incoherent and confused.

CASE STUDY REVIEW

1. What can Wanda tell Mr. Nelson, especially after noting that no records were with the elderly Mrs. Nelson when she arrived at the hospital?
2. What information would Wanda need from Mr. Nelson before complying with his request?
3. How can Wanda put Mr. Nelson at ease? What can Wanda do to help?

Summary

- Today's medical professional must have a knowledge of all sources of law.
- Administrative law regulations include many components pertinent to outpatient care.
- Contract law will determine how patients are discharged, how providers withdraw from treatment, and necessary steps to take when patients no longer require treatment.
- Tort law, a wrongful act resulting in injury, dictates a professional's standard of care and scope of practice.
- Patients are more aware than ever of their rights, especially those of confidentiality and the right to privacy, consent, and records ownership. They are likely to seek redress when they perceive their rights have been violated.
- Consent, whether informed, expressed, implied, or written, is an essential part of the patient care process. Risk management procedures and a healthy relationship between all providers and patients as well as between medical assistants and patients, and respect for the patient's rights, reduces the likelihood of any malpractice litigation.
- An understanding of the statute of limitations and the civil litigation process is helpful when there is a lawsuit.
- Providers must fulfill all public duties and comply with reporting laws.
- Patients' advance directives and powers of attorney must be identified and followed.
- Sources of information regarding state and federal laws can be obtained from the state medical society, the provider's liability insurance company, the state medical assistant society, the state attorney general's office, the Internet, and/or the public library.

Study for Success

To reinforce your knowledge and skills of information presented in this chapter:

- Review the *Key Terms* and *Learning Outcomes*
- Consider the *Critical Thinking* features and *Case Studies* and discuss your conclusions
- Answer the questions in the *Certification Review*

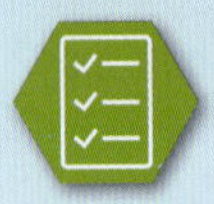
Procedure

- Perform the *Procedures* using the *Competency Assessment Checklists* on the *Student Companion Website*

CERTIFICATION REVIEW

1. What type of contract most often exists between provider and patient?
   a. Expressed
   b. Implied
   c. Privileged
   d. Civil
2. Which administrative law act prohibits discrimination in employment and is enforced by the EEOC?
   a. Controlled Substances Act
   b. Federal Age Discrimination Act
   c. Americans with Disabilities Act
   d. Health Insurance Portability and Accountability Act
   e. Title VII of the Civil Rights Act
3. What stipulation was recently added/amended to the Family and Medical Leave Act?
   a. Unpaid leave to care for a family member with Alzheimer disease
   b. Changing eligibility requirements to a time of employment of 9 months and a minimum of 935 hours worked
   c. Changing definition of spouse to recognize legal same-sex marriages
   d. Eliminating military leave provisions
4. Occasionally, a provider will be sued for an employee's negligence, even though the provider is not guilty of any negligent act. This is done on the basis of what doctrine?
   a. Res ipsa loquitur
   b. Respondeat superior
   c. Proximate cause
   d. Employer–employee contracts
   e. Regulation Z of the Employee Protection Act
5. How do the courts interpret the standard of care expected of a provider?
   a. Perform within scope of training on a par with all other providers engaged in the same medical specialty anywhere
   b. Provide reasonable, attentive, diligent care comparable with other providers in the general field of practice
   c. Exercise skill as well as possible under the circumstances
   d. Match the national norm in performance
6. What is the purpose of advance directives?
   a. They allow patients to direct how their billing is to be handled.
   b. They encourage providers to render first aid in an emergency.
   c. They allow patients to determine their choices in life-threatening circumstances.
   d. Best expressed in the POLST form, they guarantee equal treatment under the law.
   e. They give the provider power of attorney to make health care decisions.
7. What are important characteristics of a subpoena?
   a. It is a court order requesting data, an appearance in court, or both.
   b. It is sufficient to enforce a release of any type of medical record or information.
   c. It may be ignored without consequences.
   d. It allows the person being served to select a specific date or time to appear.
8. What are the four Ds of negligence?
   a. Duty, danger, damage, disaster
   b. Derelict, direct cause, damage, danger
   c. Danger, direct cause, damage, disaster
   d. Duty, derelict, direct cause, damage
   e. Duty, despair, direct cause, damage
9. Which of the following statements is true of emancipated minors?
   a. They are 18 to 25 years in age but live with their parents.
   b. They are younger than 18, are considered adults, and can consent to treatment.
   c. They live on their own but are not self-supporting.
   d. They are not married and able to work only part time.
10. Which of the following statements best describes torts?
    a. They often include battery, defamation of character, and invasion of privacy.
    b. They are always intentional in nature.
    c. They are laws to make certain the standard of care has been fulfilled.
    d. They do not include malpractice.
    e. None of these

CHAPTER 7

Ethical Considerations

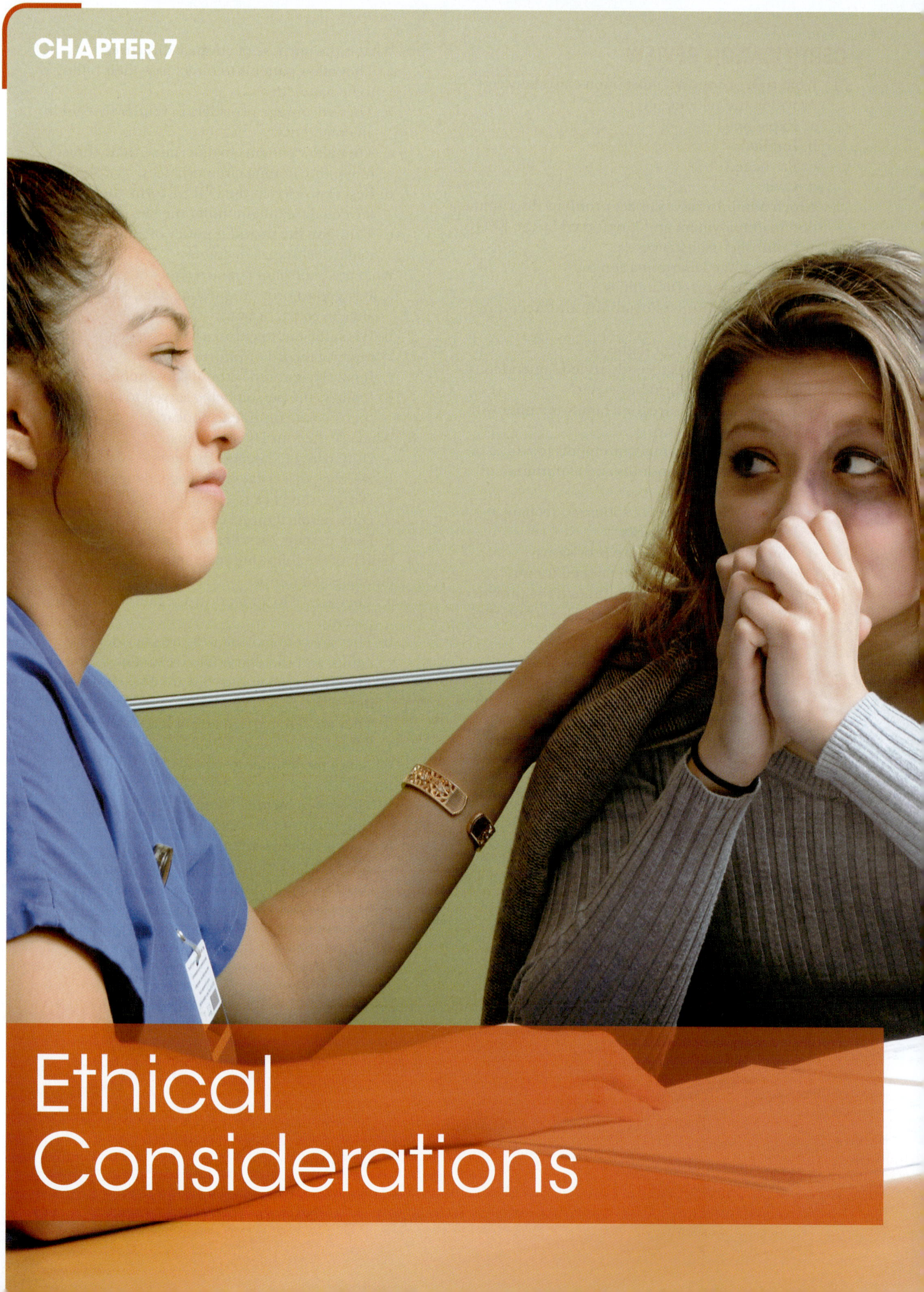

LEARNING OUTCOMES

1. Define and spell the key terms as presented in the glossary.
2. Summarize reasons for codes of ethics.
3. Paraphrase the eight characteristics of principle-centered leadership.
4. Describe the five Ps of ethical power.
5. Implement the ethics check questions.
6. Relate the five principles of the AAMA code to patient care in the ambulatory care setting.
7. Discuss the role of ethical codes in ambulatory care.
8. Critique the ethical guidelines for health care providers, giving at least four examples.
9. Summarize professional rights and responsibilities for health care personnel.
10. Categorize the different types of abuse for those individuals at risk.
11. Restate the dilemmas encountered by the following bioethical issues: (a) allocation of scarce/limited medical resources, (b) health care as a right or a privilege, (c) HIV and AIDS, (d) reproductive issues, (e) abortion and fetal tissue research, (g) genetic engineering/manipulation, and (h) dying and death.

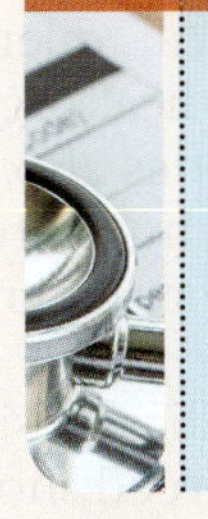

KEY TERMS

bioethics	genetic engineering	surrogates
cryopreservation	intimate partner violence (IPV)	tubal ligation
ethics	in vitro fertilization (IVF)	vasectomy
euthanasia	macroallocation	
female genital mutilation (FGM)	microallocation	

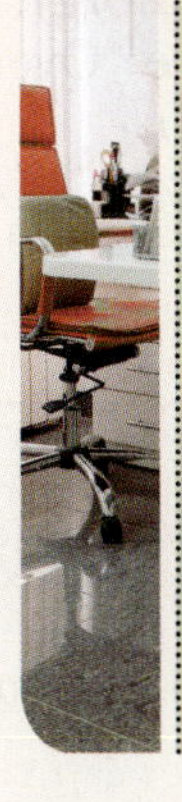

SCENARIO

Harley Navarro is a new medical assistant in a busy internist's clinic. He finished school a few months ago and is awaiting the date to take his exam to become a certified medical assistant. He is nervous and scared. All the other medical assistants are female and have many years of experience. Harley wants so much to be accepted and recognized for his skills. Today, however, he twice had a rough time taking a blood pressure reading. In fact, the provider was ready for one of Harley's patients before he was finished with the reading, and the provider stepped in to take the reading. Harley was embarrassed. His current patient is obese. His first attempt at getting a blood pressure reading failed. He gets a larger cuff for his second reading. His patient complains, however, that her arm is hurting about halfway through the reading. Harley hurries the process and takes a guess at the diastolic pressure figure, but he knows it is close.

Chapter Portal

It is impossible in today's world to function as a medical assistant without an awareness of the impact of ethics and bioethics on health care. Just as an understanding of the law and complying with the law are vital for the medical assistant, it is equally important to understand ethics and bioethics.

From Chapter 6, you have come to realize that there are many circumstances and situations that occur in health care that are guided and directed by state and federal laws. You, personally, are expected to be above reproach in all your actions in this regard. You must also work with your employer and other members of the health care team to ensure that each member of the staff functions within the law—protecting both patients and providers.

continues

Chapter Portal, *continued*

Ethics plays a huge role in such an endeavor. To function ethically demands that you never function outside the law. Ethics, however, demands something more—ethics calls for honesty, trustworthiness, integrity, confidentiality, and fairness. To function ethically, you must know yourself well and understand weaknesses and any vulnerability that might prevent you from acting ethically.

The scenario described earlier is just one situation in which medical assistants may need to reflect on their actions and be sure that they are acting ethically and within the range of their skills. Medical assistants also need to recognize the warning signs that they, or some other staff member, may be about to breach a code of ethics. Often, this kind of breach occurs when one has, or seeks to have, too much power; when one attempts to take on too much authority; or when one has too little knowledge and experience and is afraid to ask for help. When a breach seems about to occur, the individuals involved should be encouraged to step back and review their actions and the likely consequences of those actions.

ETHICS

Traditionally, **ethics** is defined in terms of what is considered right or wrong. Sometimes ethics is referred to as *morals*. However, morals refer to personal choices of conduct, whereas ethics is more of a philosophy related to making judgments about right and wrong. Professional organizations often identify their ethics in codes, which provide a set of principles and guidelines.

The American Medical Association (AMA) has established such a code of ethics called the Principles of Medical Ethics. This code can be reviewed by accessing the AMA Web site (http://www.ama-assn.org). Also published every 2 years by the AMA is The Code of Medical Ethics Current Opinions with Annotations; this document provides up-to-date information on a number of ethical dilemmas. A number of other professional medical organizations have well-established ethical codes also. They include such professions as osteopaths, chiropractors, nurses, professional coders, and emergency medical technicians.

The American Association of Medical Assistants (AAMA) has a code of ethics and a creed shown in Figure 7-1. In addition, the AAMA Mission Statement, AAMA Medical Assistant Code of Ethics, and AAMA Medical Assistant Creed appear on the AAMA Web site (http://www.aama-ntl.org). Clicking on "About" and then selecting the "Overview" link will detail these statements for you.

AAMA CODE OF ETHICS

The Medical Assisting Code of Ethics of the AAMA sets forth principles of ethical and moral conduct as they relate to the medical profession and the particular practice of medical assisting.

Members of AAMA dedicated to the conscientious pursuit of their profession, and thus desiring to merit the high regard of the entire medical profession and the respect of the general public which they serve, do pledge themselves to strive always to:

A. Render service with full respect for the dignity of humanity.
B. Respect confidential information obtained through employment unless legally authorized or required by responsible performance of duty to divulge such information.
C. Uphold the honor and high principles of the profession and accept its disciplines.
D. Seek to continually improve the knowledge and skills of medical assistants for the benefit of patients and professional colleagues.
E. Participate in additional service activities aimed toward improving the health and well-being of the community.

(A)

CREED

The Medical Assisting Creed of the AAMA sets forth medical assisting statements of belief:
I believe in the principles and purposes of the profession of medical assisting.
I endeavor to be more effective.
I aspire to render greater service.
I protect the confidence entrusted to me.
I am dedicated to the care and well-being of all people.
I am loyal to my employer.
I am true to the ethics of my profession.
I am strengthened by compassion, courage and faith.

(B)

FIGURE 7-1 (A) American Association of Medical Assistants (AAMA) Code of Ethics. (B) AAMA Creed.

The American Hospital Association replaced its original Hospital Patient Bill of Rights with a brochure that informs patients about their rights and responsibilities while hospitalized. The brochure, "The Patient Care Partnership," is available in several languages and continues to be a standard for many hospitals. Similar statements have been adapted to the ambulatory health care setting as well. See Figure 7-2 for a simple generic sample. These codes give additional guidance for making ethical decisions, taking ethical action, and further identifying patient rights and responsibilities.

There are more than 50 different codes of ethics for professional organizations, and most are related to medicine and are designed to offer guidance and direction to health care professionals.

Seven ethical codes that pertain to the entire world are pertinent for review. They include such famous codes as the Declaration of Geneva, Declaration of Helsinki, and the International Code of Medical Ethics. A listing of these codes is found by searching the Internet for "World Medical Ethics Codes." Another fascinating Web site identifies the characteristics of traditional Chinese medical ethics when you use the Internet to search for "Chinese Medical Ethics." Chinese medical ethics emphasizes self-cultivation and personal ethics of practitioners rather than a strict organizational code of ethics.

Codes of ethics bring standards of moral and ethical behavior together in one place. They assist organizations and individuals in putting words to their expected behaviors and actions. There is a benefit to such codes when they become reminders to everyone regarding appropriate conduct. Codes also can have a limiting effect, however. For instance, if an organization does not have a code of ethics, that organization is not necessarily viewed as unethical. Further, having a code of ethics does not necessarily create an ethical organization, especially if the code is mostly ignored.

Integrity

Medical assistants and medical professionals are asked to balance personal and professional areas of their lives in the middle of constant pressure and crises. At the same time, the quality of one's personal life is going to be shown in the quality of his or her service to others in his or her professional life. To be effective in the medical profession, individuals need to demonstrate maturity in both personal and professional selves to create the utmost of ethical conduct and professionalism. To do so, it is helpful to discuss principle-centered leadership and the meaning of ethical power.

PATIENT BILL OF RIGHTS AND RESPONSIBILITIES FOR AMBULATORY CARE*

As a patient, you have the right to:

Be treated with courtesy and respect, with appreciation of your dignity and without discrimination at all times.

Participate in your healthcare by receiving a prompt and reasonable response to questions and requests, receiving information concerning diagnosis, course of treatment, alternatives, risks, and prognosis.

Access your medical record and receive a copy upon request. Seek a second opinion and to know who is providing your medical services.

Confidentiality at all times and your privacy protected.

An estimate of charges for medical care.

A reasonably clear and understandable itemized bill and to have the charges explained.

Refuse any treatment.

Have your advance directive on file.

Be informed of any medical treatment for purposes of experimental research and to give consent or refuse to participate.

As a patient, your responsibilities include the following:

You are expected to provide complete and accurate personal, health, and medical history information as required.

You are expected to ask questions when you do not understand information or instructions. You are responsible for outcomes if you do not follow your care plan.

You are expected to provide accurate information regarding health insurance coverage and pay any bills in a timely fashion.

You are expected to provide a copy of an advance directive if you have one.

You have the responsibility of keeping all scheduled appointments.

You are expected to treat all health care providers with courtesy and respect.

*Compilation of several clinics across the United States; prepared by Carol D. Tamparo. CMA (AAMA), PhD.

FIGURE 7-2 Patient bill of rights and Responsibilities for Ambulatory Care.

Principle-Centered Leadership

Stephen R. Covey, a very well-known author and leadership expert, has produced an audiobook that includes collections of three of his best-selling texts. It includes *The 7 Habits of Managers*, *Principle-Centered Leadership*, and *The 4 Imperatives of Great Leaders*. Covey's original work identified eight characteristics of principle-centered leaders because he understood that leaders who know themselves and understand their principles more easily abide by a code of ethics. Consider the following questions adapted from Covey's writings as guides to how you might perform ethically in a medical setting:

- *Are you continually learning?* Do you seek training, take classes, listen to others, and learn from your peers? Are you curious? Do you realize that developing new knowledge and skills is a lifelong endeavor?
- *Are you service oriented?* Do you see your life as a mission rather than a career? Are you generally a nurturing individual who seeks service in the medical field? Can you see yourself working alongside a co-worker and pulling together with that person toward a goal? Can you put yourself in the place of others?
- *Do you radiate positive energy?* Are you cheerful, pleasant, optimistic, and positive? Is your spirit hopeful? If it is, you carry a positive energy field that allows you to neutralize or sidestep a negative energy source. Do you see yourself as a peacemaker or one who can create harmony to undo negative energy?
- *Do you believe in other people?* Can you keep from labeling, stereotyping, or prejudging other people? Can you believe in the unseen potential of others? Can you keep from overreacting to negative behaviors and criticism? Can you put aside any grudges?

The final characteristics of principle-centered leaders Covey identifies are more personal. They can help you understand yourself and how you might make ethical decisions in the medical field:

- *Do you lead a balanced life?* Do you keep up with current affairs and events? Do you know what is happening in the medical field and how that affects you? Do you have at least one confidant with whom you can be transparent? Are you physically active within your limits of age and health? Do you enjoy yourself? Do you have a good sense of humor? Are you open to communication?
- *Do you see life as an adventure?* Are you able to rediscover persons each time you meet them? Are you interested in others? Do you listen well? Are you flexible and unflappable? Does your security come from within rather than from without?
- *Are you synergistic?* Synergy is what happens when the whole of something is greater than the sum of its parts. Do you know your weaknesses? Can you complement your weaknesses with the strengths of others on the team? Can you work hard to improve most situations? Are you trusting? Can you separate the person from the problem?
- *Do you exercise for self-renewal?* In this element, Mr. Covey identifies four dimensions of the human personality that need exercise: physical, mental, emotional, and spiritual dimensions. How do you keep your body in shape? How do you keep your mind alert? Do patience, unconditional love, and accepting responsibility for your own actions keep you emotionally healthy? Do you have a way to meditate, pray, or "draw away" for a period to "fill up your spirit"?

These questions and your responses to them can give you insight into your ability to function ethically and to be successful in the world of medicine.

Covey has another book entitled *The 8th Habit: From Effectiveness to Greatness* (now available in a summary version) that discusses how individuals can be more excited about their lives and their work when they reach beyond effectiveness toward fulfillment, contribution, and greatness. Individuals who feel fulfilled and excited about their work are more apt to perform ethically than those who do not.

Five Ps of Ethical Power

Another approach to how you might act in an ethical manner comes from Kenneth Blanchard and Norman Vincent Peale, who wrote a simple but powerful little book called *The Power of Ethical Management.* In it they discuss the "five Ps of ethical power." The five Ps are as follows:

1. *Purpose.* Understand your objective or your purpose. Your purpose may change from time to time, but it is something that requires you to behave in a way that makes you feel good about yourself.
2. *Pride.* Have pride in what you do. Feel good about yourself and your accomplishments. Nurture your self-esteem while remaining humble. Be proud to be a medical assistant.
3. *Patience.* It takes time to create an atmosphere in which your objective can be obtained. Strive to believe that no matter what happens,

everything is going to work out. Expect results from yourself and your work, but refrain from demanding it "now."

4. *Persistence.* To act in an ethical manner means to strive to act in that manner all the time, not just when you want to or it seems easy to do. Winston Churchill said, "Never, never, never, never give up!" That is what persistence is. If you make a mistake, admit it, correct it, learn from the mistake, and move on, but never give up. An individual who is truly aware of his or her personal ethical power is able to admit an error, does not compromise any procedure or any technique, and does not ever put the patient at risk, even if it means facing reprimand from a supervisor.
5. *Perspective.* Keep your life and your purpose in perspective. Find time each day to maintain balance in your life (perhaps looking again at the eight questions for principle-centered individuals). Plan some quiet time, some fun time, but certainly some reflective time. The constant pressure and the crises will become overwhelming without keeping perspective.

Ethics Check Questions

Finally, when there is uncertainty about a dilemma or there is little or no experience to draw from, those striving to act in an ethical manner can perform a simple test each time there is a question about ethics. This, too, comes from Blanchard and Peale. The questions to ask are:

1. *Is it legal?* Is it against the law or any company policy?
2. *Is it balanced?* Is this the best possible approach for all concerned? Does it promote a win–win situation?
3. *How will it make me feel about myself?* Will I feel good if my decision is published in a newspaper? Will my family and co-workers be proud of my decision?

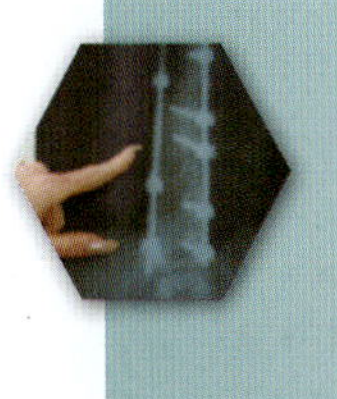

Critical Thinking

With a peer, identify one or more examples in your life when you truly did not give up on attaining your goals. Describe what you learned from that experience. How might "never giving up" help in your pursuit of a career?

These questions provide a simple yet profound guide that is easy to recall and to apply to almost any situation. They are used throughout the business world by managers and employees seeking to work and practice legally and ethically.

Ethics are not easy. Performing ethically is hard work. Being ethical means determining who you are and how you will act. Laws are more clearly defined than ethics, but acting in an unethical manner can cause as much pain and difficulty as can acting illegally. The ideas of Covey, Blanchard, and Peale give guidance, thoughts to ponder, and perhaps goals to reach. Keep them in mind both as you review the next section and as you enter into your career as a medical assistant.

KEYS TO THE AAMA CODE OF ETHICS

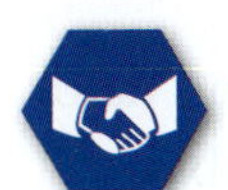

Professional

Medical assistants might consider the more salient points in the AAMA Code of Ethics (refer to Figure 7-1) and ask themselves the following questions:

A. *Render service with full respect for the dignity of humanity.*
   - Will I respect every patient even if I do not approve of his or her morals or choices in health care?
   - Will I honor each patient's request for information and explain unfamiliar procedures?
   - Will I give my full attention to acknowledging the needs of every patient?
   - Will I be able to accept people who are indigent, have physical and mental challenges, are infirm, have physical disfigurements, and who I simply do not like as equal and valid human beings with an equal right to service?

B. *Respect confidential information obtained through employment unless legally authorized or required by responsible performance of duty to divulge such information.*
   - Will I refrain from needless comments to a colleague regarding a patient's problem?
   - Will I refrain from discussing my day's encounters with patients with my family and friends?

- Will I always protect patients' medical information and records and everything included from unnecessary observation?
- Will I keep patients' names and the circumstances that bring them to my place of employment confidential?

C. *Uphold the honor and high principles of the profession and accept its disciplines.*

- Am I proud to serve as a medical assistant?
- Will I always perform within the scope of my profession, never exceeding the responsibility entrusted to me?
- Will I encourage others to enter the profession and always speak honorably of medical assistants?

D. *Seek to continually improve the knowledge and skills of medical assistants for the benefit of patients and professional colleagues.*

- Will I be willing to learn new skills, to update my skills, and seek improved methods for assisting the provider in the care of patients?
- Will I keep my credentials current and valid?
- Can I remember that I am a member of a group of broad-based health care professionals, and that my goal is to complement rather than to compete with that team?

E. *Participate in additional service activities aimed toward improving the health and well-being of the community.*

- Will I be able to serve in the community where I reside and work to further quality health care?
- Will I promote preventive medicine?
- Will I practice good health care management for myself and be a model for others to follow?

No matter how prepared, experienced, or principled one is in a chosen profession, there will still be times of great stress and concern about decisions made.

ETHICAL GUIDELINES FOR HEALTH CARE PROVIDERS

As stated earlier, it is fairly common for each professional group of medical practitioners to have its own code of ethics. The AMA's Principles of Medical Ethics and the "Current Opinions with Annotations of the Council on Ethical and Judicial Affairs" have been leaders in this field, but by no means are they the only codes. While the AMA Principles of Medical Ethics are identified in only nine principles, those principles are further identified in seven pages of specific policy issues. (Go to www.ama-assn.org and search "Medical Ethics.") The American Osteopathic Association has a Code of Ethics with 19 different sections. The American Chiropractic Association's Code of Ethics is identified in 14 sections. Other practitioners may consider their mission and policies to be their code of ethics. Some have no specific written code of ethics but rather call on their practitioners to refer to their culture as one based on ethics, mutual respect, and moral evaluation when ethical decisions are made. There are many similarities in these statements on ethics that are important for patients and medical employees. Only a few prominent statements are provided here.

Confidentiality

Providers must not reveal confidential information about patients without their consent unless the providers are otherwise required to do so by law. Confidentiality must be protected so that patients will feel comfortable and safe in revealing information about themselves that may be important to their health care. Extra caution must be taken to protect the confidentiality of any patient's data on a computer database. As few people as possible should have access to the computer data, and only authorized individuals should be permitted to add or alter data. Adequate security precautions must be used to protect information stored electronically. HIPAA has specific guidelines for computer privacy (see Chapters 10 and 13).

The following list contains examples of the kinds of reports that allow or require health professionals to report a confidence:

- A patient threatens another person and there is reason to believe that the threat may be carried out.
- Certain injuries and illnesses *must* be reported. These include injuries such as knife and gunshot wounds, wounds that may be from suspected abuse, communicable diseases, and sexually transmitted diseases.

- Information that may have been subpoenaed for testimony in a court of law.

When in doubt, it is always recommended that a provider have the patient's permission to reveal any confidential information.

Medical Records

Medical records and the information in them are the property of the provider and the patient. No information should be revealed without the patient's consent unless required by law. The record is confidential. Providers should not refuse to provide a copy of the record to another provider treating the patient so long as proper authorization has been received from the patient. Also, providers should supply a copy of the record or summary of its contents if a patient requests it. A record cannot be withheld because of an unpaid bill.

On a provider's retirement or death, or when a practice is sold, patients should be notified and given ample time to have their records transferred to another provider of their choice.

Professional Fees and Charges

Illegal or excessive fees should not be charged. Fees should be based on those customary to the locale and should reflect the difficulty of services and the quality of performance rendered. Fee splitting (a provider splits the fee with another provider for services rendered with or without the patient's knowledge) in any form is unethical. Providers may charge for missed appointments (if patients have first been notified of the practice) and may charge for multiple or complex insurance forms. Providers and their employees must be diligent to ensure that only the services actually rendered are charged or indicated on the insurance claim. Only what is documented in the patient's chart is to be billed.

There are a number of providers throughout the country who refuse any insurance payments and operate strictly on a cash-only basis. There are others who charge a yearly fee to care for a family, providing all services necessary at that flat fee. Providers, upset by the rules and regulations of insurance, find this method of payment creates a simpler form of medical practice. Providers and patients alike continue to discuss the ethics of such a move. Although providers may choose whom they wish to serve, the cash-only basis is difficult for low-income families and the poor, thereby creating an ethical dilemma.

Professional Rights and Responsibilities

As stated earlier, providers may choose whom to serve, but they may not refuse a patient on the basis of race, color, religion, national origin, or any other illegal discrimination. It is unethical for providers to deny treatment to HIV-infected individuals on that basis alone if they are qualified to treat the patient's condition. However, there are numerous instances of health care being denied to lesbian, gay, bisexual, and transgender (LGBT) individuals and those with AIDS throughout the country. Recently, lesbian mothers living in Michigan were denied care for their infant daughter because of their status. (Go to http://nwlc.org and search "Health Care Refusals" for a serious discussion of this issue.) Once a provider takes a case, the patient cannot be neglected or refused treatment unless official notice is given from the provider to withdraw from the case.

Patients have the right to know their diagnoses and the nature and purpose of their treatment and to have enough information to be able to make an informed choice about their treatment protocol. Providers should inform families of a patient's death and not delegate that responsibility to others.

Providers are expected to expose incompetent, corrupt, dishonest, and unethical conduct by other providers to the disciplinary board. It is unethical for any provider to treat patients while under the influence of alcohol, controlled substances, or any other chemical that impairs the provider's ability.

Providers who know they are HIV positive must refrain from any activity that would risk the transmission of the virus to others.

Any activity that might be regarded as a "conflict of interest" (for example, a provider holding stock in a pharmaceutical company and prescribing medications only from that company) is to be avoided. Financial interests are not to influence providers in prescribing medications, devices, or appliances.

Disaster Response and Emergency Preparedness

Medical professionals are essential at the time of any disaster, such as epidemics, floods, fires, weather-related disasters, and terrorist attacks. Care for the sick and injured is of primary concern when disaster strikes. Providers are encouraged to give their medical expertise not only to prepare for any type of disaster but to provide assistance when one occurs. Providers should consider seeking training in emergency preparedness and disaster response and lend their knowledge where it is most beneficial and effective in making certain that medical care is available during such events (see Chapter 8).

Treatment for a Culturally Diverse Clientele

Diversity

All providers are reminded to strive to provide the same quality of care to all their patients regardless of race or ethnicity. Providers must remember to eliminate biased behavior toward any group of patients deemed different from themselves. All patients have the right to participatory decision making with their providers based on mutual trust and understanding. Communication factors are to be considered and interpreters provided as necessary so that patients understand the medical information as well as any communication exchanged.

Diversity is to be encouraged in the medical profession and considered when hiring assistants. Ethnically diverse neighborhoods and clientele deserve an ethnically diverse group of medical professionals for their care. If it is not possible to employ an ethnically diverse group of medical professionals, then medical professionals who are keenly aware of and knowledgeable of the ethnic group served is of primary importance.

Care of the Poor

From the earliest history of medical treatment, care for the poor has been a concern and a goal for medical practitioners. Today that obligation is still mentioned in most ethical codes and discussions. All medical providers have a responsibility to ensure that the needs of the poor in their communities are met. Caring for the poor should be a regular part of every provider's practice and can be accomplished in a number of ways. Providers can be encouraged to take a certain number of patients on a reduced-cost basis or provide free services. Providers can volunteer their time and efforts to treat patients in reduced-cost, freestanding clinics that treat the poor or provide services to those in homeless shelters for battered and abused individuals. Providers can volunteer their time to lobbying and being advocates for those without medical coverage.

Abuse

Legal

Abuse, first discussed in Chapter 6, usually is described as neglect, physical injury, emotional/psychological/mental injury, or sexual abuse. In child abuse, there also may be molestation, sexual exploitation, and incest. Elder abuse can come in the form of any other abuse, but financial abuse is included. Stalking and rape are also considered to be forms of abuse.

All 50 states have legislation defining child abuse and mandate who is responsible for reporting such abuse. The majority of states have enacted legislation regarding the abuse of elder adults 60 years of age or older. Intimate partner (or domestic) violence is a criminal offense in some states, but whether a state requires that **intimate partner violence (IPV)** be reported depends in part upon whether a weapon is used.

Stalking is the repeated act of spying upon, following, or making contact with an individual or appearing at an individual's residence or place of employment after being asked not to. It is a crime in some states. *Rape*, also a crime of violence, is forced sexual intercourse or penetration of a body orifice with the penis or some other object. Gang rape involves several individuals. Rape is a reportable criminal act.

Medical assistants must know if their state specifically names them as reporters for abuse. A discussion should be held with medical providers and employers regarding who, when, and how the abuse will be reported and documented. It is unethical for a medical assistant to fail to report abuse simply because an employer prefers "not to get too involved." For a clearer understanding of some of the factors that constitute abuse, review Table 7-1.

It is the responsibility of medical professionals and their employees to report all cases of suspected child abuse, to protect and care for the abused, and to treat the abuser (if known) as a victim also. This is not an easy task. Abuse is not easy to witness. Although there are specific laws regarding suspected child abuse, and in most states medical assistants are mandated to report abuse, the laws are vague or nonexistent for older adults or in cases of IPV. However, whatever form the abuse takes, it is best to treat all forms of abuse in the same manner by providing a safe environment for those abused and seeking treatment for the abused and the abuser.

TABLE 7-1

DESCRIPTIONS OF ABUSE

TYPE OF ABUSE	CHILD ABUSE	ELDER ABUSE	INTIMATE PARTNER VIOLENCE
Neglect	Failure to provide basic food, shelter, care; endangering health of child	Lack of attention that causes harm; withholding basic needs; abandonment; lack of help with hygiene or bathing	Not treating a partner with respect; not recognizing the human worth of an individual
Physical abuse	Causing burns, unusual or severe bruising, lacerations, fractures, injury to internal organs; usually obvious	Assault, beating, whipping, hitting, punching, pushing, pinching, force-feeding, shaking, rough handling during caregiving, causing bodily harm or severe mental stress	Intent to harm; hitting, pushing, grabbing, biting, punching, slapping, restraining, burning; use of a weapon or one's own strength to harm
Emotional/ psychological abuse	Causing harm to child's emotional and intellectual growth; not always obvious	Actions that dehumanize; social isolation, name calling, humiliating, insulting; threats to punish; yelling, screaming	Humiliating; controlling; isolating partner from friends/ family; denying personal support and encouragement
Sexual abuse	Using a child to engage in any sexual activity; abuse not always obvious	Sexual contact without permission; fondling, touching, kissing, rape, coerced nudity; spying while in bathroom	Sexual contact without permission; abusive sexual contact; sex with one who is unable to say "no"
Sexual exploitation	Pornography, prostitution; use of child's image in media; incest or sexual activity between family members	Showing an elderly person pornographic material; forcing the person to watch sex acts; forcing the elder to undress in presence of others	Forcing a partner to engage in sexual acts with others against that partner's will
Financial abuse	Refusal to provide the basics of adequate health care or clothing	Exploitation of an elder's resources; forging signature on documents; withholding or cashing funds received	Withholding funds or basic resources; monitoring to the penny funds spent for groceries or expenses of daily living

BIOETHICS

Bioethics brings the entire focus of ethics into the field of health care and into those ethical issues dealing with all aspects of life and death. Never before in the history of medical care has bioethics been such a topic of concern. In the past, most bioethical decisions were made by physicians and esteemed members of the medical or legal profession. However, advancing technology giving patients and consumers numerous choices regarding their health now has everyone taking a more active role in bioethics.

Medical assistants will encounter ethical and bioethical issues across a total life span. A few issues are identified for contemplation and discussion.

Infants

- Imperiled newborns (seriously disabled, deformed, often premature with low birth weight) who survive with modern technology incur soaring costs of expensive intervention not always covered by insurance.

Children

- When not well fed, housed, educated and clothed, children have great need for preventive, curative, and rehabilitative health care; proper inoculations against communicable diseases; and attention to any evidence of eating disorders.
- Obesity is a health concern that is often the result of poor food choices.
- Many children live in dysfunctional families where parents are absent, abuse substances, have mental health issues, or have very little time to spend with their children.

Adolescents

- The adolescent's need for independence, changing values, and desire for peer acceptance may lead to risky sexual behavior and drug and alcohol experimentation.
- Mental health issues often interfere with normal social development, yet mental health assessment and treatment are difficult to find.
- Adolescents as young as 14 to 18 years may seek treatment for substance abuse, birth control, and even abortion without parental consent.

Adults

- It can be difficult to balance full-time employment, parenting, housekeeping, and partnering and still take care of oneself.
- War, terrorism, and an overburdened military place stress on families. Many return from service with lifelong and debilitating injuries.

Senior Adults

- Older adults have the right to dignity and privacy that is often denied when they lose their independence.
- It is often difficult for new patients to find providers who take Medicare and Medicaid, leaving them without appropriate medical attention.
- Some older adults must still choose between food on their table and the purchase of prescribed medications.
- Dementia is a growing problem that is financially exhausting and heartbreaking.
- Even with advance directives, a dying patient's wishes may be ignored.

Issues of bioethics common to the medical community are the allocation of scarce or limited medical resources; whether health care is a right or privilege; reproductive issues such as contraception, assisted reproduction, abortion, and fetal tissue research; genetic engineering or manipulation; and the many choices surrounding life, dying, and death.

Guidelines for bioethical issues are even harder to define than are guidelines for ethics, because each of the bioethical issues calls for decisions that directly affect a person's life. In some instances, the bioethical issue requires a choice about who lives and requires defining quality of life. Such dilemmas are difficult, if not impossible, to approach from a neutral point of view, even though medical professionals should strive not to impose their own moral values on patients or co-workers.

ALLOCATION OF SCARCE OR LIMITED MEDICAL RESOURCES

One issue faced daily by health care workers is the allocation of limited medical resources, or what ultimately becomes rationing of health care. Even with the 2010 Affordable Care Act (ACA), medical resources are still not available to everyone. When the administrative medical assistant determines who receives the only available appointment in a day, when patients are turned away because they have no insurance or financial resources to pay for services, when Medicare and Medicaid patients are denied services because of low return from state and federal insurance programs, medical resources are being rationed and denied.

U.S. Census data from 2014 shows that the number of uninsured Americans declined by 8.8 million the first year the ACA took effect. That is down 13.3 percent from 2013. The Census Bureau reports, however, that those states choosing not to expand Medicaid will leave millions of poor Americans without access to affordable health care.

The ACA ended some issues of rationing. The act helps more children get health coverage, ends lifetime and most annual limits on care, allows young adults under age 26 to stay on their parent's health insurance, and gives some patients access to a number of recommended preventive services such as vaccinations, influenza and pneumonia shots, and blood pressure and diabetes screenings without co-payment or deductible costs. Other reforms are in process. Hispanic and non-Hispanic black children are still more likely to not have access to health care than are non-Hispanic white children. Of note, the average waiting time by new patients for a medical appointment is 18.5 days. Older patients, many of whom have both Medicare and supplemental health insurance, have difficulty finding providers who take new Medicare patients. Providers, who can choose whom to serve, increasingly are not taking any new patients because the Medicare return dollars are most often less than the costs incurred. This dilemma can be particularly problematic when older patients move from their homes and communities to be closer to their children.

Weightier decisions might include who gets the surgery, kidney transplant, or bone marrow transplant. These allocation and rationing decisions are being made and will continue to require dedication on the part of the health care team. Rationing of health care will continue to be an issue as politicians, health care providers, and consumers struggle to balance providing access to care with curtailing costs.

Decisions made by Congress, health systems agencies, and insurance companies are termed **macroallocation** of scarce medical resources. Decisions made individually by providers and members of the health care team at the local level are termed **microallocation** of scarce resources. No matter what the level, medical assistants will be involved.

Health Care: A Right or a Privilege?

Very close to the issue of allocation of limited medical resources is the question of whether basic health care is a right or a privilege. There are many countries in the world where health care is a privilege provided only to a few either because of the availability of health care or because of one's financial resources. However, even within the United States, where the best of health care is available, there are health care professionals whose personal ideologies often lead to discrimination and denial of basic health care.

For example, consider the following circumstances. How would you choose?

- *For the available kidney.* There is a perfect match for a young mother of two or a 45-year-old gentleman (a recovering addict) with numerous body piercings.
- *For the next available pediatric appointment.* A 16-year-old who needs an athletic physical or a troubled and combative 13-year-old whose only insurance is Medicaid.
- *For artificial insemination.* A single woman desiring a child of her own or a couple who have been trying to get pregnant for 3 years.
- *Referral to a mental health specialist.* A prominent businessman suffering from depression with symptoms of bipolar disorder or a mom receiving state aid and struggling with addiction.

It is often difficult to remain neutral and wait to make decisions until all the facts are known. One continuing area of discrimination surrounds the health care issue of AIDS and HIV.

HIV and AIDS

The general public's fear and wariness of AIDS (acquired immunodeficiency syndrome) continues to cause bioethical issues. Patients who suspect they have HIV (human immunodeficiency virus) or AIDS should be tested for the virus. In fact, the CDC recommends that voluntary screening for HIV/AIDS become a routine part of medical care for all patients ages 13 to 64 years. Confidentiality must be safely guarded, however, because individuals with HIV/AIDS have been denied medical insurance, faced loss of employment and housing, and even suffered the loss of family members and friends. It is unethical to deny treatment to individuals because they test positive for HIV.

Although individuals with HIV/AIDS are to be protected, so must the public. Therefore, if providers suspect that an HIV-seropositive patient is infecting an unsuspecting individual, every attempt is to be made to protect the individual at risk. Health professionals will first encourage the infected person to cease any activity that endangers the other person. If the patient refuses to notify the person at risk, authorities can be contacted. Many states and cities have partner notification programs that will anonymously notify any person at risk, keeping the source confidential. The program informs him or her that it has been brought to their attention that he or she is a "person at risk" and provides free testing.

Reproductive Issues

Reproductive bioethical issues generally affect women more than men. A few are identified here. Most medical assistants will be faced with these issues at some time in their career, even if they are not employed in specialty clinics.

Female Genital Mutilation. The World Health Organization (WHO) reports that there are over 170,000 young girls and women in the United States who have been subjected to **female genital mutilation (FGM)**. FGM includes partial or complete removal of the clitoris (female circumcision); partial or total removal of the labia minora or labia majora; infibulation (narrowing the vaginal opening by creating a covering seal); and the pricking, piercing, or cauterizing of the genitals. These procedures are performed, in part, to enhance a man's sexual pleasure, but they destroy a woman's capacity for sexual pleasure and can cause serious infections. The practice can also cause recurring urinary tract infections, difficulties with menstruation, and pregnancy complications. FGM is illegal in this country, but can be seen in immigrants from countries such as some African, Asian, and Middle Eastern nations where it is regularly practiced.

Contraception. Birth control of any kind, other than *fertility awareness methods (FAM)* that require abstinence from sexual intercourse during ovulation, is still a taboo in some cultures and religions and becomes a bioethical dilemma. Many are opposed to any contraception that destroys a fertilized egg. Therefore, a thorough understanding of how a particular contraception works is essential for some patients.

The controversy gained attention when the RU-486 or mifepristone hormone drug became available for use in the United States in order to end an early pregnancy. In general, it can be used up to 63 days—9 weeks—after the first day of a woman's last period. Today, a primary issue is the availability of birth control to some women. In 2014, the U.S. Supreme Court ruled that employers (especially those that have a religious objection) can deny birth control as part of health insurance coverage available to their employees.

Sterilization. When permanent contraception is sought, sterilization has become the choice. It is not only used by those who simply wish to prevent pregnancy, but it may be practiced by those who prefer not to pass on a genetic anomaly. A **tubal ligation** for women and a **vasectomy** for men are considered permanent, even though there have been reversals. Some religious groups oppose permanent sterilization.

Assisted Reproduction. Assistance with reproduction is very common today. Artificial insemination, in vitro fertilization, and surrogacy are most commonly practiced.

For many individuals, *artificial insemination* is the only means by which they are able to conceive a child. Providers are called on to perform artificial insemination for couples and for women who want a child. If artificial insemination is performed, it is recommended that the signed consent of each party involved be obtained. It is also recommended that providers practicing artificial insemination by donor have several donors available for semen collection and that meticulous screening be performed before the insemination.

In vitro fertilization (IVF) is a process that has been shown to be very successful in the past decade. In IVF, the ovum is fertilized in a culture dish, allowed to grow, and then implanted into the uterus. This procedure can be used for women with blocked fallopian tubes or oviducts. Ethically, this procedure faces little controversy when a husband's sperm is used to fertilize his wife's ovum, which is then implanted into her uterus. Other procedures raise ethical concerns for some and are not addressed in law.

A woman can have a donor's egg fertilized by her husband's sperm for implantation. A woman can receive donor embryos (embryo adoption) from successfully completed IVF from two unrelated individuals. Couples who have successfully had a baby through IVF are sometimes willing to donate their additional embryos. A woman can carry an embryo created from a donor egg and donor sperm that will have no genetic relationship to her.

It is possible to screen for genetic flaws among embryos created by IVF; however, the latest medical research indicates that such analysis sometimes causes abnormalities.

Surrogacy is another method of assisted reproduction. Men have been used as **surrogates**, or substitutes, for decades with the practice of artificial insemination. Society still seems to have a more difficult time accepting surrogate mothers who are artificially inseminated by a donor and carry the fetus to term for another parent. Men sometimes seek surrogates who are able to provide them a child who represents half their genetic makeup. Women may choose a surrogate if they are unable to carry a pregnancy to term for medical or personal reasons. How should the rights of each individual in the arrangement and exchange be protected? For many of these issues, there is little protection or guidance under the law; therefore, health professionals are often required to make decisions on the basis of their personal belief systems.

Ethical questions are sometimes raised regarding assisted reproduction. Should artificial insemination and in vitro fertilization be performed for individuals who do not fit the "traditional" family model? Who will be a fit mother or father for a particular infant? Some religious faiths consider artificial insemination by donor to be the same as adultery. Who or what agency carefully protects the selection and screening process of donors and surrogates? How are donors selected? Is there a responsibility to make certain that individuals with the same father through artificial insemination by donor do not marry? Some fertility specialists recommend that a donor be chosen from a city far from where the potential mother lives and that formal adoption occur immediately when the infant is born. Some oppose in vitro fertilization because fertilized ova are destroyed if found to be genetically inappropriate. Others have great difficulty when embryos that are not implanted are often frozen for later use, but sometimes are abandoned and eventually destroyed.

Most assisted reproduction techniques were viewed as experimental and quite controversial just 25 years ago. Today, however, the procedures are widely practiced and available. Assisted reproduction is very costly and can create legal tangles for all involved if careful steps are not taken.

Abortion and Fetal Tissue Research

The issues associated with abortion and fetal tissue research will be with us for quite some time. Although the law as set forth in *Roe v. Wade* is specific on abortion guidelines, there is a continual challenge in the courts of its validity. A number of states have been successful in pressing for more restrictions regarding whether and how abortions might be performed in the second and third trimesters of pregnancy, and challenge the U.S. Supreme Court's decision in *Roe v. Wade*. However, the current law stipulates that a woman has a right to an abortion in the first trimester without interference from regulations in any state.

Medical professionals must decide whether to perform abortions within these legal parameters and under what circumstances. Providers cannot be forced to perform abortions, nor can any employee be forced to participate or assist in an abortion. Employees not wishing to participate in abortions are advised to seek employment where they are not performed.

The volatility of the issue is so strong that terrorism against some abortion clinics and their providers has made it difficult for a person wanting an abortion to receive one. Terrorism of any sort is illegal, but providers who perform abortions have been murdered, one even in a church during worship. Such terrorism points to the very passionate debate that is unlikely ever to find a common ground of agreement.

Many unanswered ethical questions related to abortion make the decision difficult for health care professionals. Should abortion be considered a form of birth control? If not, should birth control and abortion be readily available to all who seek it, regardless of age? Should insurance pay for birth control? Is it ethical to deny an abortion to a woman on welfare but provide one to a woman who has money for the procedure or whose insurance pays? Some question if *any* abortion should be legal. And, of course, the major unanswered question that must be considered by every individual is: When does life begin—at conception, when the brain begins to function, at quickening, or at birth?

The abortion issue raises the bioethical issue of fetal tissue research and transplantation. As early as the 1950s, fetal tissue research led to the development of polio and rubella vaccines. Today, fetal cells hold promise for medical research into a variety of diseases and medical conditions, including Alzheimer disease, Parkinson disease, spinal cord injury, diabetes, and multiple sclerosis. Some research indicates that fetal retinal transplants may be a successful treatment of macular degeneration, which is the leading cause of age-related blindness in the United States.

This issue is political as well as bioethical, and it changes with each major political shift in the government. About half of the states have laws regulating fetal research. Some ban research using aborted fetuses. Federal law prohibits the sale of fetal tissue and requires all federally funded fetal tissue research projects to comply with state and local laws. This issue came to light in 2015 when Planned Parenthood was accused of selling fetal tissue for profit by the Center for Medical Progress. Videos released by the Center for Medical Progress were edited, however, and Planned Parenthood can and does legally collect fees for the handling and processing of the fetal tissue. Fetal tissue research is not to be used to encourage women to have abortions; rather, the tissue would be available only after a decision had already been made regarding abortion.

While the debate related to the use of fetal tissues for research marches on, the door has opened for research using umbilical cord blood. The use of cord blood has met with little controversy. In 2005, President George W. Bush signed into legislation a federal program to collect and store cord blood and to expand the current bone marrow registry program to include cord blood. Stem cells in cord blood have shown to be beneficial. For example, they can help restore red blood cells in people with sickle cell anemia. When a small group of children newly diagnosed with type 1 diabetes were transfused with their own stored cord blood, they showed reduced severity of the disease.

Medical assistants who work in fertility clinics must at all times respect the choices made by individuals seeking artificial insemination, IVF, or surrogacy. These procedures are truly private and very personal. Anyone who feels uncomfortable with such procedures is likely to be happier finding employment elsewhere.

Genetic Engineering/Manipulation

So much is possible today in the area of **genetic engineering** and new discoveries increasingly are being made. This biotechnology can be used in the diagnosis of disease, in the production of medicines, for forensic documentation (DNA used in solving crimes), and for research. Some reasons for continuing study in this area include determining if anything can be done to prevent or cure some 4,000 recognized genetic disorders and major diseases that have large genetic components. Few individuals would not like to see a cure for certain illnesses, but there is a fear among many that genetic engineering may lead to choices that should not be made. Deciding what should be done when the unborn is determined to have a severe birth defect, manipulating genes for a more perfect offspring, and discarding defective embryos are just a few of those concerns.

When countries move past the dilemma related to the use of embryonic stem cells, a number of significant medical advances might be made. Researchers may be able to create custom-made organs to replace those that are defective or diseased. Using small pieces of muscle and tissue from individuals, reproductive organs and nasal cartilage have been successfully grown and implanted. Although it might be a wonderful thing to create a new pancreas or a semisynthetic liver to replace an organ that is no longer performing its necessary function, the greater fear of some individuals is that of cloning.

Scientists already have cloned mice, sheep, rabbits, goats, pigs, and a dog. Where does cloning stop? Will human beings be cloned if science advances further into research with stem cells? Some countries with a different political arena than the one found in the United States are moving into this area. It is interesting to note, however, that in August 2005 the General Assembly of the United Nations voted to prohibit all forms of human cloning.

Dying and Death

The goal for all health professionals is to preserve and enhance life, thus making death an event contrary to the goals of health care. Yet, death cannot be avoided. How death is faced has both legal and ethical dimensions. Legally, individuals can make choices about their death and are often encouraged to do so by health care and legal professionals. When those wishes are indicated in documents such as advance directives and when health professionals disagree or refuse to honor those wishes, a legal problem arises. (Refer to Chapter 6.)

The legal aspect was made famous by the cases of Karen Ann Quinlan and Theresa (Terri) Schiavo. Both were young women, without any advance health care directives, whose deaths were caught in battles between family members, the medical staff, and the courts. Quinlan lived for 11 years in a vegetative state after much duress with health professionals and hospital staff who believed she should be kept on a respirator. The family members of Schiavo were in legal battles for 15 years before permission was received to remove her feeding tube; she died 14 days later. When there is conflict among family and those caring for someone near death, even a well-written and executed advance directive can be challenged. Then a legal dilemma becomes an ethical dilemma as well.

Legal

Patients continue to make decisions expressing their choices in death. Oregon was the first state to pass legislation allowing physicians to prescribe medications for patients to aid in their dying. The Oregon law was voted upon and passed on two separate occasions and was challenged by the U.S. Attorney General before the U.S. Supreme Court determined that the law could stand. Voters in the state of Washington approved similar legislation November 2008. Montana, Vermont, and California were recently added to the list. Several other states are struggling with issues to allow those who are dying a death with dignity. Many patients find comfort in a law that allows them the right to choose the time and place of their own death; however, the number of individuals who choose aid in dying still is small. Some make the choice, receive the medications from their physician, and then do not use the medication. Others receive the medication, find much relief in their choice, and do take the medication. There are still others who believe that any intervention that hastens death is criminal.

Religious Opposition to Assisted Dying. While much of society supports expanded options in dying, there is a large group that is opposed to any legislation that allows a patient to make certain decisions. There are religious groups that oppose *any* aid in dying, withholding food or hydration, and/or Do Not Resuscitate orders. Today, Catholic hospitals make up 10 of the 25 largest health care networks in America, and in many communities, the only hospital is a Catholic one. Catholic hospitals have long held to the tradition of not providing medical services that contradict Catholic religious principles and will not allow their providers (many not Catholic) to perform these services. For example, Catholic hospitals will not provide emergency abortion services to a woman with life-threatening pregnancy complications, and will also deny aid in dying to patients even in those states where such services are legal. This is a good example of a conflict between the law and ethics.

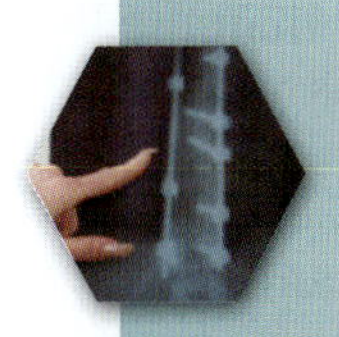

Critical Thinking

When there is conflict between what is legal and what might be considered by some to be unethical, how do you decide what action to take (see Procedure 7-1)? Could you work where abortions are legally performed? Could you deny a dying patient the right to carry out an advance directive if you did not believe in withholding food or hydration? While the law protects a woman seeking an abortion in the first trimester and allows patients to prepare very specific advance directives, what happens when the only health care source in the region does not allow either? Is this macro- or microallocation of limited resources?

The law is changing rapidly as additional states wrestle with the concept of aid in dying, but aid in dying is not **euthanasia**. The patient remains in complete control, unlike euthanasia where someone else administers the life-ending medication. Neither is aid in dying assisted suicide. These individuals want to live, but are dying from some terminal illness, and prefer a death with dignity. Many of these patients are also receiving optimal end-of-life care in hospice. For the most up-to-date information, refer to your state's legislation.

Choices available to patients who are dying create the question "What is quality of life?" Although the answer to that question is different for everyone, it is a question often in conflict with today's medical technology that can, in many instances, keep a patient alive much longer than the patient might prefer. The benefits of advanced technology will continue to be weighed against what many consider the right to die with dignity and a minimum of medical intervention.

Hospice. *Hospice* is the term used to describe either a place of residence for those who are dying or an organization whose medical professionals and volunteers are in attendance of someone whose death is imminent. The main objective of hospice is to make patients comfortable and as free from pain as possible and to allow them dignity in their deaths.

PROCEDURE 7-1

Procedure

Develop a Plan for Separation of Personal and Professional Ethics

PURPOSE:

To make a plan for circumstances when there is conflict between personal and professional ethics.

EQUIPMENT/SUPPLIES:

Paper, pen or computer

PROCEDURE SCENARIO:

A medical assistant who is also a lay Eucharistic minister (assists priest with mass and communion) must respond to a patient with end-stage pancreatic cancer requesting information regarding assisted death in Oregon.

PROCEDURE STEPS:

1. Using the Internet or Oregon's state statute on assisted death, determine the steps necessary to make assistance in death legal. RATIONALE: It is important to know the steps in this legal process to determine if they are satisfied.
2. Given this scenario, answer the ethics check questions identified in the text, and determine if and how you might assist this patient. RATIONALE: Answering these questions helps to put the emotional aspect of the scenario in perspective.
3. If you *can participate*, explain how you will proceed. If you decide you *cannot participate*, explain how you will proceed. RATIONALE: These steps aid the medical assistant in choice of words necessary in an explanation to the patient and employer.
4. Record this process and the decision you made to be true to yourself, therapeutic to the patient, and professional in all aspects of your employment.

Cardiopulmonary resuscitation (CPR), intravenous therapy, and feeding tubes are discouraged. Death is treated as a natural end-of-life experience. Death is neither hastened nor prevented.

Hospice volunteers and their counselors indicate that although many patients may choose hospice, some family members may not be as comfortable in that choice. Family members may not be ready to let go of a loved one; also, they may be uncomfortable if the hospice service is in the home rather than the hospital or a hospice facility. The latter is related to how comfortable family members are in observing or being a part of the death process. The expense of hospice is often covered by medical insurance and is less expensive than inpatient hospital care.

Medical assistants may be involved with the hospice protocol when patients of their employers are referred to and become clients of hospice.

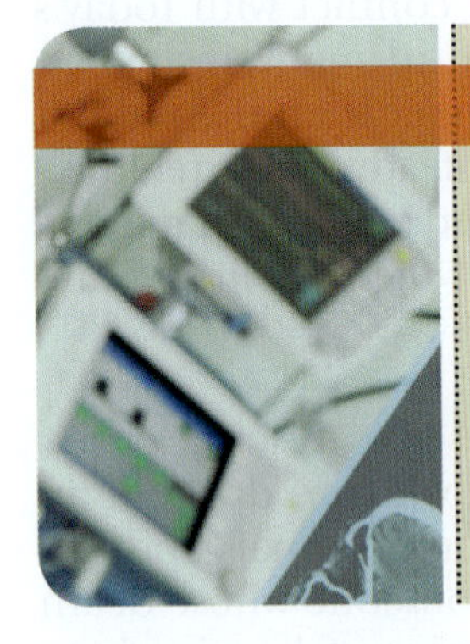

CASE STUDY 7-1

Refer to the scenario at the beginning of the chapter.

CASE STUDY REVIEW

1. If Harley's behavior does no harm to the patient, has he acted unethically? Illegally?
2. What might the office manager do if she senses Harley's lack of certainty?
3. Discuss the role of female and male medical assistants working together and how they might complement each other.

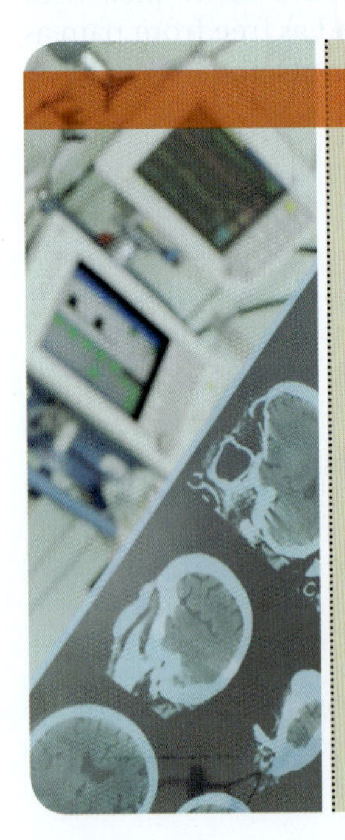

CASE STUDY 7-2

Lisa Chu is a medical assistant in the fertility clinic of a large metropolitan medical clinic and hospital. Lisa really likes her job and is delighted when parenthood is made possible for many of those seeking the clinic's advanced technology. The clinic also stores and maintains the unused frozen embryos that result from artificial insemination. She is a little alarmed when her provider-employer informs her that four of the embryos are to be destroyed. Her employer has been unable to contact the owners (now parents of more than one child from artificial insemination) for directions, and space for storage is limited. Lisa is instructed to destroy the embryos.

CASE STUDY REVIEW

1. Lisa is rather hesitant to comply with her employer's orders, so she does a little research. She discovers that most fertility clinics ask couples using **cryopreservation** to decide early in the process how to handle their excess embryos. The choices are to (1) discard the embryos, (2) donate anonymously to other infertile couples, and (3) donate to scientific research. What might Lisa do to influence the clinic's policy?
2. Can anything be done to ensure that couples do not abandon their embryos?
3. If embryos are given to other infertile couples, how is a decision made on who should have them?

Summary

- As medical technology continues to advance, a greater need for ethical guidelines is necessary.
- Providers and health care professionals at all levels must stay abreast of the issues and carefully consider all aspects before making any decision.
- Medical assistants must, however, keep the following legal and ethical guidelines in mind: (1) always practice within the law; (2) preserve the patient's confidentiality; (3) maintain meticulous records; (4) obtain informed, written consent; and (5) do not judge patients whose belief system differs from yours.

Study for Success

To reinforce your knowledge and skills of information presented in this chapter:

- Review the *Key Terms* and *Learning Outcomes*
- Consider the *Critical Thinking* features and *Case Studies* and discuss your conclusions
- Answer the questions in the *Certification Review*

Procedure

- Perform the *Procedure* using the *Competency Assessment Checklists* on the *Student Companion Website*

CERTIFICATION REVIEW

1. Typically, how has ethics been defined?
   a. It tells what is right and wrong.
   b. It determines whether an action is legal.
   c. It deals with what is the expedient thing to do.
   d. It is the best method for demonstrating professionalism in the workplace.
2. How is bioethics best explained?
   a. Biological reproduction is the main consideration.
   b. Bioethics is a new ethical dilemma.
   c. Bioethics is best explained in numerous codes of ethics.
   d. Bioethics focuses on ethical issues that deal with life and death issues.
   e. Bioethics always has to do with macro- and microallocation.
3. How is the AAMA Code of Ethics best identified?
   a. It applies only to patient rights.
   b. It is concerned with principles of ethical and moral conduct.
   c. It defines the duties the medical assistant can perform.
   d. It is intended for use by all providers.
4. When providers or medical assistants suspect child abuse, what should they do?
   a. Give the parent a warning
   b. Report it to the proper authorities
   c. Withdraw from treatment and refer elsewhere
   d. Give the child some hints on how to protect against abuse
   e. Omit the information from the electronic medical record
5. When a patient is HIV seropositive, what action should be taken?
   a. Make an immediate referral to an AIDS clinic
   b. Notify all possible unsuspecting individuals in contact with the patient
   c. Schedule appointments at the end of the day away from all other patients
   d. Protect their confidentiality while protecting any at risk
6. What does macroallocation of scarce medical resources imply?
   a. That the local health care team makes the decisions
   b. That Congress, health systems agencies, and insurance companies make the decisions
   c. That medical assistants will not be involved
   d. That patients will get the benefit of the best medical care
   e. That Medicaid patients will never be denied health care
7. Who authored the characteristics of principle-centered leaders?
   a. James R. Jones
   b. Stephen R. Covey
   c. Francis H. Ambrose
   d. Jason N. Diamond
8. What are the five Ps of ethical power?
   a. Personality, performance, purpose, pride, patience
   b. Purpose, patience, perfection, personality, procrastination
   c. Patience, purpose, pride, persistence, perspective
   d. Purpose, pride, patience, perfection, perspective
   e. Perfection, patience, perspective, personality, performance
9. Which of the following is true?
   a. A provider cannot choose whom to serve.
   b. It is unethical to charge for completing multiple and complex insurance claims.
   c. Providers and their employees cannot be forced to perform abortions.
   d. It is best to refer the poor and indigent to public health clinics.
10. When are you most likely to make ethical decisions correctly?
   a. When you do not need a clear picture of the situation.
   b. When you are emotional and passionate about the decision.
   c. When you have determined who you are and how you will act.
   d. When honesty and integrity do not influence a patient's care.
   e. When you remember to leave such decisions to your provider-employer.

CHAPTER 8

Emergency Procedures and First Aid

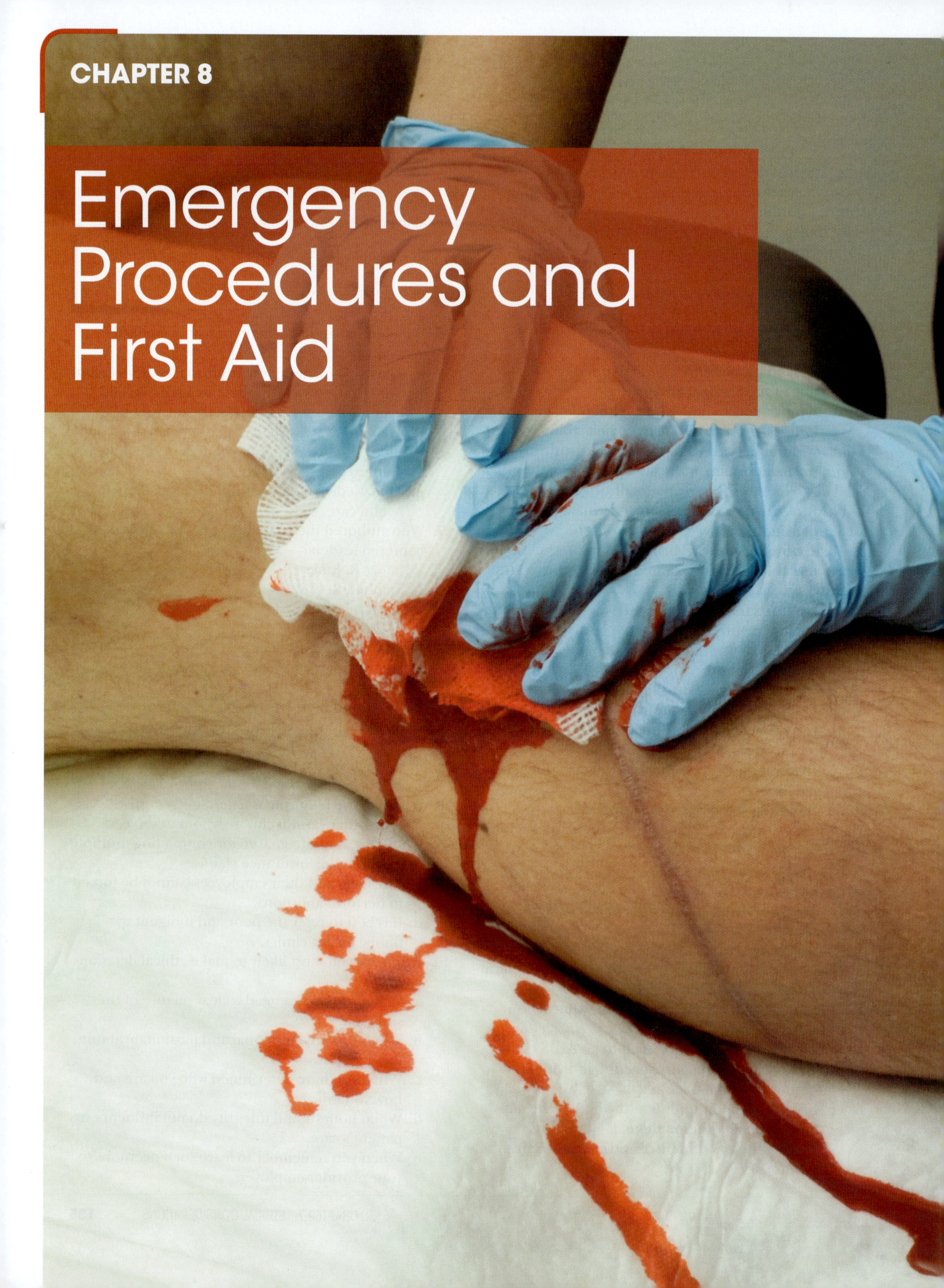

LEARNING OUTCOMES

1. Define and spell the key terms as presented in the glossary.
2. Recognize, prepare for, and respond to emergencies in the ambulatory care setting.
3. Outline basic principles of first aid and demonstrate first aid procedures.
4. Understand the legal and ethical considerations of providing emergency care.
5. Carry out appropriate interventions to prevent disease transmission considerations in emergency situations.
6. Perform the primary assessment in emergency situations.
7. Detect and care for different types of wounds.
8. Execute the basics of bandage application.
9. Discriminate among first-, second-, and third-degree burns.
10. Assess injuries to muscles, bones, and joints.
11. Summarize heat- and cold-related illnesses.
12. Explain how poisons may enter the body.
13. List the symptoms of a poisonous snake bite.
14. Recall six types of shock.
15. Detect a cerebral vascular accident.
16. Describe the signs and symptoms of a heart attack.
17. Identify potential role(s) of the medical assistant in emergency preparedness.

KEY TERMS

abrasion
anaphylactic
automated external defibrillator (AED)
avulsion
bandages
cardiogenic
cardiopulmonary resuscitation (CPR)
cardioversion
crash cart or tray
crepitation
diplopia
dislocations
dressings
electrocautery
emergency medical services (EMS)
explicit
first aid
fractures
Good Samaritan laws
hyperglycemia
hypoglycemia
hypothermia
hypovolemic
hypoxia
implicit
incision
ketoacidosis
laceration
myocardial infarction (MI)
neurogenic
normal saline
occlusion
puncture wound
rescue breathing
risk management
septic
shock
splints
sprain
Standard Precautions
status epilepticus
strain
syncope
triage
tonic-clonic phase
tourniquet
ulcers
universal emergency medical identification symbol
wounds

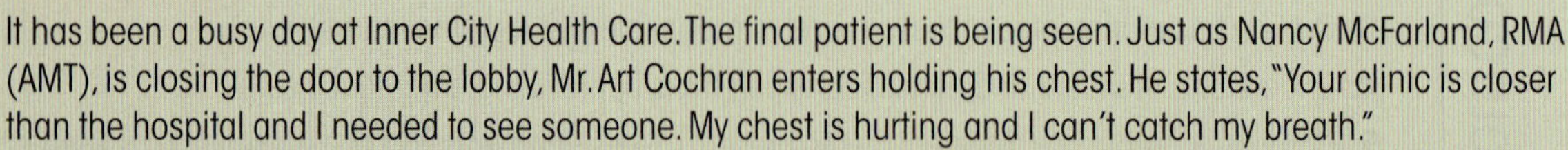

SCENARIO

It has been a busy day at Inner City Health Care. The final patient is being seen. Just as Nancy McFarland, RMA (AMT), is closing the door to the lobby, Mr. Art Cochran enters holding his chest. He states, "Your clinic is closer than the hospital and I needed to see someone. My chest is hurting and I can't catch my breath."

Based on her knowledge and experience, Ms. McFarland is aware that that Mr. Cochran is exhibiting signs of a heart attack. She remains calm, immediately notifying the provider and instructing the front desk person to call 911. Ms. McFarland escorts Mr. Cochran to a treatment room, has him lie down, and immediately takes his vital signs. As Ms. McFarland is certified in cardiopulmonary resuscitation (CPR) and first aid, she begins to take the appropriate steps to make sure that the patient is safe and cared for prior to the arrival of emergency medical system (EMS) personnel. Per the standing orders for patients with chest pain, Mr. Cochran is given a full-strength aspirin to chew and oxygen is applied. Mr. Cochran is calm and his chest pain is easing just as the EMS team arrives. It is essential to activate the EMS system as soon as possible when an emergency presents itself in a nonacute care setting. Care is then relinquished to the EMS personnel to provide further intervention.

Chapter Portal

Although the ambulatory care setting is primarily designed to see patients under nonemergency conditions, occasionally a situation will arise that requires administration of emergency care. The medical assistant is often an essential team member during a crisis situation. For the medical assistant who may need to screen or assess the patient's condition, the first and most critical step in responding to an emergency is developing the skill to recognize when emergency measures should be taken.

Some emergencies can be treated in the clinic, while others cannot, and the medical assistant must know when to initiate the request for outside help. If the emergency occurs in the ambulatory care setting, the provider usually administers immediate care. It is possible, however, that the medical assistant may be the first emergency caregiver should the provider be out of the clinic. The medical assistant also may be called on to provide care in an emergency outside the clinic environment.

This chapter acquaints the medical assistant with types of emergency situations that may occur during the course of a routine day. This chapter is merely an introduction to emergency topics and does not substitute for first aid and cardiopulmonary resuscitation (CPR) instruction taught through the American Red Cross, the American Heart Association, the American Safety and Health Institute, or the National Safety Council. Medical assistants in CAAHEP- and ABHES-accredited programs must be certified to a provider level in CPR and must be taught by instructors who are certified to teach CPR. These hands-on classes are vital teaching tools, and all medical assistants should take them on a regular basis to continually update their skills.

RECOGNIZING AN EMERGENCY

An emergency is considered any instance in which an individual becomes suddenly ill and requires immediate attention. Most emergencies develop quickly and usually without warning. They can occur unexpectedly at any time to anyone. Some may be gradual, as seen with dehydration or slow blood loss, and become an emergency over time. As you mature in your career, you will begin to develop the ability to make quick determinations about the conditions of people around you. Your experiences in medicine will allow you to assess emergency situations simply by using your senses. By using your sense of sight, you will note an abnormal coloring of the skin, an expression of pain or discomfort, or evidence of bleeding or bruising. Your sense of smell will help detect a wound that has become infected or identify the fruity breath that occurs when a patient's blood sugar is very high. Your sense of touch helps to assess a patient's pulse or the temperature of his skin. Your sense of hearing will help you recognize a wheeze or cough indicting respiratory distress. It is also essential to be acutely sensitive to any unusual behaviors such as screaming, crying, moaning, or staring blankly off in space.

In the ambulatory care setting, medical assistants may encounter a range of emergency situations requiring first aid techniques. **First aid** is designed to render immediate and temporary emergency care to persons injured or otherwise disabled before the arrival of a health care practitioner or transport to a hospital or other health care agency. Emergency situations can be minor or severe and can include:

- Choking and breathing crises
- Chest pain
- Bleeding
- Shock
- Stroke
- Poisoning
- Burns
- Wounds
- Sudden illnesses such as fainting/falling
- Illnesses related to heat and cold
- Fractures

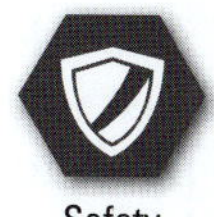

Some of these situations will be life threatening; all will require immediate care. In either case, it is critical to remain calm, to follow the emergency policies and procedures established by the ambulatory care setting, and to be well versed in first aid and certified in CPR. The patient should not be further endangered.

Responding to an Emergency

Once it has been determined that an emergency exists, it is essential to act quickly. Before making any decisions about how to proceed, it is necessary to assess the nature of the situation. Does it include respiratory or circulatory failure, severe bleeding, burns, poisoning, or severe allergic reaction?

Sometimes, it is possible that more than one type of care must be administered. As a medical assistant approaches any situation, it is imperative to begin with the CAB assessment: Circulation, Airway, and Breathing. Based on this information, the next step is to assist the provider in assessing the patient's condition so that treatment can be prioritized. When an individual experiences more than one illness or injury, care must be given according to the severity of the situation. When two or more patients present with emergencies simultaneously, screening helps determine which patient is treated first. This process is known as **triage**. Table 8-1 lists the common ordering of screening situations.

To identify the nature of the emergency and respond effectively, it is critical that the patient's overall condition be taken into consideration, including vital signs. If the patient is conscious, ask for personal identification and identification of next of kin. Try to obtain information about symptoms being experienced to identify the problem. Always check for a **universal emergency medical identification symbol** (Figure 8-1) and accompanying identification card, which will describe any serious or life-threatening health problems that the patient has. Quickly observe the patient's general appearance, including skin color and size and dilation of pupils. Check pulse and blood pressure.

TABLE 8-1

EXAMPLES OF EMERGENCY CATEGORIES

FIRST PRIORITY	NEXT PRIORITY	LEAST PRIORITY
Burns on face	Second-degree burns not on the neck and face	Fractures (simple)
Airway and breathing problems	Major or multiple fractures	Minor injuries
Cardiac arrest	Back injuries	Sprains, strains
Severe bleeding that is uncontrolled	Severe eye injuries	Simple lacerations
Head injuries	Syncope	Dehydration without change in vital signs
Poisoning	Seizure	
Anaphylactic shock	Lacerations involving multiple tissue layers	
Stroke	Hyper- or hypoglycemia	
Open chest or abdominal wounds		

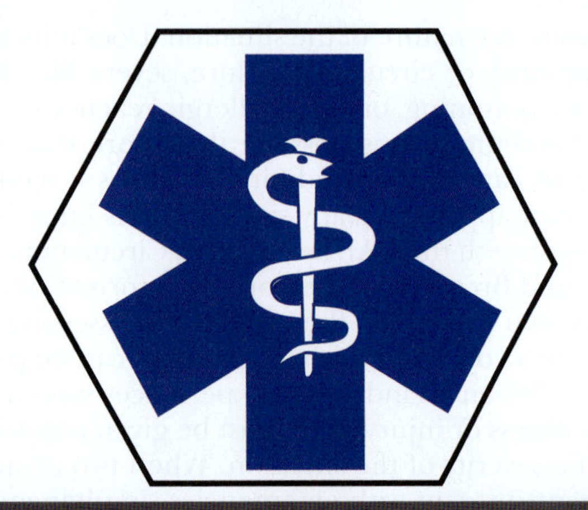

FIGURE 8-1 The universal emergency medical identification symbol.

Safety

Patient confidentiality must be maintained during an emergency situation. Take care to be mindful of those around you when an emergency situation arises, as your voice when speaking to other health care providers may be overheard by other patients. Privacy must be maintained when faxing information to the emergency department. Be sure to verify the fax number and use a fax cover sheet. Always be cautious in keeping the patient's anonymity protected.

Primary Survey

A method for assessing life-threatening injuries is known as the primary survey. Previously, this sequence was known as the airway, breathing, circulation, disability, and expose and evaluate assessment (or ABCDE assessment). In 2015, the American Heart Association (AHA) changed its recommendations so as to initiate compressions first. See the "Primary Survey" Quick Reference Guide for more information on the current assessment guidelines.

Using the 911 or Emergency Medical Services System

The **emergency medical services (EMS)** system is a local network of police, fire, and medical personnel who are trained to respond to emergency situations. This network is activated by dialing 911 in the United States. Even when preliminary emergency care is provided by the ambulatory care provider, the patient may still need to be transported to a hospital for follow-up care.

Good Samaritan Laws

Legal

When delivering or assisting in delivering emergency care, the medical assistant may be concerned about professional liability. Most states have enacted **Good Samaritan laws**, which provide some degree of protection to the health care professional who offers first aid.

Most Good Samaritan laws provide some legal protection to those who provide emergency care to ill or injured persons on a voluntary basis. However, when medical assistants or any other individuals give care during an emergency, they must act as reasonable and prudent individuals and provide care only within the scope of their abilities. Remember that a primary principle of first aid is to prevent further injury.

Although Good Samaritan laws give some measure of protection against being sued for giving emergency aid, they generally protect *off-duty* health care professionals. Also, conditions of the law vary from state to state. As part of establishing emergency care guidelines, every ambulatory care setting should understand the **explicit** and **implicit** intent of the Good Samaritan law in its state (see Chapter 6 for more information on legal guidelines).

Blood, Body Fluids, and Disease Transmission

Safety

When providing any care, including emergency care, medical assistants should always protect themselves and the patient from infectious disease transmission. Serious infectious diseases, such as hepatitis B (HBV), hepatitis C (HCV), and human immunodeficiency virus (HIV) infection, can be transmitted through blood and body fluids.

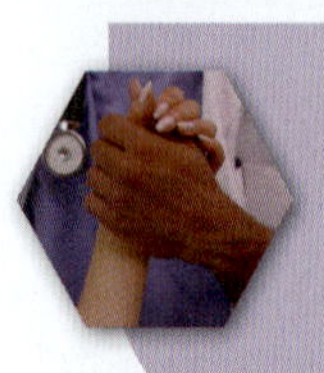

Patient Education

Alert patients to the importance of carrying the universal emergency medical identification symbol and its accompanying identification card if the patient has severe heart disease, diabetes, or other life-threatening illnesses or allergies.

QUICK REFERENCE GUIDE

PRIMARY SURVEY

Method of Assessment	Intervention	Considerations	Appropriate Action
(C) Circulation	Check carotid artery at the side of the neck below the ear.	If no pulse palpated, and if you are a trained CPR provider, initiate chest compressions.	Call for help and/or initiate 911 system. Obtain crash cart; an **automated external defibrillator (AED)** may be necessary. Initiate compressions
(A) Airway	Place face close to the patient's mouth and look, listen, and feel.	If breathing, support airway. If not breathing, first open the airway either by tilting the head and lifting the chin (Figure 8-2A) or by the jaw-thrust maneuver (see Figure 8-2B).	*CAUTION:* Do not attempt to tilt the head and lift the chin when the patient has a head, neck, or spinal cord injury.
(B) Breathing	Observe chest for rise and fall.	If no breath or only gasping, rescue breathing must be performed.	Ideally, breathing is checked simultaneously with circulation.
(D) Disability	Is the patient conscious? Responsive to questions? Pupils responsive?	Inform provider of findings. Work with provider to determine underlying causes.	Follow orders of provider to assist in delivery of care.

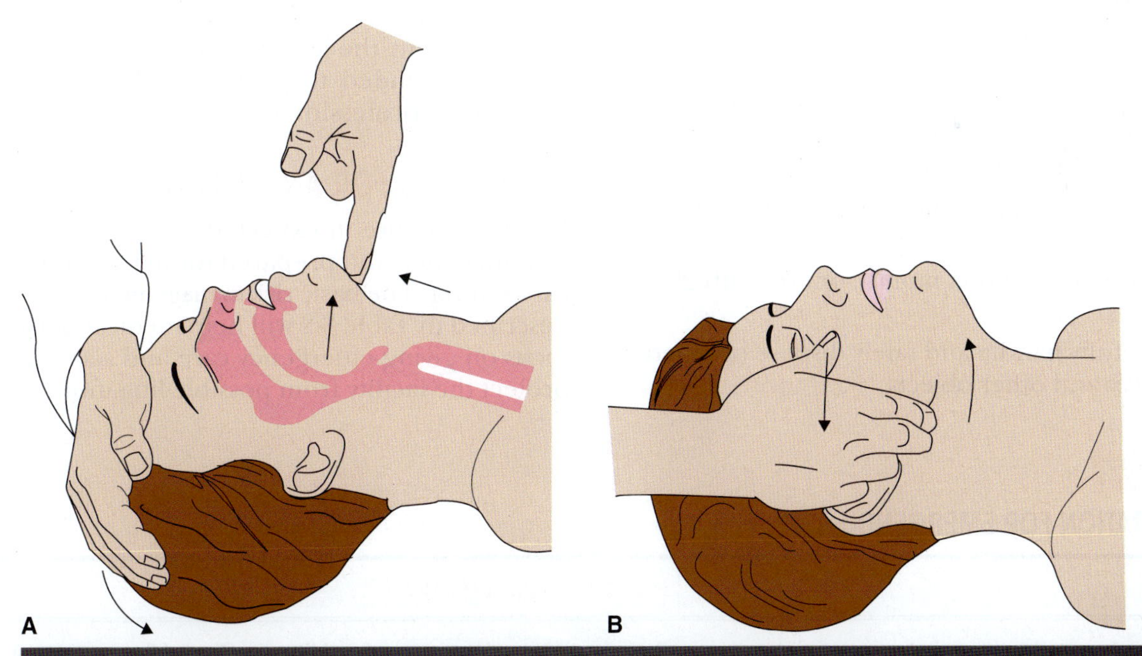

FIGURE 8-2 If the individual is not breathing, first open the airway (A) by tilting the head and lifting the chin, for victim without head or neck trauma, or (B) by the jaw-thrust maneuver, for victim with cervical spine injury. This involves placing both thumbs on the patient's cheekbones and placing the index and middle fingers on both sides of the lower jaw.

(continues)

Method of Assessment	Intervention	Considerations	Appropriate Action
(E) Expose and Evaluate	Remove clothing.	Monitor vital signs.	Initiate first aid if indicated.
	Obtain history from those accompanying the patient.	Update provider with findings.	Never leave the patient unattended.

After performing the initial assessment:

- Continuously monitor all areas of the patient's progress and keep the provider informed until EMS arrives.
- Keep the patient warm and still.
- Legs may be elevated if no indication of spinal injury.

Always remember that a medical assistant must maintain current cardiopulmonary resuscitation certification for management of emergency situations.

By establishing and following strict guidelines, the risk for contracting or transmitting an infectious disease while providing emergency care is greatly reduced.

- Always wash hands thoroughly before (if possible) and after every procedure or use hand sanitizer.
- Use protective clothing and other protective equipment (gloves, gown, mask, goggles) during the procedure.
- Avoid contact with blood and body fluids, if possible.
- Do not touch nose, mouth, or eyes with gloved hands.
- Carefully handle and safely dispose of soiled gloves and other objects.

Standard Precautions were issued by the Centers for Disease Control and Prevention (CDC) in 1996 and combine many of the basic principles of universal precautions with techniques known as body substance isolation. These precautions were reviewed and upheld in 2011 and represent the standard in infection control and are intended to protect both patients and health care professionals.

PREPARING FOR AN EMERGENCY

Emergencies are unexpected but can and should be anticipated and prepared for in the ambulatory care setting. The basic **risk management** techniques described in Table 8-2 will help medical personnel focus on giving emergency care and also will help protect the facility from possible litigation.

TABLE 8-2

PREPARATION FOR EMERGENCIES

TOOL	MEDICAL ASSISTANT'S ROLE
Policy and procedures manual	Participate in updates annually at the direction of the provider or office manager Be aware of manual's location for ease of reference
Emergency phone numbers: • EMS (911) • Poison control (1-800-222-1222)	Post in designated locations Update as necessary

(continues)

Table 8-2 continued

TOOL	MEDICAL ASSISTANT'S ROLE
Maintain supply levels	Follow established inventory listings to maintain inventory
CPR certification (see Procedure 8-1)	Recertify biannually
Safe clinical environment	Wipe up spills to prevent falls Maintain clutter-free common areas Properly store medications
Crash cart or tray (see Figure 8-3)	Locate in accessible place Once the inventory is established by the provider, perform daily check for completeness, expiration dates, and functionality of equipment Remember that only the provider can order medications or treatment

PROCEDURE 8-1

Produce Up-to-Date Documentation of Provider/Professional Level CPR

PURPOSE:

To provide evidence that one has mastered the knowledge of how to care for breathing and cardiac emergencies in adults, children, and infants.

EQUIPMENT/SUPPLIES:

Durable card provided by the training organization

PROCEDURE STEPS:

1. Attend and complete a professional level CPR training course through one of the approved organizations recognized for health care professionals, including medical assistants.
2. Photocopy your CPR card to present to your instructor and/or employer.
3. Keep the original documentation in your possession.

The Medical Crash Cart or Tray

Following is a brief list of some common supplies found on most crash carts and trays (see Table 8-3 for more information about medications found in a crash cart).

General supplies:

- Adhesive and hypoallergenic tape
- Alcohol wipes
- Bandage scissors
- Bandage material
- Blood pressure cuffs (standard, pediatric, large)
- **Tourniquet**
- Defibrillator/AED
- Dressing material
- Flashlight
- Gauze rolls
- Gloves
- Hot/cold packs
- Intravenous (IV) catheters in various sizes
- IV start pack
- IV tubing
- Needles and syringes for injection

- Glucose tabs or gel
- Penlight (with extra batteries)
- Personal protective equipment
- Stethoscope
- Syringes in 1-mL, 3-mL, and 20-mL sizes

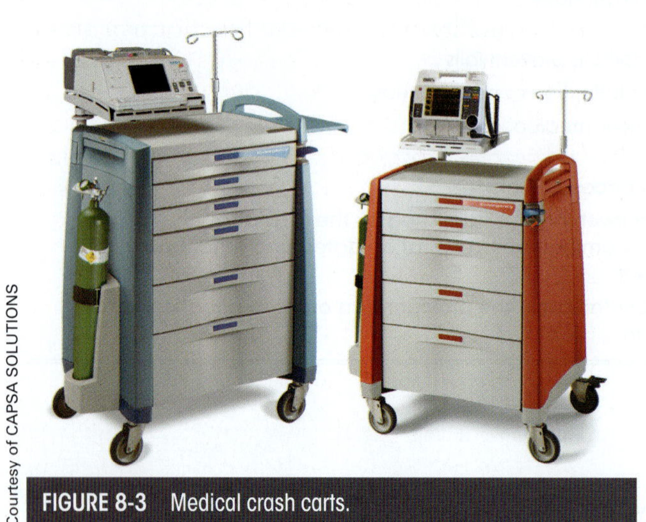

Courtesy of CAPSA SOLUTIONS

FIGURE 8-3 Medical crash carts.

Respiratory supplies:

- Airways of all sizes for nasal and oral use
- McGill forceps
- Ambu bag in infant, pediatric, and adult sizes
- Bulb syringe for suction
- Laryngoscope blades in various shapes and sizes
- Laryngoscope handles with batteries
- Nasal cannulas in infant, pediatric, and adult sizes
- 100% nonrebreather masks in infant, pediatric, and adult sizes
- Oxygen tank with Christmas tree adapter

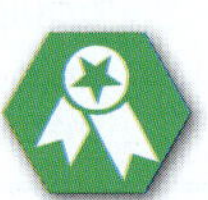

Competency

This list represents many of the supplies to be found on a well-stocked **crash cart or tray**. The medical assistant should be familiar with the equipment and medication on the crash cart or tray. Mock codes simulating various emergency situations are helpful for preparing staff members for actual emergencies.

TABLE 8-3

EMERGENCY MEDICATIONS FOUND ON A CRASH CART

EMERGENCY MEDICATIONS	USES
Activated charcoal	Poisonings
Aspirin 325 mg	Fever, heart attack
Atropine	Slow heartbeat
Benadryl	IV for treatment of anaphylactic shock
$D_{50}W$	IV solution of dextrose in water (50%) for hypoglycemia
Dextrose	Insulin reaction
Diazepam*	Antianxiety
Diphenhydramine	Antihistamine
Dopamine	Increases blood pressure
Epinephrine	Constricts blood vessels, increases blood pressure
Glucagon	Insulin reaction
Insulin	Hyperglycemia
Lidocaine	IV for cardiac arrhythmia
Narcan	Reversal of narcotic overdose
Nitroglycerin tablets, patches	Chest pain from angina pectoris
Normal saline	IV access and delivery method for emergency drugs
Pepcid 20-mg vial	Treatment of anaphylactic shock
Phenobarbital*	Sedative
SoluMedrol	IV for treatment of anaphylactic shock
Verapamil	Hypertension, angina pectoris, irregular heartbeat, tachycardia
Xylocaine, Marcaine	Local anesthetics

*Controlled substance—must be kept in locked cabinet.

COMMON EMERGENCIES

Included in this discussion of common emergencies are shock, wounds, burns, musculoskeletal injuries, heat- and cold-related illnesses, poisoning, snake bite, sudden illness, cerebral vascular accident, and heart attack.

Shock

Procedure

When a severe injury or illness occurs, **shock** is likely to develop. Shock is progressive, and if not treated immediately, most types can be life threatening (see Procedure 8-2). Once shock reaches a certain point, it is irreversible. The "Shock" Quick Reference Guide provides detail on the physiology, signs and symptoms, and treatment of shock.

Types of Shock. Shock can be defined by categories or by the underlying cause. There are several categories of shock. Cardiogenic shock is due to decreased ability of the heart to function as a pump. Another category of shock caused by decreased venous return is hypovolemic shock. High cardiac output hypotension shock is caused by underlying factors such as sepsis. Other types of shock are anaphylactic, neurogenic, traumatic, and compression of the heart. Table 8-4 describes common types of shock seen in an ambulatory care setting.

PROCEDURE 8-2

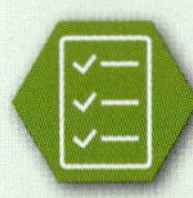
Procedure

Perform First Aid Procedures for Shock

STANDARD PRECAUTIONS:

Handwashing

Gloves

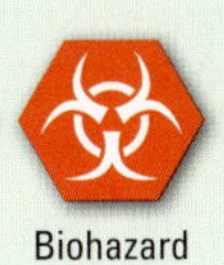
Biohazard

Gown

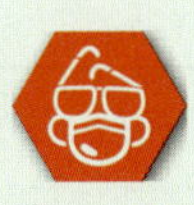
Goggles & Mask

PURPOSE:

To support and monitor the patient in shock until EMS arrives.

EQUIPMENT/SUPPLIES:

- Pillow
- Blanket
- Sterile gloves (if hemorrhagic shock)
- Clean gloves
- Gown (if hemorrhagic shock)
- Mask (if hemorrhagic shock)
- Protective eyewear (if hemorrhagic shock)
- Sterile dressing material (if hemorrhagic shock)

PROCEDURE STEPS:

1. ***Incorporating critical thinking skills when performing patient care***, notify the provider of the patient's condition immediately.
2. Activate EMS per the provider's orders.
3. Assist the patient into a reclining position. RATIONALE: This position minimizes pain and decreases stress on the body.
4. Elevate the patient's legs about 12 inches, unless you suspect head injury, spinal injuries, or broken bones involving the hips or legs. RATIONALE: This restores blood flow to the brain by decreasing the gravitational resistance.
5. As soon as possible, don clean gloves (sterile gloves if the cause of shock is hemorrhage and pressure to the wound is to be applied), and any other Personal Protective Equipment (PPE) that is appropriate.
6. Loosen any restrictive clothing or belts. RATIONALE: This allows adequate respiration.

(continues)

7. Check for pulse and respiration. If necessary, begin CPR after activating EMS or calling for assistance.
8. Control any external bleeding following steps in Procedure 8-3.
9. Assist the patient to maintain normal body temperature. Do not overheat. RATIONALE: A blanket over and under the patient can help avoid chilling.
10. ***Recognizing the physical and emotional effects on persons involved in an emergency situation***, reassure the patient.
11. Do not give the patient anything to eat or drink.
12. Ascertain that outside help has been called and stay with the patient until help arrives.
13. Obtain vital signs as soon as the patient is safely positioned. Repeat frequently, per provider's preference.
14. Assist with the transfer of care to EMS by sharing vital signs obtained.
15. If contact with blood or body fluids occurred, remove PPE and discard appropriately in biohazard waste container.
16. Wash hands.
17. Document the incident and care provided in the patient's chart.

DOCUMENTATION:

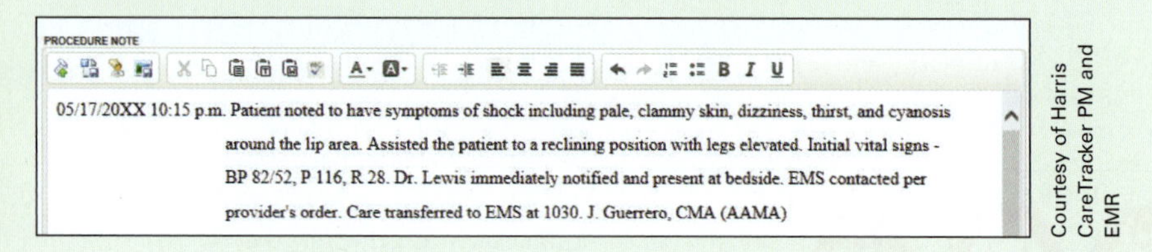
PROCEDURE NOTE

05/17/20XX 10:15 p.m. Patient noted to have symptoms of shock including pale, clammy skin, dizziness, thirst, and cyanosis around the lip area. Assisted the patient to a reclining position with legs elevated. Initial vital signs - BP 82/52, P 116, R 28. Dr. Lewis immediately notified and present at bedside. EMS contacted per provider's order. Care transferred to EMS at 1030. J. Guerrero, CMA (AAMA)

Courtesy of Harris CareTracker PM and EMR

TABLE 8-4

COMMON TYPES OF SHOCK WITH DESCRIPTIONS

TYPE OF SHOCK	DESCRIPTION
Cardiogenic	The cardiac muscle is unable to contract and adequately provide blood to the body. This can be caused by myocardial infarction, coronary artery disease, arrhythmias, or valve disease.
Hypovolemic	The body has lost blood or fluid volume to such an extent that there is not enough circulating volume to fill the ventricles. The heart attempts to compensate by increasing the heart rate.
Neurogenic	Injury or trauma to the nervous system causes loss of tone in the vessels, resulting in massive dilation of arterioles and venules. This results in a dramatic drop in blood pressure. This type of shock can be caused by brain or spinal cord injuries, general or spinal anesthesia, or pain and anxiety.
Anaphylactic	In this severe allergic reaction to substances such as drugs, blood products, contrast medium, insect or animal venom, or food products, chemicals are released that cause veins and arteries to vasodilate and decrease the amount of blood returning to the heart. Capillaries dilate and allow proteins and fluids to escape into the soft tissues, causing edema.
Septic	When overwhelming infection occurs in critically ill patients, chemicals are released into the bloodstream that cause vasodilatation and other organic products that are harmful to the organs and tissues. The vasodilation and decreased ability of the cells and tissues to utilize oxygen form the basis for this type of shock.
Respiratory	Trauma to the respiratory tract (trachea, lungs) causes a reduction of oxygen and carbon dioxide exchange. Body cells cannot receive enough oxygen.

QUICK REFERENCE GUIDE

Shock

PHYSIOLOGY

During shock, several things occur:

- The circulatory system is not providing an adequate blood supply to all parts of the body, causing a failure of normal functioning.
- The heart is unable to pump blood appropriately.
- Tissues don't receive adequate oxygenation (**hypoxia**).
- Blood flow shifts to critical organs (Figure 8-4).

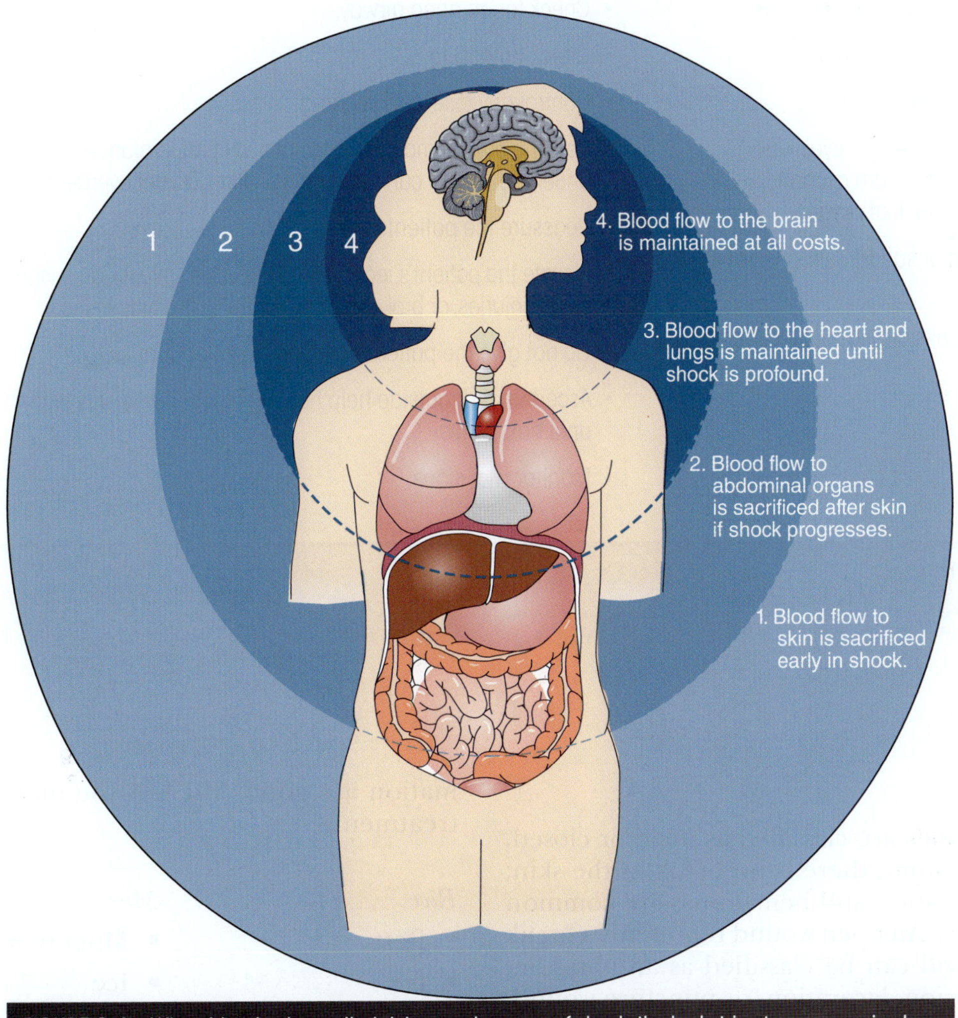

FIGURE 8-4 When blood volume diminishes, as in cases of shock, the body tries to compromise by sacrificing blood supply to the less-significant organs in order to preserve blood for the vital organs such as the heart and brain.

(continues)

QUICK REFERENCE GUIDE

Signs and Symptoms	Treatment
Learn to recognize the signs and symptoms of shock:	*To care for a patient in shock (regardless of the type), follow these procedures:*
• Patient may be restless or feel irritable. • Weakness, dizziness, thirst, or nausea may occur. • Breathing may be shallow and rapid. • Skin is cool, clammy, and pale. • Pulse is weak and rapid. • Blood pressure is low. • Area around the lips, eyes, and fingernails may turn cyanotic (blue) from lack of oxygen. • Confusion or sudden unconscious, or both. • Dilated pupils and lackluster eyes are obvious.	• Activate EMS. • Lay the patient down. This minimizes pain and decreases stress on the body. • Loosen the patient's clothing. • Check for an open airway. • Check breathing. • Control any external bleeding. • Help the patient maintain normal body temperature. A blanket over and under the patient can help avoid chilling. Do not overheat. • Reassure the patient. • Elevate the patient's legs about 12 inches, unless you suspect head injury, spinal injuries, or broken bones involving the hips or legs. • Do not give the patient anything to eat or drink. • Ascertain that outside help has been called and stay with the patient until help arrives. • Monitor vital signs.

Wounds

Typically, **wounds** are classified as open or closed. In a closed wound, there is no break in the skin; bruises, contusions, and hematomas are common closed wounds. An open wound represents a break in the skin and can be classified as an abrasion, avulsion, incision, laceration, or puncture wound. See Table 8-5 for more information on wound classifications.

A common procedure for treating a closed wound is to RICE or MICE it. It is generally thought that RICE is the preferred treatment for the first 24 to 48 hours. Once the signs of inflammation are gone, MICE is the more appropriate treatment.

Rice
- Rest
- Ice
- Compression
- Elevation

Mice
- Motion or Movement
- Ice
- Compression
- Elevation

Open Wounds. Common types of open wounds are described in the "Types of Open Wounds" Quick Reference Guide.

TABLE 8-5

CLASSIFICATION OF WOUNDS

CLASSIFICATION	PHYSIOLOGY	INDICATIONS	CONSIDERATIONS
Open	The integrity of the skin has been interrupted. Types of open wounds include: • Incision • Laceration • Abrasion • Avulsion • Puncture • Gunshot wound • Burn • Ulcer	May constitute an emergency. Needs intervention, including: • Cleaning • Debriding • Suturing • Medicating • Dressing	Represents an opportunity for microorganisms to gain entry to the body and cause an infection. May involve heavy bleeding, which will need to be controlled, probably by suturing. A tetanus injection is indicated.
Closed	The skin remains intact. Types of closed wounds include: • Hematoma or bruise • Crush injury	Cold compresses to address pain and swelling: • Protect the skin from direct application of cold • Apply cold for 20 minutes, remove for 20 minutes for the first 24 hours Warm compresses after 24 hours: • Protect the skin from the source of heat • Apply heat for 20 minutes, remove for 20 minutes for the following 24 hours	May be dangerous and associated with internal bleeding. If the pain is severe and/or was caused by a high impact, call for help and keep the patient comfortable until help arrives. Watch for symptoms of shock. Monitor vital signs.

Use of Tourniquets in Emergency Care. There has been much discussion regarding the use of tourniquets to control bleeding in the recent past. Recommendations now include the application of a tourniquet to control bleeding with the following stipulations:

- A tourniquet should be applied only if direct pressure fails to control bleeding.
- The time of tourniquet application must be clearly indicated on the device.
- Control of bleeding should be assessed and a tourniquet should be replaced by a pressure dressing if bleeding can be controlled.
- A tourniquet that is at least 2 inches wide with a windlass, ratcheting device is recommended.

If the bleeding is controlled, direct pressure is still the best method to handle blood loss.

Dressings and Bandages. After the provider has treated an open wound, it is critical to dress and bandage it properly to curtail infection. Covering of the wound is accomplished by a series of **dressings** and **bandages**.

Typically, dressings are sterile gauze pads placed directly on the wound; they often have nonstick, sterile surfaces, but they are absorbent and will soak up blood and protect the wound from microorganisms. They are often made of a gauze-type material.

Bandages, which are nonsterile, are placed over the dressing. They hold the dressing in place and are made to conform to the area to be covered. Sometimes, as in a Band-Aid, the dressing and bandage are combined. Bandage materials are selected based on the location and type of wound to be covered. Kling is a type of flexible gauze that stretches and clings as it is applied. Roller bandages (sometimes called by their brand name, Ace Bandages), such as those made of elastic, can be placed over a dressing and used to help control bleeding or swelling. Recently, there has been a rise in the utilization of self-adherent elasticized wrap known as Coban.

QUICK REFERENCE GUIDE

TYPES OF OPEN WOUNDS

	Open Wound	Description
	Incision	Wound caused by a sharp object, such as a knife or piece of glass. Incisions may need sutures. The wound must be cleaned with soap and water and a dressing applied.
	Laceration	Tears the body tissue and can be difficult to clean; therefore, care must be taken to avoid infection. If there is not severe bleeding, which in itself is a cleansing mechanism, these wounds may need to be soaked in antiseptic soap and water to remove debris. If there is severe bleeding, it must be controlled immediately (see Procedure 8-3). Lacerations with severe bleeding need suturing.
	Abrasion	A superficial scraping of the epidermis. Because nerve endings are involved, abrasions can be painful. However, they are not usually serious, unless they cover a large area of the body. Administer first aid by cleaning the area carefully with soap and water, apply an antiseptic ointment if prescribed by a provider, and cover with a dressing.
© Chaikom/Shutterstock.com	**Avulsion**	The skin is torn off and bleeding is profuse. Avulsion wounds often occur at exposed parts: fingers, toes, ear. First, control bleeding (see Procedure 8-3). Then clean the wound. If there is a skin flap, reposition it. Apply a dressing, then bandage as necessary. Note that pieces of the body may be torn away. If possible, save the body part, keep moist, and transport with the patient.
	Puncture wound	The skin is pierced and penetrated and there may be a deep wound while it appears insignificant. Usually, external bleeding is minimal, but the patient should be assessed for internal bleeding. Because a puncture wound is deep, the risk for infection is great and the patient should be advised to watch for signals of infection, such as pain, swelling, redness, throbbing, and warmth.

Some specific examples of open wounds include:

- Gunshot wounds, or ballistic trauma, which are caused by a projectile fired from a variety of firearms that inflicts damage to multiple structures. The entrance wound is usually smaller than the exit wound. Treatment is aimed at controlling bleeding, repairing damage, and preventing infection.
- Burns, which damage tissues from the skin downward into adjacent structures. Burns may be caused by direct heat, chemicals, electricity, sunlight, or radiation. Treatment varies based on the degree of injury.
- **Ulcers**, which are open cavities in the skin caused by tissue breakdown related to lack of oxygen supply to the tissues. This can be caused by vascular disease, inflammatory disorders, excessive fluid accumulation, or prolonged pressure. Treatment includes cleaning, debriding, and dressing, as well as resolution of the underlying cause.

Bandages and their applications can take many shapes and forms, depending on the type of injury and the injury site. In all cases, a bandage must be secure, but not constricting. Avoid too tight or too loose a wrap.

- Spiral bandages are useful for injuries to the arms or legs (Figure 8-5).
- A figure-eight bandage holds the dressing in place on a wound on the hand or wrist, knee, or ankle (Figure 8-6).

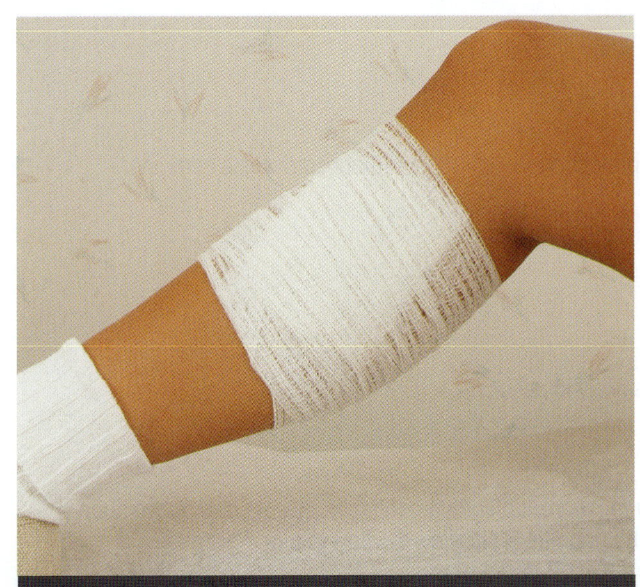

FIGURE 8-5 The spiral bandage is an option for arm and leg injuries.

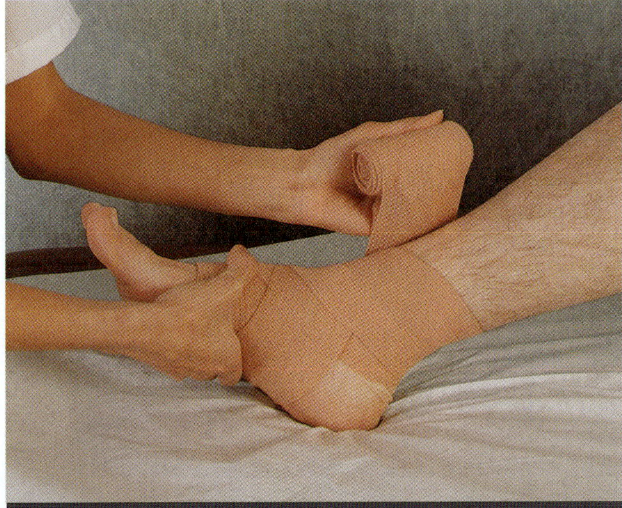

FIGURE 8-6 An elastic figure-eight bandage holds dressings in place or can be used for immobilization, as with an ankle sprain.

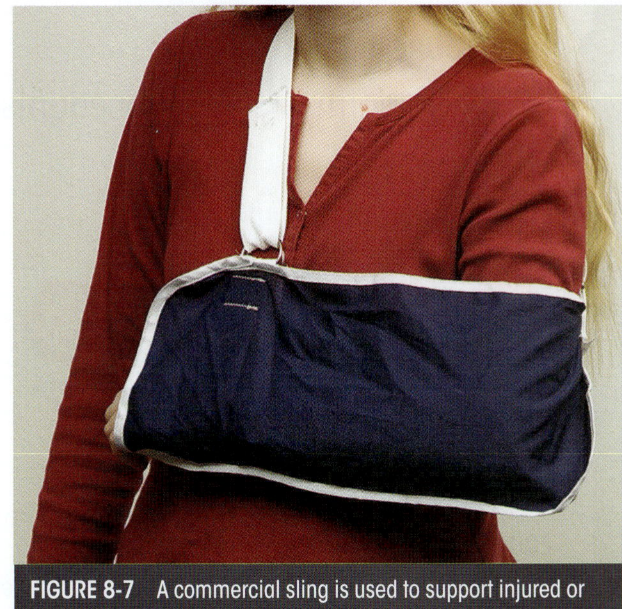

FIGURE 8-7 A commercial sling is used to support injured or fractured arms.

- Commercial arm slings are used to support injured or fractured arms (Figure 8-7). To apply, support the injured arm above and below the injury site while applying the sling.

Burns

Most burns are caused by heat, chemicals, explosions, and electricity. Critical burns can be life threatening and require immediate medical care. According to the American Red Cross, critical burns have the following characteristics:

- Involve breathing difficulty
- Cover more than one body part
- Involve the head, neck, hands, feet, or genitals
- The person sustaining the burn is a child or older adult (other than minor burns)

To distinguish critical from minor burns, it is important to understand the classifications of burns and what they mean (see the "Burn Classifications" Quick Reference Guide).

There is a formula for estimating the percentage of body surface areas that have been burned (see Figure 8-9). This formula is known as the rule of nines. In an adult, the head and each upper extremity are 9% each, the back of the trunk is 18%, as is the front (18%), each lower extremity is 18%, and the perineum is 1%.

PROCEDURE 8-3

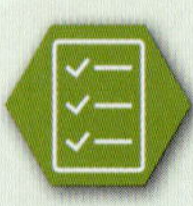

Procedure

Perform First Aid Procedures for Bleeding

STANDARD PRECAUTIONS:

Handwashing

Gloves

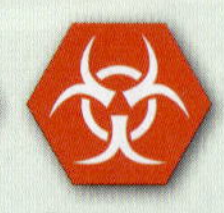
Biohazard

Gown

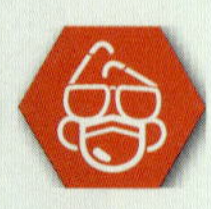
Goggles & Mask

PURPOSE:

To control bleeding from an open wound.

EQUIPMENT/SUPPLIES:

- Sterile dressings
- Sterile gloves
- Mask and eye protection
- Gown
- Biohazard waste container

PROCEDURE STEPS:

1. Wash hands.
2. Assemble equipment and supplies.
3. Apply eye and mask protection and gown if splashing is likely to occur.
4. Put on sterile gloves.
5. Apply sterile dressing and press firmly (Figure 8-8A).
6. ***Incorporate critical thinking skills when performing patient care.*** If bleeding continues, elevate arm above heart level (Figure 8-8B). RATIONALE: Raising the arm above the heart level will slow the flow of blood because it is flowing against gravity.
7. If bleeding continues, press adjacent artery against bone (Figure 8-8C). Notify the provider if bleeding cannot be controlled, ***demonstrating self-awareness in responding to an emergency situation***. RATIONALE: Pressing the adjacent artery against a bone provides solid pressure to help control bleeding.

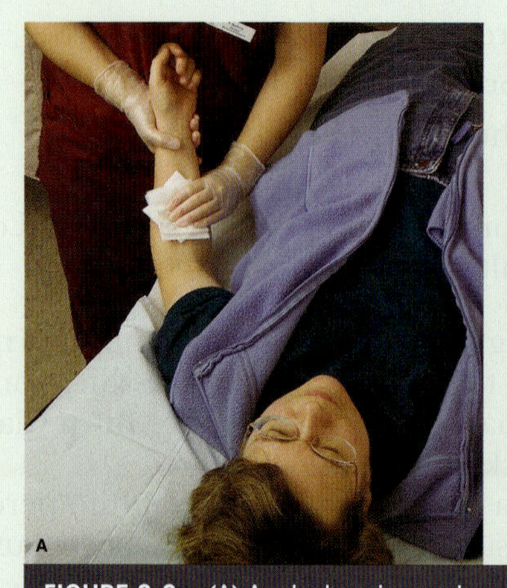

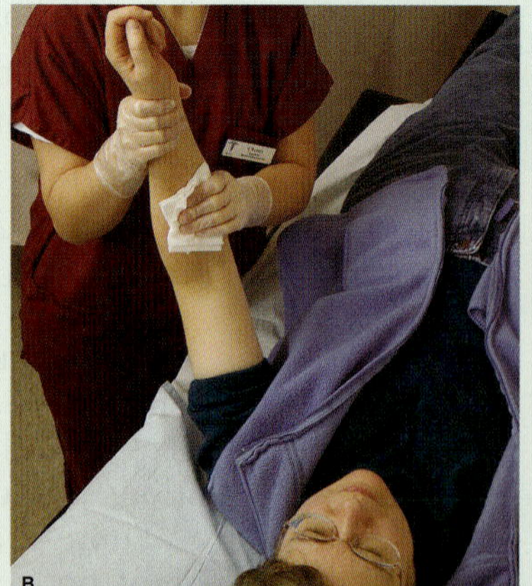

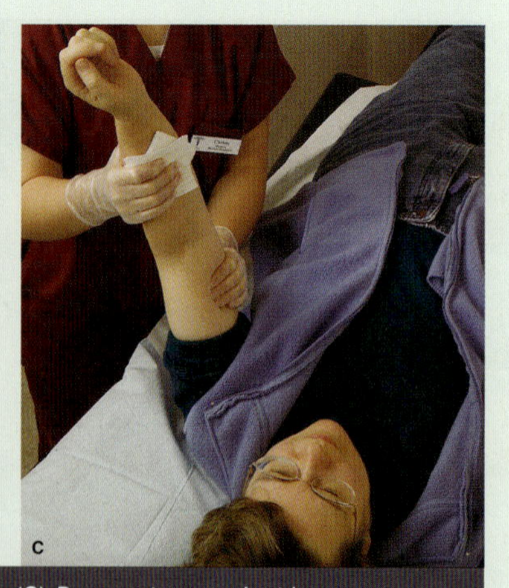

FIGURE 8-8 (A) Apply dressing and press firmly. (B) Elevate arm above heart level. (C) Press artery against bone.

(continues)

8. If bleeding still does not cease, notify the provider and continue to exert pressure on the wound with one hand while using your other hand to press the adjacent artery against bone.
9. Apply pressure bandage over the dressing.
10. Discard any waste in the appropriate container and prepare the patient for any follow-up procedure to be performed, such as suturing or stapling.
11. Remove gloves and dispose in biohazard container.
12. Wash hands.
13. Document procedure in patient's chart or electronic medical record.

CAUTION: If wound is large and bleeding is not controlled, the patient may go into hemorrhagic shock. Be prepared to call EMS immediately.

DOCUMENTATION:

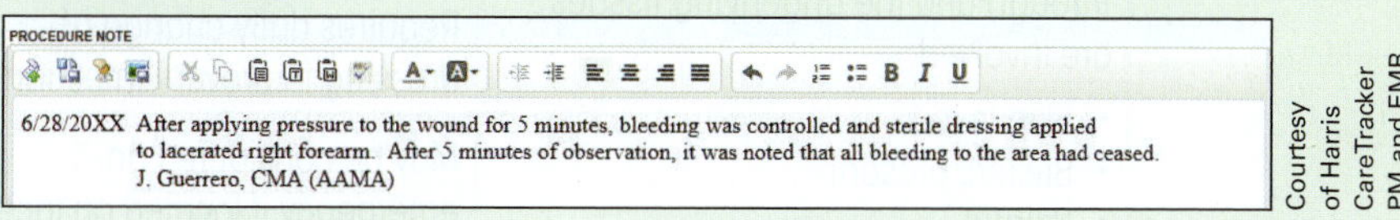
PROCEDURE NOTE

6/28/20XX After applying pressure to the wound for 5 minutes, bleeding was controlled and sterile dressing applied to lacerated right forearm. After 5 minutes of observation, it was noted that all bleeding to the area had ceased.
J. Guerrero, CMA (AAMA)

Courtesy of Harris CareTracker PM and EMR

In a child, the head, back, and front of the torso are 18% each, each upper extremity is 9%, each lower extremity is 13.5%, and the perineum is 1%.

Providers use the formula to determine the amount of body surface area that has been burned. Together with the depth of the burn, it helps the provider determine the percentage of the body that has been burned and the degree of burn. The severity of a burn can be determined and appropriate treatment given.

First Aid for Burns. First aid for burns is outlined in the Quick Reference Guide on page 155.

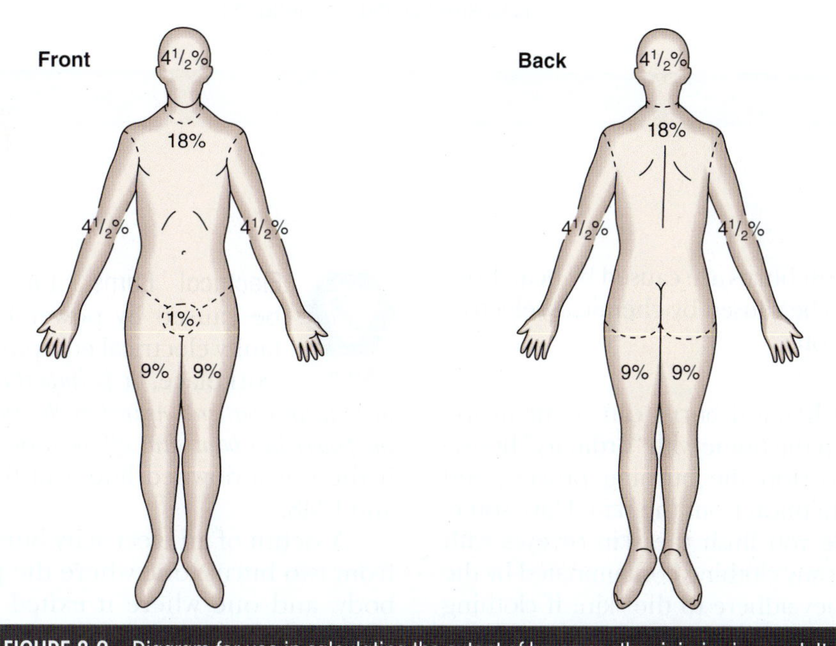

FIGURE 8-9 Diagram for use in calculating the extent of burns or other injuries in an adult.

QUICK REFERENCE GUIDE

BURN CLASSIFICATIONS

	Degree	Physiology	Considerations
© Chris Driscoll/ Shutterstock.com	First degree	Superficial, involving only the top layer of the skin: • Red • Dry • Warm to the touch • Swollen • Painful • Heals quickly without scarring	Minor unless on face, hands, feet, groin or buttocks May be considered an emergency if area involved is large enough
© Photodiem/Shutterstock.com	Second degree	First layer of skin has been burned through and the underlying tissues are involved: • Skin is red • Blisters present • Painful May take a month to heal and scarring is likely	Do not break the blisters Requires daily change of dressing to prevent infection May be considered an emergency if located on face, hands, feet, groin or buttocks, or covers a large area of the body
Courtesy of the Phoenix Society of Burn Survivors, Inc.	Third degree	Affects or destroys all layers of tissue; fat, muscle, bone, nerve: • Tissues appear charred or brown, waxy and white, raised and leathery • Extremely painful • No pain if all nerves in the area destroyed Risk of shock and loss of large volumes of bodily fluid Extensive healing time required	Emergency treatment must be sought Elevate the body part that is affected if possible Do not remove clothing if sticking to the burn Remain calm and activate EMS

Types of Burns. Most burns are caused by heat; however, burns can also be caused by chemicals, electricity, and solar radiation.

Chemical Burns. Chemical burns can occur in the workplace or even in the home with "ordinary" household chemicals. To stop the burning process, you must remove the chemical from the skin. Have someone call EMS while you flush the skin or eyes with cool water. Remove any clothing contaminated by the chemicals unless they adhere to the skin. If clothing clings to the skin, it can be cut with scissors. Do not attempt to pull clothing away from a burned area.

Safety

Electrical Burns. Electrical burns can be caused by power lines, lightning, or faulty electrical equipment in the home or workplace. *It is important to remember never to go near a patient injured by electricity until you are sure the power has been shut off, because you could be injured.* If there is a downed line, call the power company and EMS.

A victim of an electricity burn may be suffering from two burns: one where the power entered the body, and one where it exited. Often, the burns themselves may be minor. Of more serious consequence are the possibilities of shock, breathing

QUICK REFERENCE GUIDE

FIRST AID FOR BURNS

First-Degree Burn Response Guide

Questions	Responses	Action to Take	Rationale
Is skin reddened without blisters? NO ⇩	YES ⇨	Submerge in cool **normal saline** ⇨ or water for 2 to 5 minutes.	Stops burning process.
Does area involve: • Hands? • Feet? • Genitals? • Face? NO ⇩	YES ⇨	Have patient come to clinic. ⇨	These are potential danger areas and require evaluation by the provider.
Is patient: • Elderly? • Very young? NO ⇩	YES ⇨	Have patient come to clinic. ⇨	These groups are susceptible to burn complications.
Consult provider.			Provider has final decision whether patient is seen.

Second-Degree Burn Response Guide

Questions	Responses	Action to Take	Rationale
Is skin reddened with blisters or splitting of the skin? NO ⇩	YES ⇨	Submerge in cool normal saline ⇨ or water for 10 to 15 minutes if skin is intact. Use compresses if skin is broken. Do not break blisters. Do not use anesthetic creams or sprays.	Stops burning process. If blisters are broken, the area is at greater risk for infection. Creams or spray may slow healing process and increase severity of a burn.
Does area involve: • Hands? • Feet? • Genitals? • Face? NO ⇩	YES ⇨	Have patient come to clinic or go ⇨ to the emergency department.	These are potentially dangerous areas and require medical attention.
Is the area involved larger than a child's hand? NO ⇩	YES ⇨	Have patient come to clinic or go ⇨ to the emergency department.	Burns of this size are susceptible to complications.

(continues)

Second-Degree Burn Response Guide

Questions	Responses	Action to Take	Rationale
Is patient experiencing trouble breathing? NO ⇩	YES ⇨	Patient should go to emergency ⇨ department.	There may be swelling of the airways because of heat and noxious fumes.
Consult provider.			Provider has final decision whether patient is seen.

Third-Degree Burn Response Guide

Questions	Responses	Action to Take	Rationale
Does skin appear gray, black, or charred? Can muscle, fat, or bone be seen in wound? NO ⇩	YES ⇨	Tell patient or family to call EMS ⇨ immediately. Do not apply cold; do not remove burned clothing from burn area.	This is a life-threatening emergency that requires prompt attention.
Is patient experiencing: • Pallor • Loss of consciousness? • Shivering? NO ⇩	YES ⇨	Patient in shock: ⇨ Tell family to call EMS and to: • Maintain airway • Maintain body temperature • Elevate feet if appropriate • Monitor breathing Patient may need oxygen and intravenous fluids while waiting for EMS to arrive.	Need to control shock caused by fluid loss.
Consult provider.			Provider has final decision whether patient is seen.

difficulties, and other injuries. CPR often is needed in this situation.

Solar Radiation. Most "sunburns," although not advisable or good for the skin, represent minor burns. If the patient has a severe burn, however, he or she should see a provider who will cover the burn area to reduce chance of infection and protect the patient against chill.

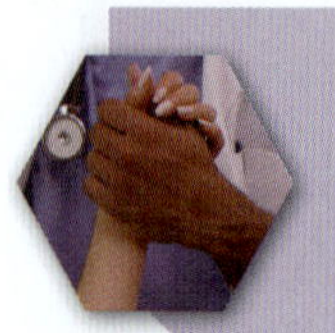

Patient Education

Some burns can be prevented. Advise patients who insist on sunbathing to protect themselves against harmful rays by using a sunscreen with 15 SPF or higher and avoiding the sun between 10 AM and 2 PM.

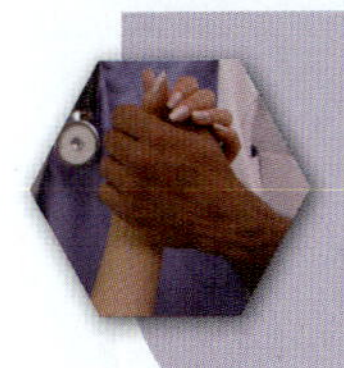

Patient Education

Advise patients not to run should their clothing catch on fire. They should fall to the ground or wrap themselves in a blanket or rug and roll on the ground to extinguish the flames. This method is known as "Stop, Drop, and Roll."

Musculoskeletal Injuries

Most injuries to muscles, bones, and joints are not life threatening, but they are painful and, if not properly treated, can be disabling. Some injuries, such as those to the spinal cord, can be quite serious and can result in paralysis. These injuries are not typically seen in the ambulatory care setting. See Table 8-6 for more information on types of musculoskeletal injuries.

Assessing Injuries to Muscles, Bones, and Joints. Sometimes it is difficult to determine the extent of an injury, especially in closed fractures. There are some assessment techniques to call on, however, to gauge the seriousness of an injury.

- Note the extent of bruising and swelling.
- Pain is a signal of injury.
- There may be noticeable deformity to the bone or joint.

TABLE 8-6

TYPES OF MUSCULOSKELETAL INJURIES

INJURY	DESCRIPTION	TREATMENT
Sprain	Injury to a joint that involves tearing of the ligaments; if minor, may heal quickly; if extensive, may require intervention Symptoms: • Rapid swelling • Discoloration at the site • Limited function	Seek medical assessment RICE or MICE as ordered by provider May require surgery Immobilize Protect from weight bearing as directed Pain management Physical therapy
Strain	Overuse or stretching of a muscle, tendon(s), or group of muscles	RICE or MICE as ordered by the provider Immobilize Protect from weight bearing as directed Pain management Physical therapy
Dislocation	Bone displaced from its normal location anatomically; usually occurs as a result of a wrenching motion	Requires urgent evaluation Radiologic imaging of affected area for diagnosis Relocation by trained professional or surgical intervention Immobilization Pain management Physical therapy
Fracture	Break or interruption of the integrity of the bone (see the "Types of Fractures" Quick Reference Guide for more information)	All fractures are emergent conditions and require urgent evaluation Radiologic imaging of affected area for diagnosis Medical intervention: setting, casting, or surgery to maintain approximation for healing Immobilization Pain management Physical therapy

QUICK REFERENCE GUIDE

TYPES OF FRACTURES

	Type	Description
Transverse Oblique	Closed fracture (simple, complete)	Complete bone break in which there is no involvement with the skin surface: • Skin intact • Discoloration of the skin • Swelling • Pain • Deformity • Inability to move affected limb • **Crepitation** (grating sensation experienced or heard when bone fragments rub together)
	Open fracture (compound)	Skin integrity is interrupted. Bone protrudes though the skin surface, creating the possibility of infection.
	Incomplete or greenstick fracture	Fracture in which the bone has cracked, but the break is not all the way through; frequently seen in children.

(continues)

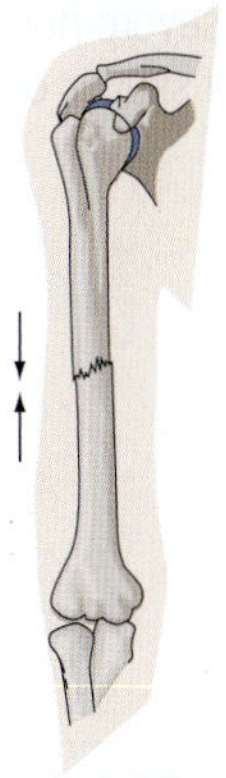	Impacted fracture	Broken ends of the bone are jammed into each other.
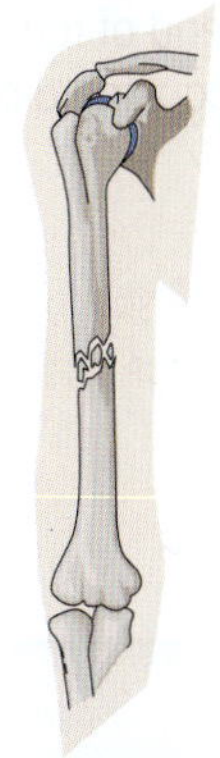	Comminuted fracture	More than one fracture line and several bone fragments are present.
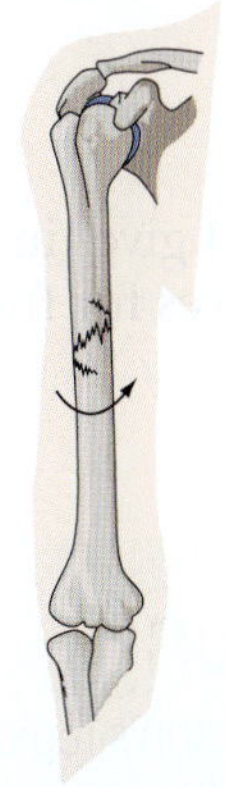	Spiral fracture	Fracture that occurs with a severe twisting action, causing the break to wind around the bone.

(continues)

	Depressed fracture	Fracture that occurs with severe head injuries in which a broken piece of skull is driven inward.
	Colles' fractures	Often caused by falling on an outstretched hand. Involves the distal end of radius and results in displacement, causing a bulge at the wrist.

- Use of the injured area is limited.
- Talk to the patient: What was the cause of the injury? What was the sound or sensation at the time of injury?

Caring for Muscle, Bone, and Joint Injuries. Most injuries to muscles, bones, and joints are treated in a similar way; some require motion, but most require rest, elevation of the injured part, immobilization, and the application of ice to the injury.

Procedure

After calling EMS (always check for life-threatening symptoms, such as breathing difficulties; bleeding; or head, neck, or back injuries), it is important to immobilize the injured area if the patient must be moved. EMS personnel use a variety of **splints** to immobilize bones and joints. Some fractures must be treated in the hospital. Compound fractures and fractures with nerve or blood vessel involvement are some examples. Most often, a fracture can be treated with outpatient care. A splint and a cast may be applied to prevent movement and to hold the fracture steady. Procedure 8-4 gives instructions for performing first aid procedures for fractures in the ambulatory care setting.

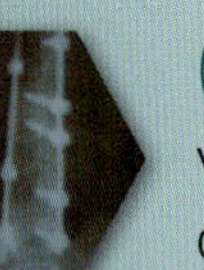

Critical Thinking

You are watching your son's regional championship baseball game and the runner from third base slides into home plate hands first. After the dust clears, it is evident that the player has sustained an injury. You are able to evaluate the player's condition and find bulging at the wrist with a definite bend in the distal arm. You work for an orthopedic office and have seen this type of injury before. What type of fracture do you suspect has occurred? What first aid measures can be implemented in a nonclinical setting?

PROCEDURE 8-4

Procedure

Performing First Aid Procedures for Fractures

STANDARD PRECAUTIONS:

Handwashing

PURPOSE:

To immobilize the area above and below the injured part of the arm in order to reduce pain, immobilize, and prevent further injury.

EQUIPMENT/SUPPLIES:

- Thin piece of rigid board; cardboard can be used if necessary
- Gauze roller bandage

PROCEDURE STEPS:

1. Wash hands.
2. Introduce yourself and identify the patient.
3. Carefully remove or cut away any clothing from the area of injury.
4. *Display a calm and professional manner* while observing the patient for swelling, bruising, difficulty moving the affected body part, pain, loss of strength, physical deformity, and symptoms of shock. *Incorporate critical thinking skills when performing patient assessment.*
5. It may be difficult to determine if the injury is a fracture, dislocation, sprain, or strain until radiologic films have been taken and interpreted by the provider. Until a diagnosis is made, treat the injury as a fracture.
6. Check the affected extremity for color, sensation, and movement.
7. If the fracture is open, apply sterile gloves and cover with a sterile gauze. Apply direct pressure around any bones. Do not attempt to force any protruding bone back into place.
8. If the fracture is closed, the injury will be immobilized by applying a splint. In order to apply the splint, follow these steps:
   a. Assist the patient into the position of greatest comfort with the least amount of movement of the affected area. RATIONALE: Not moving the extremity limits further damage to the soft tissues surrounding the fracture area.
   b. Without forcing movement, utilize a rigid splint to immobilize the extremity.
   c. The splint should be long enough to reach the joints above and below the injured area.
   d. Wrap the affected extremity with cast padding to protect from pressure and aid in comfort.
   e. Gently align the splint. Pad gaps between extremity and splint with gauze pads or other soft material. RATIONALE: Provides comfort for the patient.
   f. Secure splint to the injured extremity with an elastic bandage applied without undue pressure.
9. For a suspected fracture of a clavicle, apply a sling to support the arm and apply a wrap around the body to immobilize the arm and shoulder.

(continues)

10. For a suspected rib fracture, immobilize the rib area by applying wide pressure bandages around the area of injury.
11. Evaluate color, sensation, and movement of the affected area once the splint is applied and every 15 minutes thereafter while in your care.
12. Once the fracture area is immobilized, apply ice packs for comfort and management of swelling.
13. Elevate the area if possible.
14. Wash hands.
15. Accurately and concisely update the provider on the patient's care.
16. *Paying attention to detail,* document your findings and the procedures performed.
17. Check with the provider regarding pain medications that may be administered to the patient.

DOCUMENTATION:

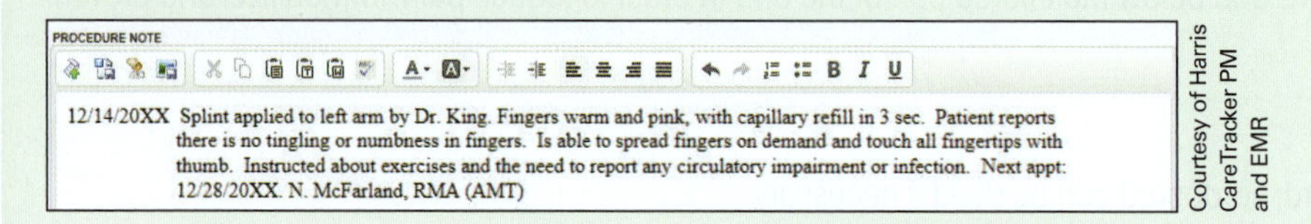
PROCEDURE NOTE

12/14/20XX Splint applied to left arm by Dr. King. Fingers warm and pink, with capillary refill in 3 sec. Patient reports there is no tingling or numbness in fingers. Is able to spread fingers on demand and touch all fingertips with thumb. Instructed about exercises and the need to report any circulatory impairment or infection. Next appt: 12/28/20XX. N. McFarland, RMA (AMT)

Temperature-Related Illnesses

The condition of patients who have been subject to extreme heat and cold can deteriorate rapidly, and either a heat- or cold-related illness can result in death. Individuals especially vulnerable to extreme exposures include the very young and very old, individuals who work outdoors, and people who suffer from poor circulation. See Table 8-7 for more information on temperature-related illnesses.

Poisoning

Poisons can enter the body in four ways: ingestion, inhalation, absorption, and injection (see the "Four Routes of Poisoning" Quick Reference Guide for more information).

Some signs and symptoms of poisoning are dyspnea, nausea and vomiting, confusion, and convulsions. The Poison Control Center (1-800-222-1222) can advise if there is an antidote for the poison (if poison is known). For many years, the treatment of choice for ingested poison was to induce vomiting by using syrup of ipecac. This practice is no longer recommended. Activated charcoal given as soon as possible is the treatment of choice for ingested poison. It is quicker and more effective.

If a patient becomes unconscious, the provider will be concerned that the patient will vomit and aspirate vomitus into the lungs; therefore, the provider may insert a flexible tube into the larynx to alleviate that possibility.

In most poisoning cases, there are specific antidotes. They work either by reversing the effects of the poison or by interrupting the pathologic process.

On occasion, there is no specific treatment and treatment will be based on the management of symptoms. A ventilator may be needed if a patient has stopped breathing. Medications that control convulsions are available, and sedatives can be administered if the patient is disturbed and restless.

Whenever a patient calls regarding poisoning or there is a suspicion of poisoning, call the Poison Control Center (1-800-222-1222) or the local emergency number and ask for instructions. Telephone numbers of the poison control center should be posted in a familiar and accessible place.

The treatment for poisoning will vary according to the source of the poisoning and must be tailored to the specific incident. The provider will have advised staff regarding specific poisoning antidotes. Generally, do not give the patient anything to eat or drink; try to determine what poison the patient was exposed to and, if ingested, how much was taken; if the patient vomits, save some of the vomitus for analysis.

Insect Stings

The medical assistant in the ambulatory care setting is likely to receive calls every summer from patients who have been stung by insects, typically yellow jackets, hornets, honeybees, or wasps. In the nonallergic patient, the sting is likely to result in localized swelling, tenderness, and slight redness.

TABLE 8-7

TEMPERATURE-RELATED ILLNESS

COLD-RELATED ILLNESS

ILLNESS	SYMPTOMS	CAUSE	TREATMENT
Frostbite	Affects extremities Skin is discolored: • Frostnip: reddened (early) • Pale, yellow, gray, or bluish (later) Changes in sensation: • Prickling (early) • Numbness (later) Joint stiffening Hardening of the skin	Prolonged exposure to extreme cold	Protect the skin from further exposure to the cold Get out of the cold Slow rewarming of the skin (for frostnip) Seek emergency medical treatment (later stages) Pain management
Hypothermia	Shivering (early) Lack of coordination Slurred speech or mumbling Confusion Dizziness	Prolonged exposure to any environment cooler than body temperature	Remove person from cool environment Remove wet clothing Cover person with blankets Monitor vital signs (VS) Provide warm beverages Activate EMS

HEAT-RELATED ILLNESS

ILLNESS	SYMPTOMS	CAUSE	TREATMENT
Heat cramps	Large muscle group cramping Common in legs and abdomen Cramps are: • Painful • Involuntary • Brief • Intermittent • Self-limiting	Excessive body exposure or exercise in hot weather	Stop exercise Rest in a cool place Drink water Increase salt intake (mix ¼ to ½ tsp of salt in one quart water) Seek medical care if progresses to heat exhaustion
Heat exhaustion	Feeling of physical exhaustion Cold, clammy skin Profuse sweating Headache Generalized weakness Thirst Nausea and vomiting Confusion Loss of consciousness	Working or exercising in extreme heat	Get out of the heat immediately Apply cool, wet towels to the body or take a cool shower Slowly drink cool water If symptoms are not relieved in 15 minutes, seek emergency medical assistance
Heat stroke	Red, dry, hot skin Weak, thready, irregular pulse	Working or exercising in extreme heat	Activate EMS Apply cool, wet towels to body Stay with patient Monitor VS

QUICK REFERENCE GUIDE

FOUR ROUTES OF POISONING

Route	Description
Ingestion	Ingested poisons enter the body by swallowing. Swallowed poisons may include medications, plant material, household chemicals, contaminated foods, and drugs.
Inhalation	Poisons are inhaled into the body in poorly ventilated areas where cleaning fluids, paints and chemical cleaners, or carbon monoxide may be present.
Absorption	Poisons absorbed through the skin include plant materials such as poison oak or ivy, lawn care products such as chemical pesticides, and other chemical powders or liquids.
Injection	Drug abuse is the most common cause of injected poisons. The stingers of insects inject poisons into the body and can be extremely dangerous and can lead to anaphylactic shock in allergic individuals.

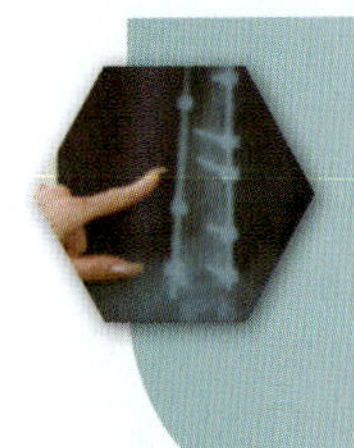

Critical Thinking

Your practice has just received poison help stickers to distribute to the parents of pediatric patients. Create an educational flyer regarding poison prevention.

The provider will recommend that these localized symptoms be managed with a topical cream and oral antihistamines. Swelling can be significant and cause for serious concern if the sting occurred in a vulnerable area of the body such as the mouth or tongue. Swelling in these locations can be frightening and dangerous because it can impair breathing. An antihistamine, administered as soon as possible after the sting, may help to curtail symptoms somewhat. Treatment of insect stings in nonallergic individuals consists of removing the stinger by scraping it off with the edge of something rigid such as a credit card or a fingernail. Tweezers can cause more venom to be dispersed into the patient's body tissues, so this method should not be used. Wash the area with soap and water, apply a cold pack to the site, and watch for a possible severe reaction.

The individual who experiences an allergic reaction or hypersensitivity to a sting needs to be seen immediately, because in severe cases a sting may induce an anaphylactic reaction that can lead to death. If allergic, individuals who have been stung are likely to experience symptoms within a half hour of the incident. Symptoms are generalized throughout the body and may include hives, itching, and lightheadedness and may progress to difficulty breathing, faintness, and eventual loss of consciousness.

For individuals with known allergic reactions, the provider will prescribe epinephrine, which patients should carry with them and self-inject should they not be able to get immediate emergency care. EpiPen is an auto-injector device that delivers epinephrine. The patient should then seek immediate emergency treatment. For individuals who present at the ambulatory care setting with an apparent allergic reaction to a sting, the provider will prescribe epinephrine, an antihistamine, and corticosteroids if necessary.

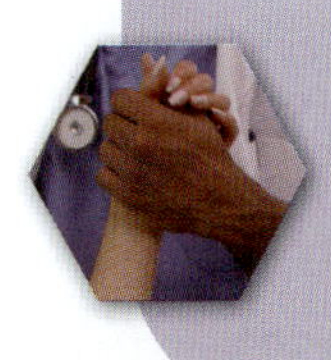

Patient Education

Remind patients who are parents of young children to remove any potential sources of poisoning from their homes or to keep such substances in locked cabinets. Also advise them to include the nearby poison control center in their list of emergency phone numbers. They should also keep activated charcoal on hand.

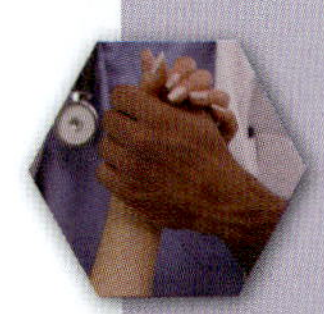

Patient Education

Snake Bite

Most snakes are not poisonous, and snakes usually will not strike unless provoked. Some poisonous snakes are rattlesnake, copper snake, cottonmouth water moccasin, and coral snake. Individuals who live in snake-inhabited areas, campers, hikers, and other outdoor lovers need to be mindful and cautious when outdoors. To avoid a possible snake bite, wear thick high boots, stay on the hiking path, do not reach down to pick up something from the ground unless you have a clear view around the area, and be careful on rocks (snakes like to live in or around piles of rocks).

Common signs and symptoms of a snake bite are rapid pulse, nausea and vomiting, severe pain, swelling, blood and fang marks at wound site, convulsions, thirst, and diaphoresis.

Emergency treatment consists of the following:

- Call for emergency help immediately.
- Wash wound with soap and water if possible.
- Immobilize body part and keep below heart level if possible.
- Cover wound with clean cool cloth.
- Monitor vital signs.
- Do not allow the victim to walk. Carry them or transport them by vehicle.

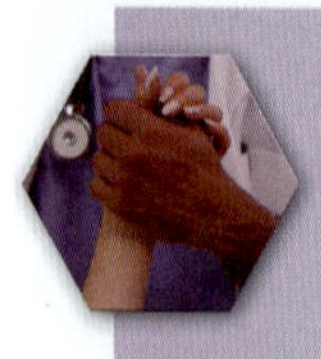

Patient Education

Advise all patients with known allergic reactions to be particularly careful when working or playing outdoors. Insects are not usually aggressive until their nests are approached; however, often these nests are not easy to detect, and an individual may approach one without being aware of its presence. Patients with allergies to insects should always wear shoes when outside; wear light-colored clothing, preferably with long sleeves and pant legs; look before taking a sip from a beverage when outdoors; and inspect lawn areas, shrubbery, and building walls periodically for evidence of stinging insect nests.

Attempt to allay patient apprehension and monitor vital signs while waiting for EMS personnel to arrive.

Sudden Illness

Sudden illness is, by definition, an unexpected occurrence. Although the cause of the illness may be unexplainable, it is important to respond sensibly and responsibly within the parameters of knowledge and resources.

Sudden illnesses include, but are not limited to, fainting, seizures, diabetic reaction, and hemorrhage (see Table 8-8).

TABLE 8-8

TYPES OF SUDDEN ILLNESS

TYPE OF ILLNESS	SYMPTOMS	CAUSE	TREATMENT
Fainting (**syncope**) (see Procedure 8-5)	May be preceded by: • Sweating • Weakness • Lightheadedness • Nausea • Disruption of sight • Ringing in the ears • Loss of consciousness	Most commonly, loss of adequate blood flow to the brain Other causes: • Emotional causes (vagal syncope) • Hypoglycemia • Severe pain • Hypotension • Dehydration • Hyperventilation	Gently lower patient into supine position Raise legs and feet above the level of the heart (if no spine or head injury) Treat the underlying causes Provide comfort measures such as loosening clothing and applying a cool cloth to the forehead Activate EMS for complex medical conditions
Seizures (see Procedure 8-6)	Absence (brief loss of consciousness) "Grand mal" or generalized tonic seizure: • Unconsciousness • Convulsions • Muscle rigidity Myoclonic seizure: • Sporadic (isolated) • Jerking movements Clonic seizure: • Repetitive • Jerking movements Tonic seizure: • Muscle stiffness • Rigidity Atonic seizure: • Loss of muscle tone	Normal brain functioning has been interrupted May be caused by: • Epilepsy • Fever • Diabetes • Infection • Brain injury	Care for the patient with medical understanding and compassion Do not restrain the patient Protect patient from self-injury: • Cushion the head • Clear the area of dangerous objects • Roll the patient onto his or her side to assist with managing fluids to prevent aspiration • Calm and comfort the patient Treat the underlying cause Activate EMS if patient is pregnant, diabetic, or injured **Do Not:** Attempt to stop the seizure even if the patient appears frightened and in pain Force anything between the patient's clenched teeth (the patient cannot swallow his or her tongue)

continues

Table 8-8 continued

TYPE OF ILLNESS	SYMPTOMS	CAUSE	TREATMENT
Diabetes (see Procedure 8-7) • Type 1 (insulin-dependent) • Type 2 non-insulin-dependent, which usually occurs in adults; in type 2, the body produces insulin in insufficient quantities)	**Hyperglycemia** (**ketoacidosis**): Dry, flushed skin • Drowsiness • Dry mouth • Intense thirst • Nausea and/or vomiting • Air hunger • Fruity breath • Weak, rapid pulse • Dimmed vision • Blood glucose > 200 mg/dL Hypoglycemia: • Pale, moist skin • Excited behavior • Drooling • Hunger • Normal or shallow respirations • Full and pounding pulse • Double vision (**diplopia**) • Blood glucose < 40 to 70 mg/dL	The inability of the body to properly convert sugar from food into energy, resulting in hyperglycemia or hypoglcemia Sugar not able to be transported into cells due to a lack of the hormone insulin	Recognize the symptoms of hyperglycemia or hypoglycemia Check blood glucose level and patient vital signs Notify the provider of findings Treat the underlying issue: If **hypoglycemia** (low blood sugar), offer the patient a high sugar content drink or snack Be prepared to administer glucose as ordered by the provider If hyperglycemia (elevated blood sugar), the provider will order insulin Activate EMS if indicated. **Note:** Provider will assess the patient prior to release; notify provider once patient has returned to homeostasic vital signs and blood glucose level
Hemorrhage (external bleeding)	Bleeding from the capillaries, veins, and/or arteries due to damage to the skin and underlying structures • Venous bleeding (blood is dark red with a steady flow) • Arterial bleeding (blood is bright red and exits the body in a pumping or spurting manner) If not controlled, will lead to shock and death	Puncture or severing of capillaries, veins, and arteries from trauma or surgical intervention *Epistaxis*. Prolonged exposure to dry air, injury, high altitude, repeated nose blowing, hypertension, or use of anticoagulant medications that easily damage the delicate mucous membranes of the nose Vaginal bleeding due to miscarriage is a rare complication, but it is a leading cause of maternal complications Vaginal bleeding might also be caused by neoplasm or trauma	Apply direct pressure Treat the underlying cause of bleeding The provider may intervene with: • Suturing • **Electrocautery** (applying controlled heat to obtain hemostasis) • Pressure dressing application To treat epistaxis: • Elevate head • Pinch nostrils for 10 minutes • Tilt head forward to prevent swallowing or aspiration of blood • If bleeding not controlled in 20 minutes, active EMS • Assist provider with cauterization or insertion of gauze packing If bleeding is associated with trauma or head injury, activate EMS To treat vaginal bleeding: • Prepare the exam room for a pelvic exam • Provide a sterile tray setup that includes a speculum • Stand by to arrange transport to an acute care setting Activate EMS Monitor vital signs Provide shock prevention measures: • Spine position • Elevate legs • Maintain airway • Maintain body temperature • Keep patient npo

continues

Table 8-8 continued

TYPE OF ILLNESS	SYMPTOMS	CAUSE	TREATMENT
Internal bleeding	Bleeding from the capillaries, veins, and/or arteries internally Lack of visible blood flow after trauma or surgical intervention The following symptoms may occur: • Rapid and weak pulse • Low blood pressure • Shallow breathing • Cold and clammy skin • Dilated pupils • Dizziness • Faintness • Thirst • Restlessness • Feeling of anxiety • Pain • Fatigue • Swelling • Abdominal board-like stiffness	Trauma that damages any internal organ Damage to any artery or vein that causes bleeding Fractures, especially of long bones Ectopic pregnancy Postoperative bleeding Alcohol abuse that results in cirrhosis of the liver causing esophageal varices	Activate EMS Monitor vital signs Provide shock prevention measures: • Place in supine position • Elevate legs • Maintain airway • Maintain body temperature • Keep patient npo

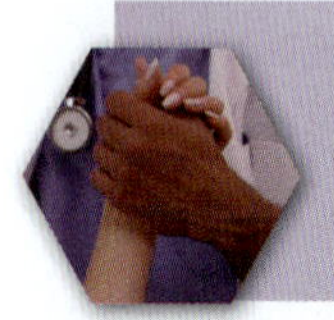

Patient Education

Advise the patient not to blow the nose for several hours after an epistaxis.

PROCEDURE 8-5

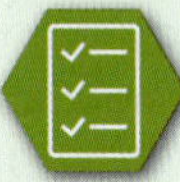

Procedure

First Aid Procedures for Syncope (Fainting Episode)

STANDARD PRECAUTIONS:

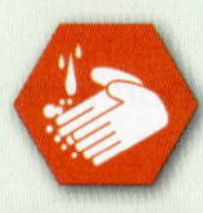

Handwashing

PURPOSE:

To provide protection from injury and administer first aid to a person experiencing a syncopal episode.

(continues)

EQUIPMENT/SUPPLIES:

- Pillows
- Blanket

PROCEDURE STEPS:

1. Be aware that if an individual that is conscious alerts you that he or she feels faint or dizzy, or when ***incorporating critical thinking skills when performing patient assessment and care,*** you note pallor and cool, clammy skin, syncope may be pending.
2. If the patient is conscious and still alert, assist him or her to a sitting position and help to bend forward, placing head between the knees until symptoms resolve.
3. If the patient has fainted or is no longer able to follow commands, position him or her on back and elevate legs. RATIONALE: This restores blood flow to the brain by decreasing gravitational resistance.
4. Loosen any restrictive clothing or belts. RATIONALE: This encourages adequate respiration.
5. Check for pulse and respiration. If necessary, begin CPR after activating EMS or calling for assistance.
6. Alert the provider to immediately assess the patient.
7. Obtain vital signs as soon as the patient is safely positioned. Repeat frequently, per provider's preference.
8. ***Recognizing the physical and emotional effects on persons involved in an emergency situation,*** provide comfort measures to the patient, such as a blanket for warmth.
9. Document the incident and care provided in the patient's chart.

DOCUMENTATION:

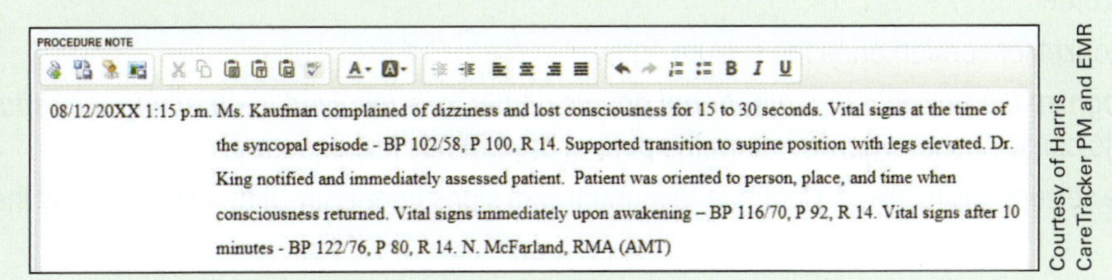
PROCEDURE NOTE

08/12/20XX 1:15 p.m. Ms. Kaufman complained of dizziness and lost consciousness for 15 to 30 seconds. Vital signs at the time of the syncopal episode - BP 102/58, P 100, R 14. Supported transition to supine position with legs elevated. Dr. King notified and immediately assessed patient. Patient was oriented to person, place, and time when consciousness returned. Vital signs immediately upon awakening – BP 116/70, P 92, R 14. Vital signs after 10 minutes - BP 122/76, P 80, R 14. N. McFarland, RMA (AMT)

Courtesy of Harris CareTracker PM and EMR

PROCEDURE 8-6

Procedure

Perform First Aid Procedures for Seizures

STANDARD PRECAUTIONS:

Handwashing

Gloves

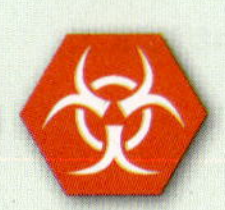
Biohazard

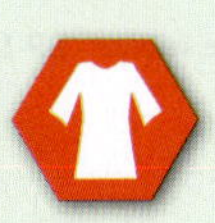
Gown

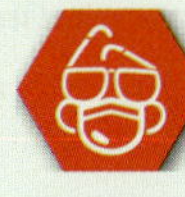
Goggles & Mask

PURPOSE:

To appropriately manage a patient physically and ensure his or her safety during a seizure.

(continues)

EQUIPMENT/SUPPLIES:

- Pillow
- Clean gloves
- Appropriate PPE
- Biohazardous waste container
- Blanket

PROCEDURE STEPS:

1. ***Incorporate critical thinking skills when performing patient assessment and care.*** If the patient is standing or sitting at the onset of the seizure, gently ease him or her to a reclining position on the exam table or on the floor.
2. Turn the patient onto his or her side to manage oral secretions to avoid aspiration.
3. Assess patient's breathing. If needed, open the airway using the head tilt or jaw thrust maneuver.
4. Call for assistance and immediately notify the provider without leaving the patient's side. Accurately and concisely update the provider on any aspect of the patient's care.
5. Apply clean gloves as soon as possible once the patient is safely reclining.
6. Clear the immediate area around the patient to avoid injury during the **tonic-clonic phase** of the seizure.
7. Place a pillow under the patient's head for support. Manage clothing by removing glasses, loosening clothing, and loosening belts.
8. Time the seizure. Seizures usually resolve in 1 to 3 minutes. If the seizure lasts 30 minutes continuously or there are two or more seizures without a period of recovery, the patient may be in **status epilepticus**. Be prepared to activate EMS on the provider's order.
9. Cover the patient with a blanket for comfort once the seizure ends.
10. Stay with the patient. ***Recognize the physical and emotional effects on persons involved in an emergency situation.*** As he or she returns to consciousness, gently inform the patient of what has just occurred.
11. Obtain vital signs once the seizure has resolved. Continue to monitor vital signs frequently at an interval set by the provider's preferences.
12. Allow the patient to rest or sleep after the procedure.
13. Document the length of the seizure and any other relevant information in the patient's chart.

DOCUMENTATION:

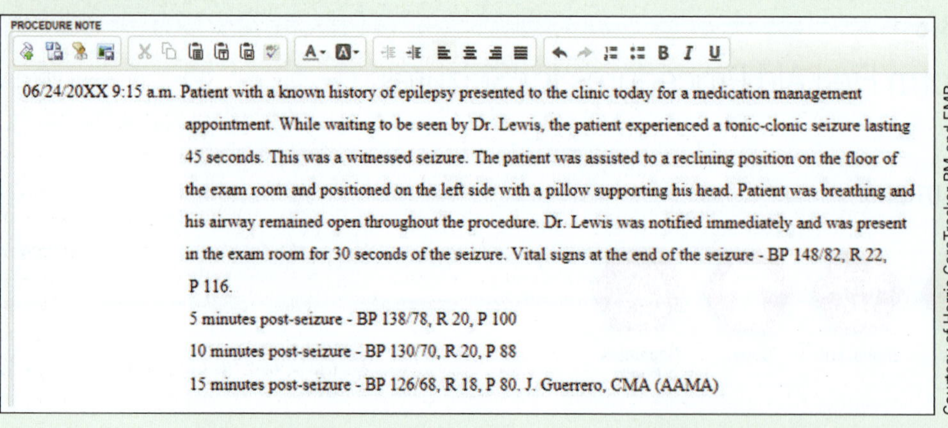
PROCEDURE NOTE

06/24/20XX 9:15 a.m. Patient with a known history of epilepsy presented to the clinic today for a medication management appointment. While waiting to be seen by Dr. Lewis, the patient experienced a tonic-clonic seizure lasting 45 seconds. This was a witnessed seizure. The patient was assisted to a reclining position on the floor of the exam room and positioned on the left side with a pillow supporting his head. Patient was breathing and his airway remained open throughout the procedure. Dr. Lewis was notified immediately and was present in the exam room for 30 seconds of the seizure. Vital signs at the end of the seizure - BP 148/82, R 22, P 116.

5 minutes post-seizure - BP 138/78, R 20, P 100

10 minutes post-seizure - BP 130/70, R 20, P 88

15 minutes post-seizure - BP 126/68, R 18, P 80. J. Guerrero, CMA (AAMA)

Courtesy of Harris CareTracker PM and EMR

PROCEDURE 8-7

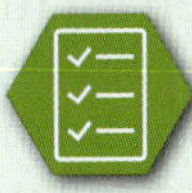

Procedure

Perform First Aid Procedures for Diabetic Emergencies

STANDARD PRECAUTIONS:

Handwashing

Gloves

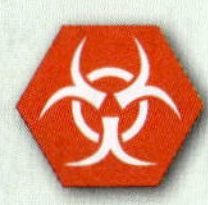

Biohazard

PURPOSE:

To appropriately assist a patient experiencing either hypoglycemia or hyperglycemia.

EQUIPMENT/SUPPLIES:

- Clean gloves
- Glucose analyzer
- Strips for glucose analyzer
- Sterile lancets
- Alcohol wipes
- 2-by-2 gauze
- Adhesive bandage
- Biohazard waste container

PROCEDURE STEPS:

1. When symptoms of hyperglycemia (ketoacidosis) or hypoglycemia are noted, have the patient sit or lie down. RATIONALE: This reduces the risk of a fall if loss of consciousness occurs.
2. Obtain vital signs.
3. Follow the provider's order for obtaining a blood glucose measurement and assemble the equipment needed to test blood glucose. ***Explain to the patient the rationale for performance of the procedure, showing awareness of the patient's concerns.***
4. Apply clean gloves and perform a blood glucose analysis.
5. Notify the provider of findings and follow provider orders.
6. ***Incorporating critical thinking skills in performing patient assessment and care,*** be prepared to offer the patient a drink that contains a high sugar content or a high sugar snack if the patient is hypoglycemic, with a blood sugar below 70 mg/dL.
7. ***Incorporating critical thinking skills in performing patient assessment and care,*** be prepared to administer insulin per the provider's order if the patient is hyperglycemic, with a blood sugar above 200 mg/dL.
8. If at any time the patient loses consciousness, place her on her side, notify the provider, and prepare to activate EMS on provider's orders.
9. Document your findings and the procedures performed.

DOCUMENTATION:

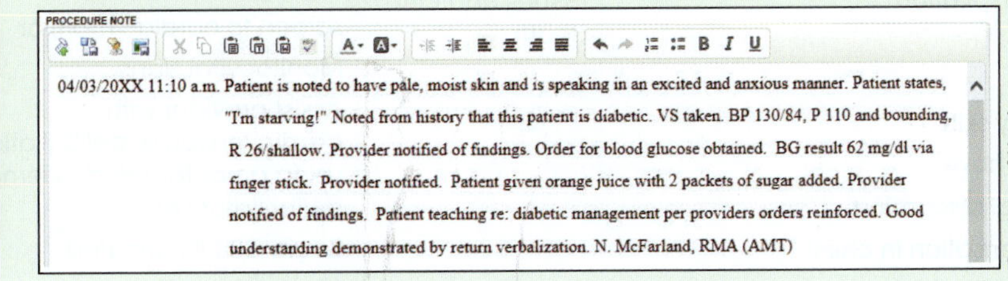

PROCEDURE NOTE

04/03/20XX 11:10 a.m. Patient is noted to have pale, moist skin and is speaking in an excited and anxious manner. Patient states, "I'm starving!" Noted from history that this patient is diabetic. VS taken. BP 130/84, P 110 and bounding, R 26/shallow. Provider notified of findings. Order for blood glucose obtained. BG result 62 mg/dl via finger stick. Provider notified. Patient given orange juice with 2 packets of sugar added. Provider notified of findings. Patient teaching re: diabetic management per providers orders reinforced. Good understanding demonstrated by return verbalization. N. McFarland, RMA (AMT)

Vascular Events

Patients sometimes present in the outpatient setting with evolving vascular events that are true emergencies. Many patients may confuse what it means to suffer a stroke or heart attack because they are unclear regarding the anatomy involved, but public education has improved in recent years to encourage rapid recognition of symptoms and treatment plans to limit the damage caused by either of these physiologic vascular events. See Table 8-9 for more information in the symptoms, causes, and treatment of vascular events.

BREATHING EMERGENCIES AND CARDIAC ARREST

Breathing or respiratory emergencies occur for a variety of reasons, including choking, shock, allergies, and other illnesses or injuries such as drowning and electrical shock. When an individual stops breathing, artificial or rescue breathing must be given quickly, for without a constant supply of oxygen, brain damage or death will occur.

When the breathing problem is accompanied by cardiac arrest, the rescue breathing must be accompanied by chest compressions. This procedure is known as **cardiopulmonary resuscitation (CPR)**. Cardiac emergencies may occur in the medical clinic because of the large number of patients who have heart disease.

In order to graduate from a CAAHEP-accredited program, medical assistants must attain provider-level CPR certification and take first aid training courses. Frequent refresher courses and recertification in CPR are necessary.

TABLE 8-9

VASCULAR EVENTS

EVENT	SYMPTOMS	CAUSE	TREATMENT
Cerebral vascular accident (CVA) or stroke	Numbness in face and extremities on one side of the body Loss of vision Severe headache Confusion Slurred speech Nausea and vomiting Shortness of breath Difficulty swallowing Paralysis	Rupture or **occlusion** of vessel in the brain interrupting blood flow to brain cells, resulting in cellular death	Activate EMS Assist patient in lying down with head turned to side to manage oral fluids Provide comfort measures Maintain airway Allow no food or drink Monitor vital signs Follow provider's orders for medication administration
Myocardial infarction (MI) or heart attack	Chest tightness or pain Pain radiating down one or both arms Pain radiating to left shoulder or jaw Rapid, weak pulse Excessive perspiration Agitation Nausea Cold, clammy skin Women may have: • Abdominal discomfort • Burning sensation in chest • Discomfort or pain in lower chest or back • Sudden fatigue • Sweating • Breathlessness	Interruption in blood flow to the cardiac muscle, resulting in lack of oxygen to tissues and cell death	Activate EMS Obtain crash cart Follow provider's orders to apply oxygen and administer aspirin and other medications Attach to cardiac monitor Monitor vital signs Assist provider with **cardioversion** or defibrillation using an automated external defibrillator (AED) Begin CPR if indicated

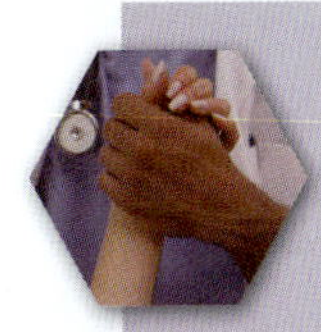

Patient Education

Lay Person CPR

- The person does not need to be certified.
- Chest compressions alone are sufficient.
- Patients are more likely to survive without brain damage with only chest compressions.
- Use 30 compressions per minute to keep blood moving to brain and heart.
- Drowning victims and smoke inhalation victims are the exception. Both need rescue breathing and CPR.

Rescue Breathing

Individuals in respiratory arrest require immediate emergency care. **Rescue breathing**, previously called mouth-to-mouth resuscitation, provides oxygen to the patient until emergency personnel arrive.

When performing rescue breathing procedures in the ambulatory care setting, it is recommended that resuscitation mouthpieces be used and that direct mouth-to-mouth (i.e., with no personal protective equipment) resuscitation never be used.

Cardiopulmonary Resuscitation

The combination of rescue breathing and chest compressions is known as CPR. Alone, CPR cannot save an individual from cardiac arrest—it represents preliminary care until advanced medical help is available to the heart attack victim.

In 2015, the American Heart Association (AHA) updated its emergency care guidelines for CPR and emergency cardiovascular care (ECC). (To review these guidelines, go to www.heart.org and search for "2015 CPR Guidelines.") The new guidelines recommend immediately beginning chest compressions rather than first opening the airway and beginning ventilations. A change in the ABC methodology to CAB was instituted in 2010 and remains the order for initiating CPR for the unresponsive patient. This change reflects the understanding that patients in cardiac arrest benefit from the return to blood flow as soon as possible. An emphasis has been placed on high-quality CPR, with chest compressions of adequate rate and depth, allowing complete chest recoil after each compression, minimizing interruptions in the compressions, and avoiding excessive ventilation.

Studies have found that if bystanders act as quickly as possible and begin CPR, many more victims could be saved. It was determined that CPR plus a shock with an AED (Figure 8-10) is the most effective immediate treatment for cardiac arrest. The AHA says that early recognition of the emergency, calling EMS, and performing immediate CPR can double or triple a victim's chances of surviving. Furthermore, the AHA says that CPR plus defibrillation (AED) started within 3 to 5 minutes of collapse can boost survival significantly. Lay rescuer AEDs are available in airports, sports facilities, airplanes, casinos, and many other locations. AEDs are becoming more readily available, are easy to use, and are very accurate. The current guidelines suggest that an AED be utilized immediately for a witnessed arrest.

The 2015 guidelines have changed the number of compressions per minute to between 100 and 120 from *at least* 100. The depth of compressions recommended is at least 2 inches. The look, listen, and feel method has been replaced by visually scanning the victim's chest for rise and fall for a period of time no longer than 10 seconds. AHA guidelines stress that compressions should begin immediately, prior to initiating rescue breathing. Table 8-10 summarizes the AHA's 2015 guidelines for CPR and defibrillation.

Immediate recognition and activation of the emergency response system once the health care provider identifies the adult victim who is unresponsive as having no breathing or no normal breathing (i.e., only gasping) is called for. Once no normal

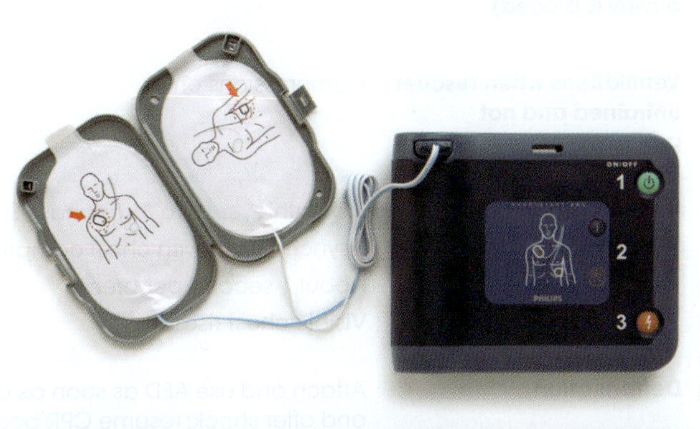

FIGURE 8-10 Automated external defibrillator.

Courtesy of Philips Healthcare

TABLE 8-10

SUMMARY OF THE AMERICAN HEART ASSOCIATION'S 2015 HIGH-QUALITY CPR GUIDELINES

COMPONENT	RECOMMENDATIONS		
Scene safety	Ensure the environment is safe for victim and rescuers.		
Recognition of cardiac arrest	Check for responsiveness No breathing or only gasping (no normal breathing) No definite pulse felt within 10 seconds (breathing and pulse check can be performed simultaneously within 10 seconds)		
Activation of EMS	**Adults and adolescents:** If you are alone and do not have a mobile phone, leave victim to activate EMS and obtain AED, and then begin CPR. If there is a second rescuer, send him or her to activate EMS and obtain the AED while you begin CPR.	**Infants and children, witnessed collapse:** Follow steps for adult and adolescent resuscitation. **Unwitnessed collapse:** Administer CPR for 2 minutes. Leave the victim to activate EMS and obtain the AED. Return to the child or infant to resume CPR, and use the AED as soon as it is available.	
CPR sequence	CAB		
Compression rate	100 to 120 per minute		
Compression depth	**Adult:** At least 2 inches (5 cm)	**Child:** At least ⅓ AP diameter About 2 inches (5 cm)	**Infant:** At least ⅓ AP diameter About 1½ inches (4 cm)
Hand placement	**Adult:** Two hands on the lower half of the sternum	**Child:** Two hands or one hand for small child on lower half of the sternum	**Infant:** Two fingers in the center of the chest (one rescuer) just below the nipple line Circle chest with hands and place two thumbs in the center of the chest, just above the nipple line (two rescuer).
Chest wall recoil	Allow complete recoil between compressions HCPs rotate compressors every 2 minutes		
Compression interruptions	Minimize interruptions in chest compressions Attempt to limit interruptions to < 10 seconds		
Airway	Head tilt-chin lift (HCP suspected trauma: jaw thrust)		
Compression-to-ventilation ratio (until advanced airway is placed)	**Adult:** 30:2, 1 or 2 rescuers	**Infants and Children:** 30:2 single rescuer 15:2 two rescuers	
Ventilations when rescuer untrained and not proficient	Compressions only		
Ventilations with advanced airway (HCP)	1 breath every 6 to 8 seconds (8 to 10 breaths/min) Asynchronous with chest compressions About 1 second per breath Visible chest rise		
Defibrillation	Attach and use AED as soon as available. Minimize interruptions in chest compressions before and after shock; resume CPR beginning with compressions immediately after each shock.		

AED, automated external defibrillator; AP, anterior-posterior; CPR, cardiopulmonary resuscitation; HCP, health care provider

*Excluding the newly born, in whom the cause of an arrest is nearly always asphyxia.

breathing has been identified, the provider then activates EMS and retrieves the AED (or sends someone to do so). Compressions should begin at this time.

More information is available from the following sources:

- American Heart Association (http://www.americanheart.org)
- American Red Cross (http://www.redcross.org)
- National Safety Council (http://www.nsc.org)
- National Institutes of Health (http://www.health.nih.gov)

Hands-Only CPR. The AHA recommends that if you witness an adult or teen suddenly collapse, call 911 and then push hard and fast in the center of the victim's chest. Further, the AHA recommends compression to the beat of the classic disco song *Stayin' Alive.* CPR can more than double a person's chances of survival, and *Stayin' Alive* has the right beat for hands-only CPR.

Once 911 has been called, you need to stay on the phone until the 911 dispatcher (operator) tells you to hang up. The dispatcher will obtain information about the type of emergency and your location. Try to be as specific as possible. This type of resuscitation is appropriate for "in the field" resuscitation in the absence of other trained personnel and emergency equipment.

SAFETY AND EMERGENCY PRACTICES

The Commission on Accreditation of Allied Health Programs (CAAHEP) believes allied health students should understand how to respond in an emergency situation, as health care professionals and citizens. Medical assistant programs accredited by CAAHEP have within their Standards and Guidelines a section requiring education regarding safety and emergency practices. Provider-level CPR and basic first aid are part of these requirements for graduation.

The Accrediting Bureau of Health Education Schools (ABHES) also has a requirement in its competencies under the heading of Medical Office Clinical Procedures.

Health professionals recognize an obligation to use their skills and knowledge in a disaster environment.

There are many kinds of mass disasters, natural and manmade. Some examples are floods, hurricanes, tornadoes, tsunamis, and earthquakes. Others are explosions, structural collapses (e.g., the 2011 Indiana State Fair stage collapse), transportation accidents, bioterrorism.

What would a large-scale disaster be like, and how could we respond? Disasters can threaten public health and safety; disrupt services (e.g., gas, water, electricity, transportation); destroy roads, bridges, homes, and other buildings; and make food and water unsafe or impossible to obtain. Law enforcement, fire departments, hospitals, and military all could be affected. There is a need for collaboration between disaster experts and health professionals to plan for emergencies.

What can medical assistants do to help? How could you use your skills without technology (i.e., if it were unavailable due to the disaster)? Some examples are assisting your neighbors at local shelters, using your first aid and CPR skills, helping out at a clinic, giving injections for mass immunizations, supporting overwhelmed providers, working with the American Red Cross, giving emotional support, and filling in at a hospital.

Competency

In addition to mass disasters, medical assistants should be prepared to respond to emergency situations in the medical clinic or a home environment. Circumstances in which a patient goes into shock, an elderly family member has a fall, or a medical clinic needs to be evacuated for a fire are examples of such emergency situations.

Medical assisting curricula may include related courses to be certain that medical assisting graduates are prepared to help during emergency situations.

In 2002, President George W. Bush asked for teams of volunteers of medical and health professionals to contribute their skills during times of need in their communities. The Medical Reserve Corps (MRC) was established (http://www.medicalreservecorps.gov), and the teams of volunteers within the MRC work with Health and Human Services of the U.S. government and the American Red Cross. The MRC is community based. Its goal is to organize and use volunteers who want to donate their time and expertise to respond to emergencies and to promote healthy living throughout the year. The MRC supplements existing emergency and public health resources. Volunteers include providers, nurses, respiratory care therapists, massage therapists, pharmacists, dentists, and a wide array of allied health professionals such as medical assistants.

The MRC volunteer units are assigned to specific geographic areas. They work with and support county and state public health departments. The main office is in the surgeon general's office in Washington, D.C.

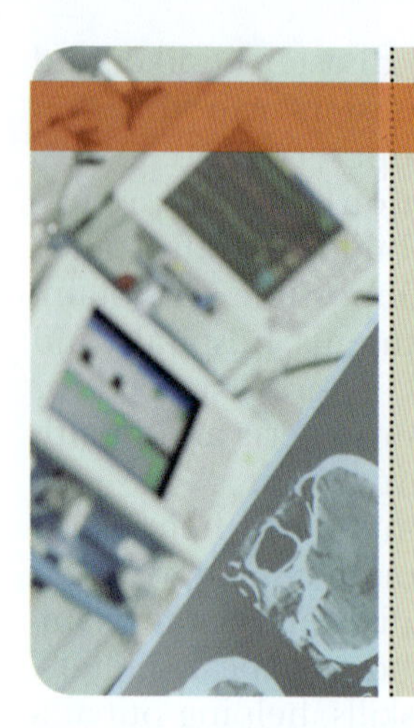

CASE STUDY 8-1

Refer to the scenario at the beginning of the chapter.

CASE STUDY REVIEW

1. Because Mr. Cochran is exhibiting symptoms of having a cardiac event, what are the first measures to be taken?
2. Why is it essential to activate EMS even though Mr. Cochran is being seen in an ambulatory care setting?
3. What questions should Nancy McFarland, RMA (AMT), ask Mr. Cochran?
4. What would be the next steps after assessing the patient if the chest pain continued and the patient lost consciousness prior to the arrival of EMS?

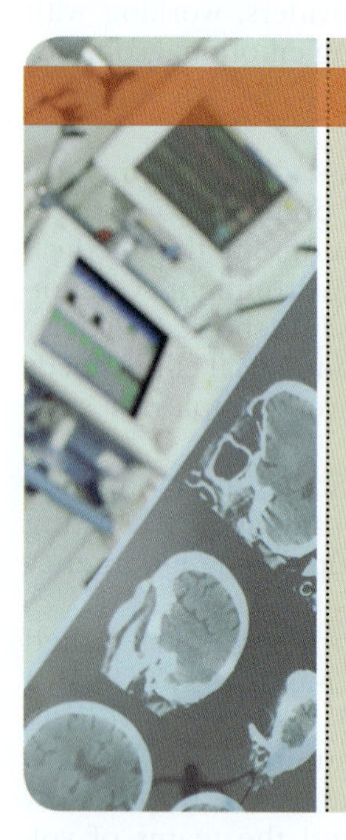

CASE STUDY 8-2

Carlette Jennings, a regular patient at Inner City Health Care, is walking her dog one morning and stops to rest on a grassy knoll, where she notices a wasp on her arm. She brushes it away, unthinking, and then realizes it has stung her. She receives two more stings and suddenly notices she is at a nest site. Carlette is now a half-hour walk from home but is not really concerned because she has never had an allergic reaction to a wasp sting. However, a few minutes after she resume walking, her palms become itchy, her ears start to burn, and she feels lightheaded. She is not having difficulty breathing. She is determined to get home and she does, at which point she notices she is covered with hives. She calls Inner City Health Care to ask whether she should come in.

CASE STUDY REVIEW

1. Joe Guerrero, CMA (AAMA), is screening calls the morning that Carlette is stung. What questions should he ask Carlette?
2. Because Carlette obviously is having a hypersensitive or an allergic reaction, she is advised to seek emergency care immediately. What first aid measures might be taken?
3. To prevent reactions to stings in the future, what patient teaching might be appropriate for Carlette?

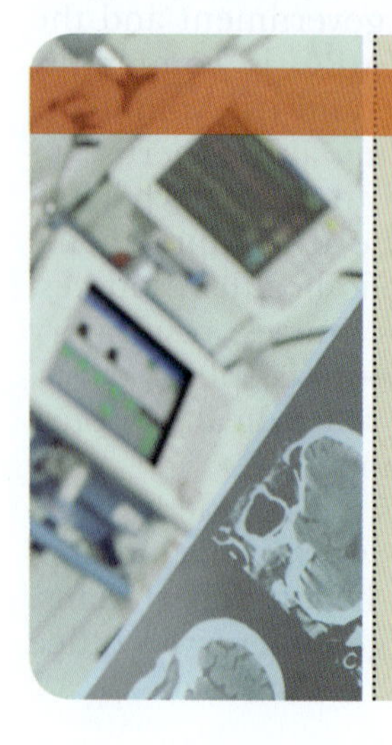

CASE STUDY 8-3

Bryan Mountjoy is a 32-year-old patient of Dr. Osborne. He has been working in the yard throughout the day, even though the temperature was over 100°F. Being so focused on the job at hand, Mr. Mountjoy has not taken in enough fluids over the course of the day. He calls out to his wife that he is feeling faint. She finds him with reddened, dry, hot skin; shallow, fast breathing; and a weak pulse. Mrs. Mountjoy calls the clinic seeking medical advice.

CASE STUDY REVIEW

1. What immediate questions should you ask Mrs. Mountjoy?
2. What would you advise Mrs. Mountjoy to do in order to receive the most appropriate level of care?
3. If Mrs. Mountjoy expresses panic, how could you help her to remain calm?

Summary

- It is crucial to be able to quickly recognize and begin intervention when an emergency occurs. These emergency situations may range from minor to severe.
- Appropriate action begins with assessment. This assessment begins with Circulation, Airway, and Breathing (CAB) as a priority.
- Response to emergencies depends on the ability to recognize an emergency immediately; being prepared to respond; knowledge of the EMS system and its activation; familiarity with the crash cart and the items that it contains; knowledge of the causes, symptoms, and treatment of the most common emergencies; CPR and AED training; and staff continuing education and certification in CPR.
- The professional medical assistant must be aware of the symptoms and treatment of common emergencies. Recognition of the various types of shock (cardiogenic, hypovolemic, neurogenic, anaphylactic, septic, and respiratory) allows early intervention to prevent an irreversible condition.
- Wounds are seen frequently in the clinic setting. Knowledge of how to provide first aid for closed and open wounds, how and when to apply a tourniquet, as well as the application of dressings are key components of the provision of first aid.
- Burns are classified as first-, second-, and third-degree burns. The physical presentation and treatment of each vary related to the degree of tissue injury.
- Orthopedic injuries include strains and sprains, as well as fractures. The goal of first aid practices is to immobilize the injured extremity to prevent further injury until radiologic evaluation and definitive treatment can be performed.
- Exposure to extreme heat or cold can be life threatening. Rapid initiation of first aid can prevent death, especially in the very young or older persons.
- Poisoning is a serious and potentially life-threatening emergency. Memorize the national Poison Control Center's phone number (1-800-222-1222).
- Other sudden illnesses such as fainting, seizures, hemorrhage, and diabetic reactions have a rapid onset and have interventions that are easy to implement. The awareness of the need to ensure the patient's safety and the knowledge of the actions that will resolve the underlying issue is the responsibility of all members of the health care team.
- Symptoms of CVA or stroke and myocardial infarction or heart attack indicate activation of EMS.
- Maintaining professional CPR certification will allow the medical assistant to recognized and initiate care for myocardial infarction.

Study for Success

To reinforce your knowledge and skills of information presented in this chapter:

- Review the *Key Terms* and *Learning Outcomes*
- Consider the *Critical Thinking* features and *Case Studies* and discuss your conclusions
- Answer the questions in the *Certification Review*

Procedure

- Perform the *Procedures* using the *Competency Assessment Checklists* on the *Student Companion Website*

CERTIFICATION REVIEW

1. Which of the following is true regarding Good Samaritan laws?
   a. They are designed to protect the public.
   b. They protect non–health care professionals.
   c. They require that all individuals providing assistance act within the scope of their knowledge and training.
   d. They protect health care professionals on the job.
2. Which of the following defines an avulsion?
   a. The skin is torn off and bleeding is profuse.
   b. There is superficial scraping of the dermis.
   c. It is a tear of the body tissue.
   d. It describes a surgical incision.
   e. All of these
3. First-degree burns are most accurately described by which of the following statements?
   a. They are the most serious burns and penetrate all layers of skin.
   b. They affect only the top layer of skin.
   c. They often leave scar tissue.
   d. They usually take more than a month to heal.
4. According to current AHA CPR guidelines, what is the order of steps for cardiopulmonary resuscitation?
   a. Airway, breathing, compressions
   b. Breathing, compressions, airway
   c. Compressions, airway, breathing
   d. Any of the steps can come first, as long as blood begins to circulate within 18 seconds
   e. None of these
5. A fracture in which the bone protrudes through the skin is called what?
   a. Greenstick fracture
   b. Compound fracture
   c. Depressed fracture
   d. Comminuted fracture
6. To control a nosebleed, it is important to take which of the following actions?
   a. Have the patient lie down
   b. Tilt the patient's head back
   c. Tilt the patient's head forward
   d. Call 911 immediately
   e. All of these
7. Which of the following is another name for a heart attack?
   a. Cerebral vascular accident
   b. Angina pectoris
   c. Myocardial infarction
   d. Stroke
8. Which of the following is the correct depth of compressions when administering CPR for adults?
   a. 1 inch
   b. 1.5 inches
   c. 2 inches
   d. 2.5 inches
   e. 3 inches
9. Exposure to extreme cold for prolonged periods can cause which of the following?
   a. Hypothermia
   b. Hyperthermia
   c. Frostbite
   d. Both a and c
10. Septic shock results from which of the following?
    a. A severe allergic reaction
    b. Overwhelming infection
    c. Trauma to the respiratory system
    d. Extreme loss of blood
    e. Hypothermia

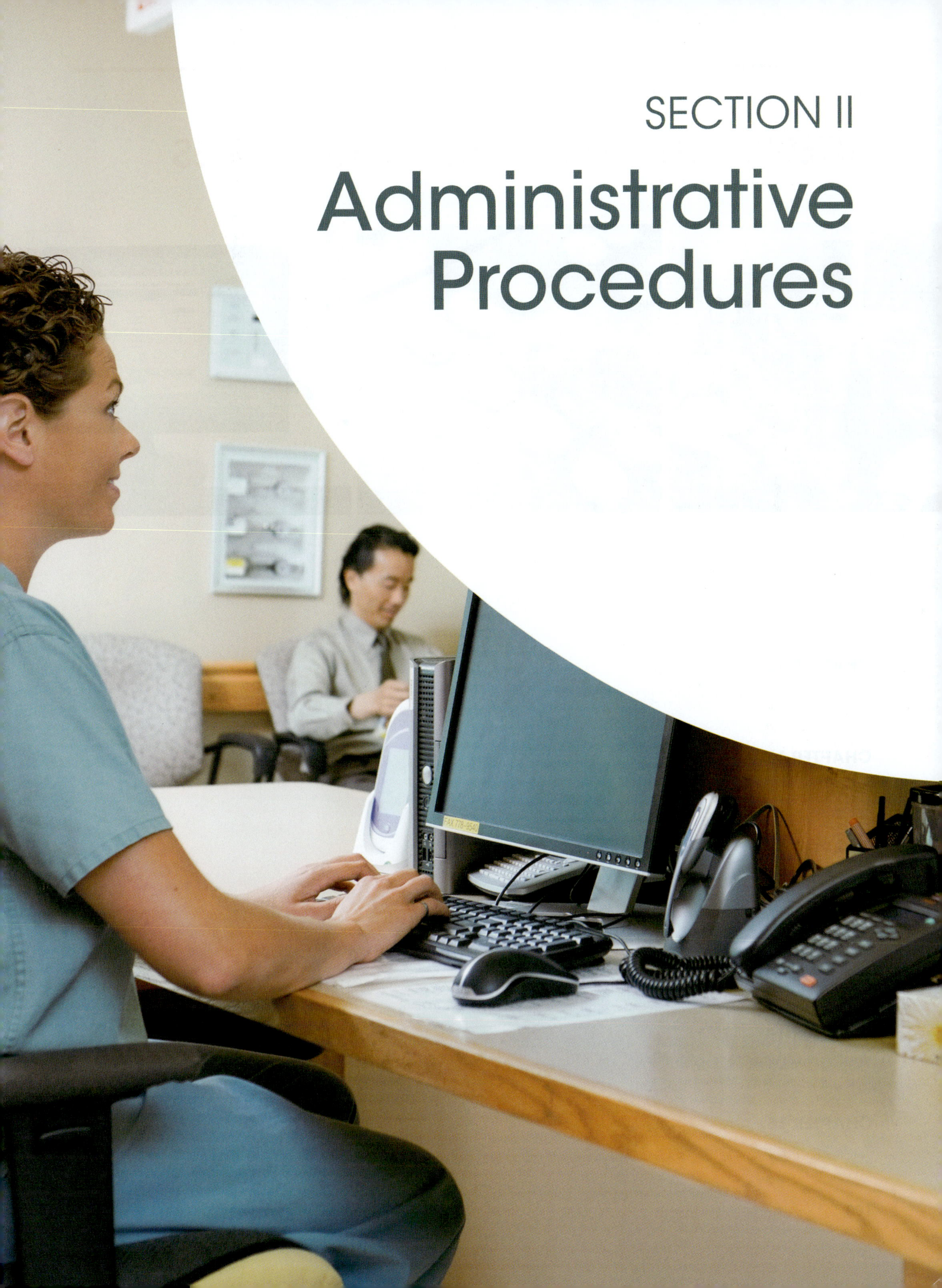

SECTION II
Administrative Procedures

UNIT IV

INTEGRATED ADMINISTRATIVE PROCEDURES

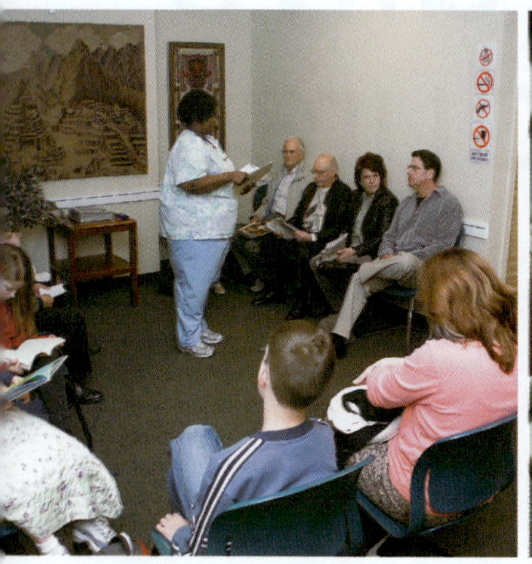

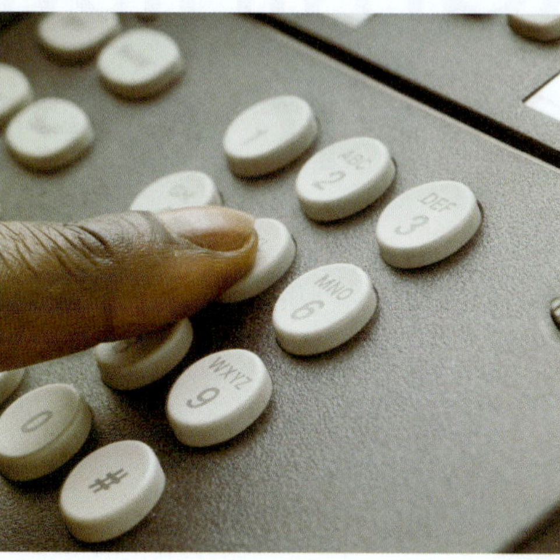

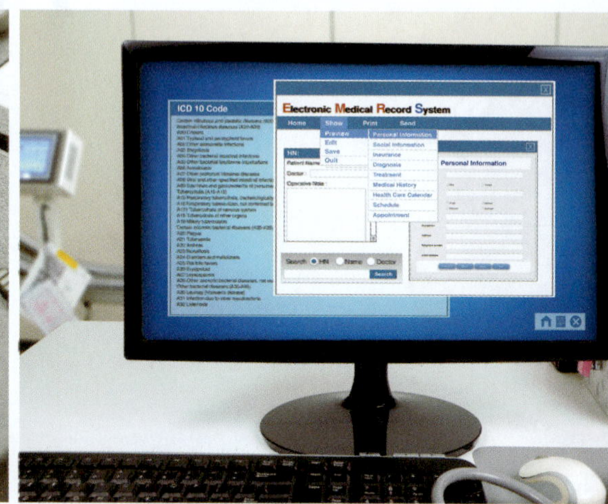

ATTRIBUTES OF PROFESSIONALISM

Medical assistants convey a great deal to patients through attitude and actions as well as empathy. A hurried or disinterested manner communicates that the patient is not a priority. Patients do not easily forget rude or insensitive staff. A hurried, disinterested manner toward patients is just as often the basis for legal action as is a negligent act.

The patient should always be made to feel worthy of attention. This validates his or her reason for calling. If you are scheduling a patient in the clinic and the phone rings, answer the call but excuse yourself first. Ask the caller to please hold for a moment. If you are on the telephone scheduling a patient and another patient walks in, acknowledge with a nod or signal that you will be right there—never let the person feel ignored. Today, patients have a variety of options for health care and tend to be much more consumer conscious of the treatment they receive.

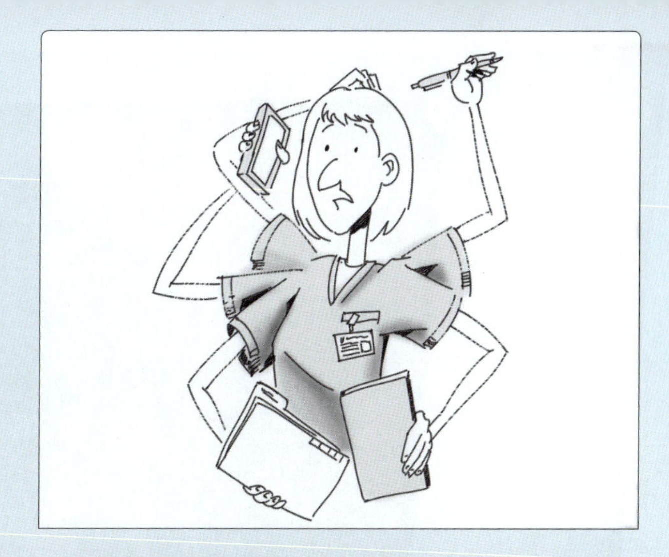

Listed below are a series of questions for you to ask yourself, to serve as a professionalism checklist. As you interact with patients and colleagues, these questions will help to guide you in the professional behavior that is expected every day from medical assistants.

Ask Yourself

COMMUNICATION

- ☐ Do I apply active listening skills?
- ☐ Do I display professionalism through written and verbal communication?
- ☐ Do I explain to patients the rationale for performance of a procedure?
- ☐ Do I speak at each patient's level of understanding?
- ☐ Do I respond honestly and diplomatically to my patients' concerns?
- ☐ Does my knowledge allow me to speak easily with all members of the health care team?
- ☐ Do I accurately and concisely update the provider on any aspect of a patient's care?

PRESENTATION

- ☐ Am I courteous, patient, and respectful to patients?
- ☐ Do I display a positive attitude?
- ☐ Do I display a calm, professional, and caring manner?
- ☐ Do I demonstrate empathy to the patient?
- ☐ Do I display sensitivity when managing appointments?

COMPETENCY

- ☐ Do I pay attention to detail?
- ☐ Do I ask questions if I am out of my comfort zone or do not have the experience to carry out tasks?
- ☐ Do I display sound judgment?
- ☐ Am I knowledgeable and accountable?
- ☐ Do I recognize the physical and emotional effects on persons involved in an emergency situation?
- ☐ Do I demonstrate self-awareness in responding to an emergency situation?

INITIATIVE

- ☐ Do I show initiative?
- ☐ Am I flexible and dependable?
- ☐ Do I direct the patient to other resources when necessary or helpful, with the approval of the provider?
- ☐ Do I implement time management principles to maintain effective office functioning?
- ☐ Do I assist co-workers when appropriate?
- ☐ Do I make adaptations for patients with special needs?

INTEGRITY

- ☐ Do I work within my scope of practice?
- ☐ Do I demonstrate respect for individual diversity?
- ☐ Do I demonstrate sensitivity to patient rights?
- ☐ Do I protect the integrity of the medical record?
- ☐ Do I protect and maintain confidentiality?
- ☐ Do I immediately report any error I make?
- ☐ Do I do the "right thing" even when no one is observing?

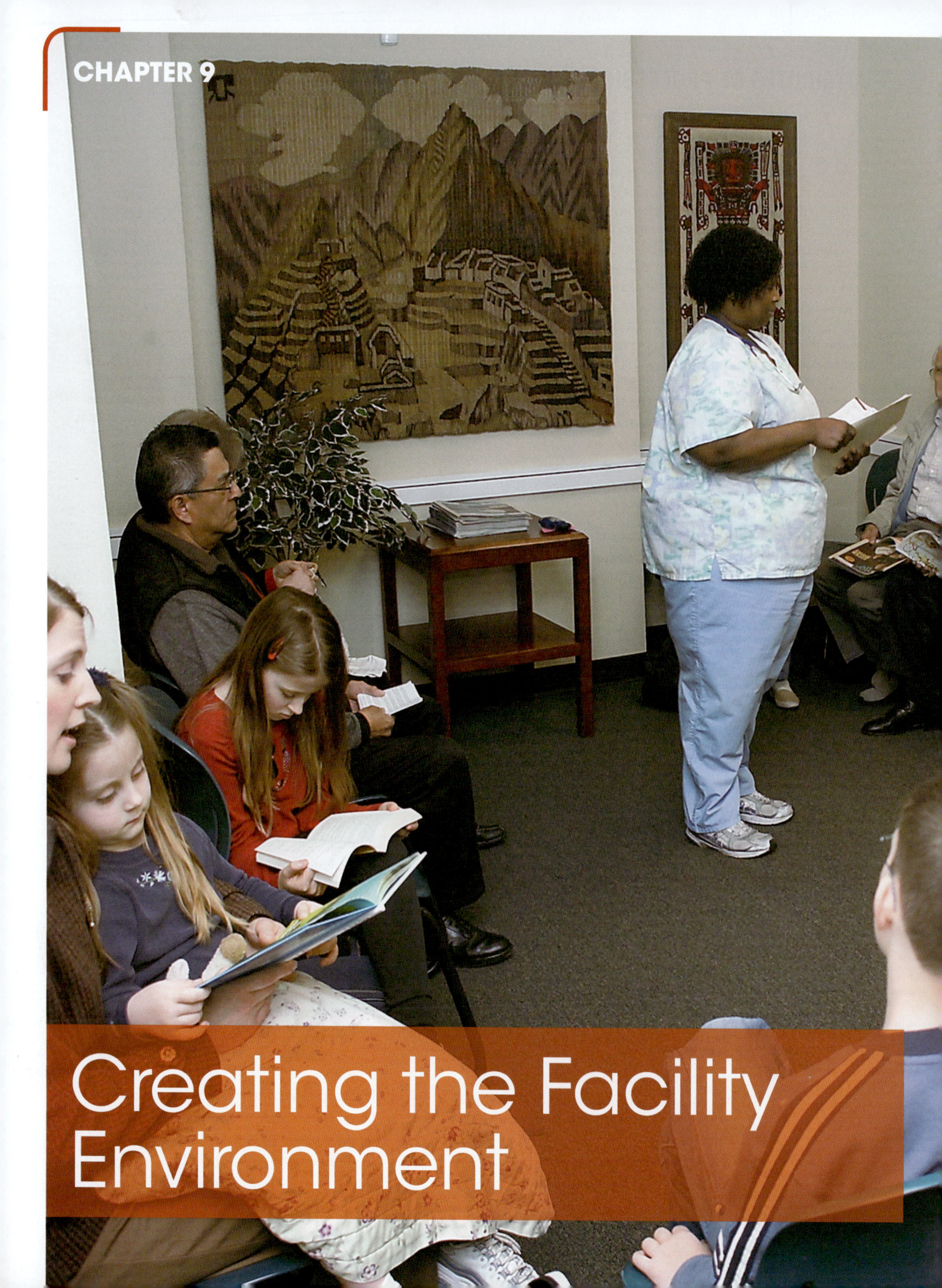

CHAPTER 9

Creating the Facility Environment

LEARNING OUTCOMES

1. Define and spell the key terms as presented in the glossary.
2. Illustrate a comfortable, welcoming, and pleasing reception area.
3. Demonstrate important personality characteristics the receptionist should possess.
4. Determine cultural aspects to consider in the reception area.
5. Discuss the needs of children in the reception area.
6. Identify how the reception area can be used for educational purposes.
7. Explain the benefits of lighting, music, color, nature, and water in a facility.
8. Interpret the role of HIPAA in patient privacy and the facility environment.
9. Determine the number of patients a reception area should accommodate.
10. Recall essential elements of the Americans with Disabilities Act.
11. Evaluate the facility for safety and emergency preparedness.
12. Develop a personal and patient safety plan.
13. Explain the components of an evacuation plan for a provider's clinic.
14. Demonstrate proper use of a fire extinguisher.
15. Review steps to take in case of a natural disaster.
16. Outline the role of the medical assistant in emergency preparedness.
17. List at least three tasks to perform when opening and closing the facility.
18. Outline characteristics of future ambulatory and outpatient health care environments.

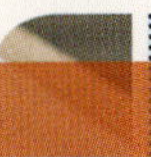
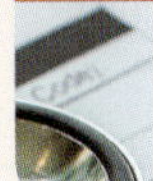

KEY TERMS

RACE
reception

SCENARIO

The design of any ambulatory setting often evolves as the needs of the clinic and patients change. At Inner City Health Care, a multiprovider family practice, the environment has always been warm and welcoming, which is particularly important because the providers see many children. However, the clinic was initially designed in the early 1980s, before the Americans with Disabilities Act (ADA) was passed by the U.S. Congress.

Once this act was passed in 1990, the clinic manager was aware of the need to comply with its mandates. In addition, the providers wanted to make all their patients, including those with disabilities, as comfortable as possible. Working with a local architect, changes were incorporated into the practice's existing space: A ramp was added outside, doorways were widened to provide wheelchair access, and new Braille signage was installed outside for patients with visual impairments. Although the changes were not without expense, the staff at Inner City Health Care willingly complied with the ADA not only because it is law but because it gave more patients better access.

More recently, while making certain the clinic protocol was in compliance with the Health Insurance Portability and Accountability Act of 1996 (HIPAA), the clinic staff took another look at the facility to ensure it was favorable in light of protecting patient confidentiality. They discovered that the reception area was seriously lacking in providing privacy and confidentiality for patient information and the entire clinic needed serious updating in many other aspects.

Chapter Portal

The environment of the medical facility contributes almost as much to a patient's well-being as does the medical attention given by providers and their medical assistants. The physical environment can foster a feeling that embraces and welcomes patients or, conversely, can cause them to feel alienated and intimidated. Numerous recent studies reveal that the physical environment of a clinic is linked to the comfort of both patient and staff. In fact, such "evidence-based design" can lead to reduced noise, improved lighting, better ventilation, and ergonomic designs with supportive work spaces and improved layout in medical clinics. These design changes make clinics safer, promote healing, lead to fewer errors on the part of staff, and reduce patients' pain and discomfort.

Dental providers have set a trend in the field of health care design. Dentists recognize that few individuals enjoy visiting the dentist and know that their patients expect to feel discomfort, pain, and extended-length procedures that are stressful. Dentists also realize that about one-fourth of the country's population refuses to see a dentist for any reason because of fear of pain and discomfort. In order to lessen patients' anxiety and to encourage patients to return on a regular basis for dental care, many dentists have turned to "spa-like" dental environments.

In this environment, patients can recline in heated chairs, are given blankets for their legs, can listen to soothing music, or may be given video headsets to watch their favorite television programs. The idea behind the entire spa-like environment is to make patients feel comfortable with their dental procedures and want to return.

Does this sound like the future of medical clinic design? Probably not, but careful observation and comparison will reveal an increasing number of medical clinics seeking to attract patients not only via high-quality medical care but also with attention to detail that creates an atmosphere conducive to comfort, confidentiality, safety, and healing. Medical providers understand that their best advertisement is a good word from patients who have had positive experiences during their medical care encounters. Closer attention to the clinic's environment and patients' personal needs might be more welcomed by patients who are not feeling well, suffering from a chronic illness, or facing a life-threatening disease.

Interior designers and experts who specialize in medical space planning advise all individuals involved in designing clinics and hospitals that patient comfort must be considered to be as important as the facility's functional utility and ease of maintenance.

CREATING A WELCOMING ENVIRONMENT

Presentation

In today's health care atmosphere, in which limited resources are being continually challenged and there are still individuals without sufficient resources to obtain proper medical care, creating a welcoming environment is essential. Creative and astute designers will tell you to consider the following concepts in fostering such an environment:

- Embrace warmth in design and in personnel
- Hide the health care's "scary" pieces from patients' view
- Create good acoustics
- Provide access to nature
- Promote health and healing
- Feed the soul

The creation of a health care facility involves many variables. Some are tangible elements, such as lighting, color choice, and furniture arrangement. Others are intangible and are expressed ways such as an administrative medical assistant's greeting and attitude toward patients. Important components of patient satisfaction are a warm and caring staff, comfortable surroundings, and the ability of patients and visitors to find their way around the medical clinic without getting lost. Convenience of access and privacy are essential. The ADA (see Chapter 6) also must be taken into account when creating any medical clinic environment by making provisions to accommodate patients who have physical challenges. HIPAA regulations (see Chapter 6) specify how a patient's privacy and confidentiality are to be protected and may also dictate medical clinic space planning. Finally, an environment that demonstrates attention to safety, the prevention of hazards, and effective response to emergency situations further enhances patient and even employee satisfaction. Together, all these elements help make an ambulatory setting the kind of environment where patients will feel comfortable and secure.

THE RECEPTION AREA

A **reception** area is just that—a place of reception. It should never be thought of as "the waiting room." The reception area is the area first viewed by the patient and this is the first opportunity to make the patient feel welcome, secure, and comfortable. First impressions are lasting. Adequate and comfortable seating, consideration for patients of all ages, proper lighting and ventilation, the use of color, noise reduction, and the influence of nature are all aspects to consider in creating the clinic environment and engaging the senses.

Space planners who specialize in medical clinics and hospitals and who have spent many hours analyzing patient flow indicate that the reception area should accommodate at least an hour's patients per provider plus a friend or relative who may accompany each patient. Another quick rule of thumb to use is 2.5 seats in the reception area for each examination room. Clinics where providers see patients without advance appointments will, of course, need a larger reception area.

Depending on the ambulatory care setting's clientele, consider the following items to help ease patients' time in any area where waiting is essential (e.g., pending laboratory results) and help take their minds off current medical problems: a table and chairs with a puzzle in progress, Internet access for busy patients attempting to work while waiting, an electronic Sudoku board, or a juice bar. Although these items are not appropriate in every setting, they certainly can be in some (refer to Case Study 9-2).

It is helpful if there is a place for patients to hang heavy coats or wet umbrellas. Accessories and artwork can easily add a special touch to a facility. Nature pictures elicit a more favorable response from patients than abstract art. Although fresh flowers might be a nice touch, they harbor microorganisms, and some patients are allergic to them. There is the tendency to use living plants in medical facilities, but silk plants and flowers also may be appropriate.

Even when the office or clinic is housed in an older building not originally constructed as a medical facility, much can be done to create an environment that enhances patient comfort. Remember to see things from the patient's point of view. If the facility is a maze of corridors where patients can easily get turned around, make certain that directions are clear and that directional signage is easily understood.

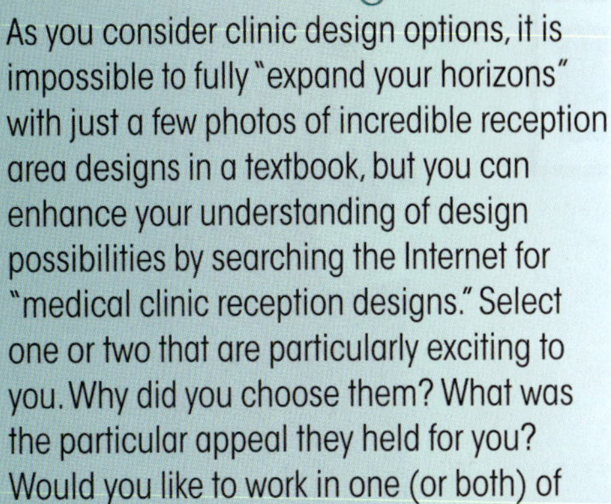

Critical Thinking

As you consider clinic design options, it is impossible to fully "expand your horizons" with just a few photos of incredible reception area designs in a textbook, but you can enhance your understanding of design possibilities by searching the Internet for "medical clinic reception designs." Select one or two that are particularly exciting to you. Why did you choose them? What was the particular appeal they held for you? Would you like to work in one (or both) of them? Justify your response.

It is worth the investment to have a professional designer who specializes in medical space planning look through the facility to make suggestions regarding color, artwork, and the general environment of the entire clinic. A designer considers the flow of patients, staff, and information; understands the focus and nature of the work of the clinic; and carefully designs the space to ensure all encounters enhance privacy and confidentiality, communication, and personal connection. What may seem like an unnecessary operational expense can result in greater satisfaction for all patients.

The Receptionist

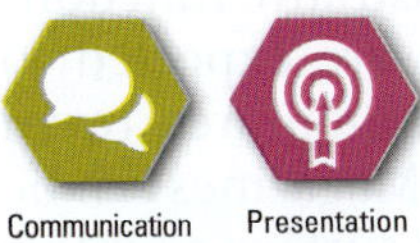

A receptionist who has a smile and genuinely friendly greeting for every patient, offers assistance, and carefully explains any waiting that might be necessary helps to create that desired reception environment. No matter how "rushed" the reception area may seem with patient activity and ringing telephones, the calm and reassuring attention of the receptionist helps set the stage for satisfied patients (Figure 9-1).

The receptionist must always keep a positive "We can help you" attitude, have a smile for each patient, and exude a genuine "We care about you" personality. This individual—who often has other duties as well—must be able to perform telephone prioritization, retrieve records, greet patients, present bills, make appointments, and log data into the computer, all the while remembering that each patient's comfort is of primary concern. All medical personnel, but especially the receptionist,

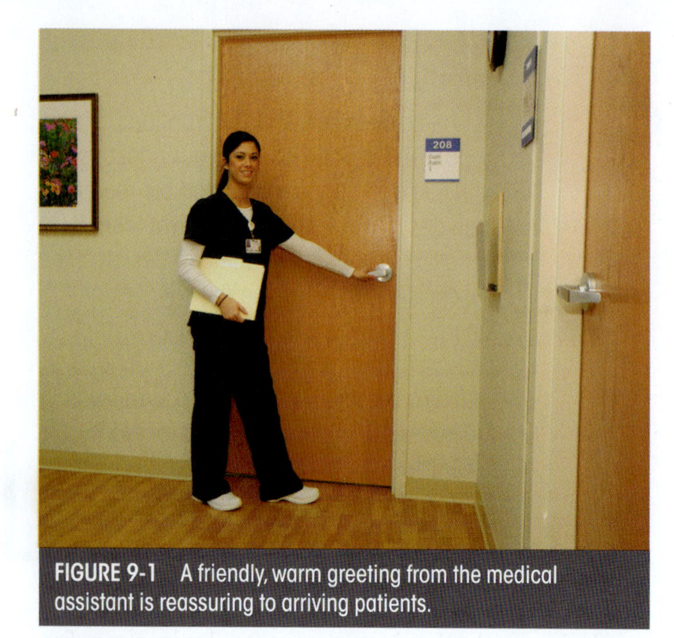

FIGURE 9-1 A friendly, warm greeting from the medical assistant is reassuring to arriving patients.

must genuinely like people and not react when patients are grumpy, irritable, or depressed and worried about an illness. Employees in the reception area of the clinic set the social climate for the interchange between patients and providers as well as the rest of the staff.

Patients who are very ill, injured, or upset should not have to wait in the reception area; rather, they should be shown to an examination room away from other patients where they can feel more comfortable. The receptionist may also have to help monitor children who may be intent on disrupting patients or whose parent is in the examination room.

Even with a number of administrative functions to accomplish, receptionists also are expected to maintain the tidiness of the reception area (even when the clinic closes for lunch). Magazines can be straightened, litter picked up, and surface counters attended to. Counters, table surfaces, and toys in medical clinics are among those most infested with microbes; therefore, they should be sanitized daily, or sometimes twice a day, especially when patients may have contagious diseases. Receptionists may be asked to remind patients that there are paper face masks in the reception area and instruct patients when they make their appointments to pick up a paper mask on arrival at the front door if they are experiencing a respiratory illness.

If there are unexpected delays in the provider's schedule, hopefully never more than 20 minutes, receptionists will notify patients of the delay tactfully and graciously and offer them the alternative of making other arrangements. The patient's time is as valuable as the provider's.

Cultural Considerations

Diversity

In consideration of cultural differences, there are some points to recall. Cultural sensitivity requires astute observation on the part of health care professionals. Keep in mind the following cultural views on health care:

- Middle Eastern and Latin cultures encourage closeness and touching, and individuals from these cultures may cluster themselves close together in the reception area.
- In general, no one likes to be touched by strangers. Cultural differences also impact the amount of space necessary for the reception area.
- In some cultures, patients are likely to bring several relatives with them to an appointment. This is especially common if the patient needs emotional support or a language interpreter. For example, Arabs, Jews, Mexicans, and Puerto Ricans tend to place greater emphasis on family care over self-care or professional care.
- Japanese patients often do not express feelings easily and expect health care professionals to make decisions about their health care, but are generally comfortable with physical closeness.
- Mexican patients believe that pain is to be endured and valued and rarely complain unless the pain keeps them from work.

Many people do not like to face other patients in the reception area and prefer anonymity. Culture aside, almost no one wants to be in close proximity to a stranger who appears to be contagious. Most are more comfortable in close quarters primarily with individuals of the same gender. Arabs may interact with health care professionals of only the same sex. While some patients are bothered by children, others find them to be a pleasant distraction. Adequate and comfortable seating affords patients their own space and respects these cultural preferences.

When Children are Patients

If the clinic treats children as patients or if children are apt to accompany adult patients, a children's area is especially helpful and appreciated. A special table and chairs for children, interactive toys (with emphasis on the interactive), and perhaps even a small television placed in a children's corner, can be provided. This area needs to be away from doors that swing or hazards on which children might be injured. A children's area should always be in sight of the administrative medical assistant or receptionist who may be charged with keeping order, especially if a parent must be seen unaccompanied by children in an examination room.

A pediatric facility that treats only children and youth might consider a particular theme for its design. Ocean murals and an aquarium are often used. Examination rooms may include examination tables designed to replicate a zoo animal. Staff in a pediatric clinic often wear bright-colored uniforms with animal prints, balloons, and similar motifs. The goal is to have much in the environment to keep children interested and enthused about their visit to the provider.

Education in the Reception Area

Many providers place appropriate educational materials for patients in the reception area. For example, new parents appreciate pamphlets related to raising children. If the provider is an ophthalmologist, the latest information on eye surgeries or new developments in contact lenses is likely to be seen in the reception area. It is also appropriate to have available in the reception area a patient information brochure that describes the services of the clinic, the function of medical staff members, measures to take in case of an emergency, and other issues that patients may need to consider (see Chapter 21 for more information on developing brochures for patient use). In some cases, the educational material may be presented in media form on a television screen.

CLINIC DESIGN AND ENVIRONMENT

Clinic environments are places where persons who are ill gather for support, diagnosis, treatment, and healing. There are a few very important factors that can make the environment more conducive to patient comfort. Some rooms in the facility, by their very nature, may cause patients to feel anxious. Recall the earlier recommendation to keep scary things out of sight. Consider a woman's discomfort when first seeing a gastroenterologist for a colonoscopy and viewing a large poster of the colonoscope on the wall. Reflect on a patient on an examination table who has on only a cloth or paper gown but must interact with the provider who is fully clothed, wearing a white lab coat and comfortably seated at a counter desk. The patient is at a disadvantage and may feel vulnerable in discussion and negotiation, contrary to the goal in medical care to empower the patient with as much control as possible (Figure 9-2).

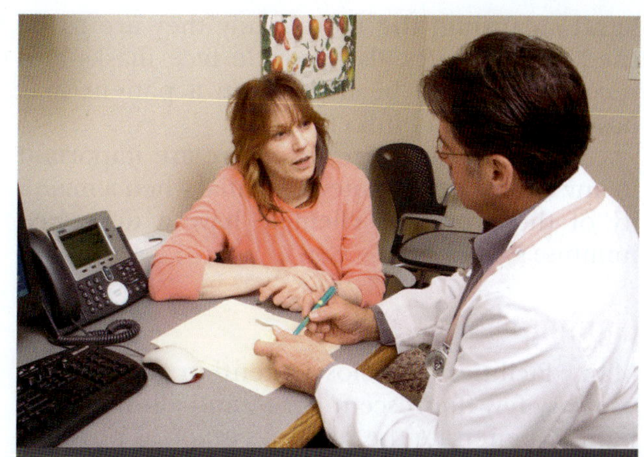

FIGURE 9-2 Patients are to be afforded as much dignity and empowerment as possible. Many patients feel more comfortable discussing conditions, treatments, or procedures face-to-face with the provider.

Ventilation and Infection Control

The risk of contracting infectious diseases due to airborne and surface contamination is high in any medical facility; therefore, proper ventilation and effective infection control measures are essential. Many patients will find offensive the common odors that can be present in a medical facility, even when the odors are from necessary antiseptics. Proper ventilation can alleviate this issue. Although ventilation systems are often overlooked in medical clinics, appropriate air filters (usually HEPA), airflow direction, and air pressure are critical elements in reducing airborne infection and are to be considered in the heating and air conditioning design of the facility.

Diligent surface cleaning and the use of alcohol-based hand-rub dispensers that are easily accessible will encourage recommended hand washing and reduce contact contamination. All areas of a clinic are susceptible to contamination and diligence is necessary to curb transmission. As noted earlier, the reception area is one of the most contaminated areas of the clinic—countertops where patients likely check in, computer keyboards, telephone ear pieces, common pens used for writing—all are examples of where microorganisms often grow and multiply. Statistics show that the easier the access to the hand-rub dispensers and sinks for hand cleansing, the more likely they are to be used Many clinics also provide face masks and recommend they be used when a patient may have a respiratory infection.

Such measures described here are important in any clinic but absolutely essential when a majority of the provider's clientele have a depressed immune system.

Lighting

Many facilities pay close attention to lighting, use very few fluorescent lights, and allow natural light to penetrate the rooms as much as possible. The use of natural light and images of nature or nature itself in the form of a garden, plants, and so on has shown to be very beneficial to both patients and staff. Sunlight is known to boost serotonin, which helps to lessen pain and depression. The goal is to provide as much peace and relaxation as possible to reduce stress and promote healing. A poorly illuminated room also may suggest poor housekeeping, dusty baseboards, soiled carpets, or faded draperies. Lighting can be soft and inviting while providing proper illumination. Note that fluorescent lighting is not used in the spaces shown in Figures 9-3 and 9-4. Ceiling can lights and lamps provide ample light for both the reception area and many of the work areas. Superior lighting in areas of any close examination, medication preparations, minor surgery, and so on helps to reduce the chance of errors.

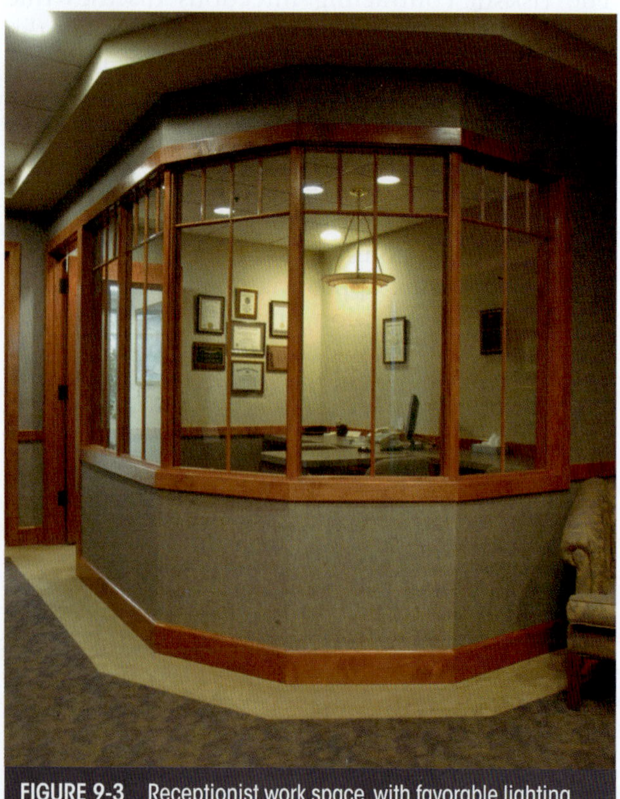

FIGURE 9-3 Receptionist work space, with favorable lighting, that provides privacy from conversations while offering a view of the entire reception area.

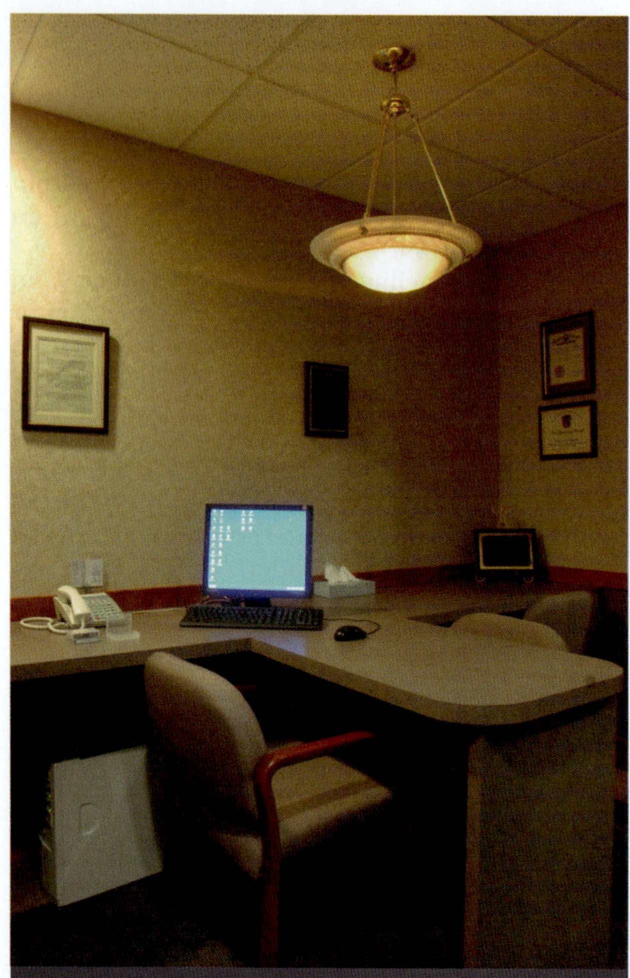

FIGURE 9-4 Small conference room adjacent to receptionist area where issues such as insurance coverage, financial arrangements, and surgical scheduling can be discussed.

Nature, Music, Water, and Color

Some clinics are designed with floor-to-ceiling windows throughout the clinic, especially in the reception area, that overlook a garden of plants, trees, and flowers as well as a waterfall or pool that attracts birds. A professionally maintained built-in aquarium can help to set a calming tone for clinic clientele. Other medical facilities are experimenting with the addition of music in their facilities. There is proof that certain melodious tunes and water sounds such as a babbling brook enhance healing. The use of these sounds

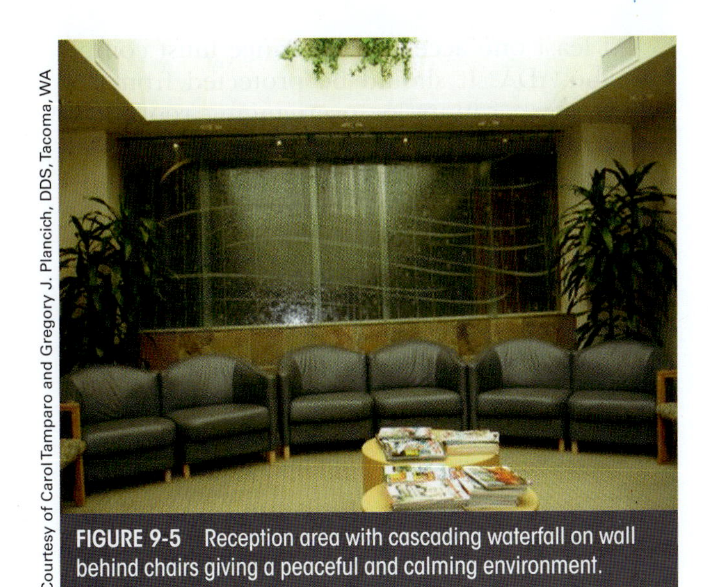

Courtesy of Carol Tamparo and Gregory J. Plancich, DDS, Tacoma, WA

FIGURE 9-5 Reception area with cascading waterfall on wall behind chairs giving a peaceful and calming environment.

reduces the time-space experience of waiting and masks the noise of electronic medical technology and even voices that might otherwise be overheard. As well as reducing stress and anxiety and refreshing the minds of patients, visitors, and caregivers, such an environment emphasizes the facility's focus on compassion and caring. Figure 9-5 shows water cascading quietly down a wall.

Color can do much to establish a comfortable environment. Greens and blues are good in areas that require quiet and extended concentration. Cool colors cause individuals to underestimate time and make heavier items seem lighter, objects smaller, and rooms larger. Warm colors with high illumination cause increased alertness and an outward orientation. The elderly adult may have difficulty distinguishing pastels because of failing eyesight. Strongly contrasting patterns and extremely bright colors can be overwhelming and even intimidating or threatening to older adults. However, bright colors and designs are quite appropriate in a pediatric clinic.

Noise Reduction

Research has shown that patients and their families are more comfortable in surroundings that provide a quiet withdrawal from the hectic pace of the outside world. The use of sound-absorbing ceiling tiles and surfaces will help reduce clinic noise. A telephone system that produces a pleasing chime is preferred to the traditional shrill ring. Staff voices that are muted and pleasant are preferred; loud laughter and teasing are to be kept to the staff room and out of the hearing range of patients. Also appreciated are appropriate and current magazines and plants or pictures of nature. The fabric and texture of draperies, upholstery, and carpet should be pleasing, comfortable, and easy to maintain as well as assist in noise reduction.

LEGAL COMPLIANCE IN THE FACILITY

HIPAA

Legal

It is necessary to ensure HIPAA compliance for protecting patient information and privacy. With this in mind, HIPAA mandates certain building features. A reception window or desk should not make the patient feel closed off from the receptionist, yet it should provide privacy for the receptionist and total confidentiality for patients, while allowing a full view of the reception area. Figure 9-3 shows an efficient working space for the receptionist while still allowing visualization of the entire reception area. Figure 9-4 shows a small conference area in the same space that can be used when issues of privacy with a patient are particularly important. This space allows for discussion about insurance coverage, billing solutions, or patient education; voices cannot be heard in the remainder of the reception area.

To ensure HIPAA compliance, some clinics have the receptionist greet patients on their arrival and then direct them to a more private area where they are checked in, their insurance or payment plan is verified, and follow-up appointments are made. The telephones are located in this more private area so conversations with callers cannot be overheard in the reception area.

In the examination room, privacy is especially important to patients. Remember that privacy implies that the patient's conversation cannot be overheard in any other part of the facility. Studies have shown that when patients fear their voices can be overheard by others nearby, they will not respond to questioning as honestly as they would if their privacy were assured. In the examination room, provide space for patients to hang their undergarments and other clothes out of view. Always ask if a patient needs help in disrobing, and always knock before entering a room. A mirror is especially helpful for dressing after the examination—one placed appropriately and large enough so that it can be used by either a short person or someone much taller.

Americans with Disabilities Act

Legal

Accessibility, or making facilities and equipment available to all users, is a major consideration when creating the health care environment. The Americans with Disabilities Act (ADA) was passed by the U.S. Congress in 1990. The purpose of this act is to provide a clear and comprehensive national mandate to end discrimination against individuals with disabilities and to bring them into the economic and social mainstream of life. In addition to accessibility regulations identified in Titles II, III, and IV, this act also provides employment protection for persons with disabilities (Title I). ADA applies to businesses with 15 or more employees; however, some states have stricter legislation applying to businesses of only 8 or more employees. Even before the ADA became legislation, most health care facilities attempted to make their premises barrier free and accessible to patients with special needs. Although many ambulatory care settings will have less than 8 to 15 employees, accessibility for all patients in all settings is important. Refer to Chapter 6, "Legal Considerations," for a more complete discussion of the ADA and its latest requirements, including the Americans with Disabilities Act Amendments Act (ADAAA).

A professional designer not only can make suggestions regarding color, artwork, and the general environment of the clinic but also can provide advice on how the facility can be made accessible to people who have physical challenges. For example, all doors and hallways must accommodate a wheelchair. Likewise, a bathroom must accommodate individuals with special needs. Signage in Braille assists patients with visual disabilities (Figure 9-6). Elevators must be provided if the facility is on more than one level.

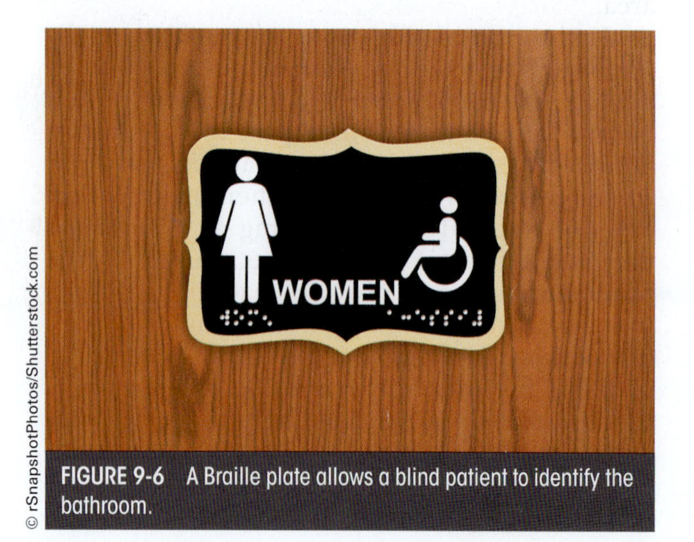

FIGURE 9-6 A Braille plate allows a blind patient to identify the bathroom.

At least one accessible entrance must comply with the ADA. It should be protected from the weather by a canopy or overhanging roof. Such entrances are to incorporate an accessible passenger loading zone. Ten percent of the total number of parking spaces at outpatient facilities must be accessible. (Visit the ADA Web site at http://www.ada.gov for more information.) Be mindful of patients whose impairments are not obvious—for example, individuals with impaired hearing or vision and individuals whose disability (temporary or permanent) may prevent them from doing certain physical activities.

SAFETY

Safety

Safety will always be paramount in any medical environment. Responsibility for a patient's safety begins the instant a patient enters the facility. Every staff member must be alert to any safety issue and be ready to offer assistance to patients at any time. Potential or current hazards are to be reported to a supervisor or provider in order to prevent or correct the hazard. On a regular basis, a safety inspection should be made of all areas of the facility. It is often best if one person is in charge of the inspection; some large clinics will have a designated safety officer. Even the smallest of clinics can maintain a checklist of safety features to be inspected on a regular basis. There are safety references throughout this text identified by the safety icon.

Creating a Safe Environment

Strict adherence to building ADA compliance identified earlier will greatly enhance a safe environment. Keep in mind that all areas must accommodate a wheelchair and provide for persons with special needs. Large multiclinic facilities often have attendants greet patients who arrive and need wheelchair assistance from their car to inside the facility. Other facilities provide parking attendants so that patients are not dropped off and left unattended while a family member parks the car.

In the facility itself, exit signs must be clearly indicated and easily seen. All restrooms should have safety bars and a pull cord that calls for special assistance when needed. The surface of all floors should be nonslippery, and all spills should be promptly cleaned and dried. A multiple-floor facility will need procedures for moving patients from one area to another or to the lower levels when elevators cannot be used. A regular inspection will check for any frayed or loose wires on equipment and uneven surfaces on floors or carpets so that immediate correction can be made.

Evacuation Procedures

Carefully identified procedures for evacuation are essential. Fire; hazardous chemical spills; power outages; earthquake; and threats of tornado, hurricane, or flood—all are examples that might necessitate evacuation of patients and all personnel. Large multiclinic facilities will have a written protocol and individuals assigned to particular areas to assist and manage in any evacuation. Smaller clinics will rely more heavily on providers and every employee for assistance. When the threat of any disaster is known, it is best to close the clinic facility for the period of the threat. Calls can be made to cancel appointments, and patients already in the facility may be directed to return home or to a designated public space prior to the event. When there is no advance warning, as in the case of earthquake or fire, clearly identified evacuation procedures are necessary.

Any necessary evacuation must include a check of every examination room, restroom, and procedure area. A wayfinding system should include easy-to-understand signs and numbers with clear directions to the exits. Special consideration is given to patients who need assistance or are in wheelchairs. Employees have the responsibility to assist patients and not leave the facility themselves until patients are safe. Any procedures that are underway, even minor surgery, must be stopped as soon as possible to facilitate the evacuation. It is important to turn off any oxygen or compressed gas systems. Never use elevators in a multistory building evacuation; always use the stairs. Close the door when an area is vacated.

Emergency Codes. There are some common emergency codes that can be helpful to understand. They are used primarily in hospitals and large ambulatory medical centers, but are applicable to any medical facility. Even though there are variations depending upon the facility, a few samples are identified as follows:

- *Code Red.* Fire emergency: Protect patients and staff from fire; it may be necessary to leave the facility.
- *Code Blue.* Adult medical emergency: Specialized personnel respond with necessary equipment.
- *Code Pink.* Infant/child abduction: Protect children and infants, block entrance and exit, notify authorities.
- *Code Gray.* Combative individual/assault: Respond to area, protect patients, notify authorities if necessary.
- *Code Green.* Bomb threat: Notify authorities of suspicious package, evacuate the building if advised.
- *Code Yellow.* Hazardous material spill: Identify unsafe exposure, safely evacuate area and protect others from exposure.
- *Code White.* Evacuation necessary: Move everyone out of the facility as quickly as possible.

Fire Safety

When there is a fire, evacuation must be considered unless the fire is quickly contained without threat to others. All employees must know where fire alarms are located and how they are activated; this is also true of fire extinguishers. Fire hazard has been decreased a great deal in medical facilities through the ban of smoking and smoking materials. Cracked or split electrical cords or plugs should be replaced, and electrical outlets should never be overloaded. If laundry is done within the facility, emptying the lint filter on the dryer after each use is a must.

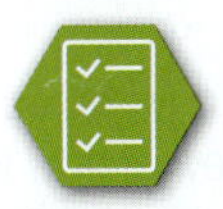

Periodically, all personnel should receive training on the use of a fire extinguisher for a small fire (see Procedure 9-1) and training for a planned evacuation when necessary. It is best remembered that fire prevention is the ultimate goal. However, if there is a fire, take the following emergency actions (**RACE**) if you are able to do so without putting yourself in danger and others are present to communicate the emergency and turn in the alarm:

- **Remove** patients and personnel from the immediate fire area if safe to do so.
- Activate the **alarm** at the fire alarm box and/or call 911. Notify other staff.
- **Contain** the fire and smoke by closing all doors to the fire area.
- **Extinguish** with proper fire extinguisher *only* if it is safe to do so, or **evacuate** as necessary.

Fire Extinguisher Safety. There are different types of fire extinguishers for different fires. The three most common are water, CO_2, and dry chemical types. A multipurpose dry chemical is suitable for fires most likely to be seen in outpatient care. Remember that all fire extinguishers should be checked periodically, usually monthly, to make certain pressure is at the appropriate level according to the manufacturer's suggestions. An extinguisher should be readily visible and not blocked by any furniture or doors. Make certain hoses and nozzles are free of insects and debris. The outside of the extinguisher should be clean and free of any oil or grease as well as any dents or signs of damage. Dry chemical extinguishers may need to be shaken monthly to prevent the powder from settling or packing. Pressure test the extinguisher periodically to ensure the cylinder is safe to use. Replace an extinguisher immediately after use. Local fire department personnel also check extinguishers and will do so in their regular facility inspections.

For more information on how to use a fire extinguisher, see the "Using a Fire Extinguisher" Quick Reference Guide.

PROCEDURE 9-1

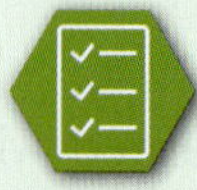

Procedure

Demonstrating Proper Use of a Fire Extinguisher

PURPOSE:

To demonstrate the ability to operate a fire extinguisher or help another person operate the extinguisher and to describe the precise steps to take to prevent errors and delay in operation.

EQUIPMENT/SUPPLIES:

Fire extinguisher

PROCEDURE STEPS:

1. Determine the type of fire extinguisher(s) on the premises. RATIONALE: The type of extinguisher will determine the kind of fires it may be able to control.
2. Examine the cylinder and carefully read any instructions supplied from the manufacturer, ***paying attention to detail.*** RATIONALE: This gives a brief review of how to operate the equipment and tells you what kind of fires to use it on.
3. Determine if you are able to handle the weight of the extinguisher, ***asking for assistance if you are unable to carry out the task.*** RATIONALE: This will tell you if you can move forward or will have to ask another to manage the extinguisher.
4. If a fire is present, ***be proactive*** by calling 911 before you discharge the extinguisher. RATIONALE: You cannot tell how quickly a fire may get out of your control.
5. Check your nearest exit. If it is blocked, ***display sound judgment*** by evacuating without discharging the extinguisher. RATIONALE: Trying to fight a fire that threatens a safe exit is dangerous and can cost a life.
6. Break the seal and turn and pull the safety pin from the handle. RATIONALE: This step is necessary before you can use the extinguisher, as it unlocks the mechanism.
7. Aim the nozzle or hose at the base of the fire and squeeze the lever to discharge the extinguishing agent. RATIONALE: The base of the fire is its source and it is vital to stop the fire at the source.
8. Standing several feet back from the fire, sweep side to side to put out the flames. RATIONALE: A side to side motion helps to put out the fire.
9. If the fire does not respond after you have used up the fire extinguisher, ***remain calm*** and remove yourself to safety immediately. RATIONALE: Do not take a chance of being caught in a fire; allow the professionals to put the fire out.
10. If the area fills with smoke, ***remain calm*** and leave immediately. RATIONALE: Smoke can be more deadly than the fire and is often very toxic.
11. Replace the depleted fire extinguisher immediately. Never leave an empty extinguisher where someone might believe it is ready for use. RATIONALE: A fire extinguisher that is fully operational and ready for use is the only kind to have in any facility.

QUICK REFERENCE GUIDE

USING A FIRE EXTINGUISHER

1. ***Call for help before extinguishing a fire.*** A fire can quickly spread to dangerous levels. The typical extinguisher should never be used on anything but small contained fires that have just started. Remember that all fires produce smoke and carbon monoxide. Some fires also produce toxic gases that often form from burning nylon in carpeting, foam padding, and so on and can be fatal.
2. ***Are you strong enough to extinguish a fire?*** Some personnel will find any commercial extinguisher too heavy to handle or have difficulty exerting enough pressure to operate it.
3. ***Check for a clear exit for escape prior to using the extinguisher.*** If the exit is at all threatened, leave immediately.
4. ***Know which type of fire extinguisher to use.*** The most common classes of extinguishers are often characterized by the class of fire—A, B, or C—or the extinguisher type—APW, carbon dioxide (CO_2), or dry chemical (Figure 9-7A).
   - *APW.* An APW (air-pressured water) extinguisher has a silver casing and is suitable for Class A fires of cloth, wood, or paper. It weighs about 25 lbs and is 2 ft tall.
   - *Carbon dioxide.* A CO_2 extinguisher is filled with pressurized nonflammable CO_2 gas. It has a red casing and a horn or spout. It is suitable for flammable liquid (Class B) and electrical fires (Class C). It should not be used on Class A fires. Weight and size vary.
   - *Dry chemical.* A dry chemical extinguisher is mainly filled with monoammonium phosphate powder that is pressurized by nitrogen. It is also known as a DC fire extinguisher. It can be used either for Class B and C fires or for Class A, B, and C fires, and will be labeled as such. It has a red casing and can weigh between 5 and 20 lbs. The dry chemical fire extinguisher appropriate for Class A, B, and C fires is the most likely choice for the ambulatory care facility.
5. ***Ready the extinguisher.***
   - Break the seal and pull the safety pin or metal ring from the handle (Figure 9-7B).
   - Squeeze the lever to discharge the fire extinguishing agent.
   - Aim for the base of the fire and sweep back and forth (Figure 9-7C).
6. ***Remember PASS to help you use the extinguisher properly: pull, aim, squeeze, sweep.***

Refer to OSHA's Web site on evacuation plans and procedures. Go to http://www.osha.gov and search for "Extinguisher Basics" to find pictures, diagrams, and more details.

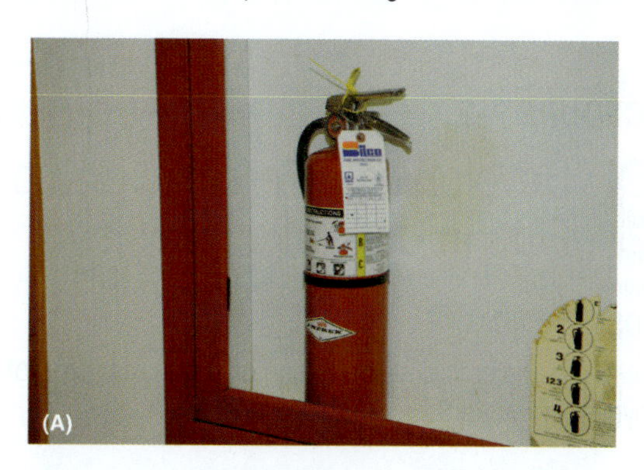

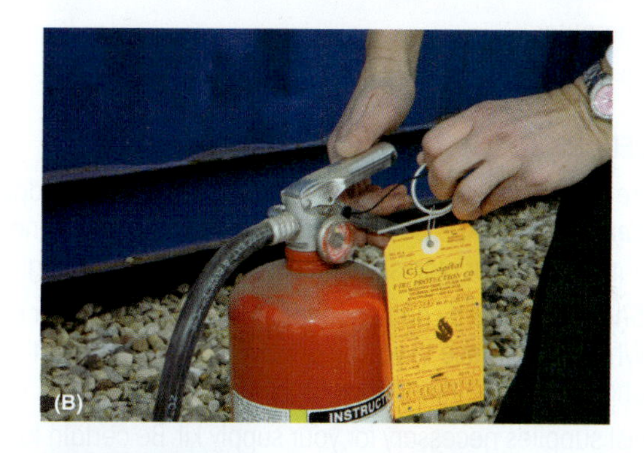

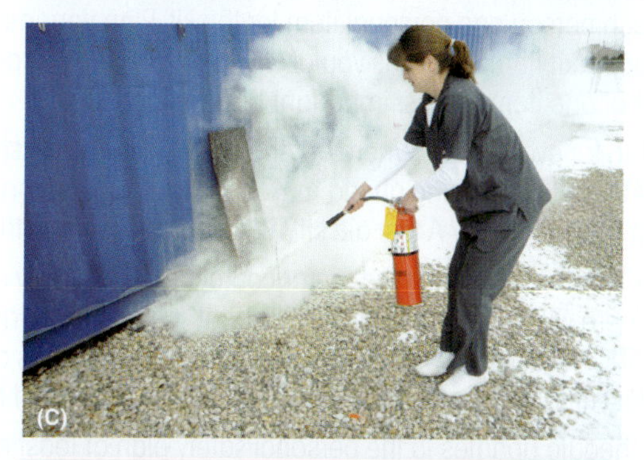

FIGURE 9-7 Operating a fire extinguisher. (A) Know the location of the fire extinguisher. (B) Pull the pin. (C) Point the hose at the base of the fire, squeeze the handle, and sweep from side to side.

Response to Natural Disaster or Emergency

Disaster can strike quickly and without warning, causing evacuation of a home or any other building. It can also confine you to a building or home. Knowing what to do and being prepared is the best protection and is your responsibility (see Procedure 9-2). A very valuable resource can be found at https://www.dhs.gov by searching for "Prepare My Family for a Disaster." This information is prepared by Homeland Security and will direct you to a number of other useful sites that have free downloadable information. There are a number of hazards to consider: floods, tornadoes, hurricanes, thunderstorms, and lightning; winter storms and extreme cold; extreme heat; earthquakes, volcanoes, landslides, and debris flows (mudslides); tsunamis; fires and wildfires; hazardous materials incidents and household chemical emergencies; and nuclear power plant and terrorism (including explosions as well as biological, chemical, and nuclear and radiological hazards) emergencies.

PROCEDURE 9-2

Developing a Personal and/or Employee Safety Plan in Case of a Disaster

PURPOSE:

In case of a disaster to develop a plan of action that promotes personal safety and can also be applied to both employees and patients in ambulatory care.

EQUIPMENT/SUPPLIES:

- Computer
- Clear plastic protector envelope for plan

PROCEDURE STEPS:

1. ***Be proactive*** by reviewing state and local recommendations for emergency preparedness. ***Pay attention to detail.*** RATIONALE: Some areas of the country are prone to particular natural disasters such as floods, tornados, or hurricanes. Your plan should be pertinent to your geographical area.
2. ***Show initiative*** by gathering family members or other employees together to discuss a disaster plan. RATIONALE: When those close to you are involved in the process, they are more likely to participate in the activity and understand the importance of the actions to be taken.
3. List supplies necessary for your supply kit. Be certain to include any special needs required in your supplies. Allow each person one personal item for the kit. Plan your needs for at least 3 days. RATIONALE: A detailed list of the supply kit items reminds you of what you will need to purchase, when items will expire or lose their usefulness, and what one item is most important to each individual.
4. Plan for evacuation. Where are the exits? Identify the safest route for exit. List the steps to take prior to evacuation. RATIONALE: Planning ahead makes it easier to function in a time of great stress. Who will be responsible for picking up the supply kit? A first aid kit? Who will turn off electricity, gas, water?
5. Determine a communication or contact plan to follow should you be separated from others during the disaster. Where will you meet? Name a "neutral" person or friend in another location who can be a telephone contact. RATIONALE: Following any disaster, the first concern is always for the well-being of your loved ones and those closest to you. Knowing how to reach one another will reduce this stress.
6. Schedule updates to the personal safety plan at least every quarter, ***developing strategic plans to achieve your goals.*** RATIONALE: This time frame allows for changes that may be necessary in the supply kit, reinforcing the safety protocol you have devised and the ability to make any other necessary changes.
7. Make certain everyone has a copy of the plan. Post a copy of your plan in a prominent place where it will be noticed regularly. RATIONALE: Unless everyone has a copy of the plan and it is posted where everyone is continually reminded of it, the plan loses its effectiveness.

While it is not the purpose of this chapter to detail responses to each of these disasters, there are some simple guidelines to keep in mind.

Every emergency plan will include information on what to do if there is no access to food, water, or electricity for some time. Most of these plans suggest creating kits to last, if necessary, for as long as two weeks but certainly never less than for 3 days. Kits can be assembled in storage bins or some other sturdy container, but should be readily accessible and regularly updated. Kits should be available for use at home, in a vehicle, and at a place of work.

In a disaster emergency it is important to pick two places for family members to meet, perhaps right outside the home or at a particular spot in the neighborhood. Decide how you will communicate with and reach others, especially family members you might be separated from during a disaster. Ask an out-of-town relative or friend to be your "family contact." It is often easier to make a long distance call than a local call. Know the location of your nearest shelter should you be required to evacuate. Make emergency phone numbers readily available to everyone. Teach everyone how to turn off the water, gas, and electricity. Keep necessary tools near gas and water shut-off valves. These safety tips are applicable to your workplace, too.

Sadly, the majority of households and places of employment do not have disaster kits. This is because it often takes a serious warning of a disaster or the experience of a disaster before individuals make the effort to prepare.

The Medical Assistant's Response to Disaster Preparedness

Competency

Because medical assistants are individuals with both administrative and clinical education, experience, and training and are able to perform emergency first aid and CPR, they can be very valuable to a community in a time of need. Individuals who respond to emergencies must not only have the skills necessary to attend to those in need, they must also be able to curb the stress they are likely to feel in order to function in a calm, yet "take control" manner. Anyone who responds in an emergency also is to be reminded of the "fallout" or "letdown" that follows a period of severe stress and/or intense care management. That is the time to have some rest to allow the body to function in a less stressful mode.

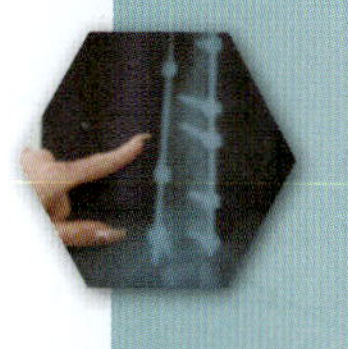

Critical Thinking

Visit the Web site indicated in this section to identify what you need to establish a disaster plan. What will you need to purchase for your supply kit for your home or car? What will be readily available to you or easy to procure? Identify special supplies you may want for any additional needs such as medications, pets, and so on. Estimate the cost of any purchases as well as any other action to be taken to establish a safety plan.

OPENING THE FACILITY

When the facility is opened in the morning, everything should be in readiness. The receptionist or administrative medical assistant, who arrives at least 20 minutes before the first patient, will make a visual check of each room to be certain it is prepared and ready for the day.

Rooms should be at a comfortable temperature, well organized, pleasantly illuminated, and spotless. The clinical medical assistant will check all necessary supplies and equipment for readiness. At all times, patient comfort and safety should be paramount.

A schedule of the day's activities is either printed for all personnel in the facility or available to all on the computer. It includes patients to be seen by the providers, meetings to be held that day, and any other information important in keeping the day's schedule running smoothly. As cancellations, no-shows, or added appointments are made, they can be changed and flagged in the schedule. If printed, this schedule can be posted in a place where staff can view it quickly, but it should never be visible to any patient. Patient charts for the day should be retrieved if not done so the prior evening. Facilities whose records are all electronic will sometimes print the latest laboratory results and information from the most recent visit to the facility for the provider to refer to when seeing the patient. The patient's information should be checked to make certain all information is up to date and accurate. The administrative medical assistant will check the answering service or machine for any telephone messages and follow up as necessary.

An effective way to check a room's readiness is to view yourself in the room as a patient. Ask yourself how you feel about being there, what mood the surroundings create for you, and whether you would feel welcome and comfortable as a patient.

CLOSING THE FACILITY

At the close of the day, each room should be checked to make certain all equipment is shut down and doors and windows are secured. Be sure that all materials of a sensitive nature are under lock and key. All file cabinets are to be closed and locked to ensure protection and confidentiality. Any drugs identified in the Controlled Substances Act list of narcotics and non-narcotics must be in a locked and secure cabinet and should also be checked when leaving the clinic. Petty cash kept on the premises must be locked in a safe container. It is best to ensure each room and area is in readiness for the next day. The day's receipts, plus a bank deposit slip, should be taken to the bank to be deposited or locked in a safe for a later deposit.

Local law enforcement officers can advise you on appropriate indoor and outdoor lighting, as well as any other security measures to take both during and after business hours.

Always contact the answering service to notify them that the clinic is closed and where and how the medical staff can be reached in an emergency.

THE FUTURE ENVIRONMENT FOR AMBULATORY CARE

Increasingly, outpatient care is claiming a larger percentage of the total health care volume than inpatient care. Outpatient/ambulatory care more often addresses chronic illness while inpatient care concentrates on acute illnesses. Moreover, there is a much greater emphasis upon preventive care and wellness than in previous decades. Much of this shift is attributed to the popularity of complementary and integrative medicine as well as the need to cut health care costs.

Another prediction is quite certain in outpatient care. The number of patients 85 years or older—who are most likely to require medical care for multiple chronic conditions—will greatly increase in the next few years. It is predicted that by 2020, almost 40% of a provider's time will be spent treating members of the population who are older adults. Although somewhat improved by the Affordable Care Act, the federal government still struggles with Medicare reimbursement policies, which do not adequately cover most costs incurred by providers when caring for this older population. Outpatient care centers will continue to struggle to provide facilities and services with environments conducive to the needs of this population.

To address this situation, the number of primary care providers willing to take new patients 65 years and older must increase. Patients will need to access their provider via convenient public transportation, take care of as many of their needs as possible in one day, and have prescriptions filled before returning home. The older population will need to navigate a wheelchair easily down corridors, into examination rooms, and into laboratories for assessment. Providers can be expected to spend additional time with older adults who will ask many questions and will be quite knowledgeable of their medical needs.

Members of the older adult's family will have an increasing presence in the care of their parents. Providers will want to give patients the opportunity for family members of their choosing to have access to their health information. HIPAA requires providers to have patients sign a release allowing their family members to be kept informed. Providers can expect family members of patients to want the very best for their loved ones, both medically and environmentally.

Discussions with older adults regarding their health care experiences reveal that their greatest frustration comes from the lack of clear instructions given by *all* health professionals, ranging from the administrative medical assistant to the primary provider. The most successful approaches to solving this dilemma include:

1. Providing clear and concise written instructions whenever possible in easy-to-read print
2. Creating an environment where movement from one department to another is not confusing
3. Making certain all patients fully understand their prescription instructions, directions for continuing care, and orders for additional tests
4. Identifying for patients under what circumstances they should report back to their primary provider for follow-up.

The goal of a medical facility and its staff should be not only to welcome and receive patients with a "we care for you" attitude but also to have patients leave the facility and staff with a sense of satisfaction related to the care received. As higher efficiency is demanded of providers and their staff members in order to reduce medical costs, thoughtful and attentive personalized care must not be forsaken.

Another prediction for the near future of health care is that the population will grow increasingly diverse. The influx of immigrants, especially in some border areas, places a great demand for bilingual providers and staff, and there is a need for health care availability in the neighborhoods where these individuals settle. These patients have many of the same needs as the older population and the four approaches above will need to be carefully adhered to.

Electronic mail (email) communication between patients and providers is now commonplace in many areas; however, patients are asked to give written permission for the transmission of information via email because privacy cannot always be guaranteed. Laboratory and radiological results can be viewed online, as can appointment reminders. Some providers offer treatment online when they understand a patient's medical history and needs. Providers may use a video chat tool such as Skype with a patient in order to discuss treatment protocols, order diagnostic services or medications, and/or schedule an in-clinic appointment.

At the same time, medical providers work diligently to decrease the number of medical errors made, and advancing technology creates new patterns of health care. Also, patients are becoming more astute consumers. These new consumers are better educated; they seek value and are comparison shoppers. They know that managed care has its limitations, and that providers can be wrong. These patients believe they know their own bodies better than anyone, and that quality of life is important. They know, too, that cost containment and the complexities of the health care system leave them vulnerable to medical difficulties if they do not take responsibility for themselves and their medical care.

Today's patients are exposed to numerous Internet sites and magazine articles that provide medical information 24 hours a day, 7 days a week. These patients arrive at their appointments with the ability to discuss potential diagnoses and treatment plans. Hopefully, the health care team welcomes this new partnership, even if health care professionals have to assist patients in weeding out some of the invalid medical information available. Providers will be continually challenged to make patients the center of their activities to provide a better experience while keeping costs reasonable.

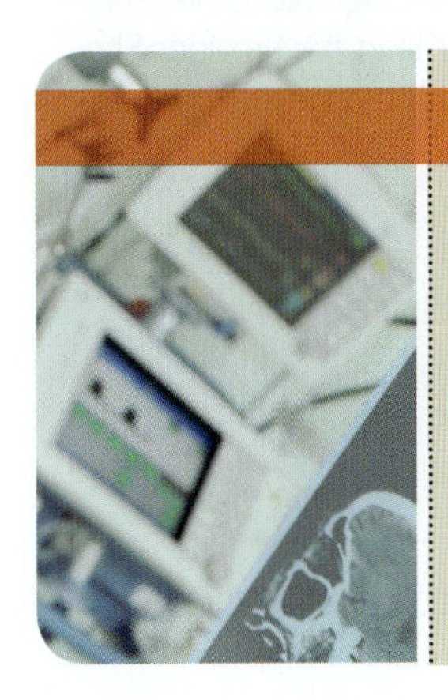

CASE STUDY 9-1

Refer to the scenario at the beginning of the chapter.

1. What is your first reaction to the environment in the medical facility described? Justify your response.
2. List as many solutions as you can to address the lack of privacy and confidentiality in the reception area. Begin with simple solutions and then move to the more complex ideas that surface in your planning.
3. How do you think patients will be affected by each of your solutions?
4. What other improvements might be considered when updating the clinic?

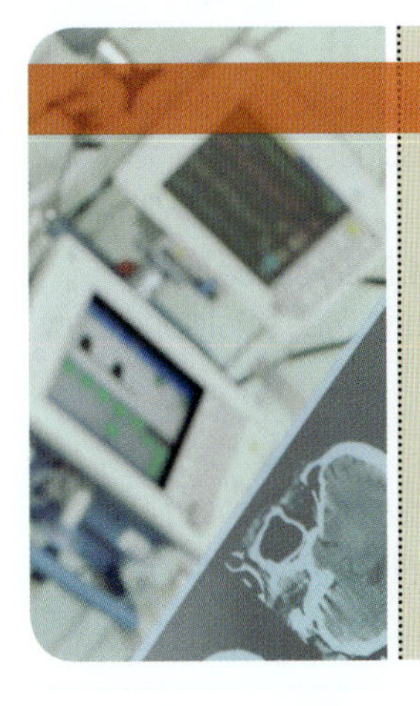

CASE STUDY 9-2

The eighth-floor orthopedic surgery department in a large metropolitan clinic has an interesting approach to patient dynamics. Providers and their assistants see patients for diagnosis and preparation for surgery. Patients often are seen in this department three to five times before and after their procedures. The staff involves their patients in the process to relieve any anxiety they might have.

Addison Burton approaches the reception desk, where he is immediately greeted and asked to wait a moment until the administrative medical assistant clears a previous patient. There is a huge box filled with slightly used tennis shoes that patients and staff are collecting for needy children and the homeless. Addison remembers he has a couple of pairs at home he could bring. After checking in, he is directed to a counter where coffee, tea, and water are available, as well as the

continues

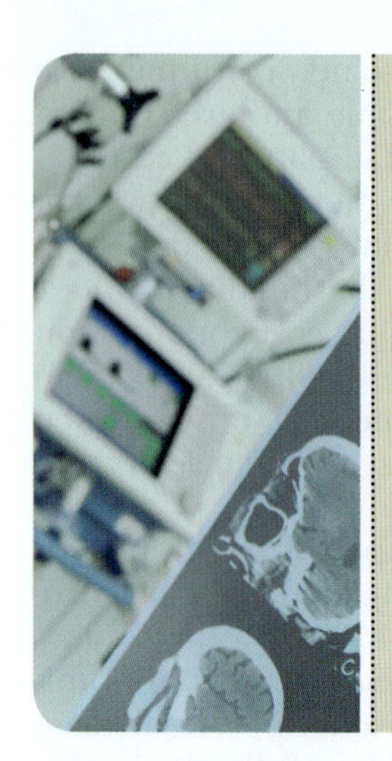

CASE STUDY 9-2 *continued*

daily newspapers. Addison can take a seat in a chair, on a couch at a window that allows him to put his feet and legs up, or at a table with chairs. The window seat gives a view of the city and a terrace garden four floors below. At the table there is an unusual puzzle being put together, and Addison takes a seat there. He is able to put four to five puzzle pieces together before being called for his appointment.

CASE STUDY REVIEW

1. When Jorja Anderson, CMA (AAMA), calls Mr. Burton to the examination room, what might the conversation be? Would this conversation help to dispel anxiety?
2. When the surgeon sees Mr. Burton for his hip problem, everyone has a good laugh—on the bottom of Addison's shoe is a puzzle piece. What kind of mood has been established for this visit?

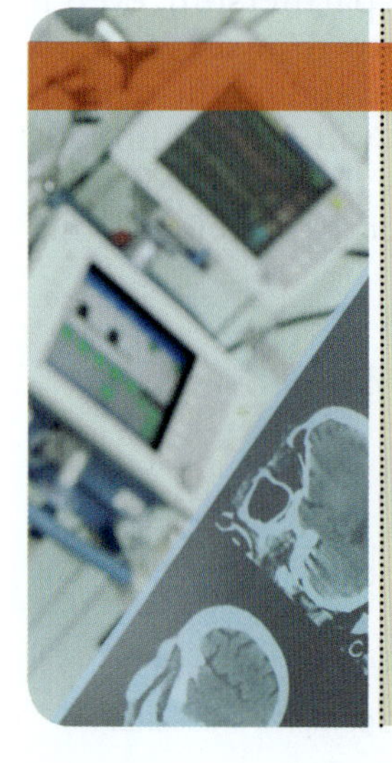

CASE STUDY 9-3

Even though she appears calm and collected on the outside, Abigail Johnson, who is about 75 years old, is quite nervous about having her annual physical. Clinical medical assistant Gwen Carr, CMA (AAMA), senses her patient's underlying tension and wants to do what she can to help Abigail relax. She knows that this patient has hypertension, suffers from occasional dizziness, and says she feels guilty about going off the diet that was designed to help manage both her high blood pressure and her diabetes. At this moment, Gwen is helping Abigail get ready to see Dr. King, her provider. She does not want to intrude on her patient's privacy but does want Abigail to relax a bit.

CASE STUDY REVIEW

1. What are some actions Gwen can take to ensure her patient's privacy?
2. In what ways can the physical environment itself become a calming influence for Abigail?
3. How will Gwen's sympathetic attitude affect her patient?

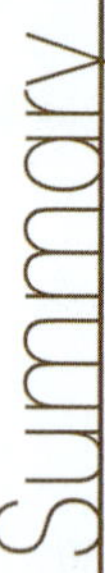

- Keep in mind that the environment in which patient care is given must promote health and healing rather than aggravate illness and feed anxiety.
- Evidence-based design will help create environments that provide effective, safe, and caring-centered facilities.
- The environment must be clean, fresh, cheerful, safe, and nonthreatening, with contemporary furnishings, appropriate colors, proper lighting, and soothing textures.
- Even if patients are not consciously aware of the message they are getting from the clinic design and environment, they are subconsciously receiving it. The clinic environment reveals things that might subconsciously undermine a patient's confidence in the provider and the health care team.
- Safety preparedness may not be obvious to patients, but its importance cannot be minimized. Every space in the facility with its appointed purpose must be designed and maintained to protect patient and employee safety, and every employee must be safety conscious every moment of the day.
- Opening and closing the facility involves a number of important steps to follow each day.
- The future of ambulatory/outpatient care will see greater demands than inpatient care. There will be increased care of people with chronic illness, an emphasis upon prevention and wellness, and cooperation with complementary or integrative therapies.

Study for Success

To reinforce your knowledge and skills of information presented in this chapter:

- Review the *Key Terms* and *Learning Outcomes*
- Consider the *Critical Thinking* features and *Case Studies* and discuss your conclusions
- Answer the questions in the *Certification Review*

- Perform the *Procedures* using the *Competency Assessment Checklists* on the *Student Companion Website*

CERTIFICATION REVIEW

1. Which of the following is appropriate for the reception area of an ambulatory care setting?
   a. Heavily scented flowers
   b. Medical journals with graphic colored pictures
   c. Dim lighting
   d. Live or silk plants
2. What is one of the goals in treating patients?
   a. Give them as much control as possible
   b. Get them in and out as quickly as possible
   c. Remind them that there is little privacy in a medical clinic
   d. Make sure they arrive on time for their appointment
   e. A full waiting room to show the success of the providers
3. What is one design element to avoid in a medical clinic?
   a. A mirror for dressing
   b. The colors green and blue
   c. Extremely bright, contrasting patterns
   d. Accessories and artwork
4. What is the ADA's primary concern?
   a. Segregating individuals according to type of disability
   b. Providing access and opportunity for individuals with physical challenges
   c. Only the work environment
   d. Getting economic benefits for people with physical challenges
   e. Making certain employees have adequate salaries
5. In any medical facility, what is the receptionist's KEY responsibility?
   a. Do not keep the provider waiting
   b. Make sure all plants are watered
   c. Greet patients in a friendly, warm manner
   d. Be efficient, even if it means ignoring patient requests
6. Which of the following statements is accurate regarding a visual check of each examination room?
   a. It is the responsibility of weekly housekeeping.
   b. It is done when opening and closing the clinic.
   c. This is a task only of the administrative medical assistant.
   d. Whoever is the last one to leave the clinic performs this task.
   e. Security is assigned this task.
7. What do space planners recommend for the reception area?
   a. Three to four seats for each examination room
   b. Seats to accommodate 1.5 hours of patients
   c. 2.5 seats for each examination room
   d. Not bringing family members to appointments
8. The ADA requires that what percentage of the total number of parking spaces in outpatient facilities be reserved for individuals with disabilities?
   a. 5%
   b. 10%
   c. 12%
   d. 7%
   e. 4%
9. What challenges will the medical environment face in the future?
   a. Increasing numbers of pediatric patients
   b. Increasing numbers of older and more diverse patients
   c. Decreasing numbers of hospital patients
   d. Decreasing government compliance
10. Which of the following is an appropriate guideline for safety in a medical facility?
   a. Be able to use fire extinguishers and have an evacuation plan.
   b. Keep an employee at the door to assist patients with special needs.
   c. Provide good quality fluorescent lights to prevent falls.
   d. Enhance proper ventilation by opening windows and doors.
   e. Call 911 to assist with any evacuation necessary.

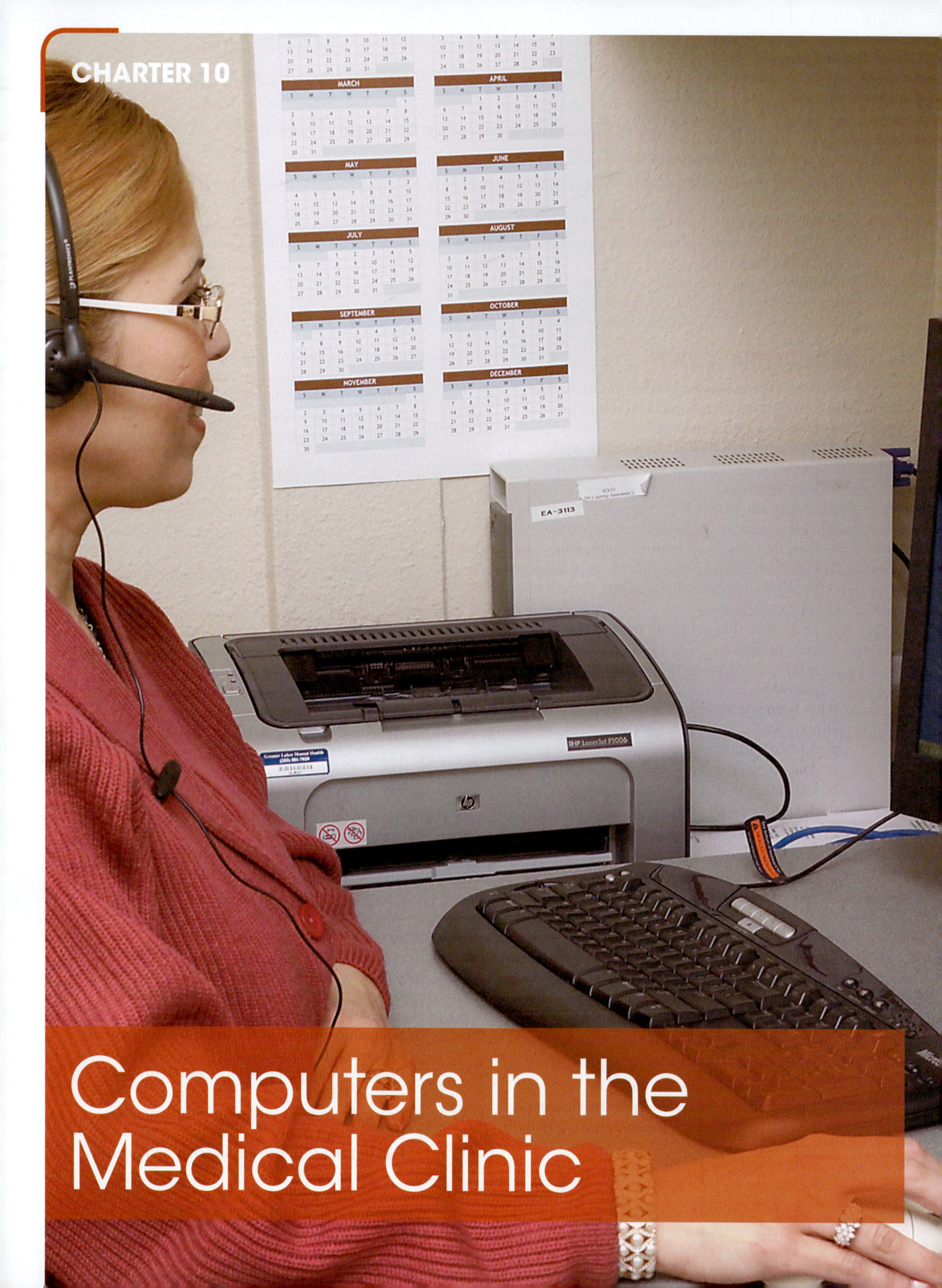

CHAPTER 10

Computers in the Medical Clinic

LEARNING OUTCOMES

1. Define and spell the key terms as presented in the glossary.
2. Identify the four main types of computers.
3. Describe the four fundamental elements of a computer system.
4. Differentiate four input devices and describe the function of each.
5. List three examples of data output devices.
6. Differentiate and discuss various types of storage devices and how they might be used in ambulatory care settings.
7. Discuss the use of flash technology and tape drives and describe how each might be used in ambulatory care settings.
8. Identify the difference between system and application software.
9. Analyze the importance of computer system documentation and how it is upgraded.
10. Differentiate the various network and connectivity technologies.
11. Analyze the principles and techniques of promoting network and computer security.
12. Discuss computer maintenance and defragmenting of the hard disc drive.
13. Differentiate between electronic health records (EHR), electronic medical records (EMR), and a practice management (PM) system.
14. Discuss principles of using electronic medical records (EMR).
15. Explain the importance of system backup.
16. Demonstrate design considerations when computerizing a medical clinic.
17. Analyze why ergonomics is important and recall at least five guidelines for setting up a computer workstation.
18. Identify guidelines for maintaining confidentiality for safeguarding personal health information (PHI) as well as electronic personal health information (ePHI) while keeping in mind HIPAA requirements.

KEY TERMS

central processing unit (CPU)
cloud computing
defragmentation
documentation
electronic health record (EHR)
electronic medical record (EMR)
ergonomics
Ethernet
firewall
hardware
input devices
Internet
license
memory
motherboard
networking
operating system (OS)
output devices
patches
phishing
practice management (PM)
program software
secure sockets layer (SSL)
server
surge protection
system backup
system software

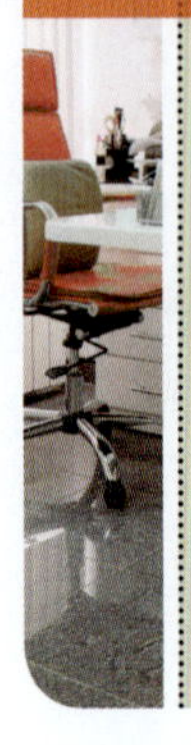

SCENARIO

Inner City Health Care, a multiprovider clinic in a large urban area, is considering a new practice management system. Clinic manager Marilyn Johnson, CMA (AAMA), has been working with the team investigating and determining specific areas of need. During meetings, Marilyn uses active listening skills and feedback techniques such as reflection, restatement, and clarification to be sure that each team member is heard and understood. The team has been charged with recommending the practice management system that best satisfies their clinic's specific needs while protecting the integrity of electronic protected health information (ePHI) and electronic medical records (EMR). All Health Insurance Portability and Accountability Act (HIPAA) security regulations must be incorporated, including the development of security audits and related policies and procedures that detect any unauthorized access to ePHI and EMR.

Chapter Portal

We interact with and rely on computers in almost all aspects of our personal lives and in the work environment. In the cars we drive, home appliances, entertainment systems, transactions with our credit or debit cards, bill paying, social networking, mobile phones, and a host of other applications, computers are at work. The medical clinic is no exception, and medical assistants will work with some form of computer whether in an administrative, a clinical, or a laboratory environment. A modern clinic could not effectively work without computers. This chapter will introduce the student to the basics of how a computer works, how it is used in the medical clinic, and some of the safeguards for maintaining confidentiality.

CATEGORIES OF COMPUTERS

Common computers can be grouped into four basic categories: supercomputers, mainframe computers, servers, and microcomputers. The following Quick Reference Guide gives the characteristics of each type of computer.

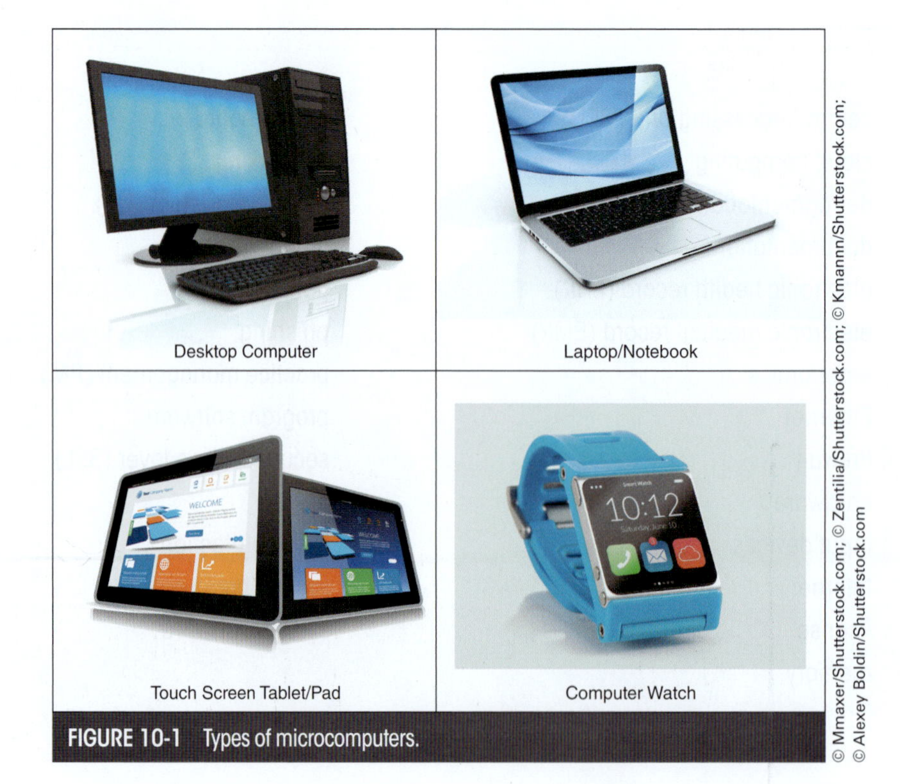

FIGURE 10-1 Types of microcomputers.

QUICK REFERENCE GUIDE

TYPES OF COMPUTERS

CATEGORY	CAPABILITY	USE	EXAMPLE
Supercomputer	Very rapid processing speed through use of multiple processors connected in parallel Computer can fill a building	Space program, medical research, weather simulation, nuclear science, and computational intensive tasks	©Timofeev Vladimir/Shutterstock.com
Mainframe computer (enterprise computer)	Large computers capable of running multiple programs simultaneously Less powerful than supercomputers Computer will fill a large room Being replaced by minicomputers	Used by large businesses and governments for accounting and client information storage	© Scanrail 1/Shutterstock.com
Minicomputer	Smaller desk-size computer with slightly less speed and power than a mainframe computer	See mainframe computer	©iStock.com/Zern Liew
Server—specialized minicomputer designed to provide program and data storage for networked microcomputers	Massive data storage capability Racks of servers can fill large buildings and consume large amounts of electricity	Data and application program storage for multiple networked microcomputers	© dotshock/Shutterstock.com
Microcomputer	Small but powerful personal computing devices designed for one user	Word processing, presentations, small databases, social networking, communication, controlling test, and manufacturing equipment	Personal computer, laptop, desktop, pads, tablet, notebook, smartphone, computer watch (see Figure 10-1)

BASIC COMPUTER ELEMENTS

All computer systems are composed of four fundamental elements (see the "Fundamental Elements of a Computer System" Quick Reference Guide). In addition to these basic elements, many support systems such as timekeeping devices, power supplies, and firewalls are part of a computer system.

Hardware

The components of a computer system that you can see, touch, or hear are referred to as **hardware**. Hardware consists of **input devices**, **output devices**, and the **central processing unit (CPU)**, as well as some firewalls and modems.

Data Storage Devices. Data storage devices are devices capable of permanently or temporarily storing digital data. Data storage device capacity is often referred to as **memory**. Together with computer speed, this area of the computer has seen the greatest improvement, with capability doubling every few years. Computers used by most of us today have no functional limitation for memory, with portable memory cartridges providing unlimited memory expansion. Data storage devices consist of read-only memory (ROM), random access memory (RAM), and data storage memory.

ROM and RAM Memory. The computer manufacturer permanently writes data or instructions into the memory on ROM chips, which are installed directly onto the **motherboard**. They contain instructions for operations such as booting the computer when the power is turned on. RAM memory is also in the form of chips and is also part of the motherboard. It provides the computer with registers in which to store in-process data. RAM memory is erased or "lost" when the computer is turned off or experiences a power failure. RAM memory is important to the user, in that a RAM capacity that is too small will cause the computer to run slow or not to run some program software.

Data Storage Memory. Data storage memory is nonvolatile, or permanent, and is not erased when the computer is turned off. It can be either read-only or read-write. Read-only data storage memory is used to store program software for loading onto the computer. CDs and DVDs have been used for this purpose, but Internet servers are increasingly used today. The following paragraphs describe several devices for providing data storage.

Mechanical Hard Disk Drive (HDD). HDDs are nonvolatile read-write storage devices consisting of a rotating metal disk coated with a magnetic material capable of locally being magnetized to store data as 0 or 1 depending on its magnetic state. The disk spins at 7,000 rpm and data is read by a head that hovers a few thousandths of an inch above the disk. The devices are subject to mechanical failure, resulting in potential loss of system software and data and should be backed up frequently. (See Cloud Storage and RAID storage for backup of data and system software.)

Solid State Drive (SSD). Solid state drives serve the same function as a mechanical hard drive, except that the data is stored on interconnected flash memory chips instead of on the surface of a metal disk with a magnetic coating. The flash memory chips are also nonvolatile and retain the data even when there is no power to them. They are less susceptible to rough treatment, although they have a limited read-write life. Except for heavy download users, however, the computer will usually become obsolete prior to the flash memory failing.

Optical Drives. Two types of optical drives are used in computers: compact disks (CDs) and digital video/versatile disks (DVDs). Currently, Internet storage and advances in flash technology are replacing optical drives.

CDs used in the computer environment are similar to those used to store music. They are used for storing both permanent and temporary records, as they have the capability to be used as read-only disks (CD-ROM), write disks (CD-R), and re-write disks (CD-RW). In addition to data storage, they are sometimes used to hold program software for installation on the computer; however, when Internet connection is available software programs are more likely downloaded directly from a server.

DVDs are identical to the DVDs used to view home movies. They look similar to CDs, except that the format for writing the data to DVDs is different, permitting storage of up to 26 times more data. Several formats for writing data are used at this time. For the system to function, it is important that the storage media, disk, and drive are of the same format.

USB Thumb Drive. Thumb drives utilize flash technology and are connected to the computer using a universal serial bus (USB 1.0, 2.0, or 3.0) port or higher performance USB serial port. The memory

QUICK REFERENCE GUIDE

FUNDAMENTAL ELEMENTS OF A COMPUTER SYSTEM

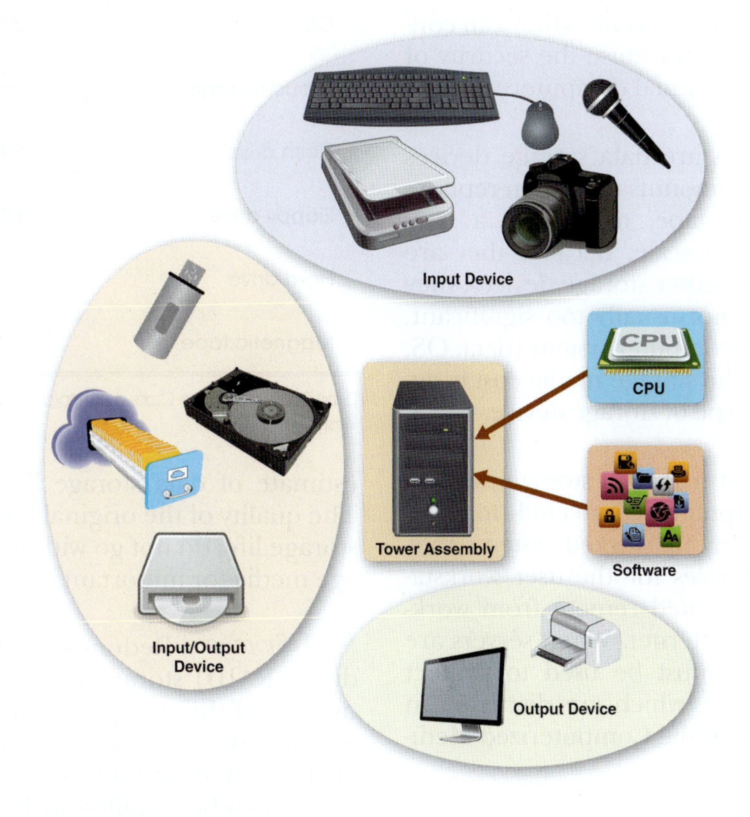

ELEMENT	FUNCTION	EXAMPLE
Input device	Device that translates analog data into a form useable by the computer microprocessor (CPU)	Keyboard, mouse, digital camera, touch screen, scanner, laboratory test equipment, server file, CD, magnetic tape
Central processing unit (CPU)	Performs mathematical computations, makes logic decisions, and controls computer functions in accord with instructions provided by system software; commonly referred to as the brain of the computer	Approximately 2-inch square microchip located on the motherboard
System software		
• Operating system (OS)	Manages computer resources	Windows 10, iOS
• Program software	Instructions for specific task	Word, Excel, PhotoShop
• Driver software	Instructions for support hardware	Printer or graphics driver
Output device	Device that displays or stores the results of operations performed on the input data by the CPU	Printer, monitor, data storage device, modem, fax machine

is nonvolatile and is slower and less reliable than the flash memory in a SSD drive. Thumb drives are about the size of a human thumb, and are useful for transferring data between computers that are not networked and for limited backup of data. (*NOTE*: Thumb drives from a nontrusted source should not be connected to a computer system as they can contain a virus that could compromise the security of the entire network or individual computer.)

Tape Drives. Tape drives are data storage devices capable of storing large amounts of data on replaceable reels of magnetic tape, much like a tape recorder but on a larger scale. Because they are much slower than many other storage devices, they are used when time is not usually too significant, such as in backing up a computer system (data, OS, and system software). The storage media cost is significantly less with this type of storage device.

Servers. **Servers** are not true data storage devices. They are pseudo-computers connected to massive hard drives. In many networked systems they become the storage devices for the user workstations. Servers may be located remote from workstations or even on the Internet. When servers are used, special protocols must be used to protect confidentiality of records, which are discussed in "Patient Confidentiality in the Computerized Medical Clinic," page 217.

Cloud Storage. Cloud storage involves storage of digital data using multiple servers in a physical facility that is frequently owned and managed by a hosting company, although it can be operated by the using organization. The servers are generally located at different locations to avoid catastrophic loss of data due to natural or man-made events. The Internet or a cable system provides the means for data transfer to the storage site. Cloud storage has many advantages over in-house data storage: Data is accessible from multiple sites, and the system requires little capital investment or technical resources by the using organization. The cloud can also host program software, freeing up computer capacity and capability requirements (see the "Cloud Computing" section on page 211).

Life Span of Stored Data. The life of stored data is dependent on the storage media, temperature and humidity, and whether the data are frequently retrieved. Assuming the media are stored under cool and dry conditions and data are infrequently retrieved, Table 10-1 provides a conservative estimate of data storage life for different media. The quality of the original media can also affect the storage life; do not go with the lowest price for storage media for important data.

TABLE 10-1

LIFE SPAN OF STORED DATA

MEDIA	ESTIMATED LIFE SPAN
CD	2 to 5 years
Cloud storage	Indefinite
Flash drive	5 to 10 years
Floppy drive	10 to 20 years
Hard drive	3 to 5 years
Magnetic tape	10 to 20 years

Data Source: Storage Craft, www.storagecraft.com/blog/data-storage-lifespan/

RAID Storage. Redundant array of independent disks (RAID) storage is a storage system that can use any of the storage media described previously. Storage devices are combined in a redundant array so that should any one device fail, a new device can be installed without shutting down the system or losing data (hot swapping).

Documentation

Computer system **documentation** consists of the manuals and **licenses** that define how many computers can use the software, and how the programs operate. Manuals explain how to execute specific functions and give the specifications for hardware, such as the frequency of the internal clock, RAM, and hard drive available memory. Although documentation is more likely to be online, it may be printed format or provided on an optical disk that contains the program or OS.

Updates to program documentation are increasingly made available on the Web site of the company providing the program, together with **patches** for glitches discovered in the basic program. The system should always be backed up prior to installing updates and patches in case they cause problems. It is recommended that this work be done when supplier technical support is available. Third-party manuals defining

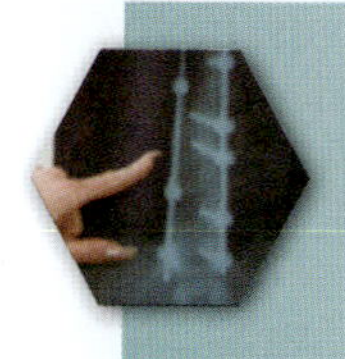

Critical Thinking

Your clinic has received legal notification requiring you to provide a list of all the software used in the practice and to show proof that all necessary licenses are current. You are successful in showing compliance, but clinic procedures were disrupted for days in meeting this court mandate. Prepare a clinic protocol designed to ensure that all software is legal and that unauthorized persons have not installed illegal software on any clinic computers.

how to use software are becoming increasingly popular and are frequently more user-friendly than documentation from the software supplier. All documentation—including licenses, recovery software, and program disks that come with the computer system; add-on hardware; and software—should be maintained in a safe location for the life of the equipment and software, and then disposed of when the system or software is phased out of use.

Hardware and Software Compatibility

The hardware drivers and **program software** of a computer system must be compatible with the **operating system (OS)**. Many program software applications share files with the operating system (OS); if there is a conflict with files having the same name, either the OS will not allow the applications program to load or it will not function properly. The documentation for most applications programs defines the versions of the operating system for which compatibility has been established and should always be checked before purchase of either a new applications program or a new version of the OS. Hardware driver requirements should also be checked for compatibility with the OS. The amount of RAM memory, CPU clock speed, and available drive storage space can affect whether a program will run satisfactorily.

Computer Networks

Networking is the electronic or optical connection of computers and peripheral equipment for the purpose of sharing information and resources.

Types of Networks. The most common networks encountered in the medical clinic are:

- Local area network (LAN)
- Wide area network (WAN)
- Internet

Both LAN and WAN are dedicated networks limited to connected computers operated by a single company, clinic, or hospital. They differ principally by the size of the geographic area covered. The LAN usually is limited to a single clinic or building, whereas the WAN covers a wider geographic area and may be linked by leased telephone lines, fiber optic cables, microwave links, or even radio. Each computer in the LAN or WAN usually has its own computing power, but it can also access other devices on the network subject to the permissions it has been allowed.

The **Internet** is a worldwide publicly accessible network of networks and computers. It differs from a LAN or WAN not only in sheer size but also in the manner of data transmission, called *protocols*. Data transmitted on the Internet are broken into packets, which are routed over different networks to the final destination, where they are reassembled for use by the client computer. If one network is inoperative the system chooses another. Data that are in transit are almost impossible to intercept, making them immune from most unauthorized users.

Connecting Networks. Connection to a network can be through either a hard-wired system or a wireless system. Hard-wired connections include standard telephone modem (dial-up), digital subscriber phone line (DSL), local area network, or through a modem using either copper wire or fiber optic cable. Wireless connections include WiFi, Bluetooth, satellite systems, and cellular technology.

Hard-Wired Connection. Hard-wired connections are often referred to as **Ethernet** connections. Connections can be made using a telephone line–type cable called a *crossover cable* between computers having an installed network interface controller. Most new computers have this feature. Hard-wired systems are capable of higher data transmission rates than wireless systems, but with advanced technology WiFi systems, the difference is not noticeable unless very large files are being transmitted.

WiFi Connection. WiFi can be used to connect computers directly or to connect a computer to the Internet. WiFi is a brand originally licensed by the Wi-Fi Alliance to describe the underlying technology of wireless local area networks (WLANs). It was developed to be used for mobile computing devices, such as laptops, but is increasingly used for more services, including Internet, voice over Internet protocol (VoIP) phone access, gaming, and basic connectivity of consumer electronics. It has a range of about 300 feet.

Because WiFi uses radio transmission, it is vulnerable to unauthorized users eavesdropping on the transmission. Measures to deter unauthorized users include:

- Suppressing the access point's (AP's) Service Set IDentifier (SSID), which is used by the AP to tell the world that it is online
- Allowing only computers with authorized media access control (MAC) addresses to join the network
- Using various encryption standards (WAP2, WAP, WEP)

WAP2 has the most sophisticated encryption and is almost totally secure. WAP encryption is the next best alternative, and WEP is better than nothing. If the eavesdropper has the ability to change his MAC address he can potentially join the network by forging his MAC to an authorized address that he determines by listening to network activity using a scanning device.

Bluetooth Connection. A technology called Bluetooth can be used to connect computers to a LAN. Bluetooth is the name given to a radio technology capable of transmitting signals over short distances (30-foot range). This means of connecting networks is primarily used to connect smartphones and microcomputers to each other and to a host computer. Because Bluetooth is a radio technology, it is vulnerable to eavesdropping, but because of the short range it is less vulnerable than WiFi. Most systems that are designed to hold personal data have built-in security in the form of a four or more digit alphanumeric personal identification number (PIN), much like the one used for an ATM at the local bank. Product owners should share PIN numbers only with trusted associates to ensure maintaining of security.

Systems Security

Safety

All systems connected to the Internet or to computers that are connected to the Internet are vulnerable to attack by hackers and require strong security measures. In the past, hackers limited their activities to those that would earn them notoriety, but that is no longer the case. Their motives have changed; they are now in it for the money. The nuisance-type attack on a computer system will always be a concern, and the theft of electronic records from a medical practice can be a virtual gold mine to a criminal hacker. Electronic theft of Social Security records of staff and patients can lead to identity theft. Theft of bank account and credit card information can result in untold consumer fraud, and compromised medical records may lead to medical insurance and reimbursement fraud.

Legal

Protection of sensitive data is a legal responsibility for any business that has such data in its computer system. The Federal Trade Commission takes enforcement actions against corporations or businesses that fail to provide adequate data security. Protection of a computer system from unauthorized access requires defense in depth. Protection can be broken into the following defenses:

- *Protocols and audits.* All medical facilities must have protocols in place to hold workers accountable for their actions while using electronic protected information (ePHI) and electronic medical records (EMR). Security audits should be randomly conducted using audit trails and audit logs that offer a back-end view of system use to ensure policies are being followed. The very knowledge that a user's actions are being recorded can act as a significant deterrent to prevent wrongdoers from committing malicious acts. The audits provide evidence of security incidents and breaches of patient privacy and help establish a culture of responsibility and accountability for patient health information (PHI). They also provide information for responding to patient privacy concerns regarding unauthorized access by family members, friends, or others. Audits are helpful in preemptively detecting new threats and intrusion attempts to the system and meeting regulatory requirements.
- *Operating system (OS).* Select an OS with the fewest flaws for hackers to use and always install the latest security fixes (patches). No OS is perfect, so diligence is the watchword.
- *Program software.* Program software has been the source of the greatest number of security vulnerabilities. As with the OS, always install security patches as they become available. Check on vulnerability ranking and select program software with the least detected

vulnerability if possible while meeting your application needs. Web browsers have the most security vulnerabilities because they are a popular gateway to access servers and spread malware.

- *Control of software downloads.* The greatest risk to computer security is the unauthorized installation of software by the computer operator. Downloaded software and data using thumb drives or from unknown Internet sites can introduce viruses and malware into the system, defeating the best **firewalls** and virus protection systems. All personnel should be made aware of this vulnerability. If possible, an information technology (IT) technician should be listed as administrator of all computers, and users should not be given authority to add software.
- *Firewall.* Protect the network with a firewall, which limits access to the system from outside.
- *Antivirus software.* Have an active, updated virus protection system.
- *Password.* Require passwords to gain access to sensitive medical and financial data. Passwords should be changed on a regular basis.
- *Training.* To avoid **phishing**, instruct personnel not to open email from unknown sources and not to go to Web sites received in an unsolicited fashion.
- *Inventory control.* Maintain strict inventory control of laptops, memory cards, and other portable devices that contain data. The best network security system in the world can be breached if a laptop is taken home and either is stolen or used with unprotected Internet access. Unknown to the user, the laptop can have programs downloaded that reveal passwords or provide a free ride into the secure system of the clinic network.
- *Data management.* Purge the system of inactive files containing sensitive data; archive or destroy them as necessary.
- *System backup.* **System backup** includes all clinic systems (data, OS, and program software) on a regular basis to permit restoration of the system in case of a catastrophic event.
- *Manual selection of WiFi access points.* Do not let the computer automatically search for and connect to the access point with the strongest signal. Hackers operate access points designed to gain access to your computer. If in doubt, check the address of the access point to be sure it represents a legitimate source or connect only to officially known access points.
- *Personal access points.* The personal access point, which is part of your network system, should be given a unique name that does not reflect the business name or the name of personnel. It should be security protected as previously described.
- 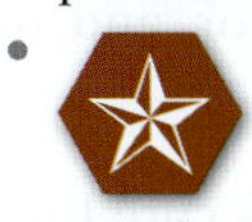
Integrity
Deactivate file sharing by your computer. Allowing files to be shared may be convenient for co-workers, but it leaves a wide open door for hackers.
- *Enable email encryption.* Enable the **secure sockets layer (SSL)** option for transmission of email by your email service provider.

Virus Protection Programs. Protection from viruses, worms, and malicious software (malware) is extremely important to prevent damage to files; unauthorized access to the files; and slowing, damage, or shutdown of the system. Viruses find their way onto a system principally through downloading materials and programs from the Internet, opening attachments from email files containing a virus, and unauthorized software. Antivirus software is one of the main defenses against computer viruses.

Antivirus software is a computer program that can be used to scan files to identify and eliminate computer viruses and malware. Most commercial antivirus software uses two different techniques to accomplish this:

- Examining files to look for known viruses by means of a virus dictionary
- Identifying suspicious behavior from any computer program that might indicate infection

In the virus dictionary approach, when the antivirus software examines a file, it refers to a dictionary of known viruses that have been identified by the author of the antivirus software. If part of the file matches a virus identified in the dictionary, the software will either delete the file or quarantine it, making it unable to spread. The program may also attempt to repair the file. The virus dictionary approach requires periodic online downloads to update the virus dictionary. The dictionary approach to detecting viruses is often insufficient due to the continual creation of new viruses.

Dictionary-based antivirus software typically examines files when the computer's operating system creates, opens, and closes them and when the files are sent or received as email. A known virus can be detected immediately upon receipt. The software can also typically be scheduled to examine all files on the user's hard disk on a regular basis.

The suspicious behavior approach attempts to monitor the behavior of all programs. If a program tries to write data to an executable program, this action is flagged as suspicious behavior, and the user is alerted and asked how to proceed.

Safety

Recognizing Secured Sites. Secure Internet sites are easily discernible by either a small padlock in the web browser window, not the Web site window itself, or by the site address (Figure 10-2). Secure sites utilize encryption and have an address beginning with *https://*. Sites that are not secure have an address beginning with *http://*, without the s.

Secure wireless sites can be identified by the same padlock next to the network name shown when your wireless device searches for a signal. When a padlock is shown, you will have to configure your device to connect to the hotspot. This is usually in the form of a password or passphrase.

Firewalls. Firewalls come in two varieties: hardware and software. Both types function in a similar fashion; namely, they establish a list of acceptable sites based on a profile the device develops of the users of the system. It will then allow these sites access to your computer. All other sites are blocked. Some firewalls limit the type of files that can be transmitted. Other firewalls cloak specific network channels, making them invisible to hackers trying to gain access to your computer. Still others monitor the content of incoming packets of data.

System Backup. Viruses, equipment failure or damage, and hacker attacks make system backup mandatory. System backup devices are basically data storage devices that store the entire contents (data, OS, and program software) of the nonportable computer memory so it can be recovered if a catastrophic system loss should occur. All clinic systems should use backup on a regularly scheduled basis. The frequency of the backup should be dependent on how much data the user can afford to lose. Magnetic tapes, optical drives, and flash drives are frequently used for this purpose. The backup is commonly done during hours when the system is not being used. Some system backup devices are automatic, requiring only that the tape or disk from the disk drive be changed in the morning and placed in safe storage. Current backup media should be stored in a secure off-site location. A backup system should be tested to ensure it is capable of restoring the computer to the initial state.

Power Outage, Electrical Surge, and Static Discharge Protection Devices. Protection devices must be an integral part of a medical clinic computer system. Computer systems should have an uninterruptible power supply, or battery backup, to prevent power outages from shutting down the system or destroying data. The power supply should also have a **surge protection** capability to prevent voltage surges on the utility line from damaging computer components. Static electricity can also be highly damaging to computers by transferring thousands of volts of electrical charge to components that are damaged by only a few hundred volts. This is the type of charge we all experience during dry weather when we get a shock from touching a grounded object and draw a spark. Synthetic clothing and walking on a synthetic fiber carpet can create static charges. To prevent damage from static discharge, grounding mats should be required at all workstations.

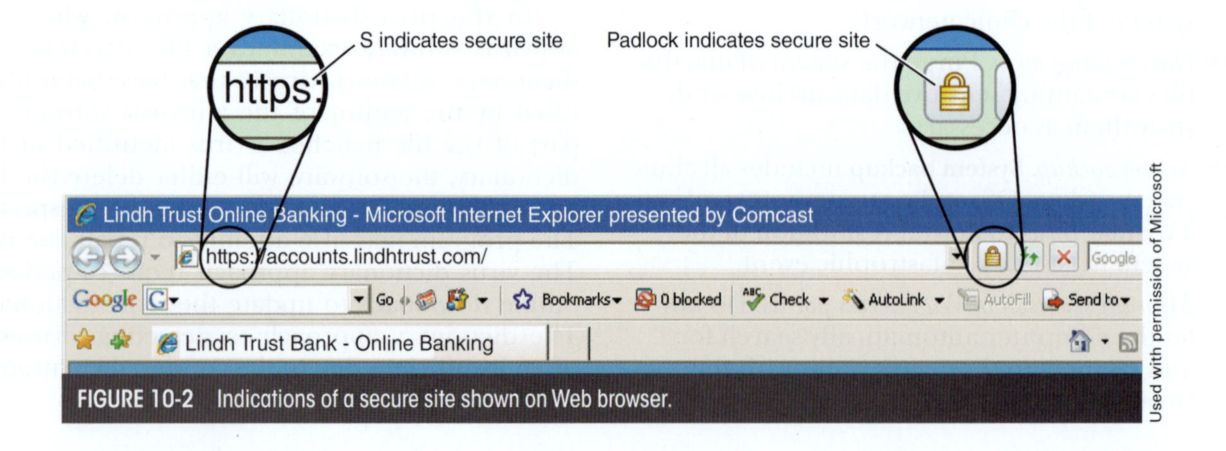

FIGURE 10-2 Indications of a secure site shown on Web browser.

CLOUD COMPUTING

While cloud storage was previously described in this chapter, **cloud computing** takes matters one step further, storing program software on servers at a hosting company so that software download is available on demand.

The cloud is like a computer rental agency where an order is placed for the applications (or apps) to be performed, such as keying in a document, or preparing graphics for a clinic bulletin board, scheduling appointments, coding procedures and billing insurance for services, and so on. The computing requirement is sent to the cloud and the app appears on the clinic monitor screen. Hardware and software updates, loading programs, or having to call the information technology (IT) person will be a thing of the past. It is all done in the cloud. The term *cloud* comes from the vision of cyberspace, where the Internet is represented by a cloud. In cloud computing, the cloud will provide all computing needs for a fixed service price on a pay-for-use basis. It will securely store data in a manner that all authorized persons in the clinic can access, and provide it as requested. This is not magic, of course; behind the service are computer resources and a management system, but the only user concerns will be availability on demand and reliability of the service. Cloud computing is made possible by the commoditization of apps, just like rental cars, airline flights, or utilities. Payment is required for only those services used. The main advantages of cloud computing are:

- Reduced cost resulting from reduction in IT personnel, hardware, software, and service hours
- Improvement in resource availability time, more secure data backup, and better disaster recovery

Some computing equipment will still be required in the medical clinic. A very basic computer and input devices capable of connecting to the Internet, as well as having a graphics capability to produce an image on the monitor, will still be necessary. A printer will still be required. Both the printer and the monitor will have to be selected to meet the requirements of the practice, just as is the case with current computing systems.

Data confidentiality will continue to be a concern to the medical community. Cloud computing services will not be without potential threats to data security, but by using encryption, virtual local area networks, and firewalls, the threats can be minimized. Multiplicity of geographical data storage can reduce the problem of data loss.

Cloud computing will be the development that makes worldwide electronic health records a reality. Electronic medical records that are accessible through a single facility or clinic using its servers are localized. Until those records are global, where anyone with authorization, regardless of their geographic location, can obtain access, electronic health records will not become a reality.

COMPUTER MAINTENANCE

Maintenance of computer systems is generally limited to cleaning the monitor screens, replacing printer ink or toner cartridges, and refilling paper trays. Other maintenance tasks that are within the capability of a computer-literate member of the health care team are file removal, disk **defragmentation**, and installation of security patches recommended by the supplier of the computer software. Defragmenting of the HDD is automatic in some OSs, and is not required with an SSD.

The HDD of a computer accumulates a host of old files ranging from old emails to obsolete programs and data files. If not removed, they use hard drive storage space and ultimately can slow the speed at which the computer stores and retrieves data. Simply right-clicking on the file with the mouse and then selecting Delete from the menu can remove these old files. After removing files, you should also empty the recycle bin. Be careful with this step, however, because once the recycle bin has been emptied, the files can no longer be recovered without extraordinary means.

When files are deleted from the hard drive, blank spaces are left on the disk. For the computer to save new files it must sort through these blank spaces. The defragmentation process removes the blank spaces similar to the way you move all the books on a shelf to one side so new books can be added to the empty side. Defragmentation is easily done using a disk defragmenter that is included with the OS. Defragmentation takes a significant amount of time and should be performed when the clinic is closed.

The medical assistant may have as one of his or her responsibilities establishing a service agreement for maintenance of computers on a periodic basis as well as any emergency repairs resulting from a major system failure. These agreements may also include personnel training and general technical support services. The medical assistant responsible for this contract should make certain that the vendor has signed the contracts required by the confidentiality protocols established by the medical clinic and that all removable data storage media have been removed and secured before hardware is taken to the service company's facility.

USE OF COMPUTERS IN THE MEDICAL CLINIC

Computers are an integral part of the medical clinic. According to 2013 CDC data, all of the hospitals and half of the clinic-based providers surveyed reported using an enhanced form of **practice management (PM)** software. PM software handles the day-to-day actions involved with a medical clinic using either an integrated piece of PM software or individual pieces of software that incorporate specific functions (Figure 10-3). Table 10-2 indicates the many tasks performed by computers.

Specialized software that ties together management of the entire practice is expensive, sometimes costing several hundred thousand dollars per application. Increased revenue resulting from improved productivity and reduction in the amount of undercoding or overcoding during the billing process have been found to more than justify the expenditure.

Electronic Records

Electronic records take two forms, **electronic health records (EHR)** and **electronic medical records (EMR)**. Both contain the same type of data, but differ in scope. EHR include all medical information from all providers and hospitals in a patient's medical universe, whereas EMR are limited to one provider, clinic, or hospital. Most records at the present time are EMR. As of 2013, CDC data showed that 78% of clinic-based providers and 60% of hospitals had adopted some form of EMR. Growth of EHR will take more time to develop and will be achieved only as the United States adopts a nationalized health care system. Such a system will allow digital health information to follow patients across the health care spectrum so that it will be available for all providers globally.

In order to satisfy legal requirements, practice management (PM) systems must demonstrate complete functionality by ensuring that the record is complete, accurate, secure, and compatible with all

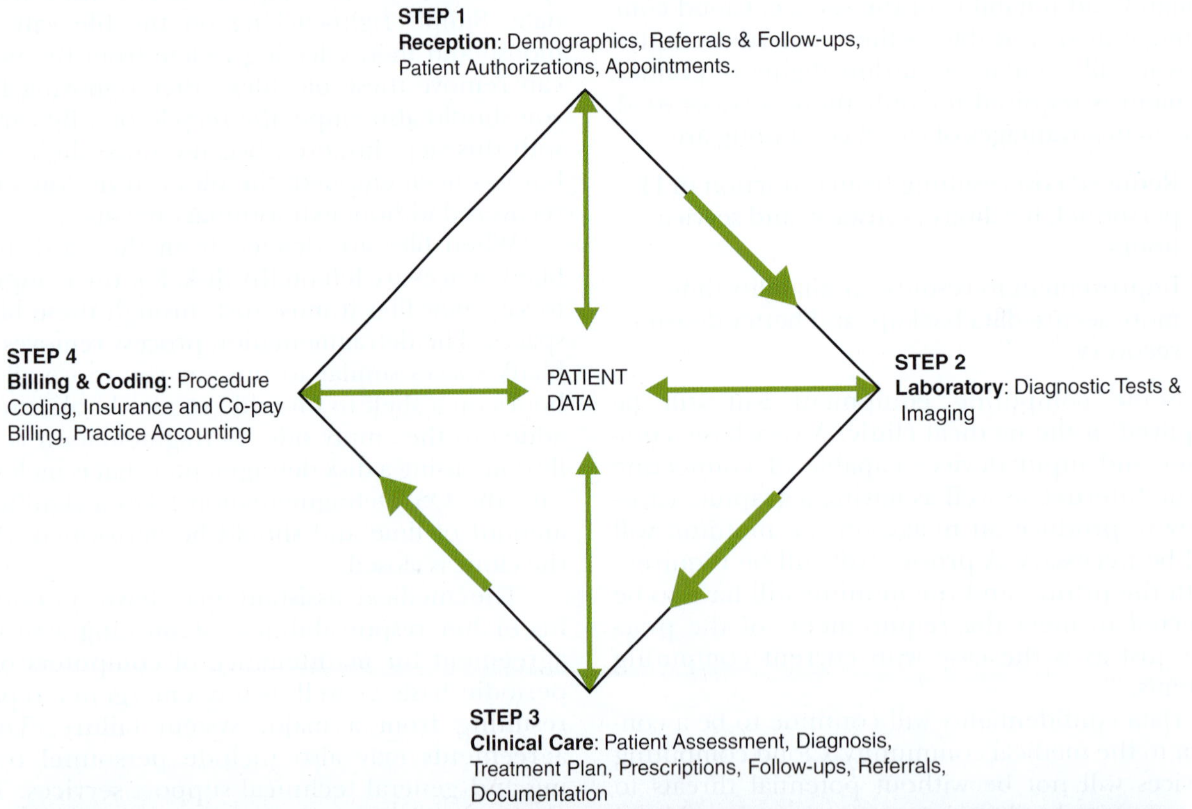

STEP 1
Reception: Demographics, Referrals & Follow-ups, Patient Authorizations, Appointments.

STEP 4
Billing & Coding: Procedure Coding, Insurance and Co-pay Billing, Practice Accounting

PATIENT DATA

STEP 2
Laboratory: Diagnostic Tests & Imaging

STEP 3
Clinical Care: Patient Assessment, Diagnosis, Treatment Plan, Prescriptions, Follow-ups, Referrals, Documentation

FIGURE 10-3 Practice management (PM) flow chart.

TABLE 10-2

THE USES OF COMPUTERS IN THE MEDICAL CLINIC

APPLICATION	TASKS
General clinic software	Patient demographics, appointment scheduling, email communication, provider referrals, follow-up directions, patient authorizations, insurance information, coding and billing procedures, accounts receivable data, accounts payable data, bank statements, monthly balance sheet (see Chapters 12 and 17)
Clinical and laboratory software	Patient assessment, diagnosis and treatment plans, follow-up lab tests and appointments, medications and e-prescriptions, scanning diagnostic tests, quality assurance data
Administrative software	Clinic protocols, personnel data, staffing requirements, job descriptions, equipment inventory and maintenance, vendors and agreements, requests for equipment and facilities (see Chapter 21)

systems from which information about the patient is obtained. The system must meet the preliminary American Recovery and Reinvestment Act of 2009 (ARRA) certification requirements of the Certification Commission for Health Information Technology (CCHIT) (http://www.cchit.org).

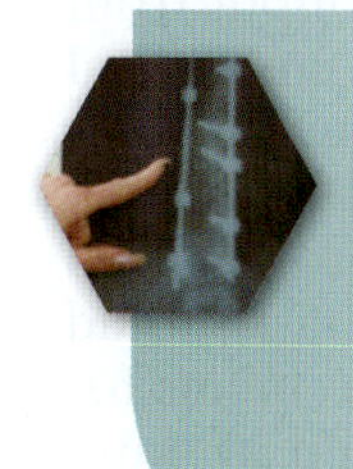

Critical Thinking

Your clinic has obtained new practice management software. List options you can think of for training clinic personnel to use the PM software effectively. Identify the pros and cons for each option.

The Virtual Medical Clinic

The revolution coming within the next 5 years is the virtual medical clinic, where patients will be treated remotely. The trend is being driven by value-based health care as part of the Affordable Care Act (ACA), in which providers, hospitals, and insurers are given financial incentives for keeping large groups of patients healthy. Prior to the enactment of the ACA, hospitals were paid when patients were hospitalized, under what is called fee for service. Health care providers are now eager to be proactive in treating anything from a cold or the flu to chronic illnesses. Insurers are providing 24/7 access to consultation by telephone, email, or Skype, with nurses providing assistance for minor illnesses and advice on when a provider should be involved. Many hospitals and large ambulatory care centers are adding urgent care options as a means of keeping down the costs of emergency care at hospital settings.

Providers are also taking advantage of wearable data-gathering platforms which remotely provide data on almost every chronic condition suffered by mankind. With this data in hand the provider can verify the patient's condition, prescribe medications, and advise the patient—all remotely, thereby increasing the productivity of the provider and reducing cost. The wearable sensors are FDA approved since they are a part of the treatment loop. Some of the illnesses/conditions for which data links are being established include epilepsy, physiological stress, grand mal seizures, sleep disorders, diabetes, atrial fibrillation, and other cardiovascular disease issues. For all of the wearable sensors the computer plays a vital role.

Computers are also being used to identify illness outbreaks such as the flu or epidemics by sampling Internet search frequency for the disease. Recent trials show several weeks' advance warning of an outbreak in a given area.

DESIGN CONSIDERATIONS FOR A COMPUTERIZED MEDICAL CLINIC

Computerization of a medical clinic requires careful consideration of the computer system, software, and physical layout of the facility. If the change to a computerized system is well planned, with input sought from all affected personnel, and with time allotted for training, the experience will be less stressful for all concerned. Involving all clinic personnel in the design of the system is extremely important because it creates a feeling of ownership and garners more willing support during the disruptive changeover period.

Software Selection

The first step in selection of software is to choose a knowledgeable and trustworthy vendor. The vendor should not only understand computers and software but also the needs of the medical clinic. A reliable vendor should be able to assist in anticipating and allowing for future needs (at least 2 years' future needs) as the medical practice grows and new diagnostic tools are introduced.

The next and most important step in developing a plan for computerization of a medical clinic is determining what tasks will be computerized and preparing specifications that will become part of the contract with the vendor. This is done in conjunction with the vendor, by seeking input from staff, and by talking with other people in medical clinics similar to your facility. Software available for each of the tasks should be identified and evaluated, preferably by actually using the programs on a trial basis. The best program for each task should be identified, and the hardware requirements for each program should be defined. Keep in mind that the program should be selected with operational commonality with all of the other software taken into consideration. Programs with similar menus and appearance on the monitor screen make training personnel much easier. Packaged programs that perform multiple tasks are commonly available. The Microsoft Office suite is an example of a packaged program that includes word processing, spreadsheet, scheduling, email, and database programs with commonality in menus and procedures. Similar programs tailored to the medical clinic are available.

Hardware Selection

Once the memory capacity (RAM, hard drive data storage capacity), CPU speed, and input and output device requirements have been identified for the software, the next step is to determine whether you are going to network. The type of network selected will be based on data transmission speed requirements and facility considerations related to running cables and the distance between computers and output devices. The hardware selected should meet or exceed the identified minimum requirements and be name-brand equipment to ensure future availability of replacement parts. If possible, get a computer system with substantially more memory than required by the software, because inadequate memory or CPU speed may restrict the ability to use future software updates or improved programs. The CPU speed should be as fast as technology permits at the time you make your purchase. The computer should also have one or more USB 3.0 ports to allow faster connection speeds. The trend is toward using more memory and requiring greater CPU speed, especially if graphic programs will be used on your system. The more memory and CPU speed you can purchase, the longer your system will be viable without replacement of hardware. The size of the monitor and screen display resolution limit should be selected to be compatible with the type of work the computer is used to perform. These requirements are necessary to achieve image sharpness and avoid eyestrain of personnel. The computer control panel display settings should also be set to match the monitor display resolution limit. Resolution is usually expressed as pixels in the horizontal and vertical dimensions of the screen. Many inexpensive computer monitors have a resolution of 1280 × 1024 and this is adequate for most clinic work. Persons doing graphic design frequently use a monitor with a resolution of 3840 × 2160, and a resolution of 3280 × 2048 is used in medical diagnostic work. For reference purposes, the most common wide-screen HD television has a resolution of 1920 × 1080 and an ultra HD screen has a resolution of 3840 × 2160. If the monitor is to be used for diagnostic work, a much wider grayscale range is required so that it can render nearly every shade of gray; the latest medical monitors offer up to 4,096 shades of gray. Color display monitors should not be used for this purpose as they have a poor grayscale response.

Scheduling the Changeover

The installation of a computer system is disruptive to the clinic routine. Not only does it take time to install the hardware and load the software, but it takes time to transfer files and data. Personnel may be intimidated by the computer and must be well trained to avoid feeling overly threatened. The installation of hardware should be scheduled during a down period such as a long holiday or vacation period. It is best to introduce the new system while continuing to use the old system. Start by transferring files and data, then when the staff is comfortable with the system and their computer skills, make the changeover. If your staff does not accept ownership for the system and is not trained and comfortable with it, disaster is almost guaranteed. The process cannot be rushed, and short-term inefficiency must be accepted as a trade-off for the efficiency that will result from a computerized medical clinic.

ERGONOMICS

Safety

Although **ergonomics** in the medical clinic is an important consideration even without computerization, specific problems must be addressed when changing over to a computerized clinic environment. Safety issues and concerns specific to the computer, if addressed, can be minimized or avoided.

Eyestrain

Eyestrain can be a problem associated with the use of computers. The computer monitor should be positioned to prevent excessive glare entering from windows or reflecting from interior lighting. Attachment of an antiglare screen to the monitor further reduces eyestrain by reducing remaining residual glare. Computer operators should take a 5-minute break each hour and focus on a distant object to prevent ocular accommodation and the headache and blurred vision associated with it. Using eye drops can minimize dry and itchy eyes. Figure 10-4 illustrates the proper positioning of the flat screen monitor to prevent glare from artificial lights in a room and incoming light from windows.

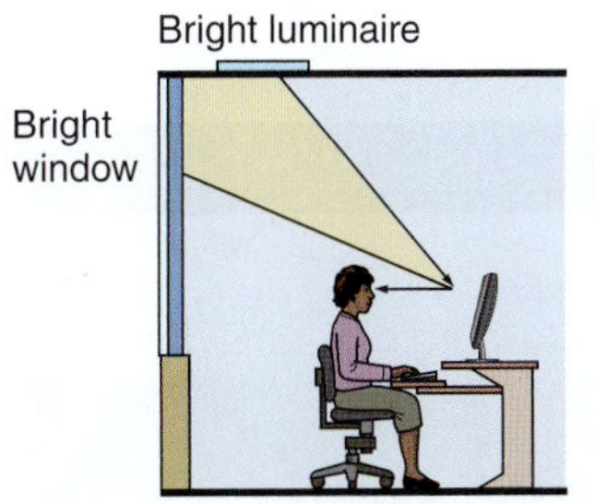

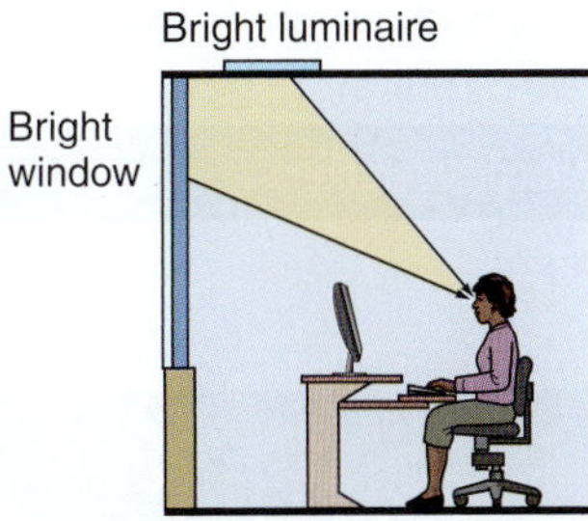

Poor location of flat screen monitor user

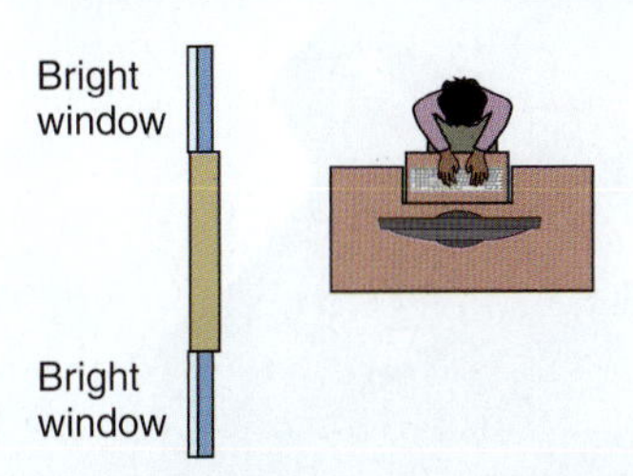

Good location of flat screen monitor user (sight line parallel to window)

FIGURE 10-4 Proper positioning of the flat screen monitor will prevent glare from incoming light from windows and artificial lights in the room.

Cumulative Trauma Disorder

The most widely known injury associated with individuals routinely using a computer is carpal tunnel syndrome. It is attributed to repetitive wrist motion. It can be prevented or the onset delayed by using a special keyboard that conforms to the natural position of the hands or by using a conventional keyboard with wrist support, as show in Figure 10-5A and 10-5B.

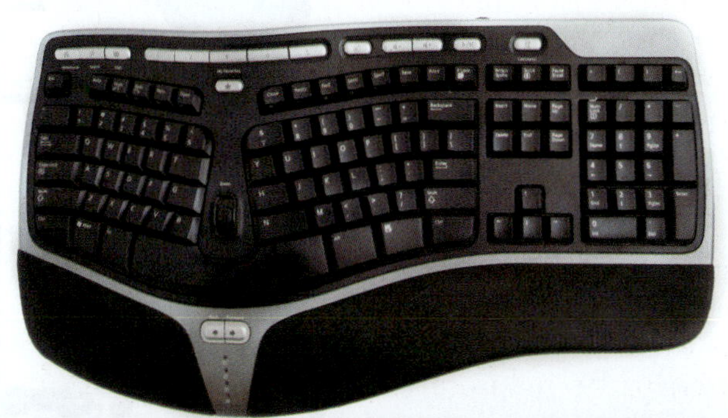

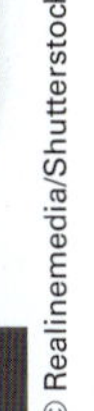

FIGURE 10-5A Ergonomic keyboard.

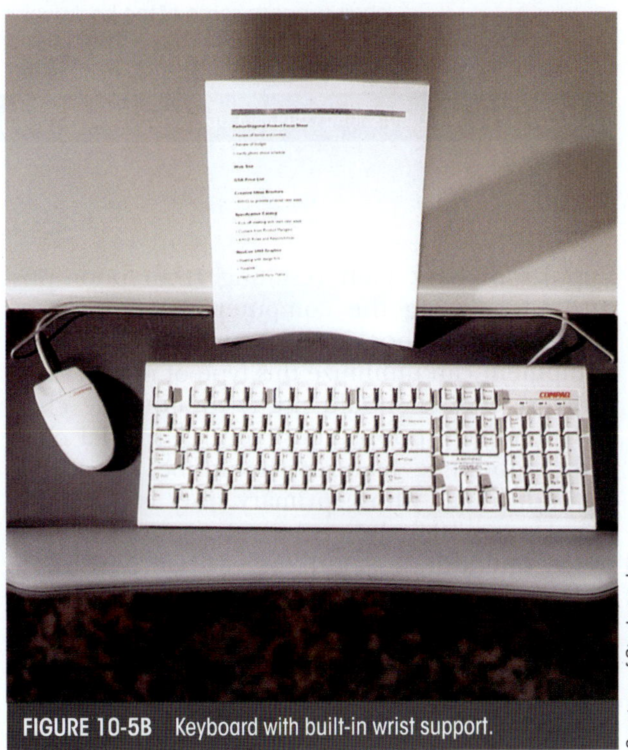

Courtesy of Steelcase, Inc.

FIGURE 10-5B Keyboard with built-in wrist support.

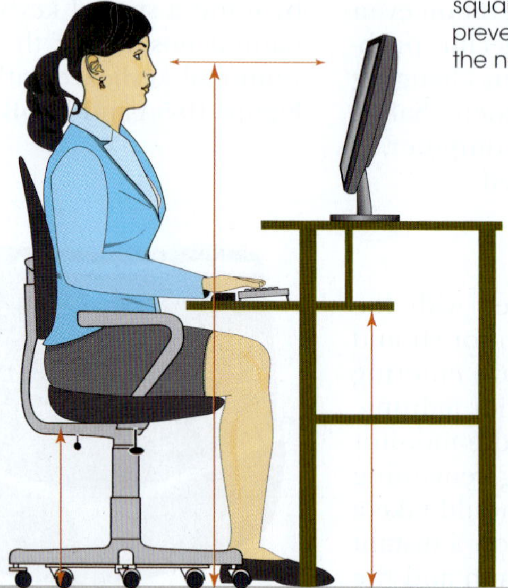

FIGURE 10-6 Recommended computer operator position with ergonomic considerations.

Posture

Reports of back pain resulting from poor posture while using the computer are quite common. Carefully choosing and setting up computer equipment can minimize this type of injury. Computer operators should use a comfortable chair with lumbar support adjustment. A special chair with ergonomic features should be considered for individuals whose primary duty is keyboarding. Figure 10-6 shows the recommended computer operator position for proper posture to prevent back strain while operating a computer. The desktop should be 28 to 30 inches above the floor with an adjustable keyboard holder allowing adjustment for individual operator body size. A footrest may be helpful in further minimizing posture problems (Figure 10-7). A document holder

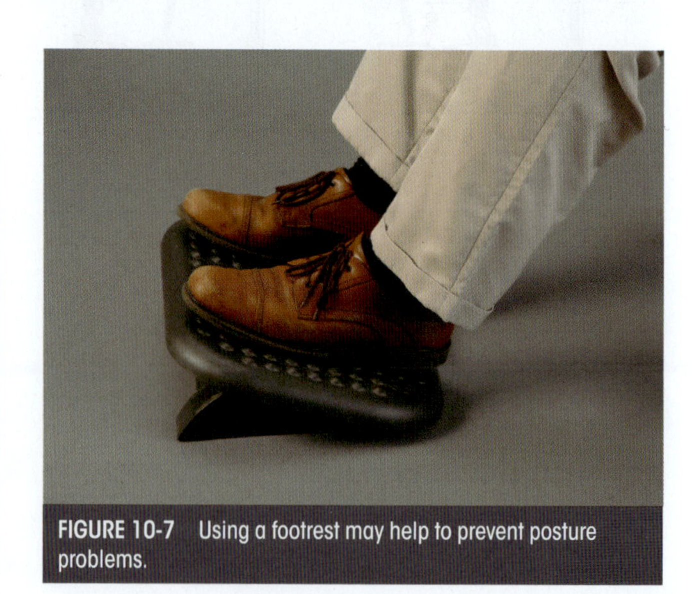

FIGURE 10-7 Using a footrest may help to prevent posture problems.

should be used to avoid excessive turning of the neck and looking downward (Figure 10-8). Operators who talk on the telephone while keyboarding or inputting data should use a headset telephone.

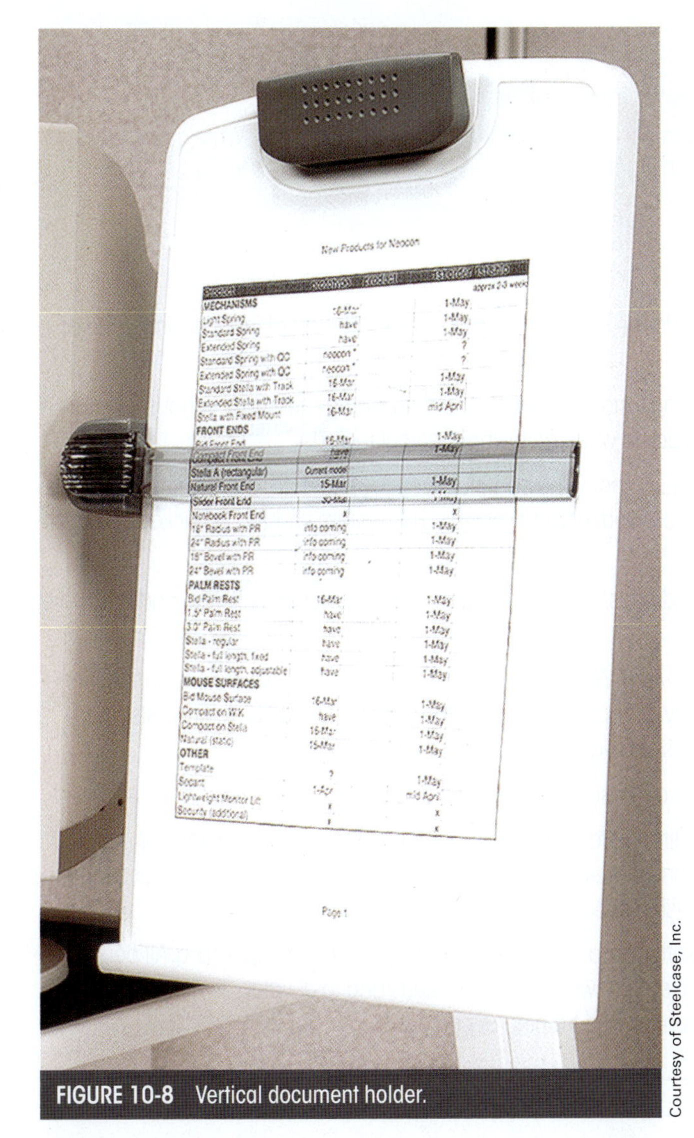

FIGURE 10-8 Vertical document holder.

Courtesy of Steelcase, Inc.

PATIENT CONFIDENTIALITY RELATED TO A COMPUTERIZED MEDICAL CLINIC

The following guidelines are in compliance with HIPAA standards for safeguarding personal health information, and provide a starting point for maintaining confidentiality of patient information:

- Confirm the patient's identity by verifying at least two of the following: clinic number, date of birth, or photo ID prior to any discussion.
- Never discuss the patient's case with anyone without the patient's permission (including family and friends).
- Safeguard computer screens and never leave hard copies of forms or records where unauthorized persons may view or access them. Restrict access to electronic databases to designated staff.
- Destroy or archive outdated or unneeded records.
- Use only secure means to send patient records or test results (for example, use password protection, encryption, official mail) and always mark information confidential with directions to destroy if misdirected.
- When using vendors or an interpreter, ensure that confidentiality protocols are in place and persons have been trained.
- Have written confidentiality protocols and provide training for personnel.

The American Medical Association (AMA) supports the adoption of standards to protect individual confidential information. To review the AMA computer confidentiality guidelines, known as Opinion 5.07, go to www.ama-assn.org and search the term "Confidentiality: Computers."

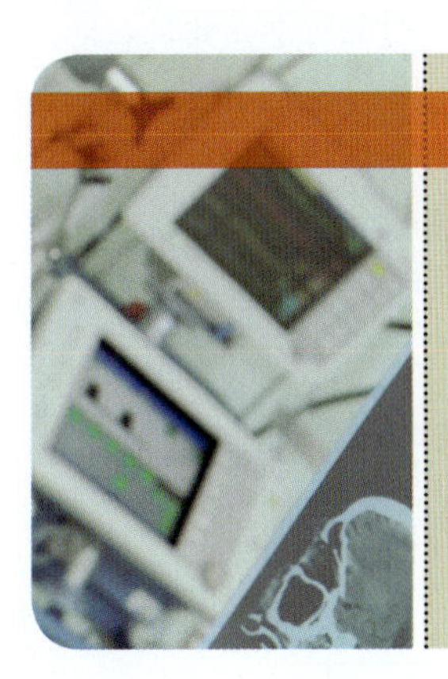

CASE STUDY 10-1

Refer to the scenario at the beginning of the chapter.

CASE STUDY REVIEW

1. How will Marilyn establish benchmarks or comparisons for computer needs?
2. Identify effective communication techniques used by Marilyn during team meetings to ensure everyone was heard and comments were understood.
3. What steps might Marilyn implement to ensure a smooth transition from a manual to a computerized system?

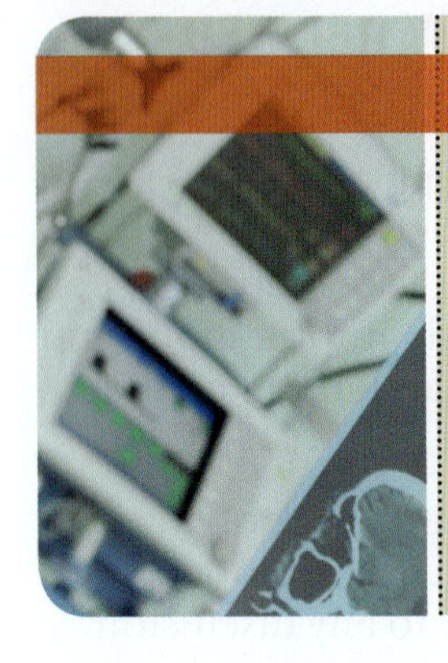

CASE STUDY 10-2

Marilyn Johnson, CMA (AAMA), who is employed by Inner City Health Care, has been given approval to computerize the clinic. Marilyn is also concerned about confidentiality issues involved with a computerized medical clinic.

CASE STUDY REVIEW

1. Identify the areas where confidentiality is most likely to be jeopardized.
2. Suggest possible solutions to protect confidentiality in each of these areas. Write a one-page summary and submit it to your instructor.

Summary

- All computer systems, from the largest supercomputer to the smallest microcomputer, consist of input devices, one or more CPUs, software, and output devices.
- The computer employs three types of memory for storing data: ROM, RAM, and data storage memory. Various forms of memory have different life spans and should be considered when archiving medical records.
- Computer software and elements of the computer system should be continually kept up to date with the latest updates and patches, and licenses and manuals should be safely filed for ready access. The system should be backed up prior to installing patches or new OS editions.
- When adding new program software or installing OS editions, compatibility with existing system software and hardware should be checked.
- Computers in the clinic may be networked using hard-wired, WiFi, or Bluetooth networks. WiFi is a wireless connection and requires security protocols to ensure confidentiality. Computers linked to the Internet should have firewalls and antivirus software loaded and kept up to date. All emails should be sent using encrypted transmission.
- Critical systems should be protected from electrical outages, surges, and static discharge.
- Computer usage in the medical clinic will typically be limited to patient demographics, scheduling, maintaining EMR, laboratory tests, billing and accounting, communication, and remote diagnosis and treatment of patients. These functions will be handled using stand-alone programs or using specialized practice management software.
- Introduction of computers or practice management software to a medical clinic requires careful planning. All personnel must be involved from the beginning to ensure the system will meet their needs and to develop ownership. Part of the planning must also take into consideration ergonomics and training of personnel.

Study for Success

To reinforce your knowledge and skills of information presented in this chapter:

- Review the *Key Terms* and *Learning Outcomes*
- Consider the *Critical Thinking* features and *Case Studies* and discuss your conclusions
- Answer the questions in the *Certification Review*

CERTIFICATION REVIEW

1. What is the best description of microcomputers?
   a. They are the fastest and most powerful computers.
   b. They handle large amounts of processing and challenge the capabilities of old mainframe systems.
   c. They are widely used in today's health care facilities.
   d. They are expensive and complex.
2. What is the best way to describe the CPU?
   a. It consists of electronic tablets with pointers, scanners, and touch screens.
   b. It is the brain of the computer system.
   c. It is often referred to as memory.
   d. It frequently is referred to as a computer program.
   e. It is also known as system software.
3. Which of the following is not considered a data output device?
   a. The monitor
   b. Printer
   c. Keystrokes, motion, and temperature
   d. Fax machine
4. What is the best definition of computer documentation?
   a. It performs a specific data processing function.
   b. It is a set of instructions that a computer follows to control computer hardware and to process data.
   c. It frequently is called the operating system (OS).
   d. It consists of the manuals and documents that define how programs or hardware operate.
   e. It is also known as a software driver.
5. Which of the following describes types of networks?
   a. Optical drives, compact disks, and digital video disks
   b. Flash drives, tape drives, optical drives, and digital video disks
   c. LANs, WANs, and Internet
   d. CDs, DVDs, and LANs
6. What is the best description of EMR?
   a. EMR are limited to one provider, clinic, or hospital.
   b. EMR include all medical information from all providers and hospitals in a patient's medical universe.
   c. EMR are used by only a handful of clinics and hospitals.
   d. EMR is a computer program that can be used to scan files to identify and eliminate computer malware.
   e. EMR are a type of CD used to store medical records.
7. What is the correct definition of ergonomics?
   a. Study of body language
   b. Granting of licenses to practice a profession
   c. Scientific study of work and space, including factors that influence worker productivity and that affect workers' health
   d. Reorganization of information on a hard disk to store files as continuous units rather than as small packets
8. The beginning point for a meaningful information security system is a comprehensive security policy that does what?
   a. Involves the use of LANs
   b. Adheres to HIPAA policies and procedures
   c. Ignores office policies and procedures
   d. Involves the use of WANs
   e. Applies phishing techniques
9. Which of the following is not an advantage of cloud computing?
   a. Cloud computing is made possible by WiFi connections
   b. Reduced costs in IT personnel
   c. Reduced hardware and software costs
   d. Important in secure data backup
10. Which of the following is not a guideline for compliance with HIPAA standards for safeguarding PHI and ePHI?
    a. Verify the patient's identity confirming two identifiers
    b. Never destroy outdated or unneeded records
    c. Never discuss PHI with others without patients' permission
    d. Have written confidentiality protocols
    e. Never leave hard copies of forms or records where unauthorized persons may view them

CHAPTER 11

Telecommunications

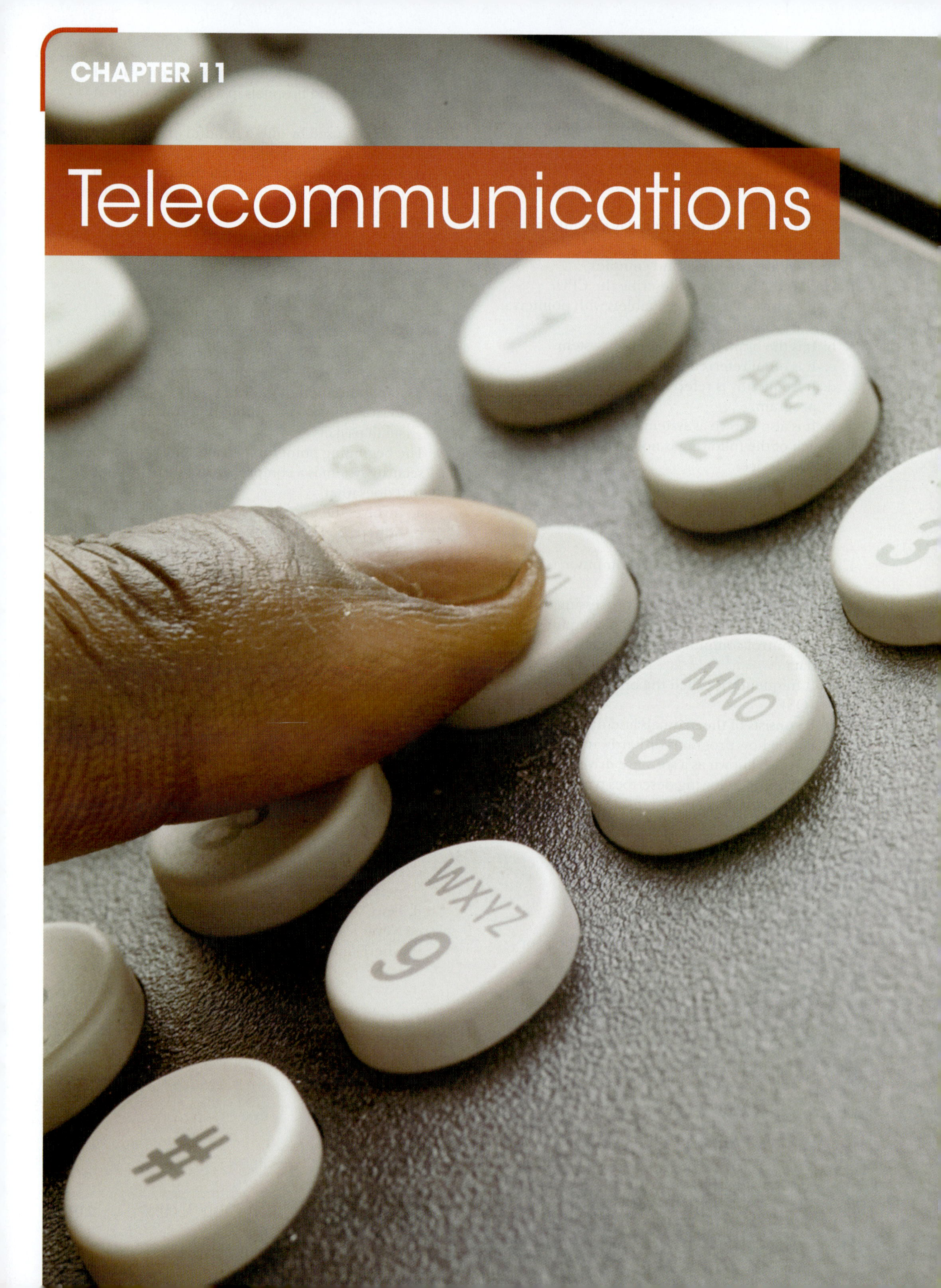

LEARNING OUTCOMES

1. Define and spell the key terms as presented in the glossary.
2. Name at least three types of calls the medical assistant can take, and state the reasons why. Name three types of calls the medical assistant should refer to the provider, and state the reasons why.
3. Discuss proper screening techniques, including six questions that should be asked during the telephone screening.
4. Discuss how calls from angry individuals should be handled in a professional manner, and demonstrate steps to follow when this type of call is received.
5. State at least five common telephone courtesies.
6. Model the proper procedure for answering incoming calls and transferring calls.
7. Describe the information every message should contain.
8. Model the proper procedure for placing outgoing calls.
9. Discuss telephone documentation.
10. Discuss the impacts of HIPAA regulations on telecommunications, including identifying ways to ensure patient confidentiality when using the telephone.
11. Identify several security measures to consider before sending a fax containing confidential information.
12. Recall several risk management considerations to address before implementing email communications.
13. Discuss VoIP telecommunications.
14. Describe email encryption and its importance.
15. Discuss the purpose of the patient portal system, including how it increases efficiency and productivity in the clinic.
16. Name at least five tasks patients can accomplish with the use of a patient portal system.
17. Define telemedicine and describe at least two patient benefits.

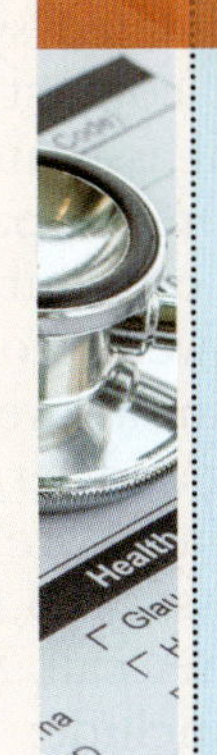

KEY TERMS

answering services
articulating
automated routing unit (ARU)
buffer words
electronic mail (email)
encryption
enunciation
fax (facsimile)
Good Samaritan laws
jargon
mHealth
modulated
patient portal systems
screening
smartphone
telemedicine
URLs (Uniform Resource Locators)
Voice over Internet Protocol (VoIP)

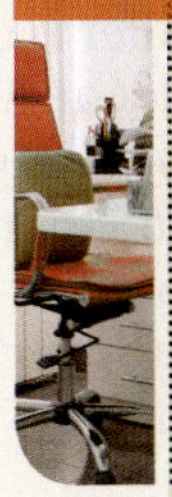

SCENARIO

At Inner City Health Care, the telephone lines are rarely quiet. Yet administrative medical assistant Ellen Armstrong, CMAS (AMT), has learned to maintain her composure when she is responsible for managing incoming calls. Ellen has in her favor a naturally warm telephone manner, but she has had to cultivate other traits so that she can represent the practice in a professional manner, help patients and other callers feel at ease, and efficiently screen or refer calls as necessary.

continues

Scenario *Continued*

Ellen has researched the three different types of Voice over Internet Protocol (VoIP) services and understands the security issues related to this type of service. Other telecommunication technologies new to Ellen include HIPAA requirements associated with facsimile (fax) machines and the use of encryption for electronic mail used in the clinic. Ellen feels organized and prepared to implement her newly acquired skills in telecommunications. To stay abreast of new telecommunication technologies, Ellen attends conferences and seminars to learn how emerging technology can be used effectively in the medical clinic.

Chapter Portal

As in many clinic settings, the telephone is the lifeline of the ambulatory care setting. By means of telecommunication, which can also include fax, wireless technology, and email transmissions, patient appointments are scheduled, referrals made, critical information related, and the practice personality conveyed.

Medical assistants, more multiskilled than ever, have a wealth of knowledge to bring to telecommunications. Over the telephone, they welcome new patients, reassure current patients, collaborate with other organizations on patient care, and calmly and efficiently deal with emergencies. They will need to draw on their resource of administrative and clinical knowledge; they will also need to cultivate a telephone personality that is warm and accessible while also being efficient and organized.

In this chapter, medical assistants will come to understand the principles basic to successful telecommunications, whether initiating or answering calls; will learn the extent and limits of their authority as medical assistants; will discover how to prepare themselves for making or receiving calls; and will be introduced to telephone systems and new technologies.

BASIC TELEPHONE TECHNIQUES

Telephone answering techniques are rapidly changing in all clinics, even the smaller single-provider practices. The medical assistant responsible for answering the telephones previously was the first contact most people had with the practice, but today the first contact is usually with an automated phone system. Just as with a human answering the phone, first impressions are lasting. The program setup in the automatic phone system should be user friendly. It is not uncommon for a person unfamiliar with a menu-driven telephone system to be unable to find the menu that applies, and it is extremely frustrating if the person cannot find a way to connect with a human operator. An option to speak with an administrative medical assistant should always be offered. An automatic answering system should begin with a message instructing the caller what to do if the call is an emergency. In most locations, the caller is instructed to hang up and dial 911. After this should be a list of menus for such items as prescription refill, billing, scheduling an appointment, and so forth. If at all possible, the menu system should only be one level deep; for example, the billing selection should not lead to another menu for Medicare, HMO, or other finance categories.

Regardless of whether the automated system or a medical assistant makes first contact with the caller, at some point the medical assistant will speak with the caller. The impression the patient forms of the practice will depend on your telephone personality and how you answer incoming calls. To create a positive impression, answer the telephone by the end of the first ring and certainly within three rings. If your station has more than one incoming line, it may be necessary to interrupt a conversation to answer another call. Some guidelines to follow in this instance include:

- Excuse yourself to the first caller by saying, "Excuse me, another line is ringing. May I put you on hold for a moment?" This should be done only once, not repeatedly during the conversation.
- When, and not before, the first caller has given permission to be put on hold, answer the second call. Determine who is calling and the nature of the call. If it is not an emergency and permission is given, place the caller on hold. Never try to quickly resolve the second call before returning to the first call.

- Return to the first caller and thank the person for holding.
- Explore the possibility of an automated message after three rings to put the calls into a waiting queue with a message that you are on another line and will answer the next call momentarily.

Telephone Personality

Presentation

First impressions are usually conveyed through verbal and nonverbal communication (see Chapter 4 for a review of these communication modes.) In telephone communications, however, personality and attitudes are conveyed only through the tone in which words are spoken and the words themselves. Remember, callers are not an interruption of your work but the reason for your job. Even in a large practice, it is rare that someone just answers the telephone and has no other duties. No matter what other duties are pressing, the primary responsibility of every employee in a medical clinic is patient care; everything else is secondary. Whoever answers incoming calls should be prepared to give the caller their complete attention.

Use a voice that is pleasant and well **modulated** (i.e., one that varies in pitch and intensity) and conveys interest in the caller's needs. Hold the handpiece correctly, about 1 to 2 inches away from the mouth, and project your voice *at* the mouthpiece, not *over* it. The use of headsets permits the mouthpiece to be positioned appropriately and frees the hands to use the computer and input information easily.

Volume, enunciation, pronunciation, and speed all have a profound effect on how you sound to the person on the other end of the line.

- Volume should be the same as when speaking conversationally.
- **Enunciation** implies speaking your words clearly and **articulating** carefully.
- Pronunciation involves saying the words correctly.
- Speed should be at a normal rate, neither too fast nor too slow. Err on the side of speaking more slowly.

Posture, the way the body is carried, also affects the voice. If the body is slumped in a chair, the diaphragm (the muscle separating the abdominal and thoracic cavities) is compressed and breathing may be restricted. Using the headset speaker with the phone promotes good ergonomic position because it decreases neck and shoulder stress by allowing you to sit up straight (Figure 11-1). If you are less tired and tense, you can focus more easily on professional alertness, which comes across to the caller in the sound of your voice.

Being organized and prepared in advance for each telephone call enables the medical assistant to respond to each caller appropriately. A pleasant vocal impression can be delivered by taking a deep breath and putting on a smile before answering the call.

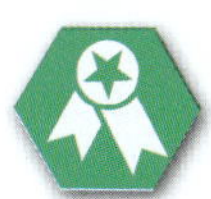
Competency

Medical assistants who enjoy their work and want to be of assistance to patients communicate enthusiasm. Enthusiasm conveys interest in the caller and projects a sincere, caring attitude that can be "heard" over the telephone (Figure 11-2). Though some callers will be upset, frightened, or even angry, the medical assistant must always be patient and in control. Some calls may be about life-threatening emergencies; medical assistants need to remain

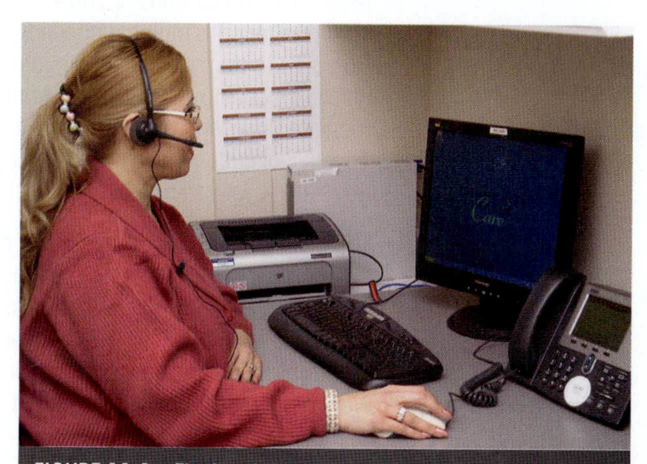
FIGURE 11-1 The headset-type telephone frees the medical assistant's hands to document and record while maintaining an ergonomic position.

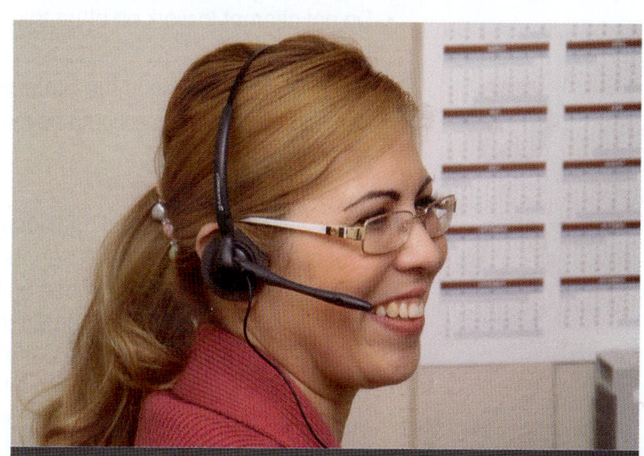
FIGURE 11-2 Tone of voice can put callers at ease during a telephone conversation.

calm to be of help to the caller, remembering their professional role as health care providers.

Professional Telephone Etiquette

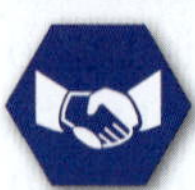

Professional

Telephone etiquette, as with all good manners, simply involves treating others with consideration. Medical assistants have chosen a profession in which care and concern for others are paramount, so it is especially important to keep the patient's feelings in the forefront at all times. Basic telephone courtesies should be kept in mind when answering any professional call (see the "Telephone Courtesies" Quick Reference Guide).

QUICK REFERENCE GUIDE

TELEPHONE COURTESIES

Communication

- Always use callers' names and titles (e.g., Mrs. O'Keefe, Dr. King) during the course of a conversation when confidentiality is assured; this shows interest in them as individuals.
- Do not use technical terms if simpler ones will convey the information adequately. Using professional **jargon**, or terminology, is an easy trap to fall into because this terminology is used daily with co-workers. Jargon often confuses people outside the profession; the goal in communication is mutual understanding.
- Do not use slang or nonstandard terms in a business setting. Slang terms may have entirely different meanings to individuals from another generation or cultural background. However, patients may use slang when they communicate. It is important not to be offended by slang terms; also, be certain that patients who use slang understand any common medical terminology you may use.
- Say "good-bye" when closing the call, and allow the caller to hang up first.

Presentation

- The "hold" button on the telephone is often misused and should be used sparingly. Never put a caller on hold until you know who is calling and why. Never place an urgent or emergency call on hold. Never put a caller on hold without asking for and receiving permission to do so. No call should be left unattended for more than 20 to 30 seconds. If it is necessary to keep callers waiting longer, go back to the caller and give the option of continuing to hold or receiving a call back in a few minutes.
- Never eat or chew gum when talking on the telephone. This impedes enunciation and is distracting to the caller.

Competency

- Pay attention to what the caller is saying and how he or she sounds. Do not interrupt or finish sentences for slow talkers. The caller may have difficulty putting some thoughts into words, but give the person a chance to explain the problem or question. Listen with empathy for the caller. Also listen to what the tone of voice expresses.
- Do not attempt to work on other things while talking on the telephone.

Integrity

- Never talk to someone in the clinic while on an open line. This is confusing to the caller, and confidential information could be inadvertently overheard.

Initiative

- When it is necessary to get additional information and call back later, let the person know when to expect the call. If for some reason the information is not available when the time for the call back arrives, call anyway to let the person know when to expect another call.
- When taking a message for someone in the clinic, give the caller an idea of when to expect a return call. If the person will be out of the clinic for an extended period, see if someone else can help or if the caller would rather wait to hear from that specific individual. Avoid promising to have someone call back when you cannot control if or when this will happen.

Answering Incoming Calls

Most calls received in an ambulatory care setting are from patients or prospective patients, but some are from other providers or medical facilities. The remaining incoming calls are from family members, salespeople, and miscellaneous others. Personal calls should not be permitted in the medical clinic because the busy lines are intended for business. Occasional personal emergency calls are appropriate.

Preparing to Take Calls. Before answering incoming calls or making outgoing calls, medical assistants should devise a simple system to keep organized throughout the hectic day of telephone communications. If the reception desk is computerized, the first step is to boot up the computer and prepare ready access to the scheduling, patient demographics, and note screens. Figure 11-3 illustrates a scheduling screen from Harris CareTracker PM and EMR. If the reception desk is not computerized, collect materials such as message pads, the master schedule book, and prescription refill request forms. Regardless of whether the reception desk is computerized, a list of frequently used telephone numbers and clinic extensions and a supply of sharpened pencils and working pens are needed. A handy reference to practice protocols would be helpful, as would a supply of new patient registration forms, release of information, and confidentiality information forms required by HIPAA.

Answering Calls. When answering incoming calls, the name of the facility should be clearly identified, as well as the name of the person with whom the caller is speaking. The name of the clinic is important because the caller wants to know the correct number has been reached. To avoid clipping off the clinic name, practice using **buffer words**. Buffer words are expendable words and may consist of introductory words, phrases, or statements such as "Good morning." They allow a caller to realize they have reached the desired number and to collect his or her thoughts.

Obtain the caller's full name and correct spelling, and ask if this is an emergency call. Ask for the caller's telephone number, street address, and date of birth (DOB). This information is necessary for retrieval of the caller's correct medical chart. Determine how you can be of assistance, and complete the call efficiently by following all established clinic protocols.

Screening Calls. One of the medical assistant's responsibilities is to screen incoming calls. The purpose of screening is twofold: (1) to be sure the caller talks to the person who will be most helpful (this is not necessarily the person asked for) and (2) to ensure the provider's time with calls is efficiently managed.

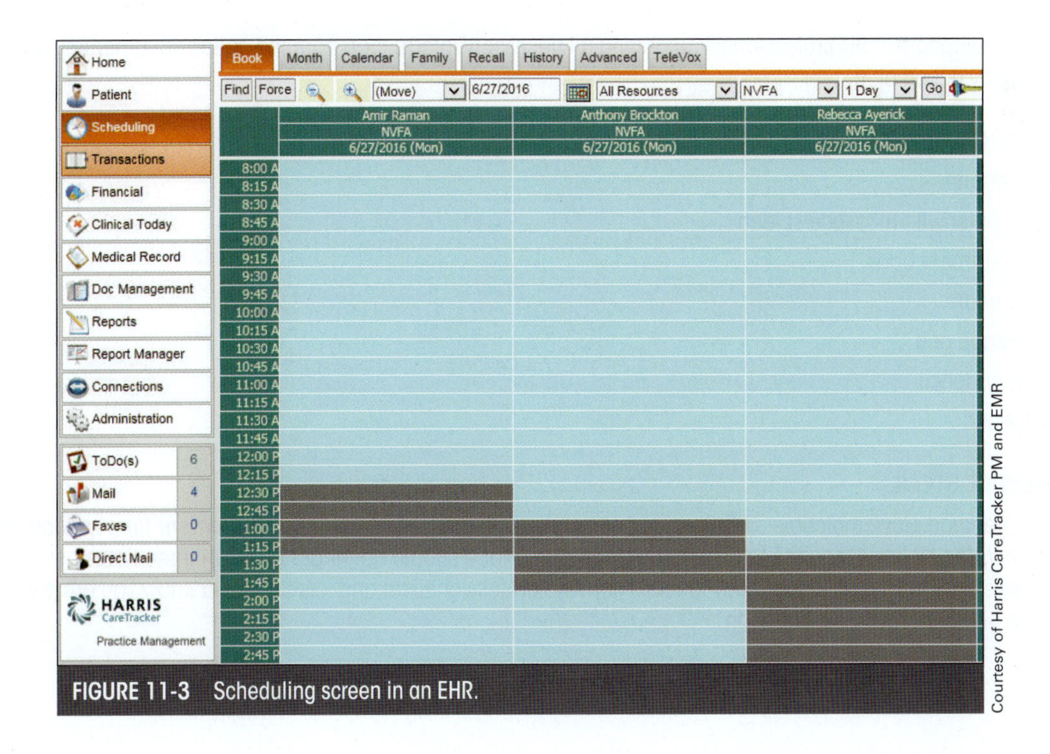

FIGURE 11-3 Scheduling screen in an EHR.

Courtesy of Harris CareTracker PM and EMR

Many people who call the clinic will ask to speak to the provider. Patients calling for appointments or with billing problems or insurance questions will sometimes ask to speak to their provider, assuming he or she is the person in charge, and therefore should answer any question or solve any problem. In most practices, this is not the case. Medical assistants and other administrative employees are equipped to deal with administrative functions; usually, providers are not involved in these procedures and sometimes may not be aware of administrative routines.

Procedure

Screening Techniques. Screening is usually a simple process of asking the caller's name and the reason for the call. There are situations, however, that will require tactful persistence to get the information needed to properly direct the caller. Sometimes callers hesitate to give information because the questions are of a confidential and possibly even embarrassing nature.

Occasionally, a caller flatly refuses to give any information or will just say, "I'm a friend." If it is a patient who refuses to give information after gentle prodding, respect the patient's privacy and take a message. If you do not know who the caller is and you are unable to get any information, take the message and give it to the provider. If the provider does not know the person, he or she can decide whether to return the call. In any event, do not argue with the caller. Be polite and professional at all times. Procedure 11-1 provides steps for answering and screening calls.

Transferring a Call. During the screening process, calls may mistakenly be directed to someone who is unable to assist the caller adequately. This call will need to be transferred to someone with more expertise in a particular area. Guidelines that ensure successful transfer of calls include:

- Get the caller's full name, telephone number, and any other situation-associated information before attempting to transfer the call.
- Determine who would be the best person to assist with this situation.

PROCEDURE 11-1

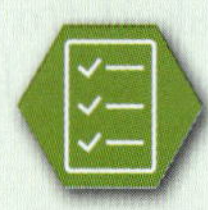
Procedure

Demonstrating Professional Telephone Techniques

PURPOSE:

To answer telephone calls professionally, acquiring all necessary information from the caller, documenting it correctly, and properly acting on it.

EQUIPMENT/SUPPLIES:

- Telephone
- Computer with message screen
- Appointment book
- Calendar
- Message pad
- Pen or pencil
- Notepad

PROCEDURE STEPS:

1. Be prepared. Have materials organized and computer with message screen up. ***Implement time management principles by*** answering the telephone promptly. The phone should not ring more than three times before it is answered. RATIONALE: Being ready for calls conveys professionalism and lets the caller know you are prepared to give him or her your full attention.

(continues)

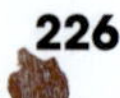

2. Introduce the clinic and yourself by answering the call with the preferred clinic greeting, speaking directly into the mouthpiece. The mouthpiece should be 1 to 2 inches away from the mouth. Sample greeting: "Good morning. Inner City Health Care. Ellen speaking. How may I help you?" RATIONALE: Use a pleasant tone of voice to convey a warm greeting. Holding the phone correctly and speaking directly into the mouthpiece aid the caller in hearing your message clearly.
3. Ask the name of the caller as quickly as possible, and ***use sound judgment*** to determine whether this is an emergency call. RATIONALE: Using the caller's name personalizes the call and acknowledges that you heard the name correctly. If this is an emergency call, follow emergency protocols.
4. ***Apply active listening skills.*** You may need additional information to assist or direct the call appropriately. RATIONALE: This gives the caller a sense that you are listening attentively while eliciting additional facts and assures that information will be transmitted correctly.
5. Repeat information back to the caller, ***using appropriate responses/feedback***. RATIONALE: This technique confirms that facts are complete and accurate. The caller also has an opportunity to hear the message and confirm that it is accurate or add something to modify or clarify the message.
6. Follow established written screening protocols for all telephone calls, ***working within your scope of practice.*** RATIONALE: Ensures that you understand your role in the health care practice and that all pertinent information is collected.
7. When using a multiline telephone as shown in Figure 11-4, it is helpful to keep a notepad by the telephone. When you answer the phone and have the caller's name, *pay attention to detail* and jot down the name, which line the caller is on, and some quick notes about the content of the call. At the end of your work shift, ***protect and maintain confidentiality*** by shredding all notepapers containing PHI. RATIONALE: Using this simple technique avoids problems if another line rings and you must put the first person on hold. Reviewing your notes allows you to accurately respond to the caller. PHI must be confidential, so disposing of notepapers properly is critical for adherence to HIPAA guidelines.

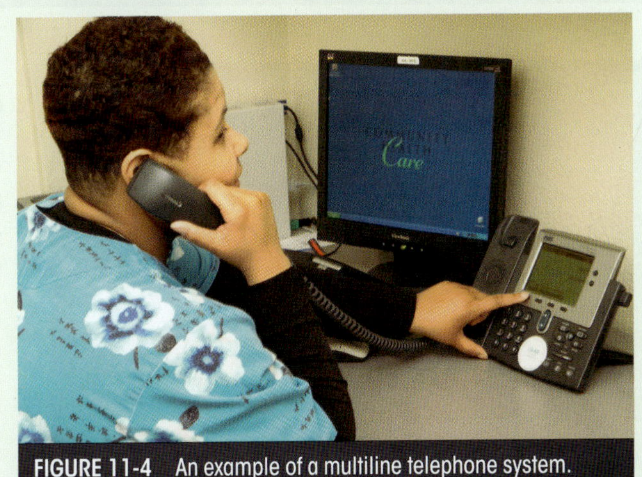

FIGURE 11-4 An example of a multiline telephone system.

8. Ask if the caller has any other questions. RATIONALE: This saves you and the caller time. It is frustrating to have to place a second call because you forgot to ask something. It also ties up the telephone lines and is not cost effective.
9. ***End the call courteously.*** Say "thank you" and "good-bye" (not "bye-bye"). Allow the caller to hang up before you disconnect. RATIONALE: Saying good-bye conveys professionalism and leaves the caller with a positive image of the clinic. Often callers think of questions just as they are ready to hang up. It is more time efficient to handle the questions immediately rather than having the caller make another call.
10. Document information and record any necessary actions. RATIONALE: This procedure is necessary for legal reasons. Remember that in a court of law, a deed not documented is a deed not done.

DOCUMENTATION:

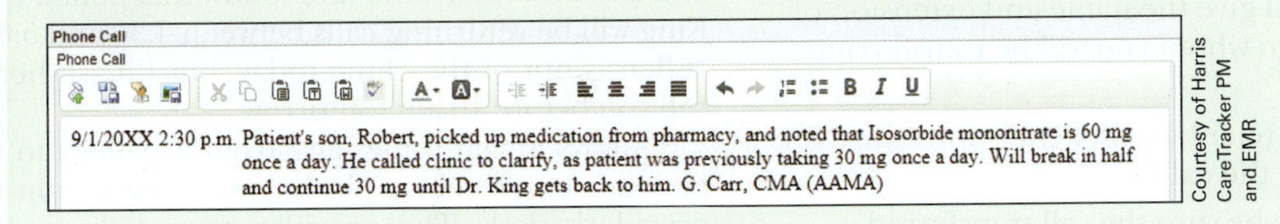

Phone Call
Phone Call

9/1/20XX 2:30 p.m. Patient's son, Robert, picked up medication from pharmacy, and noted that Isosorbide mononitrate is 60 mg once a day. He called clinic to clarify, as patient was previously taking 30 mg once a day. Will break in half and continue 30 mg until Dr. King gets back to him. G. Carr, CMA (AAMA)

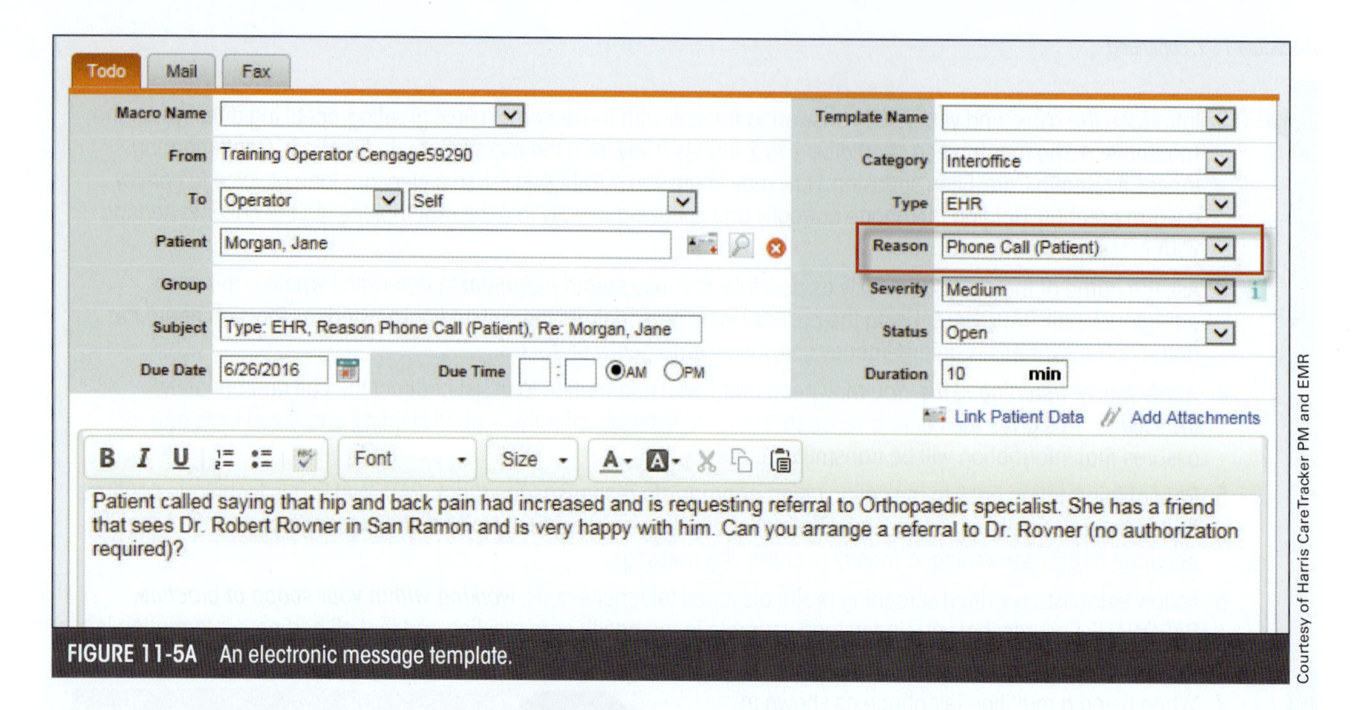

FIGURE 11-5A An electronic message template.

Courtesy of Harris CareTracker PM and EMR

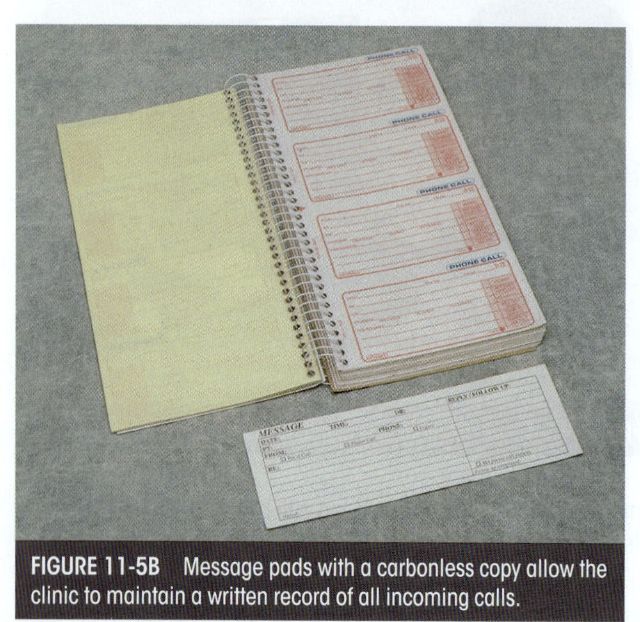

FIGURE 11-5B Message pads with a carbonless copy allow the clinic to maintain a written record of all incoming calls.

- Ask if you may place the caller on hold while you collect any pertinent data and make a call to confirm that the person best suited to assist is available.
- Return to the caller, thank him or her for holding, and give the name and extension of the person to whom you will be transferring the call.
- Follow your telephone system's procedure for transferring the call.
- Follow up to be sure the call transferred correctly.

Taking a Message. When taking messages, it is advisable to use a standard telephone message pad with a carbonless copy that allows the clinic to maintain a record of all incoming calls or the appropriate practice management (PM) screen (Figure 11-5). The information that should be recorded for *every* message includes:

1. Date and time call is received
2. Who the call is for
3. Caller's name, telephone number, and DOB
4. When the caller can be reached
5. Nature and urgency of the call
6. Action to be taken (e.g., will call back, returned your call, please call back)
7. Message, if any
8. Your name or initials (in case there are questions)

Be sure to repeat the information back to the caller to verify that you have heard and copied it correctly. When taking a message, give callers an approximate time when they might expect to receive a call back if there is an established policy and all staff understand and follow that policy. ("Dr. King will be returning calls between 4:30 and 5:00." "Ellen is out of the clinic today, but I'll ask her to call you before 10 am tomorrow.")

Always attach a message from a patient to the patient's chart before placing the message on the provider's desk. The provider cannot discuss the patient's condition or answer questions without this information. Clinics using a PM system can send and receive messages via the computer and can have immediate access to the EMR. Procedure 11-2 identifies the steps and rationales in taking a telephone message.

Ending the Call. Ending the telephone call is as important as answering the call promptly. Bring the conversation to a courteous close and repeat any pertinent information back to the caller. ("Your appointment is scheduled for Friday, January 12, at 9 AM with Doctor King.") Pause just a moment to see if the caller has any additional questions. If not, say "Good-bye." Never use slang terms such as *bye-bye, see you later*, or *so long*. These terms do not reflect a positive professional image. You should always stay on the line until the caller hangs up. The caller might think of something else he or she wanted to ask or verify, and staying on the line gives the caller the opportunity to verbalize a thought rather than having to call back.

ROUTING CALLS IN THE MEDICAL CLINIC

The administrative medical assistant staffing the reception desk is responsible for greeting each patient, whether in person or via telephone, with a warm, friendly response. Incoming calls in the

PROCEDURE 11-2

Documenting Telephone Messages Accurately

PURPOSE:

To record an accurate telephone message and follow up as required.

EQUIPMENT/SUPPLIES:

- Telephone
- Message pad
- Black ink pen
- Notepad
- Medical record if available
- Clock or watch

PROCEDURE STEPS:

1. Answer the telephone following the steps outlined in Procedure 11-1. RATIONALE: Being prepared and answering the phone promptly with the preferred clinic greeting prepares the medical assistant mentally to focus on the caller's needs. Using a pleasant tone of voice conveys a warm greeting.
2. Use a message pad, or document directly into the EMR. ***Pay attention to detail*** when requesting the following information:
   - Date and time call is received
   - Full name and correct spelling of person calling, and daytime and evening telephone numbers, including area code and extension when appropriate
   - Date of birth, clinic number, or social security number to verify correct patient
   - Who the call is for
   - The reason for the call
   - The action to be taken
   - The name or initials of the person taking the call

   RATIONALE: Complete and accurate information is necessary to respond to the caller's requests efficiently.

(continues)

3. Repeat the above information back to the caller. RATIONALE: Verifies that the information was recorded accurately and allows the caller to acknowledge that the message is correct.
4. If the call is from an established patient or concerns an established patient, pull the medical record/chart and attach the message to it before delivering the message to the intended individual. When using EMR save the message and forward it to the intended recipient. RATIONALE: Information about the patient is available should it be needed, and any required documentation can efficiently be made in the chart.
5. Maintain the old message book with all carbon copies intact. RATIONALE: Documents all telephone calls received by the clinic. This information could be useful in determining the need for additional telephone lines into the clinic.

DOCUMENTATION:

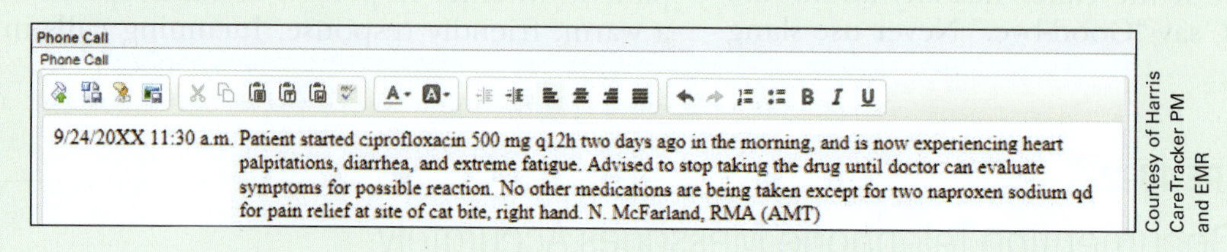
Phone Call

Phone Call

9/24/20XX 11:30 a.m. Patient started ciprofloxacin 500 mg q12h two days ago in the morning, and is now experiencing heart palpitations, diarrhea, and extreme fatigue. Advised to stop taking the drug until doctor can evaluate symptoms for possible reaction. No other medications are being taken except for two naproxen sodium qd for pain relief at site of cat bite, right hand. N. McFarland, RMA (AMT)

Courtesy of Harris CareTracker PM and EMR

medical clinic typically are routed by the administrative medical assistant according to subject and who can best respond. The administrative medical assistant, as well as clinical medical assistants, must always follow the provider-approved protocols when screening and responding to telephone calls. Table 11-1 illustrates examples of routing calls in the medical clinic.

Types of Calls the Medical Assistant Can Take

Keep in mind that, no matter how experienced, the medical assistant has definite limitations of authority and knowledge. Most calls can be handled by the knowledgeable medical assistant, but there are situations that only the provider should manage simply because the provider ultimately is responsible for what happens in the practice. Examples of calls the administrative or clinical medical assistant can take are as follows:

1. *Established patients.* When an established patient calls to set up an appointment, record the patient's name, daytime telephone number, and the reason for the appointment.
2. *New patients.* Require the same information for as the established patient plus some additional information, including:
   - Address
   - Age/DOB
   - Employer
   - Insurance carrier, HMO, Medicare, and any secondary insurance

TABLE 11-1

ROUTING CALLS IN THE MEDICAL CLINIC

ADMINISTRATIVE MEDICAL ASSISTANT	CLINICAL MEDICAL ASSISTANT	PROVIDER
Scheduling appointments	Scheduling tests and procedures	Other providers
Changing appointments	Prescription refills	STAT reports
Cancelling appointments	Progress reports	Provider's family
Fees and billing questions	Radiological and lab reports	Request for test results (positive)
Insurance questions	Patient referrals	
Information requests	Request for test results (negative)	
General questions about practice	Complaints about medical service	
Salespeople	Salespeople	

- Insurance ID numbers of subscriber or policy holder
- Name of insured (self, spouse, or parent)
- Name of referral source

This information serves as a source for the establishment of the chart and may lead to a discussion regarding payment of fees. Information for both new and established patients should be entered into the PM system or appointment book if not a computerized clinic.

3. *Scheduling appointments.* A major portion of telephone communications is spent scheduling patient appointments. (See Chapter 12 for detailed information on patient scheduling and rescheduling.)
4. *Scheduling patient tests.* Scheduling tests for patients can involve a great deal of coordination. Often appointment times need to be arranged among providers, the patient, and the facility where a test may be conducted.
5. *Billing questions.* Billing questions can be involved and complex, and medical assistants should be prepared to answer questions by retrieving information on the patient's insurance and billing status.
6. *Insurance information.* Calls will come from patients about insurance, as well as from insurance carriers and HMOs with questions about patients or their treatment. Prior to responding to insurance carrier requests for patient records, authenticate that the call is from the carrier using established clinic protocols and ensure that a signed release of information form is on file.
7. *Requests for prescription refills.* If a patient or family member is requesting that a prescription be refilled, medical assistants may take the call. However, they may not authorize a refill or tell the patient that a prescription will be refilled without the provider's approval. Most clinics ask that the patient call his or her refill requests directly into the pharmacy; the pharmacy then calls or faxes the provider's clinic for approval. Messages taken on these calls should be attached to the patient's chart or entered into the PM system and given to the provider for review and for permission to refill. When the provider approves the refill, the pharmacy may be called with an approval. Some practice protocols give authority to the CMA and RMA to refill standard medications with appropriate guidelines, for example, oral contraceptives or maintenance drugs, such as blood pressure medications, among others.

Procedure 11-3 identifies the steps for calling a pharmacy to refill an authorized prescription.

8. *Receiving routine progress reports.* Frequently, providers will ask patients to report on their progress. If the patient is doing well, it is acceptable for the medical assistant to take that information on a message form or enter the message into the patient's EMR.
9. *General information about the practice.* People may call requesting information about hours, location, financial protocols, or areas of practice.
10. *Salespeople.* The medical clinic should have policies regarding the scheduling of pharmaceutical and medical supply representatives.

Today, many medical clinics take advantage of options offered through their computerized PM system when responding to telephone calls. The medical assistant will screen calls and forward messages to other personnel as "tasks." These tasks or messages can go back and forth between administrative and clinical medical assistants as necessary, or they may include the provider if his or her professional judgment is required to handle the call. An example of this screening procedure is as follows: (1) The administrative medical assistant answers a call from a patient wishing to have a prescription refilled. (2) The administrative medical assistant collects all of the pertinent information and sends a message to the clinical medical assistant. (3) When checking the patient's chart, the clinical medical assistant sees there are no additional refills authorized by the provider. (4) The clinical medical assistant forwards the pertinent information to the provider. (5) The provider, having complete access to the EMR of the patient, authorizes the refill, documents the order, and sends the notice to the clinical medical assistant. (6) The clinical medical assistant calls or sends a fax to the pharmacy to authorize the prescription refill.

Types of Calls Referred to the Provider

Providers have many demands on their time: surgeries, hospital rounds, patient appointments, documentation, and consultations with other providers, to name a few. Therefore, their time is extremely valuable, and misuse of time impacts the clinic in many ways. It is important to carefully screen calls going to providers to ensure that they receive only the calls that are necessary.

PROCEDURE 11-3

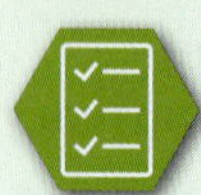

Procedure

Calling a Pharmacy to Refill an Authorized Prescription

PURPOSE:

To notify a pharmacy to refill an authorized prescription.

EQUIPMENT/SUPPLIES:

- Patient's chart
- Provider authorization to refill prescription
- Drug name, dosage, and instructions for when and how to take the medication
- Pharmacy name and telephone number
- Telephone

PROCEDURE STEPS:

1. Receive patient's request for a prescription refill. Follow appropriate telephone techniques. RATIONALE: Appropriate telephone techniques demonstrate consistent customer service.
2. Obtain the following information from the patient and include it on the message form or EMR message screen:
   - Patient's full name and correct spelling, and patient's DOB
   - Telephone number where the patient can be reached
   - Name of medication and how long patient has been taking it
   - Patient's symptoms and current health condition
   - If patient is a child, ask his or her weight
   - History of this condition (last clinic visit)
   - Treatments the patient has tried
   - Any known allergies
   - Pharmacy name, telephone number, and address if a chain

   RATIONALE: This information is needed by the provider for assessment as to whether a prescription will be refilled, if something else should be prescribed, or if the patient needs to be seen by the provider.
3. Attach the completed message to the patient's chart or EMR and give it to the provider. RATIONALE: The provider may wish to review the patient's history before refilling the prescription.
4. After the provider has responded, review comments in the chart by the provider. If the refill is authorized, call the patient's pharmacy with the refill information. Ask the pharmacy to repeat the information back to you. RATIONALE: Verifies the pharmacy has recorded the prescription accurately.
5. ***Paying attention to detail,*** document in the patient's chart the date and time the prescription was called to the pharmacy and the pharmacy address. Verify that the correct drug, dosage, and dosage instructions were provided to the pharmacy. RATIONALE: Provides accurate documentation in the patient's chart.

DOCUMENTATION:

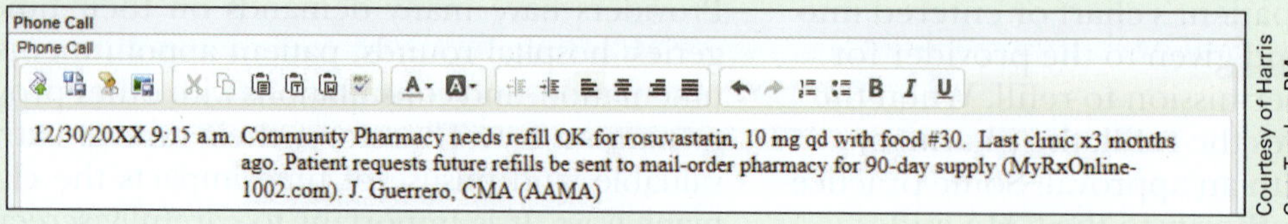

Courtesy of Harris CareTracker PM and EMR

Examples of calls that should be referred to the provider include the following:

1. *Other providers.* When other providers call, always ask if they need to speak to the provider immediately or if they would like a call back. Be sure to ask if the call is regarding a specific patient; if so, attach a message to the chart.
2. *STAT reports.* In most cases the provider will only initiate STAT reports when the results are needed immediately.
3. *Provider's family.* Most providers will have an established protocol related to calls from family members. Family members generally do not call unless it is necessary, so in most cases their calls are put through directly.

Many other calls coming into the clinic may require the provider's professional judgment. Generally the majority of these calls can be handled with the PM system task/message feature. When the provider has a minute between patients, he or she can respond or provide specific instructions.

Special Consideration Calls

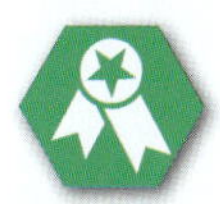
Competency

Answering the telephone in an ambulatory care setting places the medical assistant in contact with a variety of callers: those needing referrals to other facilities; emergency calls; and callers who may be angry, older, or speak English as a second language. As a professional, your goal is to treat every individual with courtesy and respect and to respond to their queries appropriately or to transfer the caller to another team member who can assist.

Initiative

Referral Calls to Other Facilities. If it is necessary to refer the caller to someone outside the clinic, such as to a laboratory or another provider, be sure to tell the caller:

- Why he or she should speak to someone else
- The telephone number to call (be sure to include the area code and extension)
- Who, specifically, to speak with at that number
- What information to have ready when he or she makes the call
- When to call
- If you would like a call back after the other contact is made

Legal

Emergency/Urgent Calls. The medical assistant must be careful when handling emergency or urgent calls to ensure that he or she works within the scope of his or her education and training. Donald A. Balassa, JD, MBS, Executive Director and Legal Counsel for the AAMA, states: "Procedures which constitute the practice of medicine, or which state law specifically delegates to licensed professionals to perform, may not be delegated to unlicensed professionals such as medical assistants." Therefore, prior to screening calls the medical assistant should always direct the caller to call 911 if the caller believes he or she may be experiencing a life-threatening emergency. Every attempt should be made to obtain the caller's name and telephone number before assisting with making the 911 call if it appears the person is confused or unable to dial for himself or herself.

Screening is the act of evaluating the urgency of a medical situation and prioritizing the call. Telephone screening is one of the most important functions for the person answering the telephone. Telephone screening requires skill and experience. An urgent condition is one that requires medical intervention that can be handled in a timely manner at an ambulatory care center.

To determine if a call is truly a medical emergency, keep a list of provider-approved questions near the telephone to assist in evaluating the situation. Standard screening questions can determine the nature of an emergency. Not all questions are appropriate to every call; suitable questions depend on the nature of the situation. Screening questions to ask may include:

- What happened?
- Who is the patient? (Ask name and age.)
- Is the patient breathing?
- Is there bleeding? How much? From where?
- Is the patient conscious?
- What is the patient's temperature?
- If the patient ingested something:
  - What did the patient take?
  - How much?
  - Are there poison or overdose instructions on the bottle?

Screening does not only pertain to emergency calls. Screening techniques can also help determine when a patient with symptoms should be seen by asking the caller questions such as:

- How long have you had the symptoms?
- Is there any fever?
- Are you taking any medications?

This information helps determine whether an appointment should be scheduled immediately or if it can wait a few days.

Legal

The practice should periodically review procedures for handling emergency/urgent calls. If a clinic situation involves a great deal of telephone screening, the staff should enroll in an advanced first-aid course. This will enable all participants to more accurately give instructions or to handle these calls if there is no provider in the clinic at that moment. In service training provided by the providers is a great tool to make telephone screening run smoothly. Remember, you should only render aid *within the areas of your training and expertise.* **Good Samaritan laws** do not cover paid employees, only uncompensated situations. All ambulatory settings should also post a list of numbers to be used in case of emergencies, such as the poison control telephone number.

Procedure

Angry Callers. Medical assistants will probably have occasion to speak with callers who are upset or angry. Although these calls eventually may need to be referred to the clinic manager or the provider, medical assistants need techniques for managing problem calls.

Competency

The first priority is to defuse the situation. This cannot be accomplished if you become upset or angry. As a professional, it is important to remain calm and in control at all times. Like most skills, defusing a difficult situation becomes easier with practice (see Procedure 11-4).

Older Adult Callers. Several issues may arise when dealing with older adult patients, such as impaired hearing, confusion, and an inability to understand procedures or technical information.

Do not assume that all older adults are senile or hard of hearing. This is a dangerous pitfall into which many people stumble.

If the individual has a hearing impairment, speak more slowly, more clearly, and a little louder

PROCEDURE 11-4

Procedure

Handling Problem Calls

PURPOSE:

To handle calls in a positive and professional manner while providing necessary comfort, empathy, and information to the caller to resolve the problem.

EQUIPMENT/SUPPLIES:

- Telephone
- Message pad
- Pen or pencil

PROCEDURE STEPS:

1. Answer the call as outlined in Procedure 11-1.
2. Remain calm and avoid becoming upset with an angry caller. Let the caller say what needs to be said without interruption (unless it is a medical emergency requiring immediate action). RATIONALE: Permits the caller to express concerns without having to repeat information or possibly forget something important.
3. Lower your voice both in pitch and volume. RATIONALE: Has a calming effect on an angry caller.
4. ***Listen to and acknowledge*** what the caller is upset about. Paraphrase information to verify that you have understood the problem. RATIONALE: Lets the caller know you are truly listening and have understood the problem.
5. ***Be courteous, patient, and respectful.*** Use the words "I understand" and show that you are interested in hearing the caller's concerns. RATIONALE: This does not necessarily mean you agree with the caller, but rather that you are willing to empathize and at least accept that, from a particular point of view, there is a reason to be upset.
6. Do not take the call personally. RATIONALE: It is the situation that made the caller angry; you have not done so.
7. Offer assistance. RATIONALE: Ask what you can do to help, and then follow through.

(continues)

8. Document the call accurately and properly. RATIONALE: Complete documentation promotes risk management and prevents lengthy litigation experiences.
9. When dealing with a frightened or hysterical caller, ***display a calm, caring, and professional manner*** by speaking in a soothing voice; use a slower, lower tone than normal. RATIONALE: This often has a calming effect on the caller.
10. If the call is an emergency, begin screening procedures as needed and ***attend to any special needs of the patient.*** RATIONALE: Have a list of screening questions at hand to refer to or instruct the caller to dial 911. Be sure you have the name and telephone number for follow-up.
11. Always have the caller repeat the instructions you provided. RATIONALE: People who are upset may not hear or comprehend much of what is said. Your instructions may deal with an emergency situation; thus it is important they are clearly understood.
12. Finalize and follow through on action to be taken, whether it is confirming emergency medical personnel are on the scene or scheduling an emergency appointment. RATIONALE: Ensures quality patient care.
13. Always report problem calls to the provider or clinic manager at once. RATIONALE: This will ensure appropriate action is taken, and it is important for risk management purposes.

DOCUMENTATION:

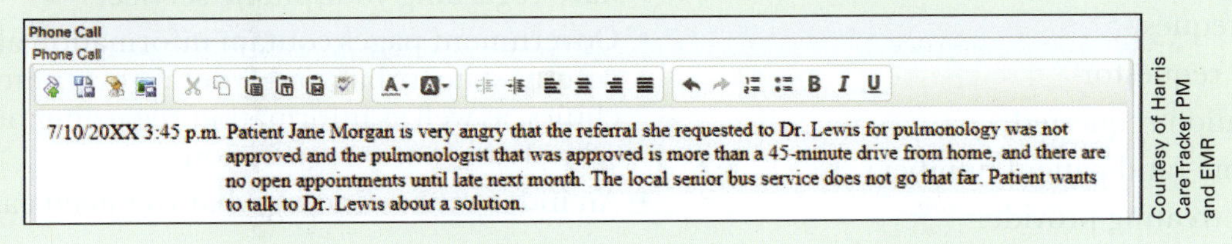
Phone Call

Phone Call

7/10/20XX 3:45 p.m. Patient Jane Morgan is very angry that the referral she requested to Dr. Lewis for pulmonology was not approved and the pulmonologist that was approved is more than a 45-minute drive from home, and there are no open appointments until late next month. The local senior bus service does not go that far. Patient wants to talk to Dr. Lewis about a solution.

Courtesy of Harris CareTracker PM and EMR

than normal. Do not shout. If you are uncertain that the person has heard everything, ask if there are any questions, or ask the person to repeat information back to you.

If the person has difficulty understanding you, simplify the information; ask frequently if there are any questions; and try to explain in simple, concrete terms. At times, if it is difficult to communicate with an older adult patient, someone from the patient's family should be given certain information. Discuss this option with the clinic manager or provider first, and be sure signed documentation is on file.

Diversity

English as a second Language Callers. In any clinic, it is possible to have contact with many patients whose primary language is not English.

It is extremely helpful to have at least one person in the clinic who is bilingual. For the nonbilingual medical assistant, certain techniques may help when communicating with all but totally non-English-speaking patients.

- A patient who does not *speak* fluent English may still *understand* as well as anyone. Do not assume that individuals with strong accents cannot understand you.
- Speak at a normal volume; raising the voice does not increase the other person's ability to comprehend.
- If the other person has difficulty understanding, speak more slowly. Avoid complicated words when simple ones will express the meaning just as well.
- Ask the person if clarification is needed. Be willing to review the information again.
- Be patient.

If these techniques are not successful, it is the responsibility of your provider-employer to supply an interpreter.

TELEPHONE DOCUMENTATION

Requests for medical information over the telephone should be discouraged. A provider or facility that needs the information to treat the patient usually places an emergency request. A call back verification procedure should be implemented for this type of request. Request the caller's name and telephone number, and state that you will call back with the necessary information. Then call back to verify the identity of the caller and provide or fax the information. It is important to follow this procedure

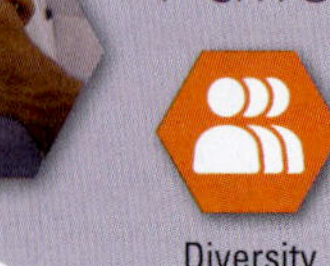

Patient Education

Patients who have difficulty with English may be confused by medical terms. Listen to the terms the patient uses and use those terms during conversation with the patient. Avoid using abbreviations without first explaining what they mean.

during routine telephone interchanges that take place between facilities/provider clinics and laboratories seeking test results or consult findings.

Legal

All telephone requests for medical information should be documented either in a log reserved for that purpose or in the patient's medical record. This information is important to protect yourself and the medical practice in case of litigation. Documentation includes the following:

- Date of the request
- Name of the requestor
- The information requested
- Patient's name (and patient number)
- Name of the treating provider
- The information released
- To whom the call was referred (if applicable)

When a patient telephones the clinic to request prescription refills, is displeased with medical treatment, or expresses some form of a complaint, documentation of the call should always be recorded in the medical chart. Follow established clinic protocols when handling each and every telephone call. Document every call you have with a patient, including all pertinent information.

USING TELEPHONE DIRECTORIES

The medical assistant should have on hand in the clinic a variety of print and online telephone directories and be skilled in their use. The telephone directory contains an organized, accurate, and complete listing of the name, address, zip code, and area code with telephone number for most individuals with telephone service. Often, the pages within the directory are color-coded; residences are listed on white pages, business numbers on blue pages, and advertisements on yellow pages. The front pages of many directories contain other useful information such as:

- Information related to emergency and nonemergency numbers is provided.
- The Internet guide makes it easy to get online.
- An information guide and consumer tips provide a variety of free facts and answers about the things you want to buy and the services you need.
- Community pages provide attraction, event, and general-interest information unique to a particular geographic area. Often, maps are provided on these pages.
- Phone service pages answer questions you may have regarding your phone service.
- Government pages contain information about county, state, tribal, and federal government clinics, as well as information regarding public schools and voter registration.
- An index makes finding what you need easy.

While print telephone directories are still being published and distributed, it is becoming more popular to use Internet resources as the general public becomes more savvy with digital devices.

There are many types of online resources available, in the form of business directories, local listings, and search engines that will list web links for any key word or topics requested. This includes extensive information on local, state, and federal government sites, as well as a wealth of resources for finding people, places, events, and maps, beyond what the printed directory is able to offer.

Most medical centers and hospitals produce their own directory. These directories list important telephone numbers specific to that facility. Examples of information available within these directories include:

- Community education services
- Nurse counseling service/nurse line
- Main hospital/facility telephone number
- Automated operator
- TTY line for the hearing impaired
- Medical center departments
- Medical staff, including department and photo of providers and their names with credentials

Some of these publications list providers who no longer maintain their active/associate privileges at the facility. Often, a map of the facility is included within the front or back pages. Large facilities also may produce supplements to maintain current information.

COMMUNITY RESOURCES

Community resources are assets in a community that are available in the form of people, organizations, and locations that offer support and assistance to the needs of a certain population and improves quality of life. Often, there are patient needs that go beyond the capabilities of the clinic environment. In such situations, the clinic and its staff can provide guidance as a patient navigator and recommend, refer, or facilitate connecting the patient to the available resources that best meet their needs. In many cases, patients may be unaware that there are community resources that can aid them, as most are dealing with health related issues that may be new to them and their families.

It is a good idea to have community resources specific to the needs of the patients related to the clinic's speciality gathered and available for easy reference. Brochures, phone numbers of contacts, and other useful information can be given out when needed. Representatives of service providers can provide materials, and some insurance carriers will have social or case workers that work with certain plans to assist the clinic with covered services and facilities from within a network. The Internet can provide a plethora of information on local resources and downloadable information or applications.

Examples of types of community resources for health care include adult day care, assisted living facilities, Alzheimer's support, cancer care, counseling services, crisis hot line, disability services, HIV/AIDS, home health agency and in-home treatment, hospice, medical equipment and supplies, mental health services, nursing homes, pain management, psychiatrists, senior citizens' services, Spanish/Hispanic services, substance abuse services, support groups, transportation, utilities assistance, veterans services, victims' services, and youth services.

Procedures 11-5 and 11-6 provide direction on creating a list of community resources, and providing patient referrals to these community resources.

PROCEDURE 11-5

Developing a Current List of Community Resources Related to Patient Health Care Needs

PURPOSE:

To use research tools to assemble a list of current community resources as a referral resource for patient health care needs.

EQUIPMENT/SUPPLIES:

- Internet access and search engine
- Telephone directory
- Hospital directory
- Pen or pencil
- Notepaper and binder

PROCEDURE STEPS:

1. Assemble research tools and equipment. Select three types of community resources discussed in the "Community Resources" section of this chapter. RATIONALE: Researching community resources will be based on the specialty practice and needs of the patients receiving services at the clinic. Select three of particular interest to you.
2. For each type of community resource selected, gather information and organize your data in a useful table for patient reference. Include name of resource; a brief description of the services or assets available; phone number, address, contact names if applicable; Website address; special instructions, if applicable; and other pertinent

(continues)

information. RATIONALE: Information given to patients should be accurate and as complete as possible to promote ease of use and compliance by the patient seeking services.

3. For each type of community resource selected, verify the information gathered and request further documentation and brochures, and ensure the resource is up to date with the latest data. RATIONALE: Services, location, and contacts often change and can become outdated. Periodically verifying and updating information will keep resources relevant for patients.
4. Create a binder for the clinic staff as a reference of the community resources researched. Organize the data in a Word table or Excel spreadsheet and print copies as a patient handout. RATIONALE: Community resources should be easily accessible for staff reference and made readily available to patients as the need arises.

PROCEDURE 11-6

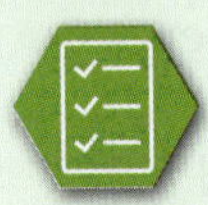

Facilitating Referrals to Community Resources in the Role of a Patient Navigator

PURPOSE:

To use a list of current community resources as a referral resource to facilitate referrals by guiding patients with information.

EQUIPMENT/SUPPLIES:

- Internet access and search engine
- Telephone directory
- Hospital directory
- Pen or pencil
- Referral sources from Procedure 11-5

PROCEDURE STEPS:

1. Using the referral sources from Procedure 11-5, offer the patient one of the resources by discussing services and assets, contact information, Web address, and other pertinent information gathered on the resource that is useful to the patient. RATIONALE: The patient or patient's family may need to be coached and advised when community resources are required. Assisting with contact information, other details, and feedback will help guide the patient where needed.
2. Verify the information with the patient, and then document the referral. Follow up in 48 hours by placing a call to the patient. RATIONALE: Documenting the referral in the patient record allows for follow-up with the patient, and offers a reminder to the staff of the resources given to the patient.
3. Print the referral information documented in the patient record to give to the patient.

PLACING OUTGOING CALLS

When making calls for the medical clinic, whether to patients, health care facilities, or other providers, know what information is needed and have it at hand before making the calls. For example:

- If arranging for a patient to receive care at another facility, have the patient's health record and insurance information available. Determine provider instructions as to the diagnosis and type of care (specific tests, radiographs, and so on) that need to be ordered.
- If calling insurance companies for claim follow-up, gather copies of all claim forms and

medical documentation so you can answer specific questions regarding each claim.

- If scheduling meetings or outside appointments for clinic providers, have their schedules in front of you.

Legal

Arrange to make outgoing calls from a telephone in a location that is free of distractions. If the calls concern patients (whether about bills, insurance, or care), it is mandatory that the calls be made from a telephone where you cannot be overheard by other patients or people in the reception area.

Always choose a time when calls can be made without interruption. Do not make outgoing calls while covering incoming call responsibilities.

It is best to establish a routine for making various types of outgoing calls. Most clinics call the next day's patients to confirm appointments near the end of each day. Collection and insurance calls, as well as pharmacy callbacks, are usually done either before the clinic is open for patients in the morning, during the period from noon to 2 PM when the clinic is closed for lunch, or after the last patient has been seen.

PLACING LONG-DISTANCE CALLS

Most long-distance calls medical assistants make are likely to be direct dialing calls, that is, calls placed without the help of an operator. Many business phone packages used in the clinic will include free or low-cost long distance calling. There may be times when operator-assisted calls are necessary, although the use of these types of calls are less common. These can include:

- Person-to-person calls
- Conference calls
- International calls
- Collect calls

Conference calls may be local or long distance and are convenient for communicating or discussing information with several individuals at the same time. Each person involved in the conference call must be notified about specifics regarding the date and time, and any special instructions related to the call. Many clinics have conference call capabilities on their telephone or computer systems.

International direct distance dialing (IDDD) is available in many parts of the Unites States. Additional numbers or codes may preface the international access, country, and city codes when using IDDD. Station-to-station calls may be dialed following this sequence:

- Dial the international code 011
- Dial the country code
- Dial the city code
- Dial the local telephone number
- Press the pound sign (#) button if the telephone is touchtone

It may take up to 45 seconds after dialing any international code for the ringing to begin. The Internet posts frequent updates on international call procedures and country and city codes.

When making a long-distance call out of the area code, it is possible that a time zone change may occur (Figure 11-6). When scheduling the day's calls, it is important to keep in mind the location of the call and plan accordingly. Time zones in the United States include Pacific, Mountain, Central, and Eastern times and usually span a three-hour difference. If it is noon in New York, it is 11 AM in Illinois, 10 AM in Arizona, and 9 AM in Washington state.

Many conventional telephone companies, wireless services, and Internet providers are competing for long-distance business. Judging the offers and services of long-distance companies can be a complex task, but a wise choice can save a clinic hundreds of dollars a year or more in telephone charges. It is important to analyze the medical clinic's long-distance requirements and then make comparisons among several long-distance companies. Company representatives usually are more than willing to discuss their services in light of specific needs to help you comparison shop. The decision of which service to use will usually be made by the providers and the clinic manager with feedback from all employees.

LEGAL AND ETHICAL CONSIDERATIONS

Legal

Two of the most important issues in the medical setting are patient confidentiality and the right to privacy. Respecting the confidentiality of all patient information

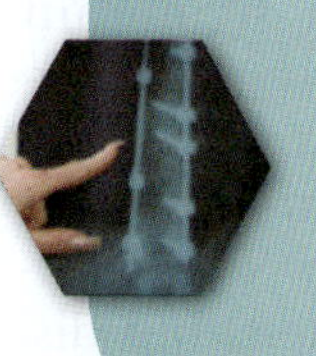

Critical Thinking

Your clinic is located in Seattle, WA, and you are calling Charleston, NC. What are some important considerations before placing the call?

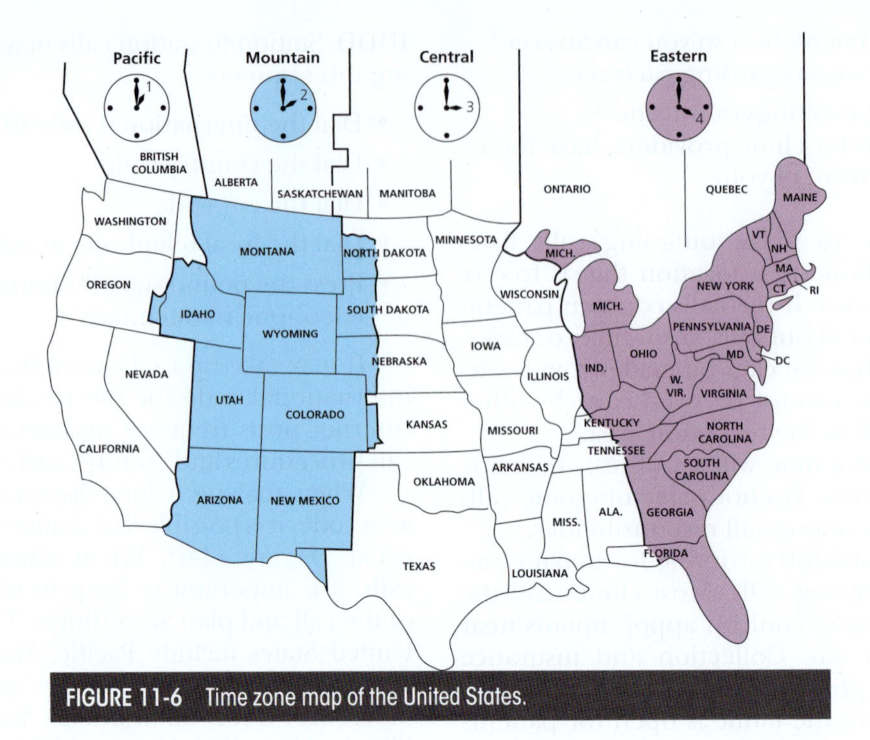

FIGURE 11-6 Time zone map of the United States.

is a legal and ethical obligation. No information about patients is to be discussed outside the clinic, with family or friends, or with other patients. All notes that may be jotted down on paper during telephone calls must be disposed of following clinic protocols. In most cases, this means shredding the notes. Violations of confidentiality leave you and your provider open to lawsuits. More importantly, they are violations of patient trust.

Integrity

When calling patients, whether to discuss treatment or finances, do so with respect for the patient's privacy at all times. The front desk is certainly not the place to make collection calls when other patients are in the reception room. Either make calls from another location or choose a time when other patients cannot overhear you. Always be aware of the surroundings and who may be able to overhear conversations.

There are many situations when individuals will call the clinic to discuss a patient. Parents, spouses, grandparents, other relatives, significant others, employers, and friends often will have questions about a patient's condition or finances. Usually these people are asking questions out of genuine concern and a desire to help. The information they request may seem harmless, but discussing anything about a patient can turn into an ethical and legal issue.

To ensure patient confidentiality and practice sensible risk management, never discuss a patient with:

- The patient's spouse or family, without specific permission and a signed release
- The patient's employer
- Insurance carriers, HMOs, or attorneys without a signed release
- Credit bureau/collection agencies (reporting a patient to a credit bureau or collection agency is a violation of confidentiality if medical information is disclosed)
- Other patients
- People outside the clinic (friends, family, acquaintances)

When necessary for medical or administrative reasons, you can discuss a patient with:

- Members of the clinic staff as necessary to the patient's care
- The patient's insurance carrier or HMO, if you have a signed release
- The patient's attorney (usually in accident or Workers' Compensation cases), if you have a signed release
- The patient's parent or legal guardian, except concerning issues of birth control, abortion, HIV, or sexually transmitted disease (check

the laws in each state regarding minors' right to privacy)

- Another health care provider (provider, laboratory, or hospital) that is providing care to the patient under orders from the patient's provider
- Referring provider's clinic

HIPAA GUIDELINES FOR TELEPHONE COMMUNICATIONS

The following guidelines should be followed when communicating information to patients by telephone:

- Determine whether the patient has requested confidential communications. Specific instructions should be provided to staff members on how to determine whether the patient has requested and been granted special conditions for keeping communications with the medical practice confidential.
- If the patient has not requested confidential communication, the patient should simply be called at the standard phone number contained in his or her records. If the patient has requested confidential communications and has provided an alternative telephone number, care should be taken to ensure that only the alternative number is called.
- The caller should identify himself or herself by name and say that he or she is an employee of the medical practice (use the complete official name of the practice).
- If the patient is not available, it is acceptable to leave a live or recorded message asking the patient to return the call. Leave the telephone number, and if the medical practice is returning a call made by the patient, it is acceptable to state this in the message that is left for the patient. However, it is important that the message does not contain any medical information or mention the purpose of the call. Never leave a message containing test results.
- When the patient is contacted, it is acceptable to discuss his or her medical information over the telephone. It is critical, however, that test results and other protected health information (PHI) *not* be given to anyone other than the patient or a person designated as the patient's representative.

AMERICANS WITH DISABILITIES ACT (ADA)

Safety

The ADA requires that communication procedures are available for persons with disabilities. Combined with HIPAA requirements, this presents a challenging situation in dealing with patients who are deaf or hearing impaired. The act requires that health care providers give effective communication alternatives using auxiliary aids and services that ensure that communication to people with hearing loss is equal to others without this disability. This includes patients as well as caregivers of patients, guardians, or spouses.

Alternative devices or services include interpreters for individuals with a language problem, assistive hearing devices, note takers for individuals who have difficulty writing, written materials, and so forth. The health care provider can choose the device as long as the result is effective communication. The patient who is deaf or hard of hearing should be consulted on which device he or she finds to be most effective. The cost of alternative devices or services cannot be billed to the patient. The expense must be charged against the overhead of the clinic or practice.

Telephone service for patients who are hearing impaired is required by the ADA. Many individuals who are hearing impaired, deaf, or speech impaired may use a teletype (TTY) or telecommunication device for the deaf (TDD). These devices transmit a keyed-in message via the telephone network just as a voice message would be sent if spoken. The recipient of the message reads the keyed-in message on the TTY's text display. A TTY or TDD device is required at both ends of the conversation in order to communicate. In addition, Internet chat capability that can replace TTY or TDD devices is readily available online.

TELEPHONE TECHNOLOGY

Though much of this chapter has been dedicated to the interpersonal nature of telephone communications, astute medical assistants will also investigate and become knowledgeable about the technology of telecommunications.

Ongoing advances in telecommunications have had a tremendous impact on how the staff of a medical clinic communicates both within the clinic and with patients, hospitals, and others outside the clinic. These advances include telephone systems with automated routing units, Voice over Internet Protocol (VoIP), electronic transmissions (fax and email), and cellular phones.

Automated Routing Units

Many hospitals and larger ambulatory care settings have **automated routing unit (ARU)** telephone systems to manage heavy telephone traffic. The system answers the call, and a recorded voice identifies departments or services the caller can access by pressing a specified number on the touch-tone telephone. If callers indicate they are having a medical emergency, the system can be programmed to immediately route calls to the medical assistant. This saves patients with immediate medical problems from waiting during busy telephone times.

Most automated telephone systems have electronic mailboxes so the caller can leave a message if the person they are calling is unavailable. In many ARU systems, selecting any of the numbered choices often gives the caller a second, third, or fourth menu of choices. If the caller does not select an option, the ARU will usually switch the call automatically to a live operator.

A disadvantage with ARU systems is that the recorded voice may be difficult to hear, especially for older adults or patients who are hearing impaired. Many patients may not understand the recorded options. Clinics with an ARU system should provide to all patients an information sheet explaining their options when calling the clinic and how to get through to the clinic quickly in an emergency.

Answering Services and Machines

One responsibility of the clinic manager/medical assistant is to ensure that patient calls are answered after clinic hours, both in the evenings and on weekends. Although in smaller ambulatory care settings it may not be possible to have staff on telephone duty 24 hours a day, nonetheless calls must be answered and messages taken. **Answering services**—typically staffed by a live operator—and answering machines are two methods of taking calls after hours.

Many ambulatory care centers favor answering services because a live operator is reassuring to patients and other callers. These services also can provide flexibility in routing calls and locating the provider for emergencies. Typically, fees for answering services are by the month or by the number of calls.

Answering machines are convenient but perhaps less reassuring for the caller. The machine must be checked frequently for messages should an emergency occur. Sometimes, the message may leave a telephone number where the provider can be reached, but this system is likely to be cumbersome, because too many nonemergency calls may be directed to the provider. If an answering machine is used, the message often contains a number, other than the provider's, that callers can use for emergencies. That call is answered by a live operator who then screens and refers the call appropriately.

Voice over Internet Protocol (VoIP) Telecommunications

Voice over Internet Protocol (VoIP) is a rapidly growing form of telecommunication. The biggest advantages to VoIP are price and flexibility. On the surface, a VoIP phone seems like a common landline telephone, but VoIP services convert a voice into a digital signal that travels over the Internet or a virtual private network. When calling a regular telephone number, the signal is converted to a regular phone signal before it reaches the destination. VoIP calls can be made directly from a computer, a special VoIP phone, or a traditional telephone connected to a special adapter wherever there is broadband connectivity.

Three different types of VoIP services are in common use:

- *Analog Telephone Adapter (ATA).* The ATA allows connection through a standard telephone using a computer or network connection. The ATA is an analog-to-digital converter. It takes the analog signal from a traditional phone and converts it into digital data for transmission over the network. VoIP providers usually bundle the ATAs free with their service.
- *IP Phone.* These specialized phones look just like normal telephones. They have an RJ-45 Ethernet connector in place of the standard RJ-11 telephone connectors. IP phones connect directly to the cable router with all the hardware and software included. Special WiFi phones allow making VoIP calls from any WiFi hotspot. These devices have all of the security problems associated with WiFi (see Chapter 10).
- *Computer to Computer.* This was the original VoIP form of telecommunication. Several companies offer free or very-low-cost software that can be used for this type of VoIP service. Aside from an Internet-connected computer with audio card, microphone, and speakers, nothing else is required. Except for a normal

monthly ISP fee, there usually is no charge for computer to computer calls regardless of distance. This type of VoIP can be vulnerable to security problems depending on the security of the URL employed.

Most VoIP providers bundle call waiting, caller ID, three-way calling, repeat dial, return call, and call transfer with the service plan.

Some of the disadvantages of VoIP telecommunications are as follows:

- Most VoIP services do not work during power outages.
- Emergency services through 911 may not be available.
- Directory assistance/white page listings may not be available.

VoIP Security. Small and medium-sized organizations are increasingly adopting VoIP technology. With the increased popularity of this technology, the likelihood of attacks by cyber criminals increases. A cybercriminal attack on a VoIP service could mean the criminal eavesdrops on conversations; interferes with audio streams; or disconnects, reroutes, or even answers other people's phone calls.

VoIP is part of the Internet and is susceptible to disruption of service and spam just as are other Internet services. A potentially more serious security problem with VoIP, however, is eavesdropping on sensitive conversations. Hackers can eavesdrop on unprotected media streams and intercept VoIP packets to obtain sensitive information by reassembling the packets into speech. One way for hackers to do this is through a man-in-the-middle attack, where a third party spoofs the unique hardware address (MAC address) of the two speaking parties, forcing the IP packets to flow through the hacker's system. Although eavesdropping is not just a risk for VoIP telecommunications, the nature of IP networks makes access to the phone conversations much easier. Eavesdroppers no longer need to physically put a tap into a phone line; they can simply gain access from a laptop connected to the network. A hacker breaking into a VoIP data stream has access to more calls than he or she would with a traditional telephone wiretap. As a result, the hacker has a much greater likelihood of getting useful information by tapping a VoIP data stream than from monitoring a traditional phone system. Another security compromise possible with VoIP is intercepting a genuine call to a bank and rerouting it to a bogus bank teller.

The following are a few of the safeguards that can be used to provide in-depth protection to a VoIP system:

- Use dedicated VoIP phone instruments (having a digital certificate), not a *softphone.* A softphone uses software for making telephone calls over the Internet on a general purpose computer.
- Use a stateful packet inspection (SPI) firewall. This type of firewall technology ensures that all inbound packets are the result of an outbound request.
- Ensure that VoIP service providers have security in place for their internal systems.
- Update security patches for computer operating systems and VoIP software.
- Encrypt voice traffic.
- Use a virtual private network (VPN) to separate the data stream from the public Internet over which it travels. This is accomplished by connecting to a server that is set up to communicate with your device using an encrypted data flow. Any data that may be intercepted by a nearby hacker is rendered totally useless unless the encryption code is known. Most corporations use VPNs they operate, and VPN-for-hire firms are available to provide servers to small organizations and individuals. In the case of VPN-for-hire servers, the connection between your device and the Internet is secure; however, the connection between the server and your traffic's destination is not.

Facsimile (Fax) Machines

Fax machines are common in ambulatory care settings as they are used to send reports, referrals, insurance approvals, and informal correspondence. A **fax** is a **facsimile** transmission sent over telephone lines from one fax machine to another or from a modem to a fax machine. A fax can be sent as easily as putting the document in the machine, similar to the way a document is put in a copy machine, and dialing the receiving telephone number. There are other issues involved in using the fax, especially when sending patient information. Several legal and confidentiality issues should be considered before sending any communications by fax. These include obtaining proper records release authorization, using fax machines in secure and not publicly accessible areas only, using a cover sheet with a confidentiality warning, and confirmation of the receiving fax number, with a follow-up call to verify arrival at proper destination.

HIPAA requires all medical practices to implement technical measures to protect against unauthorized access to protected health information (PHI) when it is transmitted over electronic telecommunications networks. Two security measures must be addressed: the integrity of the information transmitted, and the vulnerability of the information to unauthorized use or disclosure.

When information is transmitted over public networks, static and other less benign problems can introduce errors into the information. The security rule requires the implementation of security measures to verify the integrity of the information that is transmitted.

Information transmitted over public networks may be intercepted and used by unauthorized users. In some cases, the interception can be deliberate to access sensitive information. In other instances, the interception may be the result of error by the person making the transmission. For example, a person sending a fax dials the wrong number and sends information to an unintended recipient.

The security rule requires implementation of a mechanism to encrypt PHI when appropriate. Encryption requires the cooperation of both parties to the transaction, and the encryption methods are specified in any agreement between the parties.

With the increasing use of electronic records, much of the information that was sent between medical facilities by fax is now being accessed through secure, digital means.

Each medical facility involved in a particular transaction will need to have access to the same system, and as electronic software becomes more wide-spread in use, this will be more easily possible. The required data are obtained faster and under more secure circumstances because they are contained in the EHR.

Additionally, if the medical record is not accessible between facilities, patients can now be given their records on digital media, such as a DVD or flash drive, containing documents, digital images, and other necessary data that can easily be taken to the next provider that needs to review this information. Even uploaded large files, such as images, can be shared between business associates using secure file sharing systems over the Internet.

Electronic Mail (email)

Electronic mail (email) involves the process of sending, receiving, storing, and forwarding messages in digital form over computer networks. Email is a non–real-time method of communication—it permits us to leave a message at our convenience and allows the recipients to read and respond at their convenience. Emails can be sent to multiple people at the same time, something a traditional telephone call does not allow. Keep in mind, however, that there is a professional email etiquette that must be adhered to. It is not acceptable to forward email messages without the permission of the original author, and caution must be taken to avoid sending information that is not appropriate in a professional setting.

Composing email is similar to composing any written communication. Just as a letter or memo has a particular format, the email transmission should also follow a format style. The subject line should be brief and clearly identify the content of the email body.

If your message is in response to another piece of email, your email software probably will preface the subject line with *Re:* (for "regarding"). If your email software does not do this, it would be polite to key in "RE:". If your message is time critical, starting with "URGENT" is appropriate. If you are referring to a previous email, you should explicitly quote that document to provide context.

If a message is to be sent to several parties, individual email messages may be sent to each, thereby protecting their privacy. In many instances, however, it is useful for parties involved in a group "conversation" to be aware of who the other participants are. In this case, all of the addresses may be included on the same email message. Sending a "bcc," or blind copy, also protects the privacy of your email because it does not show to whom else the message was sent.

The body of the message should contain short and clear sentences. In trying to be brief and to the point, however, it is important to not leave out important facts or information. Remember also that some email software only understands plain text. Italics, bold, and color changes should be used sparingly. Some software recognizes **URLs (Uniform Resource Locators)**, more commonly known as Web site addresses, in the text and makes them "live" so they can be clicked and opened. Because different software recognizes different parts of the address, if you include a URL in your email message, it is much safer to use the entire address, including the initial http://. See the following Quick Reference Guide for additional email etiquette.

The advantages of using email as a means of communication include:

- Asynchronous communication—both parties need not be available at the same time for communication to take place
- Providers and patients can prepare, leave, read, and respond to messages at times that are convenient
- Can be used to automate certain tasks such as sending out appointment reminders or normal reports of laboratory results
- Creates a documentation trail of interactions between provider and patient
- Some patients may be more forthcoming using email than in face-to-face discussion
- Reimbursement for time spent receiving and responding to clinical email may be billed under the Online Medical Evaluation section of the Current Procedural Terminology reference (see Chapter 17). Codes should be checked for changes and updates annually for these services. As of January 2016, modifiers have been introduced, to be used with CPT codes. The current CPT and Healthcare Common Procedure Coding System (HCPCS) codes that describe a telehealth service are generally the same codes that describe an encounter when the physician and patient are in the same location.
- Modifiers are being used to describe the technology used in a Telehealth encounter. One of these modifiers should be used to distinguish between an encounter that has taken place by telecommunication, as opposed to the provider and patient being at the same site. These modifiers are—GQ (Via Asynchronous Telecommunications systems) and—GT (Via Interactive Audio and Video Telecommunications systems).

The disadvantages of email communications include:

- Lack of real-time interaction and feedback
- Lack of body language or vocal inflection, which may lead to misunderstanding
- May not be suitable for time-sensitive material because determination of when the message will be delivered or read cannot be assessed

Safety

Encryption of Email. To prevent possible compromise of medical data when using email, **encryption** renders the transmission essentially secure. Encryption of email can be accomplished in several ways: The email service provider can employ TLS (transport layer security) protocol or its predecessor, SSL (Secure Socket Layer). The email will automatically be encrypted for transmission. The URL address will display the *https* prefix and a padlock icon when the email provider uses this protocol (see Figure 10-3). If the provider does not use this protocol, the sender can initiate encryption by obtaining and using a digital ID. Digital IDs, sometimes referred to as certificates, allow recipients to verify that an email was actually sent by the intended person. Because forging, hijacking email addresses, and even hackers intercepting email is common, a digital ID can be used to encrypt messages, hide their content, and protect the email as it reaches its destination.

If the e-mail service provider used in the clinic does not already provide Digital ID, follow the instructions provided by the service to turn on this feature, when available. At many businesses, the system administrator will provide and set up emails for office use with encrypted email. Most email service providers are working toward encrypting messages sent to and from servers. TLS is being adopted as the standard for secure email, and most of the well-known providers, such as Outlook, Google Mail, and Amazon, have already implemented this encryption technology, either TLS, SSL, or both.

Patient Portal Systems

Patient portal systems are secure online Web sites or applications combined with other software, such as an EMR, that allow patients to have convenient 24-hour access to interact and communicate with their health care providers. Because the patient uses a login and password, the portal environment is much more secure compared to using regular email. The area for communications is usually set up much like the standard email interface most people are now accustomed to, including buttons to compose (write), send, and read messages.

A patient portal system may be available as a standalone Web site, offered and administered as a service by vendors to health care providers. Other portals can be integrated directly into the existing Web site of the clinic or hospital, and yet others are application modules that can be added to the EMR. These patient portal systems are becoming more popular to use, as they offer the capacity to utilize patient health information in a secure manner via the Internet.

QUICK REFERENCE GUIDE

EMAIL ETIQUETTE

Most organizations implement etiquette rules for the following reasons:

- Professionalism: Using correct grammar, spelling, and language conveys a professional image.
- Efficiency: Email is a more effective means of communication.
- Protection from liability: Appropriate, business-like language in all email communications limits liability risks.

Remember that an email message is not delivered with body language. A great deal of human communication comes from nonverbal signals such as facial expressions and tone of voice. These cues help make the message clearer. The following etiquette rules promote professionalism, efficiency, and protection from liability:

- Use proper structure and layout. Use short paragraphs and blank lines between each paragraph. When making points, number or bullet each point. Keep it brief, but give pertinent details.
- Do not attach unnecessary files.
- When sending attachments is necessary, tell the recipient the format of the attachment. If a large attachment must be sent, call the recipient first to be sure his or her Internet service will accept it.
- Do not overuse the high priority option.
- Do not overuse Reply to All. Use this feature only when your message needs to be received by everyone. Do not copy a message or attachment without permission. You could be infringing on copyright laws.
- Use a meaningful subject. This helps the recipient focus immediately.
- As a courtesy to your recipient, include your name at the bottom of the message. The recipient may not know that the return address belongs to you.
- Do not write anything you would not say in public.
- Do not write in CAPITALS. If you write in capitals, it seems as if you are shouting.
- Do not send flame emails; that is, insulting messages designed to cause pain, as when someone "gets burned."

When confidential or privileged material is sent via email, it should include a disclaimer stating that any review, retransmission, dissemination, or other use of the material is prohibited. It should also state that if the message is received in error, the recipient should contact the sender and delete the material from the computer. See the example below:

This message is a privileged and confidential clinical communication intended solely for the person to whom it is addressed. If you are not the intended recipient, please be advised that any disseminating, copying, or distributing of this message is strictly prohibited. If you received this message in error, please forward it back to the sender.

Providers and patients are realizing the benefits of using a portal system in terms of increasing efficiency and productivity. Clinics are reporting reduced costs in mailing referrals, lab results, and other correspondence. Reduced phone calls to the clinic for routine requests and inquiries have also been realized. The ability for staff or providers to respond to patients at a time of convenience, and redirecting tasks as required to medical assistants, billing specialists, or other providers has its benefits. Below is a list of health information patients can view, as outlined by the Health IT Standards Committee at www.healthit.gov:

- Recent doctor visits
- Discharge summaries
- Medications
- Immunizations
- Allergies
- Lab results

In addition to exchanging email with the health care team, patients may also be able to do the following tasks in the portal:

- Request prescription refills
- Schedule nonurgent appointments
- Check benefits and coverage
- Update contact information
- Make payments

- Download and complete forms
- View educational materials

As is usually the case with similar technology, the patient portal system can have some drawbacks. The patient must provide information to the clinic so that a registration password, or token, can be issued. This will allow the patient to set up a secure login and password and create an account. Some patients can forget to follow through with the process upon arriving home from the clinic, and for others, having to track multiple family members, such as individual children, becomes difficult with so many logins. Another drawback comes for patients who have multiple providers. A person with a PCP and a few specialists due to complex health issues may very well have many portals that are not integrated, causing a disconnect with continuity of care. This is an area that may be addressed in the future, and become more standardized, especially with EMR modules.

One concern providers may have is that they will be overwhelmed with email messages, patients not adapting to the patient portal, or communication issues between patients and providers. Table 11-2 lists some common concerns, many of which are actually unfounded, based on studies done on the current patient portal systems in use today.

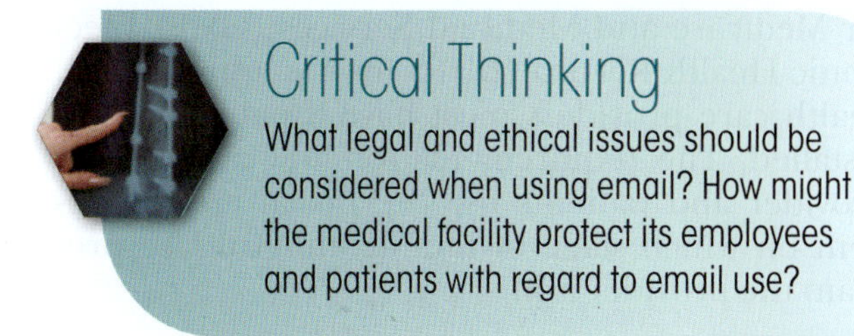

Critical Thinking

What legal and ethical issues should be considered when using email? How might the medical facility protect its employees and patients with regard to email use?

Patient portal systems also factor in where Meaningful Use is concerned. Meaningful Use encourages providers to switch from paper charts to electronic records. If a provider provides services to Medicare or Medicaid patients, that provider may be eligible to qualify for the Meaningful Use program. For providers that do not participate, Medicare penalites began in 2015. Medicare offers incentive payments for adopting electronic health records. These incentive payments are equal to 75% of Part B allowed charges up to an annual maximum. In contrast, those providers that do not comply will be penalized starting at 1% of their Part B Medicare reimbursements, increasing each year to the 5% maximum.

There are three stages to the implementation of the Meaningful Use program. In order to have met the 2014 requirements of the Centers

TABLE 11-2

COMMON CONCERNS WHEN USING PATIENT PORTAL SYSTEMS

CONCERN	FACTS
Providers will be flooded with email messages from patients.	Rather than being inundated with messages, providers report increased efficiency and appreciate being able to respond to patients at their convenience. Evaluation studies find that telephone volume decreases when secure messaging is introduced.
Patients may use messaging inappropriately.	Studies find that the communication content of patient messages tends to be appropriate, addressing non-urgent care issues. Best practice is to educate patients about when and how to use secure messaging.
Providers will be unable to bill time for communicating with patients on the portal and the practice will lose revenue.	Portal features have been found to provide cost savings by decreasing indirect and direct labor costs, such as mailing costs for lab results, online billing questions versus telephone, online appointment scheduling, and online appointment reminders.
Patients will be confused or upset by information contained with the EHR.	Best practices for displaying test results include providing a brief explanation and guidance for any follow-up along with the results.
Patients won't adapt to using a patient portal.	A majority of consumers favor using online tools to communicate with providers, obtain lab results online, and make appointments. Medical practices have had success in getting a wide range of patients—including the elderly, lower income, and those with chronic illnesses—to use a patient portal.

Source: HealthIT.gov

for Medicare and Medicaid Services (CMS) Electronic Health Record (EHR) for Meaningful Use, health care providers must have a patient portal installed. The requirements for how actively the provider and patients use the portal are dependent on which stage of the Meaningful Use program the provider is in.

Legal and Ethical Issues. When using email or communicating within a patient portal, it is important for providers and staff to remember that the same ethical responsibilities to patients must be adhered to as for other types of encounters. The same standard of professionalism must also be satisfied. Along with the convenience offered through digital communications come some risks. Fortunately, following specific guidelines can minimize risks to a level considered acceptable by many practices.

Legal

Patients who meet criteria for digital correspondence established by the practice should be identified, and an informed consent form should be signed by each patient desiring this mode of communication. The form may be part of the form used for handling release of PHI or may be part of the registration process for the patient portal. The form should provide instructions to the patient in the secure use of email, the security risks involved, and practice policies for communication. As discussed, a disclaimer absolving the practice in the event of patient noncompliance or technical failure in the system is recommended. The original signed form should be filed in the patient chart and a copy given to the patient for his or her records.

A procedure should be established to automatically respond to patients' email messages informing them they have been received. Patients should also be requested to respond to your messages acknowledging their receipt.

DOCUMENTATION

From: *Elizabeth J. Parker*
Sent: *Tuesday, July 20, 20XX 8:55 am*
To: *Dr. King [King@doctor.com]*
Subject: *Prescription refill*

Please call in a prescription refill for my thyroid medication. The pharmacy is Inner City Pharmacy and the phone number is 890-271-2600. The prescription number is RX6437350 and I have enough pills for three days ______________________________

Telemedicine, Video Conferencing, and mHealth

The remote delivery of health care by means of telecommunications is referred to as **telemedicine**, also known as telehealth. Video conferencing is a method of having an interactive encounter with a patient in a remote location using two-way video and audio transmission. For patients, this means having access to medical professionals and services, no matter their geographic location, which offers them the potential to receive care that may not be available locally. Providers can now make virtual house calls, conduct consultations, and monitor ICU and emergency department patients, in cooperation with on-site staff. For patients with mobility issues, who are incarcerated, or who are otherwise unable to afford travel or to physically do so, the possibilities of expanding access to medical care through video conferencing are exciting.

In addition, providers using video conferencing have the opportunity to not only access expanded information and training, they also have the ability to collaborate with other professionals in the latest medical developments and techniques, or obtain assessments before moving forward with a patient care plan. The potential for professionals to improve quality of care, outcomes, and benefit to patients by sharing expertise and knowledge beyond the local hospital or clinic will eventually transform how health care is delivered.

mHealth, or m-health, stands for *mobile health*, a term that refers to the practice of medicine supported by mobile devices. The term *mHealth* is most commonly used when referencing the specific use of mobile devices, such as smart phones, tablets, and other portable devices, for health services. According to the analyst firm Berg Insight, the number of people monitored using mobile telecare systems in Europe and North America was about 450,000 at the end of 2015. Growing at a compound annual growth rate (CAGR) of 40%, this number is expected to reach almost 3.4 million by 2021. In addition, as smart phones and tablets continue to become commodities available around the world, especially in more poor regions or those just recently gaining access to the Internet, there will be more opportunities for much needed medical care and resources to reach these areas virtually by connecting patients and health care providers remotely.

An added benefit is the cost saving potential of telemedicine, for both providers and patients. A current challenge is getting insurance companies to adopt this technology and have a consistent reimbursement system for telemedicine options. Many are slow to adopt what is considered relatively new or unproven health care delivery methods. Medicare will consider reimbursement only for patients in rural areas or medically underserved areas, and then only for video conferencing. However, as the projected mass use of mHealth devices continues to grow worldwide, eventually insurance administrators will need to start integration of and payment for telemedicine services.

PROFESSIONALISM IN TELECOMMUNICATIONS

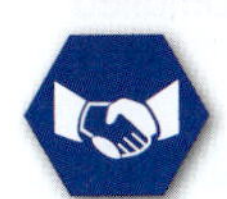

Professionalism in telecommunications is crucial in the medical clinic environment. The way in which the telephone is answered conveys either a message of a sincere desire to help or a message of interruption. Callers expect to have the phone answered in a professional manner and their concerns addressed promptly. Forwarding calls to someone else in the clinic who is more specialized in the topic of the caller's questions and following up to see that the situation was resolved provide evidence of a responsible attitude and of being a team player. One should always be courteous and diplomatic and work within the scope of one's education, training, ability, and legal boundaries.

Remember that personal telephone calls, other than emergency calls, should be avoided during working hours. When speaking with patients or other health care members, slang terms should not be used. Never eat or chew gum while answering the telephone. When completing a call, say "good-bye" and allow the caller to hang up before you do.

Additional attributes of professionalism include using appropriate guidelines when releasing information. Confidentiality guidelines must always be followed, with awareness of any ethical or legal responsibilities. Documentation is mandatory for follow-up care and for any legal implications. Continuing education is important to stay on the leading edge of new technologies being implemented in the area of telecommunications.

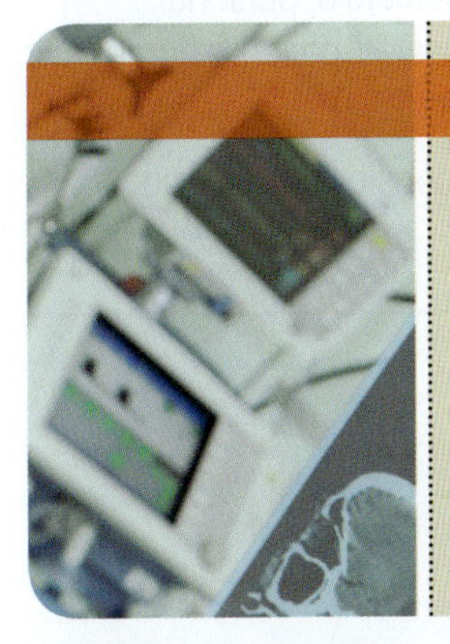

CASE STUDY 11-1

Refer to the scenario at the beginning of the chapter.

CASE STUDY REVIEW

1. Recall ways to maintain composure when handling and screening incoming telephone calls.
2. Describe the three types of VoIP services and identify safeguards that can be used to provide in-depth protection to a VoIP system.
3. Discuss HIPAA requirements related to fax machine use and PHI.
4. What is encryption, and how is it used with email communication?

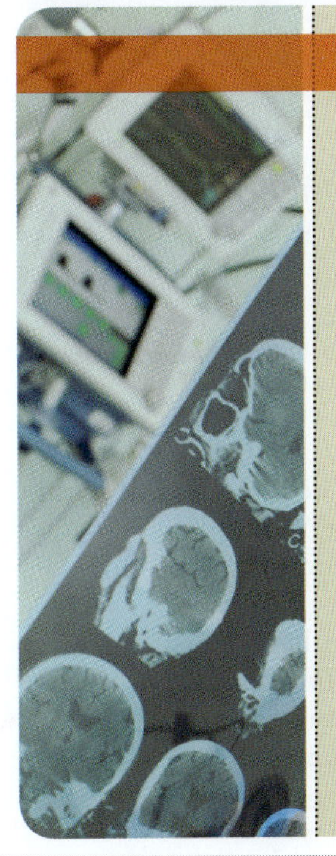

CASE STUDY 11-2

Nancy McFarland, RMA (AMT), a clinical medical assistant at Inner City Health Care, receives a telephone call from Claussen-Mason Laboratories requesting medical information about patient Juanita Hansen. Nancy is told by laboratory personnel that the information is needed to perform the tests scheduled by Dr. King. Wanda is not familiar with this request and asks if she can check the chart and return a call to the laboratory (callback verification procedure).

CASE STUDY REVIEW

1. What information will Nancy need from Claussen-Mason Laboratories?
2. What is the purpose of the callback verification procedure?
3. After the verification has been established, what should Nancy do?

DOCUMENTATION:

In the log reserved for telephone documentation, the following entry could be made based on Case Study 11–2.

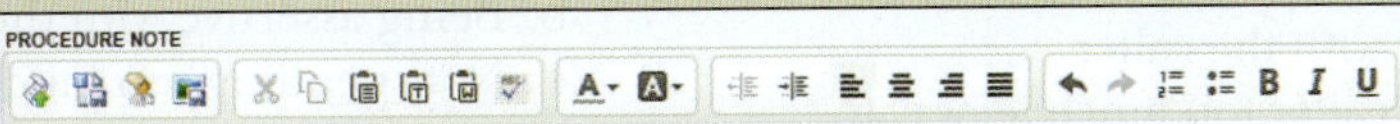
PROCEDURE NOTE

07/16/XX 4:00 p.m. Claussen-Mason Laboratories requested previous laboratory findings from Qwik Lab for Juanita Hansen, patient number 306-30-7840. Juanita is a patient of Dr. King. The information was released to Janet Bailey, employee of Claussen-Mason Laboratories, as directed by Dr. King. N. McFarland, RMA (AMT)

Courtesy of Harris CareTracker PM and EMR

Summary

- By means of telecommunication, which can also include fax, wireless technology, and email transmissions, patient appointments are scheduled, referrals made, critical information related, and the practice personality conveyed.
- Medical assistants are to be prepared for incoming and outgoing calls.
- The medical assistant must be familiar with basic telephone techniques, project appropriate tone and personality, and maintain telephone etiquette and courtesies.
- Effective screening techniques must be used, so that each caller is directed to the area or individual best able to assist him or her. Screening promotes good use of time and resources for those receiving calls, by redirecting to those better able to handle the call, or by collecting further information so that a response can be obtained and addressed at a more appropriate time.
- Proper telephone techniques include transferring calls with the data necessary to follow through, and taking detailed messages, so that the respondent has complete information for returning the call.
- The medical assistant will take a variety of calls, and must know the proper responses or actions to take, as agreed to by the provider-employer or clinic manager. This facilitates routing of calls correctly and establishes a "put through" list of the types of calls to be referred to the provider immediately.
- The medical assistant will also handle special considerations calls, including placing calls to facilities outside the clinic, using clear and direct language; maintaining proper composure and action when receiving emergency phone calls; dealing with older adults or those that speak English as a second language; and defusing and assisting angry callers.
- Proper documentation of messages should be completed, and care must be taken with requestors of personal information. Basic data gathered should include name of the requestor, the information requested, patient's name (and patient daytime or mobile number), name of the treating provider, and the information released.
- The medical assistant must understand email use in the clinic, and the legal and ethical responsibilities for using it, adhering to the same standards as for other encounters.

Study for Success

To reinforce your knowledge and skills of information presented in this chapter:

- Review the *Key Terms* and *Learning Outcomes*
- Consider the *Critical Thinking* features and *Case Studies* and discuss your conclusions
- Answer the questions in the *Certification Review*

- Perform the *Procedures* using the *Competency Assessment Checklists* on the *Student Companion Website*

CERTIFICATION REVIEW

1. How can the medical assistant create a positive first impression over the telephone?
   a. Using the hold button sparingly
   b. Being authoritative with the caller
   c. Not permitting the caller too much leeway to speak
   d. Working while talking on the telephone
2. What telephone personality techniques convey an effective telephone personality?
   a. Volume, enunciation, pronunciation, and control of speed
   b. Being assertive with the caller
   c. Not spending too much time talking
   d. Referring all calls to the provider
   e. Talking in a distracted manner

3. When transferring a telephone call, what guidelines will not ensure the successful transfer of the call?
   a. Determining who would be the best person to assist
   b. Following your telephone system's procedure for transferring the call
   c. Following up to be sure the call transferred correctly
   d. Getting the caller's name and telephone number is not necessary
4. How should the medical assistant handle a problem from an angry caller?
   a. Take it personally
   b. Listen calmly to the upset person
   c. Become upset to identify with the patient
   d. Ask emotionally charged questions to calm down the patient
   e. Put the caller on hold
5. What is the proper callback verification procedure?
   a. It should never be documented.
   b. It should always be documented.
   c. It should sometimes be documented.
   d. It is not appropriate in the ambulatory clinic setting.
6. What is an example of an inappropriate security measure when using the fax to send PHI?
   a. Have a signed form authorizing the release of PHI before releasing the information
   b. Faxed messages should only be sent to telecopiers that are located in a secure area
   c. A cover sheet containing warning of confidential information is not necessary when faxing
   d. Always recheck before sending the fax that the correct telephone number was selected and entered correctly
   e. After faxing, call the person who is receiving the fax and confirm that it was received
7. What is the definition of screening telephone calls?
   a. It is the act of evaluating the urgency of a medical situation and prioritizing the call.
   b. It is expressing oneself clearly and distinctly.
   c. It is using expendable words while answering the telephone.
   d. It is the ability to be objectively aware of and have insight into others' feelings, emotions, and behaviors.
8. When are TTY and TTD devices used in the clinic?
   a. By individuals with hearing and/or speech impairments
   b. When most individuals are placing long-distance calls
   c. When using smart phones
   d. When using facsimile machines
   e. Never
9. Which example does not apply to the use of clinical email to or from the patient?
   a. Clinical email to or from patients should be treated differently than telephone messages or letters
   b. Print and file the initial message and any reply to clinical email in the patient's chart
   c. Have a written agreement of understanding signed by all patients using clinical email
   d. Use clinical email protocols in the clinic procedure manual
10. How does the medical assistant provide privacy when making telephone collection calls?
    a. By ensuring no other patients can overhear details of the call
    b. By selecting a private location to place collection calls
    c. Collection calls made at the front desk during office hours are always acceptable
    d. Collection calls are always handled by a collection agency
    e. Both a and b

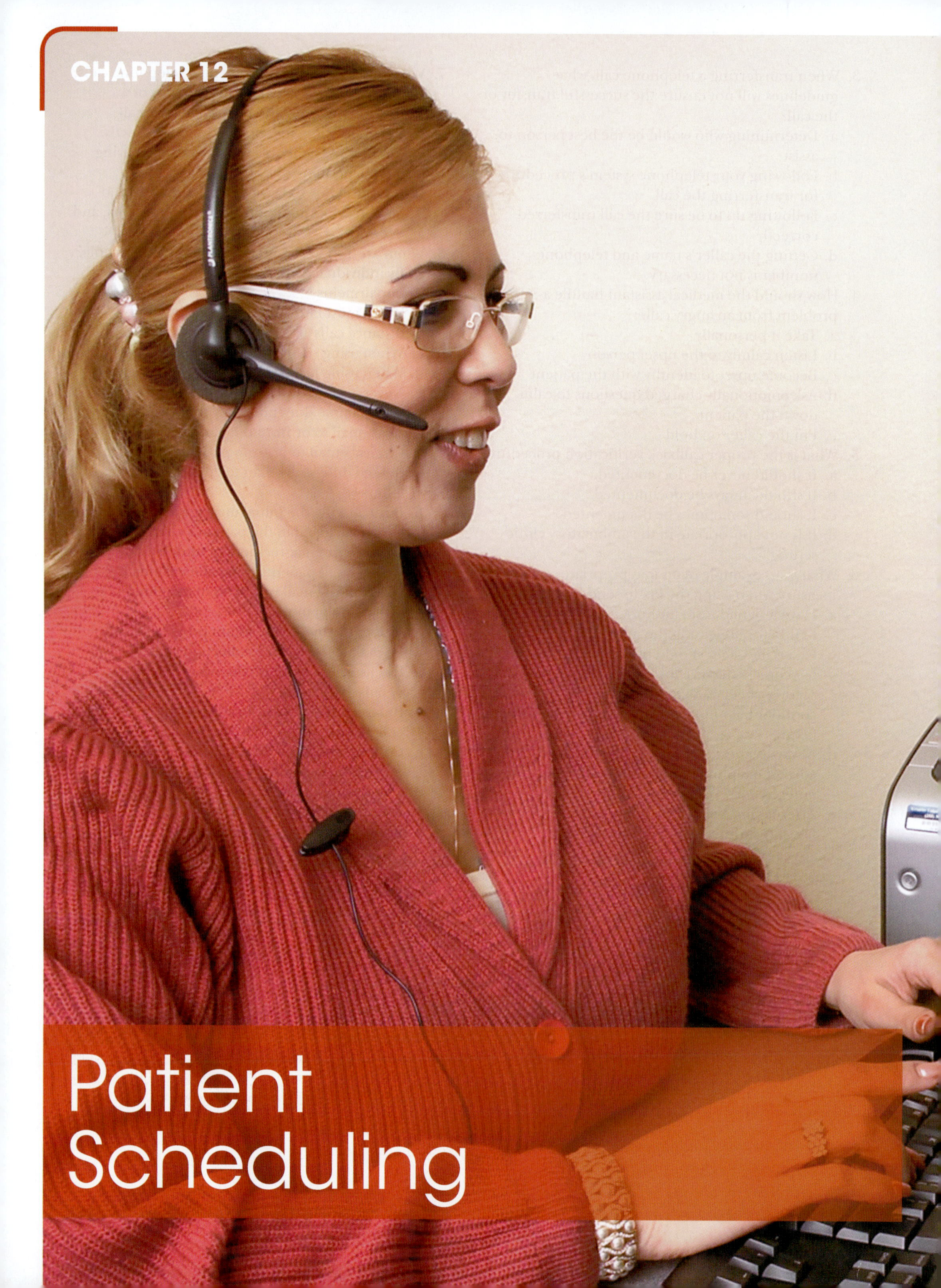

CHAPTER 12

Patient Scheduling

LEARNING OUTCOMES

1. Define and spell the key terms as presented in the glossary.
2. Identify pros and cons of six major scheduling systems.
3. Describe the guidelines in scheduling appointments.
4. Explain the importance of screening in scheduling patient appointments.
5. Review proper cancellation procedures and explain the legal necessity of documenting cancellations.
6. List and define three types of reminder systems.
7. Choose an appropriate appointment scheduling tool and describe its advantages.
8. Establish a matrix for the upcoming quarter for a provider.
9. Check in patients using a daily appointment sheet.
10. Schedule appointments using a manual system and an electronic system.
11. Schedule outpatient procedures and inpatient admissions.
12. Explain why there is a move toward online scheduling and DIY appointments using EMR and patient portals.

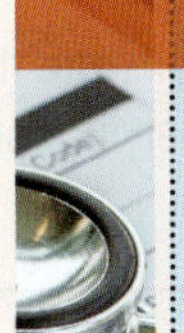

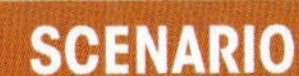

KEY TERMS

cluster scheduling
double booking
encryption technology
matrix
modified wave scheduling
practice-based scheduling
screening
stream scheduling
wave scheduling

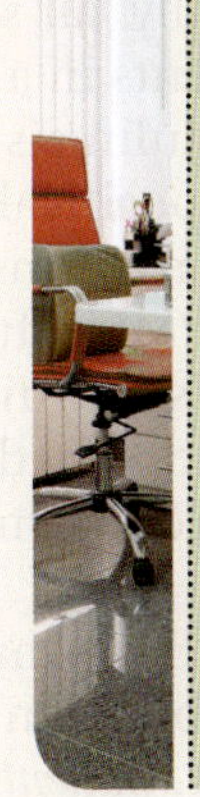

SCENARIO

At Inner City Urgent Care, medical assistant Walter Seals, CMA (AAMA), is responsible for efficient patient flow. Because Inner City is an urgent care center, patients are seen as walk-in appointments, on a first-come, first-served basis unless there is an emergency situation. Inner City also operates specialty care clinics, and these clinics require scheduled appointments. Walter has found that the clustering system is most efficient for these specialized care clinics, with certain days dedicated to certain procedures.

Because of the high volume of patients and the need to coordinate multiple provider schedules, Walter's job is not an easy one. However, Inner City is computerized, so paperwork is easy to generate as appointments are made, canceled, or rescheduled. And although Walter manages a smooth patient flow, he makes it a point to remain flexible to accommodate patient needs and keep stress to a minimum.

Chapter Portal

Patient scheduling has undergone many changes. A medical appointment is most often scheduled over the telephone or in person. Information technology allows appointment scheduling through secure online access using the clinic's Web site or patient portal system. However the appointment is made, the medical staff will need the patient's home telephone number and will want the number of the cellular phone that often accompanies the patient

continues

Chapter Portal, continued

or is used in place of a landline telephone. In the case of online appointment requests, the patient's email address is necessary. If online appointment scheduling is available at the clinic, the medical assistant may ask if the patient has a computer and is willing to use the computer for online appointment scheduling.

Patient scheduling is an integral part of the daily workload for medical assistants, whether in large family practices, urgent care centers, or sole proprietor clinics. Scheduling becomes more complicated if providers are practicing in more than one location and traveling between them. Scheduling patients can be stressful, especially if the telephone rings constantly and the medical assistant is unable to provide patients a convenient appointment.

Although patient appointment scheduling may seem like a routine function, a smooth patient flow often determines the success of a day in the clinic. A variety of administrative skills are used in the performance of this vital function. By effectively scheduling patients to fit a particular practice, it is possible to make profitable use of provider and staff time.

In addition, efficient patient flow pleases the patient. A common patient complaint is the time spent waiting in the reception area or the examination room. Most patients appreciate a clinic that recognizes the value of their time. Accordingly, these patients do not hesitate to advertise their experience (good or bad) to friends and families—a fact of great significance to any medical setting.

In addition to the required administrative skills, medical assistants involved in scheduling patients must put into practice their best interpersonal and communication skills. Scheduling an appointment may be the first contact patients have with the medical facility. They remember and value the treatment they receive from the time of first contact. The personality of the clinic is always reflected in the treatment and respect given to patients.

Whether scheduling is done online, through a computerized system, or in the paper appointment book (rare these days), practitioners and their staff must remember the importance of that first impression and make it satisfying for patients.

TAILORING THE SCHEDULING SYSTEM

Competency

The patient population of each medical facility will determine the best method for scheduling appointments. A surgeon's clinic will have a much different flow of patients than a pediatrician's clinic. The key is to customize the system to best accommodate the practice. Primary goals in determining this should include:

- A smooth flow of patients with a minimal amount of waiting time
- Flexibility to accommodate acutely ill, STAT (or emergency) appointments, work-ins, cancellations, and no-shows

Medical providers may feel uncomfortable if their days are not busy with patients or they experience idle time. It is also true that patients want access to their medical providers when needed and prefer not to wait several days to be seen. There is no one perfect scheduling style, and some facilities may even be unable to identify their style of scheduling by name. One thing is certain, however; patients, providers, and their staff will know when scheduling is not working successfully.

SCHEDULING STYLES

There are a number of methods for patient scheduling. The best method for a practice is the one that effects good patient flow and proper utilization of staff and physical facilities and meets the needs of the provider(s). Traditionally, all scheduling was done by writing appointments in a book by hand. Increasingly, however, scheduling is done using computer software designed specifically for that purpose or using scheduling programs that are part of practice management (PM) software. Keep in mind that even the most sophisticated computerized system will fail if the scheduling style does not comfortably fit the predetermined and necessary patient flow.

It is important to note that some clinics may use terminology that makes a distinction between types of hours kept in a clinic. For instance, *patient hours* may be used to indicate the hours patients are seen by providers in the clinic. *Office hours* may indicate when the clinic is open. For example, a clinic may have office hours of Monday through Friday, 8 AM to 5 PM and be closed on Wednesday afternoons. However, patient hours are Monday mornings and afternoons, Tuesday afternoons, and Thursday and Friday mornings. Whenever the clinic does not have patient hours, the staff customarily will be at the clinic completing the many tasks of the practice.

Some clinics ask patients to sign in as they arrive. Some legal authorities believe that the only infallible way to prove patients have kept a medical appointment is to have them sign their name upon arrival and give the time. The Health Insurance Portability and Accountability Act (HIPAA) has ruled that patients can be asked to sign their name upon arrival as long they are not asked to provide any other personal information, such as address, telephone number, Social Security number, or clinic identification number. HIPAA has also ruled that patients cannot be forced to sign if they feel uncomfortable in doing so. A word of caution is important here. The patient's right to privacy ensures that patients do not see confidential information (such as the reason for the visit) of other patients. HIPAA regulations have caused facilities to be more cognizant of patients' rights to privacy and confidentiality.

If the setting and circumstances indicate that a sign-in sheet for patients is the most efficient means of checking in patients, forms can be purchased that meet the privacy and confidentiality expectations of patients.

Figure 12-1 illustrates a carbonized pack with perforations that allows a patient to sign in giving the necessary information. The patient is instructed to remove the top ticket, leaving the information on the bottom form only. The next person to sign in does not see the information of the previous patient. In cases where complete confidentiality is required, this type of ticket also has a number in the upper right-hand corner. The medical assistant can call the patient by number, instead of by name, in environments where this may be necessary.

Open Hours

In open hours scheduling, patients are seen throughout a particular time frame, for example, 9:00 AM to 11:00 AM or 1:00 PM to 3:00 PM. Patients are seen on a first-come, first-served basis. Many clinics frequently choose this method because they are able, by their nature, to maintain a steady flow of patients. A sign-in sheet is often helpful with open hours scheduling, because patients are seen on a first-come, first-served basis. It is important to remember that a sign-in sheet can never replace a warm, welcoming greeting from the administrative medical assistant to set the tone for care given that day.

Double Booking

When the **double booking** method is used, two or more patients are given a particular appointment time. This method is limited to a practice that can attend to more than one patient at a time. For instance, Maria Jover and Jim Marshal are both given a 9:30 AM appointment. Ms. Jover requires a complete checkup including lab tests, vitals, and provider visit. Mr. Marshal is being seen for suture removal. While the staff conducts the lab tests on Ms. Jover, the primary care provider can see Mr. Marshal. Obviously, this method requires a precise accounting for time, rooms, and adequate staff. A good rule to remember is that if patients consistently have to wait for staff to attend to them, double booking is not a wise choice of scheduling method.

Clustering

The **cluster scheduling** method involves grouping or categorizing similar types of visits or procedures on particular days or blocks of time. Cluster scheduling is sometimes referred to as *specialty scheduling*, or **practice-based scheduling**. It is popular in clinics where groups of patients require similar visit types and are scheduled during these predetermined times.

Examples would include an OB/GYN clinic, where all prenatal checks are scheduled so that two to three patients come in every 15 or 30 minutes. The medical assistant generally will handle the vitals sign, weight, and other pertinent information, and the provider can check in on patients and focus on those that turn out to not be routine, have problems, or are more complex cases that require attention.

Another example would be a day or time block set aside by surgeons for postoperative checks. Most of these follow-up visits involve making sure incision sites are clean and healing well, and that the patient is following all medication and therapy

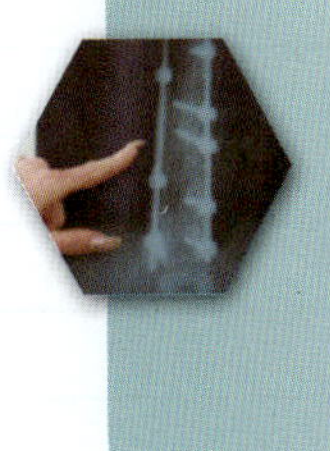

Critical Thinking

When a sign-in sheet is used for patients but the administrative medical assistant is assisting the other staff members when patients arrive, what can be done to create an atmosphere that welcomes patients and puts them at ease?

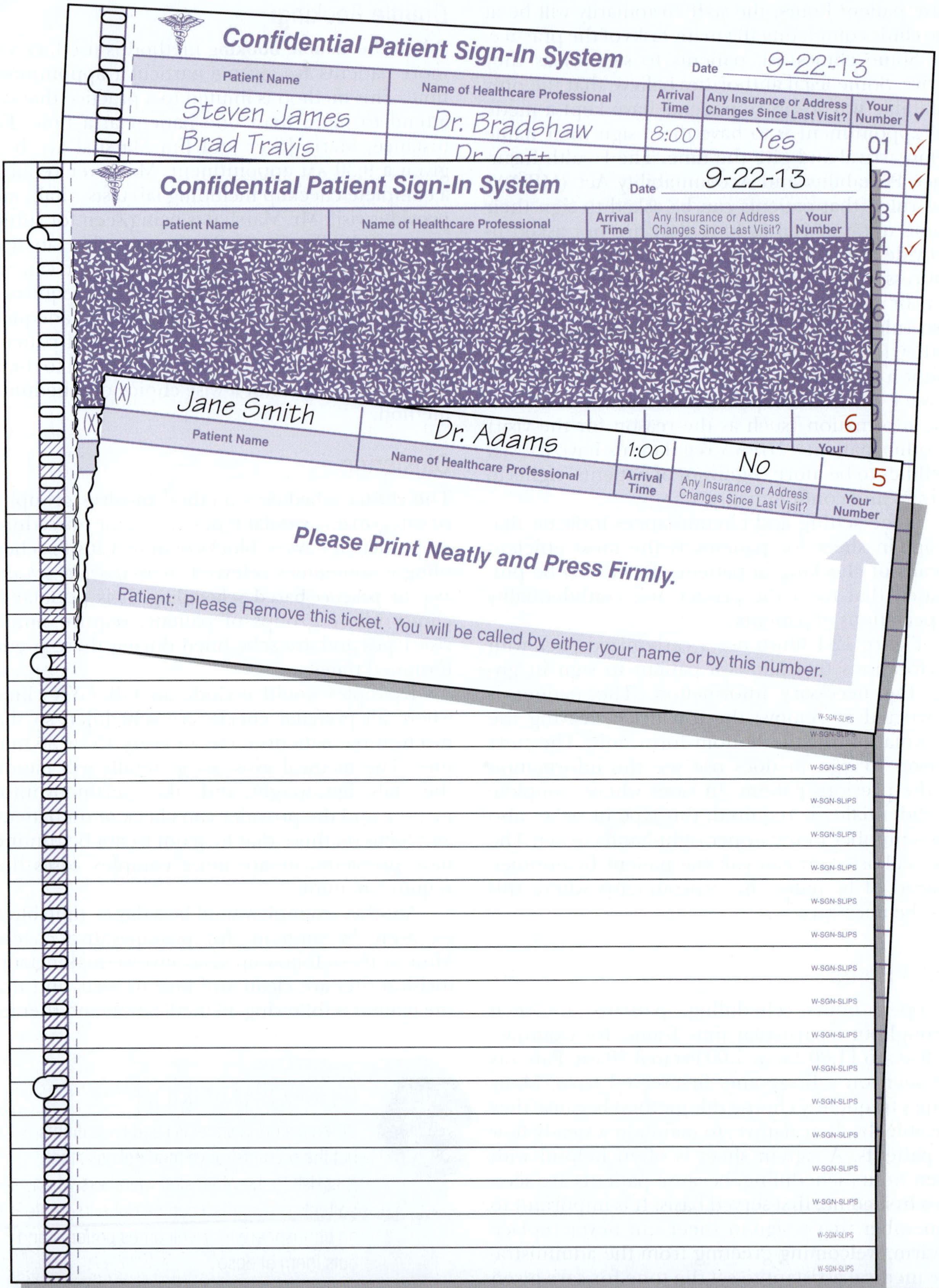

Confidential Patient Sign-In System

Date 9-22-13

Patient Name	Name of Healthcare Professional	Arrival Time	Any Insurance or Address Changes Since Last Visit?	Your Number	✓
Steven James	Dr. Bradshaw	8:00	Yes	01	✓
Brad Travis	Dr. Cott			02	✓

Confidential Patient Sign-In System

Date 9-22-13

Patient Name	Name of Healthcare Professional	Arrival Time	Any Insurance or Address Changes Since Last Visit?	Your Number
(X) Jane Smith	Dr. Adams	1:00	No	6

Patient Name	Name of Healthcare Professional	Arrival Time	Any Insurance or Address Changes Since Last Visit?	Your Number
(X)				5

Please Print Neatly and Press Firmly.

Patient: Please Remove this ticket. You will be called by either your name or by this number.

W-SGN-SLIPS

FIGURE 12-1 Confidential patient sign-in system that offers privacy. A patient can be called by the number of the ticket or by name.

orders and progressing as expected. Again, these visits are normally quick and routine. Clustering allows a higher volume of patients to be seen comfortably. This can be very convenient for the patient, taking away long wait times for what might be a 5- or 10-minute post-op check.

There are many creative ways for certain specialties to utilize cluster scheduling. Having similar patients together also offers opportunities for patient education. Presenting videos or information sessions on particular procedures or conditions can optimize everyone's time. This could include initial visits for bariatric surgery, where patients will be evaluated and need to complete a battery of required assessments or meetings before surgery can be approved or scheduled.

It is important for the clinic to maintain an atmosphere of individualized care, and avoid an assembly-line feel. Staff, rooms, and resources will need to be carefully planned to keep the larger volume of patients flowing efficiently.

Wave Scheduling

Wave scheduling is another method that can be used effectively in medical facilities that have several procedure rooms and adequate personnel to staff them. Using the wave scheduling system, patients are scheduled only in the first half hour of each hour. For example, three patients may be given the time of 11 AM. Generally, the first one to arrive is seen first. If they all arrive on time, the one who is most ill is usually seen first, and there will be a waiting time for the other two patients. Depending on the practice, some administrative medical assistants will be instructed to schedule three patients at the top of the hour and another two or three patients at the bottom of the hour (e.g., 11:30 AM). Patients who do not understand this system of scheduling may become irritated if they discover that another patient has the same appointed time with the same provider. This method takes into account that there will be no-shows and late arrivals. It can also accommodate work-in appointments. However, it does require personnel who are able to prioritize patient problems precisely when establishing the appointments.

Modified Wave Scheduling

Modified wave scheduling is a variation of the wave method where patients are scheduled in "waves." In this method, two or three patients are scheduled at the beginning of each hour, followed by single appointments every 10 to 20 minutes the rest of the hour.

A variation of this method assesses major and minor problems. Major time-consuming problems are seen at the beginning of the hour (e.g., new patients). Minor problems are seen from 20 minutes past the hour to half past the hour (e.g., follow-ups, bandage changes, and other minor procedures), and walk-ins (e.g., a child with a 103°F temperature) are accommodated at the end of the hour. Again, good screening will determine the success of this method.

With both the clustering and wave methods, empty or unscheduled periods can be used to catch up on other responsibilities.

Stream Scheduling

Stream scheduling is perhaps the best known and most widely used scheduling system. When this system works as it should, there is a steady stream of patients at set appointment times throughout the workday. There could be, for example, a 30-minute appointment at 9:00 AM; a 15-minute appointment at 9:30 AM; and a 15-minute appointment at 9:45 AM. Each patient is assigned a specific time. This can best be accomplished by establishing realistic time guidelines for particular types of appointments, such as 45 minutes for consultations, 15 minutes for immunizations, and 30 minutes for hearing tests.

Online Scheduling

As technology advances in health care, so does the concept of self-scheduling patient appointments. New self-scheduling software that integrates with electronic health record software is available, and not just for smaller or specialized practices with small or no staff. Larger practices are realizing higher efficiency, decreased phone calls, and happier patients by allowing do-it-yourself (DIY) appointments.

In this age of people reserving tables at restaurants, hailing a taxi, or buying groceries right from their smart phones, the demand for self-scheduling of routine doctor appointments is more prevalent. Currently, many clinics are using *patient portals*, which may include either appointment requests or self-scheduling modules (see Chapter 11).

A patient portal is a secure Web site that provides a patient with 24-hour access to his or her health care information for a particular practice. Popular functions include communicating via email with the health care team, obtaining test results, requesting medication refills, and many other capabilities, such as requesting or scheduling

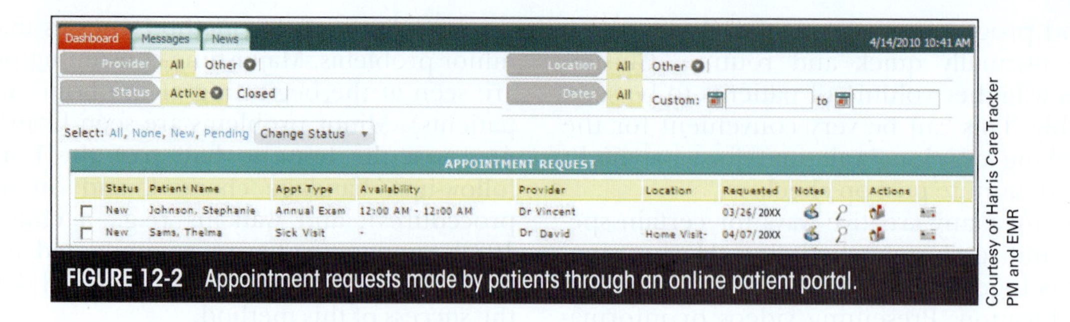

FIGURE 12-2 Appointment requests made by patients through an online patient portal.

Courtesy of Harris CareTracker PM and EMR

appointments. Some portals will allow a patient to request an appointment, and a staff member will schedule it and send a confirmation back to the patient (Figure 12-2). Others enable the patient to select a date, or the next available date and time, and self-schedule an appointment.

Consider a recent survey by Accenture, a business services and consulting company, which shows 77% of patients think that the ability to book, change, or cancel appointments online is important. A rapid explosion in the use of digital solutions for DIY appointment scheduling will radically alter the U.S. health system marketplace over the next 5 years. Accenture research predicts that by the end of 2019, there will be 66% of U.S. health systems offering digital self-scheduling and 64% of patients will book appointments using digital tools. Nearly 38% of appointments will be self-scheduled, representing almost 986 million appointments.

ANALYZING PATIENT FLOW

When reviewing the current scheduling practice, a simple analysis can maximize a clinic's scheduling practices. This entails looking at appointment times, patient arrival times, the actual time a patient is seen, and the time a visit is completed. A simple grid chart can be produced for a given period, for example, 1 to 2 weeks (Figure 12-3). In addition, monitor and chart the number of no-shows and cancellations. An electronic scheduling system can automatically provide the detail necessary to analyze the effectiveness of patient scheduling. It has the capability of indicating the scheduled time for specific procedures, for each provider, and for each service given to the patient.

This analysis will provide a clear picture of patient flow and whether personnel are being used efficiently. The data will assist in estimating how many patients to schedule and realistic time frames for particular problems or procedures. If the staff is scheduling return patients every 15 minutes yet the analysis shows these visits average 24 minutes, then the scheduling method needs adjustment. This may mean either allowing more minutes for follow-up visits or building in slack time when no appointments are made.

PATIENT FLOW ANALYSIS

February 2, 20XX — **Dr. King**

Patient Name	Length of Appt.	Appt. Time	Time Seen	Time Out
Martin Gordon	15	10:20	10:22	10:45
Jason Jover	45	11:20	11:20	12:30
Nora Fowler	30	1:00	1:25	1:45
Jim Marshal	15	1:30	1:50	2:10
Herb Fowler	60	2:45	2:15	3:25

FIGURE 12-3 Patient flow analysis helps a practice determine realistic time frames for appointments.

Develop a simple list of commonly scheduled visits with time estimates for each. This procedural sheet will be particularly useful when training new employees or when temporary help is used for scheduling. A list of commonly scheduled visit types with set duration times can also be set up when using an electronic scheduling system (Figure 12-4).

Waiting Time

One of patients' frequently voiced frustrations with medical clinics is excessive waiting time. Obviously, emergencies and other unexpected

Appointment Type	Group	Duration	Active
Established Patient CPE	All	30	Y
Established Patient Sick	All	15	Y
Follow Up	All	15	Y
Lab	All	15	Y
MA Visit	All	15	Y
New Patient CPE	All	45	Y
New Patient Sick	All	45	Y
PAT	All	60	Y
Pap Smear	All	30	Y
Procedure	All	30	Y
X Ray	All	15	Y

Add New | Build Schedule | Show All

FIGURE 12-4 Most practices have a list of typical types of visits with time estimates.

Courtesy of Harris CareTracker PM and EMR

interruptions cannot be anticipated. However, there are certain measures the medical assistant can take when attempting to keep the schedule on target. If patients are kept waiting, it is a good strategy to explain the reason for the delay and give patients an estimate of how long the delay will be. *Never* ignore the delay hoping patients will not notice; doing so may even increase perceived waiting time. Find ways to make patients comfortable while they wait; for example, provide an appropriate choice of reading materials (or in the case of children, activities). If a delay can be anticipated—for example, if the provider is called away for a baby delivery or surgery—attempt to contact patients before they leave home to reschedule the appointments.

If the delay is likely to be a half hour or longer, provide patients with options, for example:

1. Offer patients the opportunity to run an errand, having them return at a specified time.
2. Offer to reschedule appointments for another day, or later that day, or to see another provider in the practice if possible.

In any case, remember that good customer relations dictate your willingness to acknowledge the inconvenience to the patients, and do attempt to provide an acceptable solution. Remember also that some patients simply will not appreciate any efforts to apologize for a delay, in which case you must continue to act professionally toward them.

LEGAL ISSUES

Information provided in any patient scheduling system may be used for legal purposes. A case of malpractice or questions regarding a provider's availability may require a copy of the daily schedule. It might become necessary to identify how many times a particular patient was a no-show or canceled an appointment, never calling to reschedule. The appointment schedule could verify that a patient was seen and treated on a particular day, thus affirming the information in the patient's record. A patient sign-in sheet may serve this purpose, also.

All computerized systems provide a permanent record of patients seen, and any alterations to that schedule are saved and are shown when a printout is produced. If an appointment book is still used, the staff will have to make certain there is a permanent record or daily appointment sheet that indicates cancellations, work-ins, urgent care needs, and no-shows. Any changes to the daily appointment sheet are to be made in pen; therefore, there will be no question regarding accuracy.

Taking the time to accurately and consistently document all aspects of patient care makes a statement about the providers in the practice and their staff and reflects positively on the presumed quality of patient care.

INTERPERSONAL SKILLS

Scheduling appointments requires interpersonal skills. Medical assistants convey a great deal to patients through attitude and actions as well as empathy. A hurried or disinterested manner communicates that the patient is not a priority. Because patients are often distraught or anxious when making appointments, it is extremely important to reduce rather than increase anxiety. Also, the medical assistant who schedules appointments may be the first contact a patient has with the clinic; patients do not easily forget rude or insensitive staff. A hurried, disinterested manner toward patients is just as often the basis for legal action as is a negligent act.

If any form of online scheduling is used, be certain that it is user friendly, has a rapid response time of no more than 24 hours, and provides patients an option if the online scheduling proves unsatisfactory for any reason. Make certain that staff are ready for online scheduling and that those responsible for assignments and backups are carefully prepared. It is important that patients not be made to feel inadequate if they choose not to use online scheduling.

The patient should always be made to feel worthy of attention. This validates his or her reason for calling. If you are scheduling a patient in the clinic and the phone rings, answer the call but excuse yourself first. Ask the caller to please hold for a moment. If you are on the telephone scheduling a patient and another patient walks in, acknowledge with a nod or signal that you will be right there—never let the person feel ignored. Today, patients have a variety of options for health care and tend to be much more consumer conscious of the treatment they receive.

GUIDELINES FOR SCHEDULING APPOINTMENTS

Whether completed by manual methods or computer technology, the process of scheduling appointments for patients and other visitors to the clinic involves a number of variables, including (1) the urgency of the need for an appointment; (2) whether the patient is a referral from another provider; (3) recording methods for new and established patients; (4) implementation of check-in, cancellation, and rescheduling policies; (5) use of reminder systems; and (6) accommodating visits from medical supply and pharmaceutical company representatives.

Screening Calls

Urgent calls will need to be screened or assessed, before they can be scheduled. **Screening** calls is defined as the person making the appointment determining the actual urgency of that call and how the patient can best be scheduled. This requires both communication skills and medical knowledge, especially details specific to the clinic itself according to the practice specialty.

Appropriate questions will be asked to determine the actual urgency. Is the patient in immediate need of medical assistance? Is there any bleeding? If so, where? How profuse is the bleeding? Are there chest pains? How intense is the pain? Is the pain localized? How long have the symptoms been present? The medical assistant needs to determine whether this is a life-threatening matter, or whether the problem is urgent in the patient's eyes but not a medical emergency. Precise information will help to determine the critical or noncritical nature of the call.

In screening the patient's urgency of care, be tactful in questioning and avoid making the patient feel that the need is insignificant. If questioning indicates this is a medical emergency, follow the policy for having the patient seen (whether it be an emergency appointment or referral to the emergency department). If referral to the emergency department or a call to 911 is necessary, make the call for the patient, being certain you have the correct address and telephone number available. Such a referral minimizes disruption to patients being seen in the ambulatory care setting. If it is determined that the best method in handling this emergency is to see the patient in the clinic, let scheduled patients know of the emergency and offer them the opportunity of rescheduling or waiting until the emergency has been resolved. A built-in slack time of 30 minutes in the morning and 30 minutes in the afternoon can provide some flexibility in last-minute emergency scheduling. If it is determined that the situation is not an emergency, work the patient into the schedule as the situation warrants and time allows, and make certain the patient is comfortable with the scheduled time. Be sure to leave the patient with the understanding that you have done your best to address the situation. (See Chapters 8 and 11 for more information on screening.)

Referral Appointments

One of the primary sources of patients for any provider is referrals from other providers. This is especially true in a managed care climate, where patients usually must have a referral from their primary care provider and where providers are part of an HMO network. It is important that these appointments be given special consideration and that referred patients are given an appointment as soon as possible.

Adequate information needs to be obtained to determine the urgency of scheduling. If the referring provider or clinic staff calls directly, the situation can be assessed at that time. However, if the referred patient calls, it is best to obtain necessary records and information from the referring provider's clinic to determine the urgency and appropriateness of an appointment. Often, the referring provider's clinic has initiated a referral authorization from the patient's insurance and this is forwarded to the appropriate provider. The patient also receives a notification that the referral was approved, and to which doctor. The notification may be sent to the patient by regular mail, a patient portal system, or other secure method.

If the patient does not know if a referral authorization has been obtained, or the authorization has not been received, it may be necessary to direct the patient to ask the referring provider for authorization. In some cases, the medical assistant will need to call the referring provider's clinic to obtain more information before an appointment is scheduled. Assure the patient that an appointment will be scheduled upon receipt of the authorization, and then follow up as required.

Recording Information

Patients can be sensitive to the amount of information they are required to provide to make an initial appointment. Keep the information as simple as possible and obtain only essential information. It should be tailored to fit the practice; for example, an obstetrician and a pediatrician will have different questions for the first-time patient.

When patients schedule an appointment online via the clinic's Web site, they are directed to a patient preregistration and health history that can be completed online prior to coming to the facility. The information provided in this format is often more detailed than what is obtained over the telephone. Nevertheless, the following basic items should be obtained from a new patient:

1. The patient's full legal name (with the correct spelling)
2. A daytime telephone number
3. The reason for the visit
4. The referring provider, and when relevant, if a referral authorization has been obtained
5. Date of birth
6. Type of insurance
7. Insurance identification and group numbers

In privacy, repeat this information back to the patient to ensure accuracy. The critical determination is whether the information is essential to the first contact or whether it can be obtained at the time of the visit.

An established patient, someone who has already been seen in the clinic, should be required to provide only the following information:

1. Full legal name
2. Chief complaint or reason for the visit
3. A daytime telephone number
4. If the patient has not been to the office in more than six months, or if it is the first quarter of the year, confirm whether address or insurance information have changed and update where needed.

When the information is recorded, print legibly and accurately if using a manual system and key in the information if using a computer system. Check for accuracy in either system. Record the appointment as soon as it is made—never rely on memory.

When scheduling an appointment time, ask the patient what day and time is most convenient and then make the appointment for the first available time stated. If possible, provide the patient with a choice of appointment times. Finally, confirm that the patient clearly understands the date and time of the appointment; be sure to repeat the date and time to ensure that both of you have recorded the same information. If the patient is making the appointment in person, provide an appointment reminder.

Scheduling an appointment for the clinic's available times for anyone with an extremely busy schedule can require a great deal of patience. If the patient requests a particular appointment that is not possible, courteously offer an explanation.

Many ambulatory care settings, especially those specializing in family practice and pediatrics, provide alternative hours for scheduling appointments. Having evening appointments at least one day a week or Saturday morning appointments can be helpful for individuals whose work schedule does not permit weekday appointments.

Appointment Matrix

Procedure

Before appointments can be scheduled, the times a provider is not available will need to be blocked out. This is called establishing the **matrix**. The matrix provides a current and accurate record of appointment times available for scheduling patient visits. Clinic hours are noted with times blocked when the facility is closed. Provider's schedules, vacations, holidays, hospital rounds, and any responsibilities that make providers unavailable for appointments are recorded. The matrix of the scheduling plan might include slots for patients who need to see only staff members for their appointment; therefore, times when they are unavailable are important to the matrix. Any evening or weekend appointment slots available also are noted (see Procedure 12-1).

Typically, when using an electronic system for scheduling, the program will search through a database of appointments, find an open appointment, and allocate an appointment time according to your instructions. These instructions can include finding an open appointment with a specific time length, on a specific day, or within a

PROCEDURE 12-1

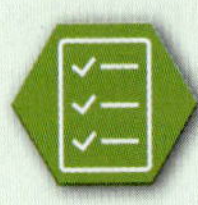

Procedure

Establishing the Appointment Matrix

PURPOSE:

To have a current and accurate record of appointment times available for scheduling patient visits.

EQUIPMENT/SUPPLIES:

- Paper appointment scheduling system or computerized PM system
- Provider and staff schedule

PROCEDURE STEPS:

1. Block off times in the appointment scheduler when patients are not to be scheduled. Ideally, the whole year can be mapped out to avoid scheduling patients when the provider has other commitments or when the clinic is closed.
   a. In paper system, make an *X* through these time slots. This establishes the matrix.
   b. In a PM system, open the scheduling module and block the time slots patients are not to be scheduled by date and time.

   RATIONALE: Identifies visually when patients cannot be scheduled for an appointment.
2. Indicate all vacations, holidays, and other clinic closures as soon as they are known. It may be helpful to indicate absences that might affect patient scheduling; for example, the vascular laboratory technician is gone April 20–23, so no Doppler procedures will be scheduled. RATIONALE: Informs all staff members of absences from the facility and indicates when these members are not available to see patients.
3. ***Paying attention to detail,*** note all provider meetings, hospital rounds, appointments, conferences, vacations, and other prescheduled provider commitments. If the provider has routine items, such as a Medical Society meeting that is always held on the first Thursday of the month at 7:00 PM or daily hospital rounds at 8:00 AM, write these in. RATIONALE: Informs all staff members of prescheduled commitments when a provider is unavailable to see patients.
4. If the clinic has a scheduling system for certain examinations or procedures (e.g., all cast removals are done in the morning before 10:30 AM), these can be color coded with highlighters in a paper system. In a PM system, use the method specific to the software to assign either color, room assignment, or staff assignment for special procedures and equipment. By utilizing these methods, it is easily and quickly evident where particular types of appointments are available to be scheduled. RATIONALE: Allows all staff members to see at a glance where certain examinations or procedures can be scheduled. The color-coded highlighting helps prevent errors in establishing such specific times for certain procedures. The completed matrix provides proof of the completed task.

specified time frame. Once the appointment time is confirmed with the patient, patient data are keyed in, and the appointment is automatically scheduled.

Telephone Appointments

Procedure

More appointments are made by telephone than by any other method. Remember the guidelines for appointment scheduling and appropriate screening of all calls to determine urgency and need, and to follow your provider-employer's instructions regarding patient referrals for appointments. Make certain that you get all the necessary information from the patient when the appointment is made. Procedure 12-2 provides practice for telephone appointments. The professional manner in which telephone appointments are made for patients sets the tone for their satisfaction with the clinic, its providers, and their care.

Patient Check-In

Procedure

Records of patient appointments serve a legal purpose. Establishing a procedure for checking in appointments simplifies tracking the arrival of patients (see Procedure 12-3). This is particularly true in

PROCEDURE 12-2

Procedure

Making an Appointment

PURPOSE:

To schedule an appointment, entering information in the appointment schedule according to clinic policy.

EQUIPMENT/SUPPLIES:

- Telephone
- Paper appointment scheduling system or computerized scheduling PM system

PROCEDURE STEPS:

1. In a private and quiet location, answer the ringing telephone before the third ring. Identify the facility and yourself. RATIONALE: Assures the patient calling that he or she has the correct number; sets the tone for the conversation. The private location ensures that others will not hear any information said during the telephone call.
2. As the patient begins to speak, make notes on your personal log sheet of the patient's name and reason for the call. RATIONALE: Makes certain you are focusing on the call and will not have to ask the patient to repeat something you missed.
3. ***Applying active listening skills***, determine whether the patient is new or established, the provider to be seen, and the reason for the appointment. RATIONALE: Provides necessary information to determine when the patient should be seen and how much time will likely be necessary.
4. ***Discuss with the patient any special appointment needs***, and search your appointment schedule (using appointment book or the appointment search feature in the PM system) for an available time. RATIONALE: Tells the patient that his or her needs and the needs of the clinic are essential to this conversation.
5. Once that patient has agreed to an appropriate time, enter the patient's name in the schedule.
   a. In a paper system, enter last name first, followed by the first name, telephone number (home, work, or cell), and the chief complaint (reason for the visit).
   b. In a PM system, use the patient selection feature and select the patient to be scheduled. Select the date, time, and provider using the software, and enter the reason for visit where indicated.

   RATIONALE: Provides necessary information for staff to pull a record or to make a chart; chief complaint helps identify the length of time to allot for the appointment. The telephone number provides immediate information without having to pull the chart should there be a need to change the appointment.
6. Repeat the date and time for the appointment, using the patient's name. Provide any necessary instructions about coming to the facility. RATIONALE: Confirms the appointment date and time with the patient and gives information about how to get to the facility.
7. ***End the call politely***, perhaps saying, "Thank you for calling. We will see you at 3:45 PM Monday. Good-bye."
8. Make certain you transferred all necessary information from your telephone log to the appropriate appointment schedule. Draw a diagonal line through your notes on the log. This indicates you have completed the task.

multiprovider settings where patients are attended by a number of staff before, or instead of, seeing the primary care provider.

As mentioned earlier, more than one method can be used to check in patients. A sign-in sheet might be used, especially in a facility with open hours scheduling. The administrative medical assistant can place a check mark (usually in red) by the patient's name in the appointment book or make an indication electronically in scheduling software (Figure 12-5).

The check-in procedure serves the additional purpose of alerting the staff when a patient has arrived and is available to be seen. Communication among the administrative medical assistants and the clinical medical assistants is important for a smooth patient flow and to save time for both patients and providers (Figure 12-6).

PROCEDURE 12-3

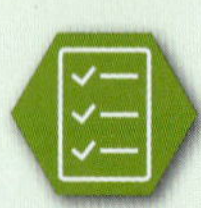

Checking in Patients

Procedure

PURPOSE:

To ensure the patient is given prompt and proper care; to meet legal safeguards for documentation.

EQUIPMENT/SUPPLIES:

- Patient chart
- Black ink pen
- Required forms
- Check-in list or appointment book
- Computerized scheduling PM system, if applicable

PROCEDURE STEPS:

1. The previous evening or before opening the ambulatory care setting, prepare a list of patients to be seen.
   a. In a paper system, either type the names of the patients and scheduled times with provider name and photocopy for each area of the clinic that requires it, or photocopy the page of the appointment book for reference purposes. Charts for patients are then pulled and prepared for visits.
   b. In a PM system, create a schedule or reference sheet using the appointment scheduler. Each PM system will have a feature for producing this sheet. Distribute the reference sheet to each area of the clinic that requires it. If charts are used in the clinic, they are pulled and prepared for visits.

   RATIONALE: Provides a patient list to use as a guide through the day's schedule; charts are ready before patient arrival. If the task is left to the last minute, it may not get done.
2. Check charts or electronic patient records to see that everything is up to date, ***paying attention to detail***. Gather necessary letters, test results, and other data that will be needed during the patient's visit. RATIONALE: Ensures that providers and staff have all the necessary data before seeing a patient.
3. ***When patients arrive, acknowledge their presence.*** If you cannot assist them immediately, gesture toward a chair; thank them for waiting as soon as you are available. RATIONALE: Patients feel welcomed, their time is valued, and their presence is noted.
4. Check in the patient and review vital information, such as address, telephone number, insurance, and reason for visit. Be certain to ***protect the patient's privacy*** by reviewing this information where doing so cannot be overheard by others. RATIONALE: Ensures that you have the latest personal information regarding your patient; provides patients with the privacy and confidentiality to which they are entitled.
5. Use a pen to check off the patient's name from the Reference Sheet if one is used for the permanent record. If the PM system has a check-in feature, input the patient's arrival. RATIONALE: Ensures that there is a permanent record of the patient's arrival in the facility for an appointment. Provides documentation for later referral if necessary.
6. Politely ask the patient to be seated and indicate the appropriate wait time, if any. RATIONALE: Provides direction to the patient and indicates how long a wait might be.
7. Following clinic policy, place the chart where it can be picked up to route the patient to the appropriate location for the visit. RATIONALE: The patient's chart is in readiness when the clinical medical assistant, laboratory personnel, or provider is ready for the patient.

DAILY APPOINTMENT WORKSHEET

Thursday, August 21

8:00	Hospital Rounds		
9:15 ✓	Chris O'Keefe	30 minutes	Immunizations
9:30 ✓	Jim Marshal	15 minutes	Blood pressure check
10:00	Martin Gordon	60 minutes	PE/lab work
11:00	Nora Fowler	30 minutes	URI
11:30	Lunch break		
12:30	Dentist Appointment, Dr. Schleuter		
2:00	Maria Jover	30 minutes	Suspicious rash
2:45	Meet with drug rep regarding new beta-blocker agents		
4:00	Joseph Ortiz	30 minutes	Choking problems

A

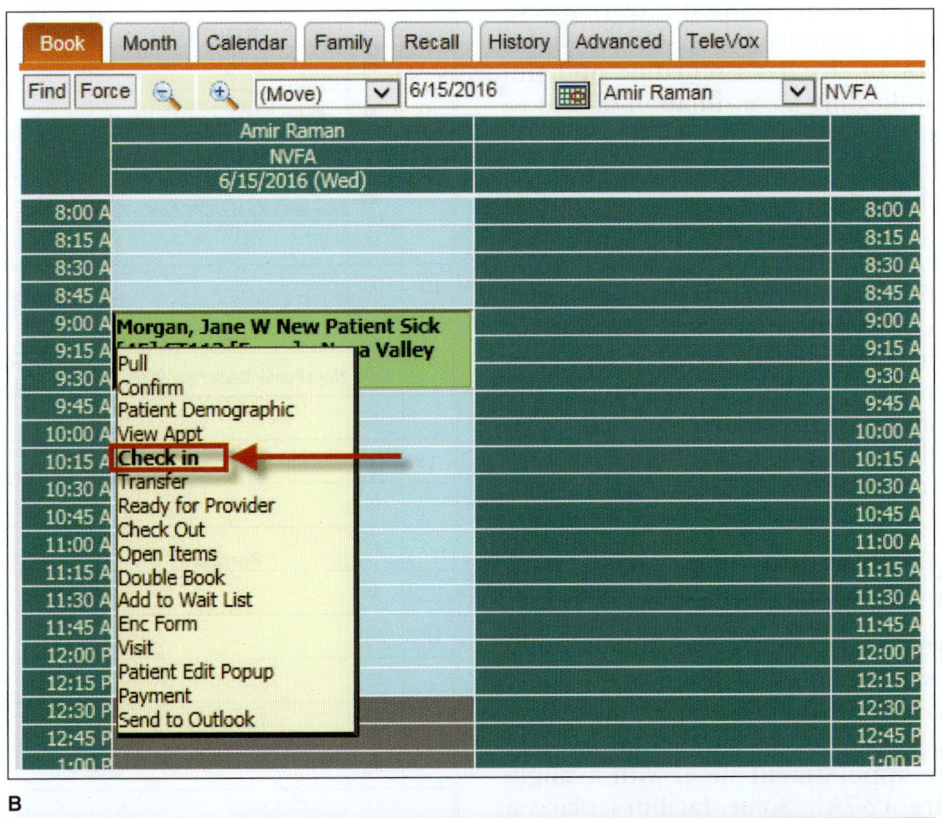

B

FIGURE 12-5 (A) Daily appointment worksheet (manual). (B) Checking in a patient using an electronic scheduling system.

Courtesy of Harris CareTracker PM and EMR

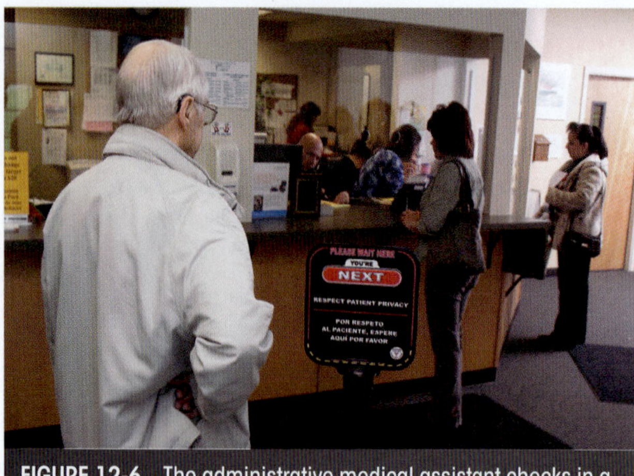

FIGURE 12-6 The administrative medical assistant checks in a patient and keeps the patient check-in list current.

Computer scheduling systems include a space to indicate when a patient arrives for an appointment. Some clinics use the printed activity schedule to check when patients arrive. Other clinics rely upon a copy of the day's schedule and the patient's chart indicating a consultation or visit to legally verify the patient's presence in the clinic.

Unfortunately, even the best of electronic systems may fail temporarily. In that case, the manual system is used as a backup. If the day's schedule has already been printed, it can be used to monitor the patient flow and to check in patients. It may also serve as adequate information for any work-in patients to be accommodated that day. However, for appointments to be made in the future, the administrative medical assistant may have to return a call to the patient when the computer is back up and running properly.

Patient Cancellation and Appointment Changes

Procedure

A permanent record of no-shows should be designated on the appointment sheet with a red *X* or some other distinctive mark. Cancellations should be marked through on the appointment sheet with a single red line (Figure 12-7A). Some facilities place a notation next to the patient's name. Computer scheduling will also provide an area to indicate no-shows and cancellations. No-shows and cancellations should always be noted in the patient's individual chart (Figure 12-7B). Again, it is imperative that the provider's care of the patient be thoroughly documented. Should a patient develop complications and claim a provider was unavailable, the daily appointment sheet and chart would document the patient's failure to show.

Occasionally, patients do not arrive for an appointment because they simply forgot, or sometimes they come on the wrong day or at the wrong time. That can happen simply by human error or

MONDAY, NOVEMBER 23

		Dr. King	Dr. Lewis
7	00		
	15		
	30		
	45		
8	00	Hospital	
	15		Surgery
	30	Rounds	
	45		
9	00	Abigail Johnson - Black	Lenore
	15	Diabetes Check/466-2964	McDonell
	30	Marge O„Keefe/CPE/296-7234	
	45		
10	00		Joseph Ortiz/New Pt/462-1121
	15		
	30	Nora Fowler/Back Pain/466-2234	~~Maria Tover/Stomach Problems/292-2104~~
	45		
11	00	~~Jim Marshal/CPE/763-2067~~	Maria Tover/Stomach Problems/292-2104
	15		
	30	Partners	Partners
	45		
12	00		
	15		
	30		
	45		
		Lunch Meeting	Lunch Meeting
1	00	Matt. Hanes/Consultation/763-3284	Boris Bolski/New Pt./466-8156

FIGURE 12-7A Multiprovider clinic where providers' commitments and no-shows are marked with a red *X* and cancellations are marked with a single red line.

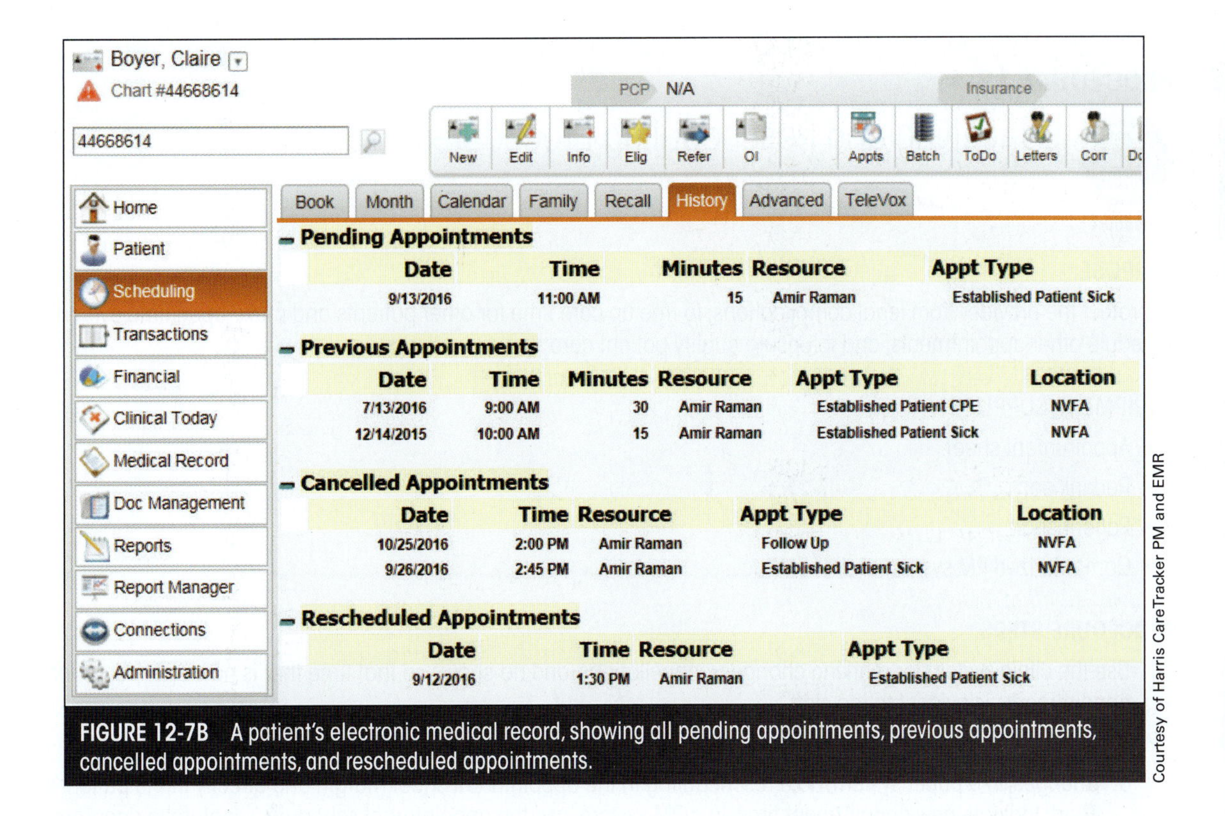

FIGURE 12-7B A patient's electronic medical record, showing all pending appointments, previous appointments, cancelled appointments, and rescheduled appointments.

Courtesy of Harris CareTracker PM and EMR

miscommunication. However, if one patient begins a pattern of getting the dates and times mixed up or forgets the appointment entirely, the primary care provider should be made aware of the fact. Sometimes, a pattern of missed and mixed-up appointments is a first sign that the patient may be experiencing memory loss and mental confusion.

Many clinics have established firm policies for multiple no-shows and cancellations. The general rule is that after three no-shows or cancellations in a row, the provider will review the records. For the provider to adequately treat a patient, the patient's cooperation is necessary. A no-show pattern may indicate that the patient is not truly committed to assisting in treatment. If a patient routinely cancels or does not show, the provider may write a letter terminating services and explaining why the provider is discontinuing care. This should be sent by certified mail, return receipt requested, to ensure that the patient received the notice (see Chapter 6 for more information on termination of services). Procedure 12-4 outlines the proper cancellation procedures.

Although software programs differ, cancellations are typically performed by deleting the patient's name from the time slot; if the appointment is to be rescheduled, the name is then keyed in to the appropriate time, usually the first time open for other appointments.

When canceling appointments by computer, be certain that the program maintains a list of canceled appointments including patient name, date, and time. This documentation is necessary for legal purposes. Also, be certain to record canceled appointments in the patients' charts.

Reminder Systems

When patients are reminded of their scheduled appointments, it results in a greater rate of fulfilled appointments. Give patients appointment card reminders when appointments are made at the medical facility. Those cards may easily be

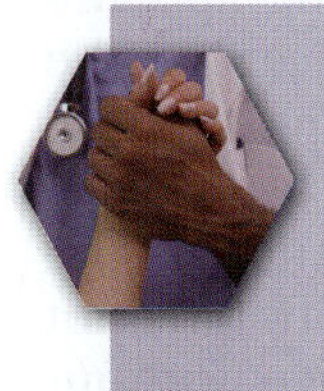

Patient Education

Encourage patients to participate in their health care by keeping appointments or by notifying the clinic that they need to reschedule. Some cancellations are unavoidable, but gentle reminders and a two-way provider–patient relationship encourage responsible patient behavior.

PROCEDURE 12-4

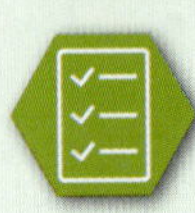
Procedure

Cancelling and Rescheduling Procedures

PURPOSE:

To protect the provider from legal complications; to free up care time for other patients and make open time evident to schedule other appointments; and to ensure quality patient care.

EQUIPMENT/SUPPLIES:

- Appointment sheet
- Red ink pen
- Patient chart
- Computerized PM system and/or EMR

PROCEDURE STEPS:

1. Use the clinic system for marking changes, cancellations, and no-shows so that time that is now open for other appointments is evident to the staff.
2. Indicate on the appointment sheet all appointments that were changed, canceled, or no-shows:
   a. *Changes.* In a paper system, note rescheduling in the appointment sheet margin and directly in the patient's chart; indicate new appointment time. In a PM system, use the appointment scheduler's feature to document changes to the patient's record. RATIONALE: Notifies all staff of a schedule change; documents same information in patient's chart or EMR.
   b. *Cancellations.* In a paper system, enter a note on both the appointment sheet and the patient's chart. Draw a single red line through canceled appointments. Date and initial cancellation in the patient chart. In a PM system, use the appointment scheduler's feature to cancel (and if applicable, reschedule) the appointment to document the cancellation in the patient's record. RATIONALE: Notifies staff of a schedule change; documents cancellation in patient's chart or EMR, thus identifying a change in the patient's plans. A cancellation may initiate a follow-up call from a staff member to determine the reason for the cancellation.
   c. *No-shows.* In a paper system, enter a note on both the appointment sheet and the patient's chart. Date and initial notations in the chart. No-shows can be indicated with a red *X* on the appointment sheet. In a PM system, use the appointment scheduler's feature to indicate a no-show to document the missed appointment in the patient's EMR. RATIONALE: Notifies the staff of a schedule change; documents the no-show in the patient's chart or EMR. Provides a reminder to a staff member to follow up on the reason for the no-show.

tucked in a wallet and forgotten, however. Many clinics notify patients the day before the appointment with a reminder via their choice for the communication—telephone, text message, or email.

Legal

Keep in mind that the reminder is confidential information and should not be left on a recording device without the patient's express permission to do so. (When initially seeing the patient, obtain a number where a personal message could be left.) Finally, reminders can be mailed. This would be most appropriate for patients who come in on a regular basis (e.g., once every 6 months).

Scheduling Pharmaceutical Representatives

Some medical facilities schedule time with representatives of pharmaceutical and medical supply companies. On the other hand, there are some medical clinics that refuse to see any pharmaceutical representatives. When representatives are seen, however, they can provide a valuable service to providers and staff, and with clear guidelines regarding when and how often representatives can visit, a working partnership can develop. Providers may set aside a specific time during the week to meet with these representatives; generally, a time allotment of 15 to 20 minutes is sufficient for these appointments. Some representatives try to establish a standard appointment once a month. If this is a representative your provider desires to see on a regular basis, that policy can be helpful to both the provider and the representative.

SCHEDULING SOFTWARE AND MATERIALS

No matter what materials and which methods are used, the proper tools will enable patient scheduling to be a smoothly functioning, easily documented process. Materials needed for scheduling should be customized to the ambulatory care setting. For instance, a smaller practice may prefer a manual method involving appointment books; a large urgent care–type setting will use a computer program for patient scheduling that may be part of a practice management (PM) software program.

Appointment Schedule

An appropriate appointment schedule system is essential to any medical practice in the ambulatory care setting. Each clinic has unique needs in its physical facility and for its staff. The physical arrangement of the scheduler, including the various combinations of time allotments, must be determined. Some have major headings for hours with minor spaces for 15-minute intervals, others have 10-minute intervals, and still others only hour intervals. An appointment sheet is necessary for both legal risk management and quality management purposes. Copies of the daily appointment sheet, also known as a *reference sheet*, are made available to the doctors, medical assistants, and any other staff members. Using the daily appointment sheet, it is easy to check in patients as they arrive and to indicate no-shows and cancellations. Indicating the check-in and checkout times can be useful for quality management purposes. More importantly, the daily appointment sheet enables all staff members to see the total scheme of the day's patient flow.

If a provider works between two clinics or a hospital and clinic, it is helpful to have this appointment schedule transferred to a handheld computer device for immediate referral. If a handheld computer is not used by the provider, reduce the dimensions of the appointment schedule sheet to pocket-size for the provider's easy access. Generally, if the provider makes hospital visits before coming to the clinic in the morning, this schedule is printed the previous evening before closing.

These daily appointment sheets can also be used to include other provider commitments such as meetings and visits from pharmaceutical representatives. Such a complete record of time ensures that no patient appointments will be booked when, in fact, the provider is not available.

Computer Scheduling Software

Even the smallest of medical facilities today will benefit from the use of information technology. Numerous software programs for the ambulatory care setting require only basic computer hardware that can save time for providers and their staff members. Other programs are more sophisticated and may require on-site technical support.

Some scheduling software programs will schedule resources, equipment, examination rooms, and specialty staff, as well as patients and providers. Some will show co-payments due, authorization expiration dates, and insurance expiration dates. They can select the next available appointment, search for appointments by provider, copy and paste appointments, and specify minimum time increments between appointments. The staff can view multiple schedules daily, weekly, monthly, or even yearly. Reminder notes can be created for both providers and patients.

Computerized scheduling systems that are a component of a complete practice management facility, including medical records, are able to indicate no-shows and cancellations in the system and the patient's chart at the same time. Facilities that are partially computerized will still want to indicate patients who do not keep their appointments on the daily worksheet and in the patients' medical records.

Online systems can handle prescription refill requests, patient–provider email messages, and laboratory results. Some will allow patients to update insurance data and complete registration forms. All of the online systems are done within the provider's Web site, which includes security measures and sophisticated **encryption technology**. Therefore, security is less of a concern.

With America's ongoing goal of giving patients increased access to their electronic health record (EHR) and Congress pushing to have prescriptions transferred electronically, electronic scheduling has become the "entry" to the entire field of computerized medical information. Employers in ambulatory care settings who make certain that patients understand computerized scheduling, who have put time and effort into determining the best program for their use, and who have trained their staff well will not be disappointed with the outcome. Whatever system is chosen, keep in mind that the patient's time, the staff's time, and the provider's time are extremely valuable. The goal is to manage that time as efficiently as possible.

INPATIENT AND OUTPATIENT ADMISSIONS PROCEDURES

Often, patients are scheduled for either outpatient or inpatient hospital admissions or for special procedures performed in another facility. These appointments are most likely made while the patient is present in the clinic and has just been seen by the provider. Have a calendar handy for visualization of the days discussed. If the patient has their agenda on hand, this is especially helpful. If not, the appointment may need to be scheduled at another time.

Outpatient procedures may include endoscopy examinations and specialized radiologic examinations such as Computerized tomography (CT), magnetic resonance imaging (MRI), mammography, and bone scans. If a patient prefers to make his or her own arrangements for a procedure, advise the patient the following information is necessary:

- Name, address, and telephone number of patient
- Name of provider ordering the procedure
- Name of the procedure and preoperative diagnosis
- Name of patient's insurance, ID number, and Social Security number

If required, follow up in a day or two to make certain the procedure has been scheduled (see Procedure 12-5). In addition, please be certain that the patient has been given and understands any special instructions that must be followed prior to the procedure. This might include, but is not limited to, fasting (no eating or drinking after midnight, or a specified time); withholding the consumption of certain medications (such as anything that can interfere with the anesthesia); having a spouse or loved one available to speak with the provider and staff; or not using lotions, oils, or powders prior to the procedure.

Generally, a real service is done for the patients and staff when the medical assistant schedules

PROCEDURE 12-5

Scheduling Inpatient and Outpatient Admissions and Procedures

PURPOSE:

To assist patients in scheduling inpatient and outpatient admissions and procedures ordered by the provider.

EQUIPMENT/SUPPLIES:

- Calendar
- Black ink pen
- Computerized PM system and/or EMR
- Telephones
- Referral slip
- Patient's calendar or schedule (helpful, but not critical)
- Provider requests/orders regarding procedures/admissions being scheduled

PROCEDURE STEPS:

1. In a private and quiet location, discuss with the patient the inpatient admission or outpatient procedure ordered by the provider. **RATIONALE: Helps the patient identify the time necessary for this appointment and the reason for it.**
2. If required, seek permission from the patient's insurance company for the procedure or admission. **RATIONALE: Clearly identifies for the patient who is responsible for the bill and how it is to be paid.**
3. Produce a large, easily read calendar and check to see if the patient has one also. **RATIONALE: Visualization of the calendar is easier for determining available time for the appointment. Patient's calendar further identifies available days and times for the appointment(s).**

(continues)

4. Place telephone call to the facility where the appointment is to be scheduled. Identify yourself, your provider, the clinic from where you are calling, and the reason for the call. **RATIONALE: Alerts the receiver of the call that a provider's office is calling to schedule an appointment.**

   NOTE: The more familiar the medical assistant is with the specific procedure to be scheduled or a specific type of hospital admission, the easier it is to make certain the patient has all the information necessary. It can be helpful for medical assistants to discuss such arrangements with specialty clinics and hospitals.
5. ***Displaying sound judgment***, identify any urgency. Request the next available appointment for the particular type of appointment to be scheduled and provide the patient's diagnosis. Identify any time that is not possible for the patient. **RATIONALE: Tells the receiver how quickly an appointment is to be made, for what reason, and if any dates or times are not possible.**
6. As a time is suggested, confer with the patient for an immediate response.
7. Once the appointment has been scheduled, provide receiver pertinent information related to the patient (e.g., full name, insurance information, Social Security number, telephone number). **RATIONALE: Provides essential information to secure the appointment for the proper patient.**
8. Request any special instructions or advanced data necessary for the patient. **RATIONALE: Helps to ensure that a smooth transition is made from the provider's clinic to the facility where the referral is made and provides the patient with any special instructions.**
9. Complete a manual referral slip, or use the PM or EMR system to enter the referral for the patient; send or fax a copy to the referral facility. **RATIONALE: Ensures that the patient, the referral facility, and the patient's chart have a copy of the reason for the appointment, any specific instructions, and the date and time of the appointment.**
10. If an immediate hospital admission is to be made, ***attend to special needs of patient*** by providing him or her time on the telephone to call family members to make arrangements to receive personal items and any other arrangements necessitated by the appointment. **RATIONALE: Provides patients a little time to notify family members and make necessary arrangements.**
11. Place a reminder notice to yourself on the calendar or in a tickler file. **RATIONALE: To check to make certain the appointment was completed and a report is received from the appointment facility.**
12. Document the referral in the patient's chart. A copy of the referral slip and all pertinent data are to be included. Document in the chart when the appointment is completed and a report is received from the referral facility. Date and initial.

DOCUMENTATION:

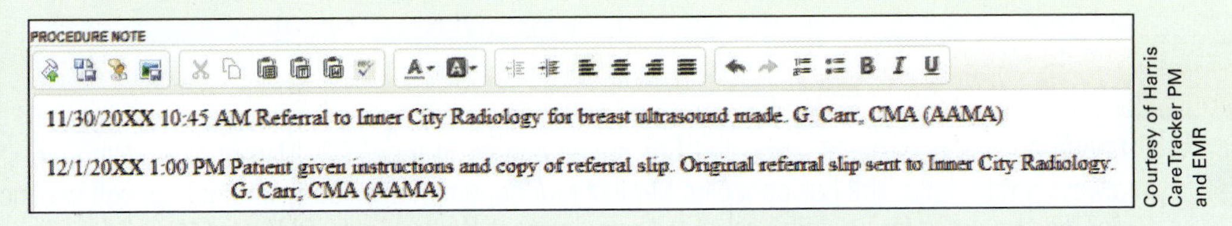
PROCEDURE NOTE

11/30/20XX 10:45 AM Referral to Inner City Radiology for breast ultrasound made. G. Carr, CMA (AAMA)

12/1/20XX 1:00 PM Patient given instructions and copy of referral slip. Original referral slip sent to Inner City Radiology. G. Carr, CMA (AAMA)

Courtesy of Harris CareTracker PM and EMR

the procedure. With the patient present, place a telephone call to the facility where procedures are to be performed. Identify yourself, your provider, and the clinic from which you are calling. Identify any urgency to the request and ask for the next available appointment. As dates and times are discussed, your patient is able to give an immediate response. Consider travel time for your patient and whether there is apt to be any uncomfortable pre-examination procedure that might make travel difficult. Be certain to advise the patient if someone is needed to provide transportation home after the procedure. Often, there is a paperwork follow-up that indicates the nature of the illness and the reason for the specialty examination. Your employer will tell you if a phone response to the examination is required, or if it is acceptable to wait for the written test results.

Once a date has been established, make certain the patient knows the correct date and time, as well as how to get to the place where the examination is to be performed. Inform the patient how and when he or she will receive test results.

Scheduling inpatient admissions to the hospital is similar. However, the provider may want the patient in the hospital as quickly as possible. Call the preferred or designated hospital. Expect to provide pertinent patient and insurance information required by the hospital. Assist the patient in determining whether it is permissible to return home for some personal belongings and to make home arrangements or whether admission is immediate. Some large facilities have a surgery scheduler to make all these arrangements. In primary care, the medical assistant will do this kind of scheduling.

When a surgery is being scheduled, the medical assistant must sometimes coordinate several entities. Arrangements must be coordinated with an assistant in the surgeon's clinic, with the hospital or outpatient surgery center where the surgery will be performed, and occasionally for scheduling specialty equipment and personnel to be available, as well as with the patient's schedule. If any one of these entities is not available at the time requested, the process needs to begin again and can become quite convoluted. If the scheduling of the surgery is especially complex, the medical assistant should consider obtaining the patient's scheduling preferences and limitations and letting the patient go home to be contacted later when all the parts are in place.

Be sensitive to the patient's needs at this time. Scheduling a specialty examination or a hospital admission is rarely a convenience. More likely it is a great inconvenience to the patient, even when necessary. Anything that makes the scheduling more accommodating or pleasant for the patient will help in creating a beneficial atmosphere for all involved.

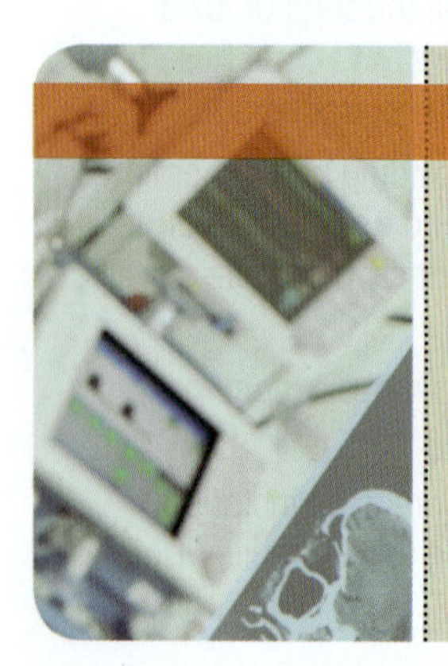

CASE STUDY 12-1

Refer to the scenario at the beginning of the chapter. It appears that this clinic has a smooth-flowing scheduling system and that Walter Seals has everything under control.

CASE STUDY REVIEW

1. What personal traits might Walter need to possess in order for this scenario to be true?
2. What factors, if any, might make the scheduling at Inner City Urgent Care work well?
3. If clients are seen on a first-come, first-served basis, how does the clustering system work if patients need to be referred to one of the specialty care clinics?

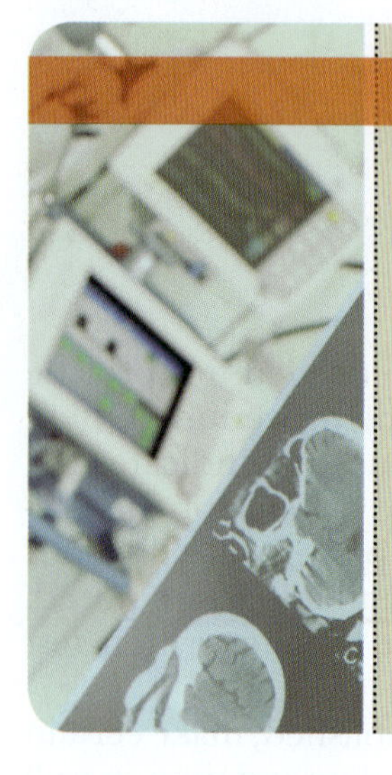

CASE STUDY 12-2

Rhoda Au has persistently canceled her appointments at Inner City Urgent Care. Although she always reschedules, she has canceled her last four appointments. Today, she did not call to cancel nor did she arrive for her fifth scheduled appointment. Walter Seals, CMA (AAMA), who is responsible for scheduling and patient flow, is concerned that Rhoda is canceling because she is afraid to come in for some reason. Rhoda has been a patient for a few years now, and she was always responsible about keeping her appointments.

CASE STUDY REVIEW

1. From the point of view of the urgent care center, why should Walter be concerned that Rhoda is canceling appointments? What action might be taken?
2. From the patient's point of view, why should Walter be concerned?
3. How should Walter record these cancellations and no-shows?

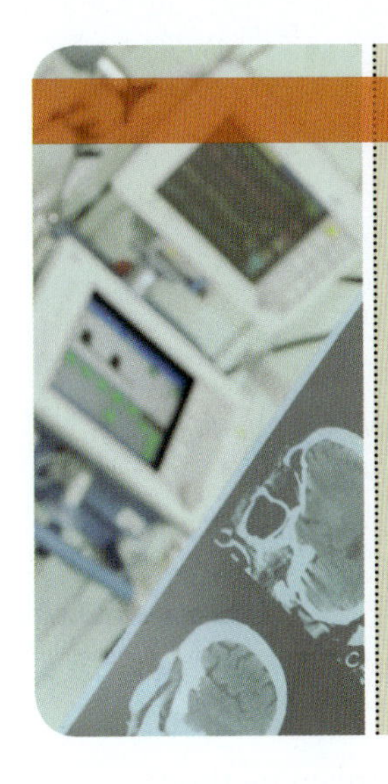

CASE STUDY 12-3

Nancy McFarland, RMA (AMT), is a clinical medical assistant at Inner City Health Care. In the past 3 weeks, Nancy has been doing phone screening, primarily because the clinic has been so busy and the providers believe screening calls will help. In fact, Nancy discovered that the administrative medical assistant is screening quite well, but that there does not seem to be sufficient appointment slots to meet the patient demand.

CASE STUDY REVIEW

1. What might be done to determine whether there is a better scheduling style to fit the current demands?
2. What happens when professional staff, providers, and patients view this medical facility as "too busy"?
3. What are some solutions that you can identify?

Summary

- Medical assistants involved in scheduling patients must put into practice their best interpersonal and communication skills. Scheduling an appointment may be the first contact patients have with the medical facility. They remember and value the treatment they receive from the time of first contact.
- Scheduling has undergone changes, and can be done in person, over the telephone, and using technology for online appointments.
- Scheduling can be stressful, especially when other office tasks are pressing at the front desk. The medical assistant must apply good organizational skills, a calm composure, and effective communication.
- Tailor the scheduling system to the needs of the type of practice, provider habits, and availability of equipment and staff with a focus on minimizing patient wait times. The ability to add unexpected visits for acute illness, add work-ins, and adjust for cancellations is important.
- The various scheduling styles include open hours, double booking techniques, clustering, wave scheduling, modified wave scheduling, stream scheduling, and online scheduling.
- The medical assistant must obtain key information required for scheduling, including the urgency of the need for an appointment and whether the patient is a referral from another provider; understand recording methods for new and established patients; implement check-in, cancellation, and rescheduling policies; use reminder systems; and coordinate visits from medical supply and pharmaceutical representatives.
- Use proper screening techniques to obtain basic information about new and established patients when scheduling appointments.
- The medical assistant must know how to use an appointment matrix, both in a manual and an electronic scheduling system, and apply this matrix to the needs of the practice and patients.
- Familiarize yourself with scheduling for inpatient and outpatient admissions procedures.

Study for Success

To reinforce your knowledge and skills of information presented in this chapter:

- Review the *Key Terms* and *Learning Outcomes*
- Consider the *Critical Thinking* features and *Case Studies* and discuss your conclusions
- Answer the questions in the *Certification Review*

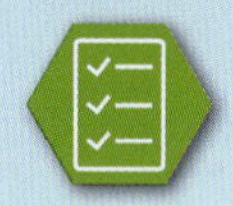

Procedure

- Perform the *Procedures* using the *Competency Assessment Checklists* on the *Student Companion Website*

CERTIFICATION REVIEW

1. Which of the following is one of the legal guidelines for appointment scheduling?
   a. It should be recorded only in pencil.
   b. It should be current, accurate, and saved as documentation.
   c. It should be left on the front desk for patient viewing.
   d. It should be recorded only in red ink.
2. What is the definition of screening patient calls?
   a. It involves taking only emergencies.
   b. It is assessing the urgency of a call and need for appointment.
   c. It means sorting appointments by specialized procedure.
   d. It should only be performed by providers.
   e. Schedule the patient on a first-come, first-served basis.
3. How should representatives from medical supply and drug companies be scheduled?
   a. They should only be seen as a last resort.
   b. They should not be scheduled, but seen only if the provider has time.
   c. They can provide a valuable service and should be scheduled for short visits.
   d. They have complex information to communicate and need 1-hour appointments.
4. What is the definition of the double-booking method?
   a. It gives two or more patients the same appointment time.
   b. It keeps patients waiting unnecessarily.
   c. It is never the system of choice.
   d. It is purely for the provider's convenience.
   e. It is a way for the provider to see two patients at the same time.
5. What is a description of the stream method?
   a. It gives patients appointments as they walk in.
   b. It schedules appointments at set times throughout the workday.
   c. It only works in sole-proprietor clinics.
   d. It refers to streamlining paperwork for each appointment.
6. Why is it necessary to have daily appointment sheets?
   a. They indicate when providers and staff take lunch.
   b. They provide a permanent record for legal risk management and quality management.
   c. They are available only in computerized scheduling.
   d. They tell the staff which patient to see first.
   e. Both a and b
7. Why is analyzing patient flow important?
   a. It can maximize a clinic's scheduling practice.
   b. It often reveals why patient flow is not efficient.
   c. It may indicate a change in pattern for patient scheduling.
   d. All of these
8. What is the most important principle used in tailoring the scheduling system?
   a. Always schedule in ink.
   b. Schedule for the patient's convenience.
   c. Be flexible and sensitive.
   d. Referral patients are first.
   e. Double book the first appointment of the day.

9. What is the best way to approach a patient who must wait for an appointment?
   a. It is best to say nothing about the delay.
   b. Explain the delay and offer options when possible.
   c. Find ways to make the patient comfortable.
   d. Both b and c

10. Which of the following is true of scheduling outpatient procedures?
   a. It is best done by patients who understand their availability.
   b. It is coordinated and completed by the clinic's staff.
   c. It is an important way to enhance patient satisfaction.
   d. The patient cannot understand the urgency or the need for the procedure.
   e. Both b and c

CHAPTER 13

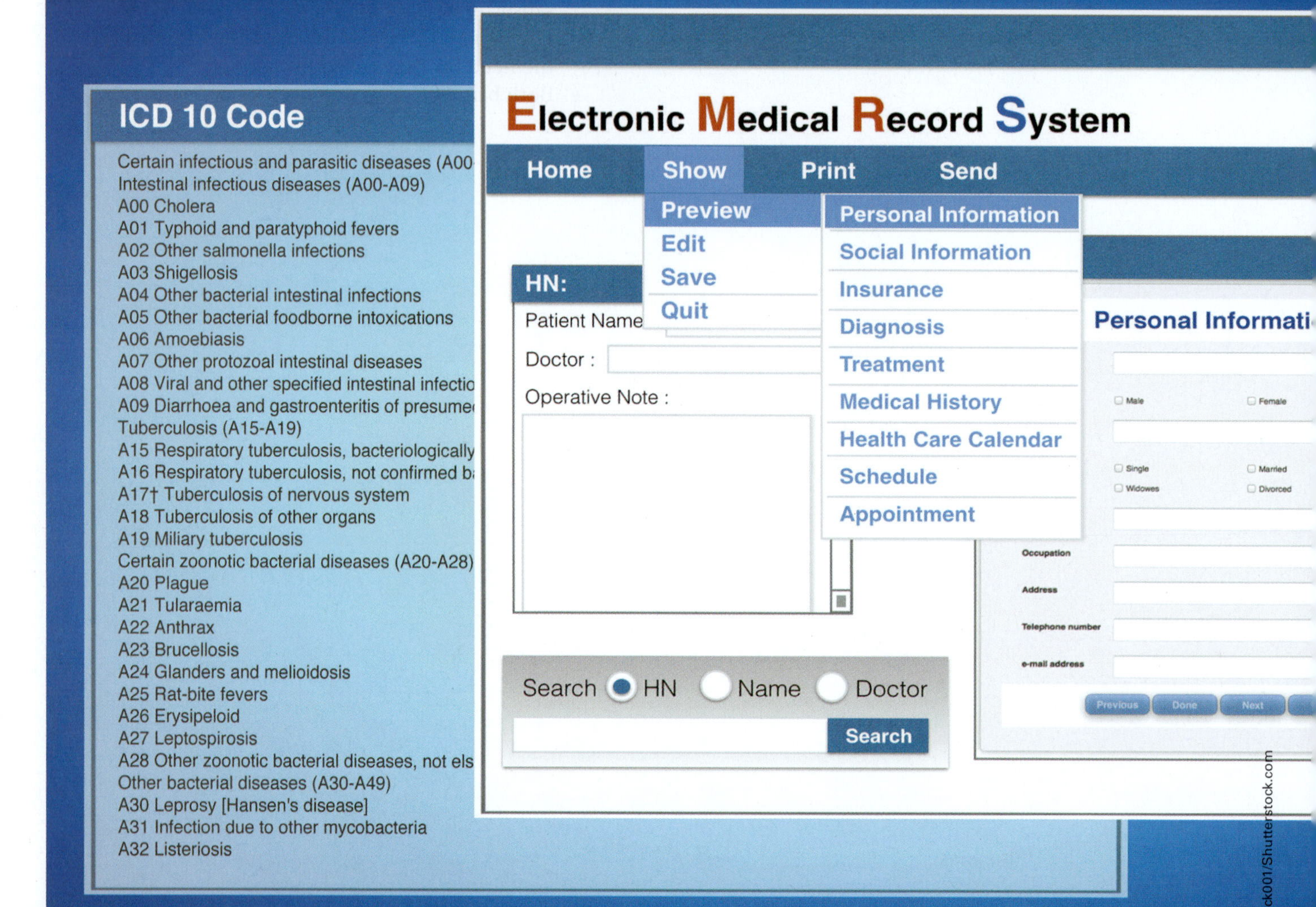

pandpstock001/Shutterstock.com

Medical Records Management

LEARNING OUTCOMES

1. Define and spell the key terms as presented in the glossary.
2. List the purpose of medical records.
3. Discuss the ownership of medical records.
4. State the reasons for accurately maintaining ambulatory care files.
5. Describe how and when information is released from the medical record.
6. State the pros and cons of the manual medical record and the electronic medical record.
7. Correct a medical record, manually and electronically.
8. Recall eight common supplies used in medical records management.
9. Identify the rules described under Basic Rules for Filing.
10. Describe the five steps commonly used when filing any documentation.
11. Name the two filing systems most often used in the clinic setting.
12. State the purpose of cross-referencing.
13. Recall four common documents kept in the patient's medical record.
14. Discuss storage and purging of medical records.
15. Describe electronic medical records and their usefulness to the clinic.
16. Discuss confidentiality and privacy as related to medical records.
17. Explain HIPAA security standards for electronic medical records.

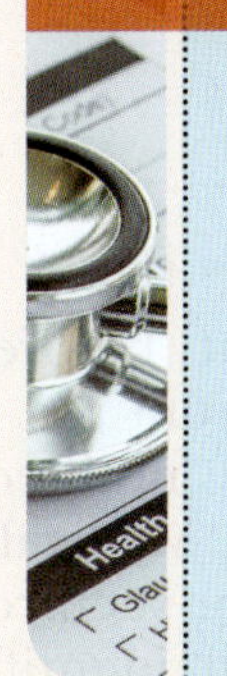

KEY TERMS

accession record
caption
cross-reference
indexing
key unit
meaningful use
out guide
problem-oriented medical record (POMR)
purging
SOAP/SOAPER
source-oriented medical record (SOMR)
tickler file
unit

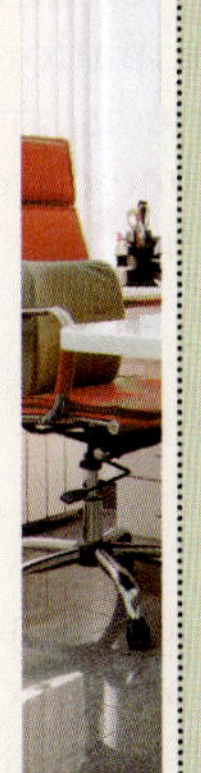

SCENARIO

Consider a situation that might arise at multiprovider Inner City Health Care. Patient Juanita Hansen was seen on Tuesday morning by Dr. Lewis for acute stomach pain. She was given a thorough examination and sent for appropriate testing that afternoon. She was then scheduled to return to Inner City on Friday to see Dr. Lewis.

After she was seen Tuesday morning, Juanita received an upper and lower gastrointestinal series; the results were then sent to Dr. Lewis's clinic. However, Nancy McFarland, RMA (AMT), the medical assistant, attached the results to the wrong patient's file. Friday arrived and Juanita came back to Inner City for her appointment, anxious to know the results of her tests. Dr. Lewis reviewed Juanita's medical record and realized the patient's test results had not been filed correctly.

This left Dr. Lewis with an anxious patient. Nancy McFarland is off today, so the provider checks with the other medical assistants on duty. They have no knowledge of the test results. The act of not properly filing Juanita's test results causes undue stress for the provider, medical assistants, and patient.

Chapter Portal

Every medical facility generates a large amount of information. Business, insurance, personnel, and financial records must be maintained. Supplies and equipment records must be managed. Licensures and certifications must be current. Some records are kept for the life of the practice. The greatest bulk of information, however, comes from patient medical records. A vital function of any medical facility is the maintenance of patient records identifying the care given. Medical assistants, both administrative and clinical, will spend a fair amount of time managing patients' records. Medical records potentially record all medical data about an individual from birth until death.

Even in medical facilities where patient records are managed electronically, there are ample paper records to be stored and retrieved manually. A number of functions essential to proper records management are discussed in this chapter. A clear understanding of the proper methods used to manage the records in a medical facility is an important and necessary skill for medical assistants.

Chapter 10 defined electronic medical records (EMRs) as those coming from a single medical practice, hospital, or pharmacy. When EMRs from multiple sources are combined into one database for a patient, the term electronic health record (EHR) is used.

THE PURPOSE OF MEDICAL RECORDS

The primary purposes of medical records in the clinic are to:

1. Provide a base for managing patient care
2. Provide interoffice and intraoffice communication as necessary
3. Determine any patterns that surface to signal the provider of patient needs
4. Serve as a basis for legal information necessary to protect providers, staff, and patients
5. Provide clinical data for research

OWNERSHIP OF MEDICAL RECORDS

Legal

State statutes have ruled that medical records are the property of those who create them. The information within the medical record, however, belongs to the patient, and that information is always to be protected with the utmost privacy and confidentiality. Patients can be allowed access to their medical records, ask for notes or information to be added to their files, and request that certain information not be included in their files.

Integrity

Providers who include their patients in their medical record keeping foster trust and respect with their patients. For example, a provider who enters patient data into the electronic patient record while sitting at a computer monitor in the examination room beside the patient has the opportunity to explain that the information is entered now so there is no room for error in reporting or in the provider not accurately recalling the patient information if entered at a later time. Care should be taken when discussing sensitive information that may be of concern to the patient and requires strict confidentiality. For example, such diagnoses that involve psychiatric, infectious, or serious illness are areas where patients may feel that disclosure to certain entities, such as co-workers, employers, or even family members can be of concern. Respecting these concerns and taking the proper steps to assure the patient of their privacy is of utmost importance.

AUTHORIZATION TO RELEASE INFORMATION

Legal

It is recommended that before any information is released from the medical record, the patient be notified and written approval received. Medical facilities will have appropriate forms for such release of information. The form should identify the reason for the release of information and what information is specifically requested. Only that information should be released. This does not include the release of information to a patient's chosen insurance carrier. A number of different methods exist to release that information. For some insurance carriers, the release is granted when the patient accepts the insurance coverage. For others, a yearly release form must be signed by the patient.

MANUAL OR ELECTRONIC MEDICAL RECORDS

Today's medical environment has a mixture of manual, or paper, medical records and the electronic form of medical records. Some medical providers continue to have difficulty with including the necessary information that is considered vital in documentation for further enhancing the transition to EMR. Key medical data have been either improperly documented or have been omitted from some patients' records, which can create numerous compliance and billing issues when corresponding with insurance companies. By becoming more specific in documentation, providers will ensure that all of a patient's data is included in the electronic record and further enhance the transition to EMR. During his presidency, President George W. Bush announced his Health Information Technology Plan, which included the goal of ensuring that most Americans would have electronic health records by 2014. Planned projects included transmitting X-rays and laboratory results electronically to providers for immediate analysis and standardizing electronic prescriptions, decreasing errors in patient care.

Consider the following advantages and disadvantages of both types of records:

MANUAL MEDICAL RECORD

ADVANTAGES	DISADVANTAGES
• Currently established and understood • Easier to protect confidentiality • No worry of computer malfunction	• Can be used by only one person at a time • Easily misplaced or misfiled • Equipment and storage space required • More susceptible to error

ELECTRONIC MEDICAL RECORD

ADVANTAGES	DISADVANTAGES
• Multiple users are possible • Not easily misplaced or misfiled • Errors less likely • Patterns and data more easily accessed • Quickly available in emergencies • Office storage space not required • Legible, organized patient documentation • Improved medication management • Improved quality of care	• Needs protection to prevent loss of data • Expensive to establish and maintain • May require on-site assistance • Can require up to 12 weeks for staff to prove productive after installation

In 2009, President Barack Obama signed the American Reinvestment and Recovery Act (ARRA). This law provides numerous incentives for providers and hospitals to make the transition to EMR. As mentioned in Chapter 11, **meaningful use** is a Centers for Medicare and Medicaid (CMS) program that awards incentives for using certified electronic health records (EHR) to improve patient care. To achieve meaningful use and avoid penalties, providers must follow a set of criteria that serve as a road map for effectively using an EHR. Meaningful use encourages providers to switch from paper charts to electronic records, improves efficiency, and will earn incentives for providers. Medicare reimbursement penalties for lack of participation began in 2015, and it is expected that other health insurance carriers will follow suit in the coming years in an effort to transition away from the use of paper records. For more information on meaningful use and its stages, go to http://www.healthit.gov and search for "Meaningful Use."

For the time being, not all clinics have fully computerized their medical records. Compliance issues may involve cost, labor, and time involved in transferring over data to an electronic medical record system. Although there are compelling reasons for providers to make the switch, the process has been slow, and will still require some time in the next decade to fully implement the changes.

No matter what stage of the transition a clinic is in, the management of the medical records must provide easy retrieval of information. All documentation must be complete and correct. Wording must be easily understood and grammatically correct. How corrections are made in the chart, how documents are removed from or added to the chart, and the format of the chart must be predetermined and understood by all users of the information.

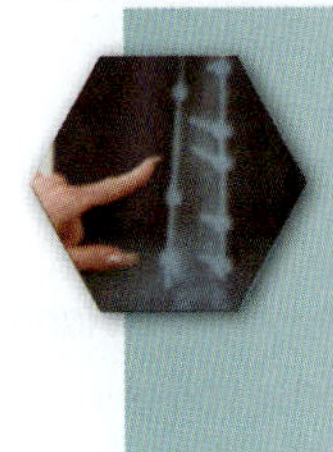

Critical Thinking

Your clinic is planning to implement an electronic medical records system. What steps must you take to ensure the transition goes smoothly? What factors should be considered when selecting an EMR system? How does the implementation of such a system affect overall patient care?

THE IMPORTANCE OF ACCURATE MEDICAL RECORDS

Accurate medical records are essential to patient care in any health care setting. One incorrect digit in a patient's Social Security number causes reimbursement problems. An incorrect address or telephone number or a misspelling of a name makes it difficult to contact patients about test results and prescription refills. Medical treatment documentation errors are even more disastrous and can cause serious medical problems for patients. Patient files are critical to the facility's smooth functioning and are important when referring the patient to outside specialists with whom the facility may need to coordinate care. Each treating primary care provider must be aware of tests, procedures, and diagnoses. Maintaining a conscientious record of patient care is also absolutely essential in controlling the costs of medical care.

Medical records management is also important because of the legal issues that every medical clinic and health care professional must face today. The standard in court is that if there is no record of any piece of information related to a patient and that patient's care and treatment, then it did not happen. The question to ask yourself about any piece of information is: "Does this relate to the patient's care, and should it be in the chart?" To be prepared in the event of medical litigation, you must document all medical treatment. No matter how competently a provider has performed treatment, if a written record cannot prove how and what was done, there is no basis for a defense in a court of law.

Creating Paper Charts and Electronic Records

The patient's medical chart is prepared on or before the day of the patient's first visit to the medical facility. Paper charts require the assembly of appropriate file folders, divider pages labeled with identifying tabs, and a number of essential forms to be completed by the patient. Included forms provide demographic information, social and family medical history, previous surgeries, HIPAA guidelines, and release of information details. Often, paper charts include adhesive twin prong fasteners to ensure that sheets of paper are securely held within the chart. Electronic patient medical records are prepared in much the same manner with the exception being that all information is stored electronically. Patient information that is collected via the paper route will have to be scanned and entered into the record. The EMR will provide an orderly arrangement of patient information according to the particular software design or a predetermined plan selected by the providers and their staff. Procedure 13-1 provides guidance on creating a patient medical record.

PROCEDURE 13-1

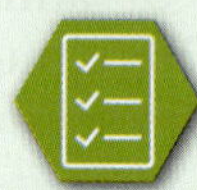

Establishing a Medical Chart or Record for a New Patient

PURPOSE:

To demonstrate an understanding of the principles for establishing a medical chart or record.

EQUIPMENT/SUPPLIES:

For Paper Charts

- File folder used in the facility (flip-up or book-style)
- Divider pages used in the facility (SOAP/SOAPER laboratory reports, HIPAA information sheets, and so forth)
- Adhesive twin prong fasteners for divider pages
- Twin hole punch for twin prong fasteners
- Selected tabs to identify folder and divider pages
- Demographic patient information completed before or at the first appointment

(continues)

For Electronic Charts

- Computer
- EHR program
- Demographic patient information completed before or at the first appointment

PROCEDURE STEPS:

For Paper Charts

1. Assemble all supplies at a desk or table. RATIONALE: Everything is in one place for efficient use.
2. Punch holes in the manila file folder and any necessary divider pages. RATIONALE: Creates holes for the twin prong fasteners.
3. Affix the adhesive twin prong fasteners. RATIONALE: Places fasteners as appropriate for material to be attached.
4. Assemble the divider pages dictated by the practice and the clinic policy in the proper location of the chart over the twin prong fasteners. RATIONALE: Ensures that items are placed in the same place as in all other charts in the facility.
5. Securely fasten twin prong fasteners over the divider pages. RATIONALE: Ensures that no pages will fall out of the chart.
6. Index and code the patient's name according to the filing system to be used (i.e., alphabetic, numeric, or color). RATIONALE: Determines where the chart will be placed.
7. Affix appropriately labeled tabs to the folder cut. RATIONALE: Prepares the chart for patient information.
8. Transfer demographic data in black ink pen or affix the demographic divider sheet to the inside front cover of the chart. RATIONALE: Identifying patient information is readily available inside the chart cover.
9. Affix HIPAA required information to the chart, after it has been read and signed by the patient, as determined by clinic policy. RATIONALE: Ensures that this task is not omitted.
10. Place prepared chart in proper location for pickup by the provider or clinical medical assistant. RATIONALE: Signals to all staff that the chart is ready for the patient's visit.

For Electronic Charts

1. Access EMR or PM system to be used and open a new patient record.
2. Enter demographic information provided by the patient.
3. Enter insurance information provided by the patient.
4. Review the information entered and confirm accuracy.
5. Save the patient's record and close out of it when complete.
6. Print and obtain HIPAA-required information after it has been read and signed by the patient, and file or scan to the EMR as determined by clinic policy.
7. Print documents and encounter form, or mark the daily appointment sheet for pickup by the provider or clinical medical assistant.

Correcting Medical Records

The medical record must be readable and accurate; however, errors do occur and may not be discovered immediately. Any corrections necessary to a paper medical record should be corrected using the following method: draw a single line using a red ink pen through the error, make the correction, write "Corr." or "Correction" above the area corrected, and indicate your initials and the current date. The red line through the information indicates the "error" portion of the report. The words "Corr." or "Correction" by the correction indicate the change. The date and initials identify when the correction was made and by whom. Obliterations should never occur. When the medical record becomes the center of attention in malpractice litigation, forensic experts will be able to tell if a record has been tampered with or if information or pages have been added later. When not properly done, altered records become a detriment to any provider's defense in court.

Errors discovered immediately after the fact in an electronic medical record are corrected

ADDENDUM
Pt requests referral to Dr. Robert Rovner for orthopedic evaluation.

FIGURE 13-1 Addendum added to electronic progress note.

differently. Each EMR has its own method of handling corrections and tracking them, often with a log that identifies the person making the correction, date, and time. In addition, it is customary for only certain staff members to be able to alter or correct medical records; therefore, access may be restricted for this purpose. Generally, a correction is made in an EMR using the Edit function, which does not change the original entry, but adds an addendum with the corrected information (Figure 13-1).

If a correction is necessary of any information after either a paper chart or an electronic chart has been sent to another provider or facility, make a copy of the corrected information and send it to the provider or facility as quickly as possible.

TYPES OF MEDICAL RECORDS

Whether patient charts are kept manually or electronically, there are common threads that run throughout medical records. How material is stored within records is important. The choice of method must be in accordance with how the information needs to be accessed and used for each individual clinic. No one method is best. In the examples that follow, arrangement of materials is also discussed.

Problem-Oriented Medical Record

The **problem-oriented medical record (POMR)** places in a prominent location vital identification data, immunizations, allergies, medications, and problems. The problems are identified by a number that corresponds to the charting relevant to that problem number, that is, bronchitis #1, broken wrist #2, and so forth. If the patient returns in 9 months with recurring bronchitis, the same number (#1) is used.

The patient chart is then further built by adding a numbered and titled section for each problem the patient experiences, for example, bronchitis #1, broken wrist #2. Figure 13-2 shows an example of a POMR.

Each problem is then followed with the **SOAP** approach for all progress notes:

S Subjective impressions

O Objective clinical evidence

A Assessment or diagnosis

P Plans for further studies, treatment, or management

Some medical facilities have added variations to the SOAP approach, creating **SOAPER** or the SOAPIE. These additional charting tools can be especially useful in providing additional information more specific to the practice and specialty requirements:

Added to SOAPER:

E Education for patient

R Response of patient to education and care given

Added to SOAPIE:

I Implementation of the plan (what was done)

E Evaluation, indicating whether care is effective, or results

This process makes the chart easier to review and helps in follow-up of all the patient's medical needs. The SOAP/SOAPER/SOAPIE approach also allows medical personnel to be aware of the patient's current medications. Starting and resolution dates for each problem also are noted on the tracking page. Figure 13-3 shows SOAP note documentation in a paper chart.

Internists, family practitioners, and pediatricians use the POMR system more commonly than do specialists because they see their patients for a variety of problems over a long span of time. It is commonly used in manual medical records as well as EMRs.

A number of medical supply companies produce various formats for POMR manual charts. There are flip-up folder styles and book-style folders with twin prong fasteners to hold paper documents in place. Divider pages may come with tabs that are preprinted to specific needs or have adhesive labels that can be printed on a printer exactly as you want them. Sometimes, the inside front and back covers are printed with information to be filled in. These areas are often used to provide essential personal information such as name, address, telephone numbers, insurance information, and responsible party. Over a period of time, however, because the information changes, entries on the inside cover are less desirable. A patient demographic form can be attached to the inside cover. It can be updated annually and changed easily. In a prominent place, usually on the inside front cover, is the word *ALLERGIES*

Problem and Medication List

Patient Name: **DOB:**
Allergies: **Pharmacy #**

Date	Dx #	Chronic Problems	Dx #	Chronic Medications	Date	Refills					
					Start	Date					
					Stop	Initials					
					Start	Date					
					Stop	Initials					
					Start	Date					
					Stop	Initials					
					Start	Date					
					Stop	Initials					
					Start	Date					
					Stop	Initials					
					Start	Date					
					Stop	Initials					
					Start	Date					
					Stop	Initials					
					Start	Date					
					Stop	Initials					
					Start	Date					
					Stop	Initials					

Preventive	Date	Date	Date	Date	Date	Date
History Update Every 2 Years						
Breast Exam (plus Self-Exam)						
Mammogram						
DEXA						
Diabetic Blood Sugar Monitoring						
Diabetic Foot Care						
Diabetic HbA1c						
Diabetic LDL						
Diabetic Retinal Exam						
Diabetic Proteinuria						
Fasting Glucose						
Lipid Panel						
Pap/Pelvic						
Prostate Exam, PSA						
Rectal Exam						
Sigmoid/Colonos						
Stool for Occult Blood						
Testicular Exam (plus Self-Exam)						

Immunizations

Vaccination	Schedule	Date	Date	Date	Date
Hepatitis	As appropriate				
Influenza	At risk—q1y				
Pneumovax	At risk X 1				
Td Booster	PRN—q10y				

Education

	Date	Date	Date	Date
Advanced Directives/ Power of Attorney				
Alcohol/Drug Use				
Birth Control/Menopause				
Diabetes				
Diet				
Exercise				
Smoking				
Stress				

FIGURE 13-2 A sample patient problem and medication list that also provides space for dates and details of preventive actions, patient education, and immunizations as well as for the patient's pharmacy phone number.

in big letters (often preprinted in red). Any allergies that patients have are listed here. Also prominently displayed should be any forms the patient has signed granting release of information, as well as any forms signed to comply with HIPAA regulations.

The problem list may be entered on a divider flap or on specially printed paper. Other dividers may be used for laboratory reports, progress notes, history and physicals, hospital admissions, and medications. Depending on the practice and the wishes of the provider, tab dividers are available for consultations, correspondence, insurance data, hospital notes, pathology reports, and electrocardiogram reports. The problem list is most likely the first divider used, followed by laboratory reports and progress notes, usually in the SOAP format.

SOAP is easily adapted to the EMR. There are a number of methods of indicating SOAP in the EMR. (See the example in Figure 13-4.) For a look at different models, use a computer search engine to key in "SOAP Charting in EMRs." You will be able to compare a number of examples.

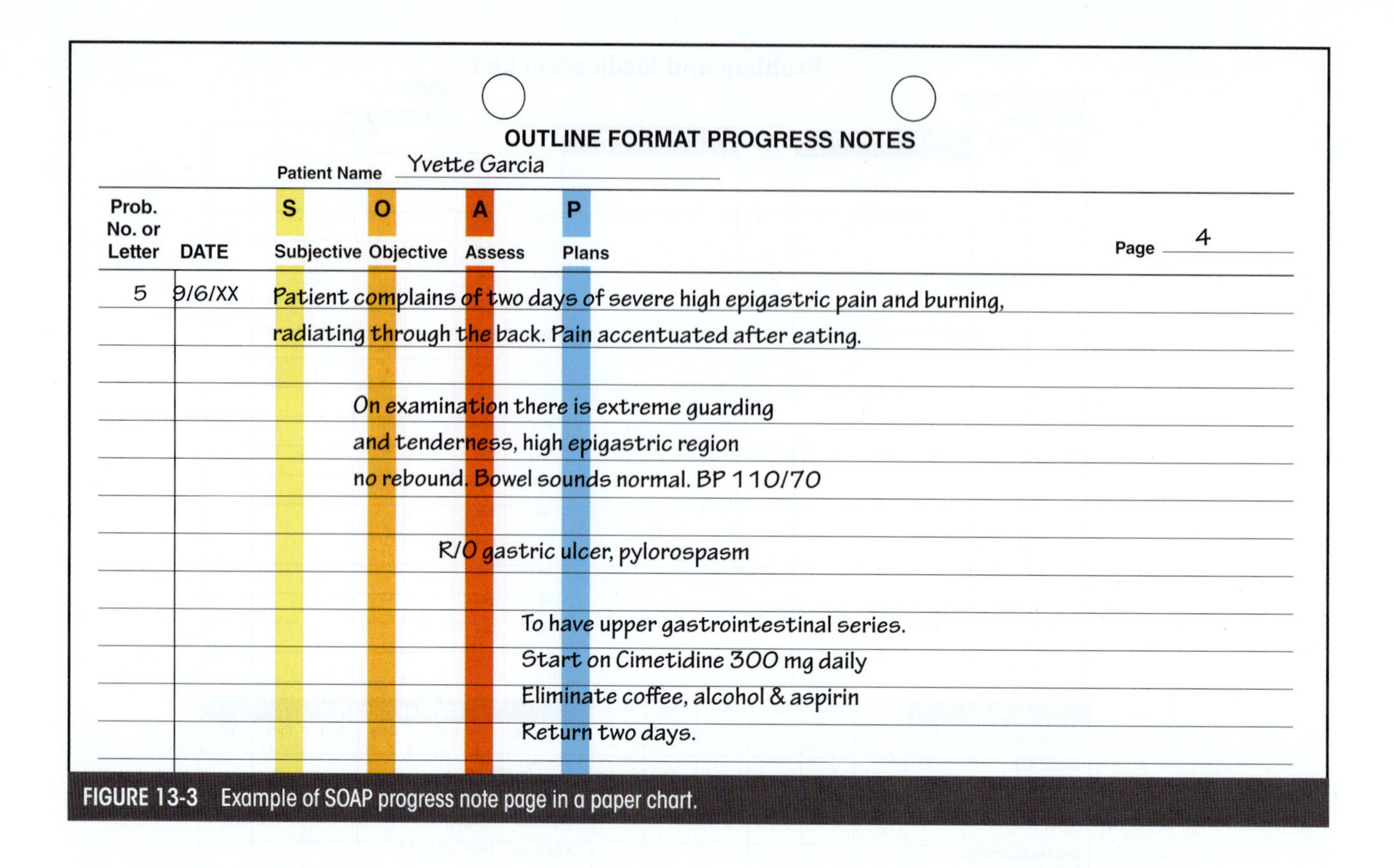
OUTLINE FORMAT PROGRESS NOTES

Patient Name Yvette Garcia

Page 4

Prob. No. or Letter	DATE	S Subjective	O Objective	A Assess	P Plans
5	9/6/XX	Patient complains of two days of severe high epigastric pain and burning, radiating through the back. Pain accentuated after eating.			
			On examination there is extreme guarding and tenderness, high epigastric region no rebound. Bowel sounds normal. BP 110/70		
				R/O gastric ulcer, pylorospasm	
					To have upper gastrointestinal series. Start on Cimetidine 300 mg daily Eliminate coffee, alcohol & aspirin Return two days.

FIGURE 13-3 Example of SOAP progress note page in a paper chart.

Ms. Sabrina Katherine Lake DOB 12/23/1977
01/29/XX

Subjective	Pt states, "I've been feeling very tired and weak for the past month," LMP 01-15-XX very heavy flow. Exam: 6 # Wt loss since last visit 12/19/XX.
Objective	BP 112/70, Hb 10.4, Hct 31%. Decrease in muscle strength, pale.
Assessment	R/O anemia.
Plan	CBC with diff sent to lab, return in 1 week.

FIGURE 13-4 An example of the SOAP method of charting in an electronic record.

Source-Oriented Medical Record

The manual **source-oriented medical record (SOMR)** groups information according to its source; for example, from laboratories, examinations, provider notes, consulting providers, and other sources. Facilities use this method because it makes different types of information quickly accessible. A fastener folder is used that contains several partitions with their own fasteners. This allows for a separate section for laboratory reports, pathology, progress notes, physical examinations, and correspondence to be filed chronologically within each section. In the SOMR system, many providers use the SOAP method to record their chart notes.

The organization of the SOMR is quite similar to that of the POMR chart with the one exception that the SOMR does not have the problem list. Also, the SOMR may continually add sheets of identifying information with appropriate sections in the chart rather than transferring any data. Many EMR software packages use either the POMR or the SOMR format and are easily adapted to a particular provider's practice.

Strict Chronological Arrangement

Using strict chronology, data are filed strictly with the most recently charted materials to the top of the folder. For instance, a patient is treated from 2008 to the present. To locate information recorded in 2009, it is necessary to flip through the chart until the material for the year 2009 is located. This method makes it difficult for a provider or medical assistant to quickly assess a patient's clinical picture. This type of arrangement may seem confusing, but it may fit a specialty clinic such as a dietitian, radiologist, or physical therapist where patients are usually seen on a short-term basis.

EQUIPMENT AND SUPPLIES

Three primary types of file cabinets are used in medical clinics where manual files are stored: vertical, lateral, and movable. For more information on the types of filing cabinets and filing supplies, see the "Filing Equipment and Supplies" Quick Reference Guide.

BASIC RULES FOR FILING

Regardless of the type of filing system used, alphabetizing is the key to organizing all files and charts. It is necessary to know more than just the alphabetic order of the letters *A* to *Z*. Thus, certain indexing rules have been developed by the Association of Medical Records Administrators (AMRA) to facilitate the alphabetic process in maintaining files in the medical clinic.

Indexing Units

There must be an organized method of identifying and separating items to be filed into small subunits. This is accomplished with the use of **indexing** units. A unit identifies each part of a name. In this process, each **unit** is identified according to unit 1 (the **key unit**), unit 2, unit 3, and so forth, with each segment of the filing label identified. This process can be applied to individual names, organizations, or clinics. Accepted filing rules describe how to assign unit numbers to each element.

Example: Annette Barbara Samuels

Unit 1	Samuels
Unit 2	Annette
Unit 3	Barbara

When working in a medical setting with patient charts, the patient's legal name is always used for the chart rather than a nickname or abbreviation. If the clinic has a practice of calling patients by preferred names, a note of name preferences and nicknames may be noted on the chart. However, the filing label should use the proper name.

Example: The following items to be filed would be assigned units as illustrated:

	Units Assigned		
	1	2	3
Cole Blanche Little	Little	Cole	Blanche
Wayne Lee Elder	Elder	Wayne	Lee
Kelso Medical Supply	Kelso	Medical	Supply

Filing Patient Charts

Rule 1. The names of individuals are assigned indexing units, respectively: last name (surname), first name, middle, and succeeding names.

	Units Assigned		
	1	2	3
Jaime Renae Carrera	Carrera	Jaime	Renae
Lee Allen Au	Au	Lee	Allen
Bill Hugo Schwartz	Schwartz	Bill	Hugo

Rule 2. Names that include a single letter are indexed as the legal name and are placed before full names beginning with the same letter. "Nothing comes before something."

	Units Assigned		
	1	2	3
J. Larson	Larson	J	—
James R. Larson	Larson	James	R

Rule 3. Foreign language prefixes are indexed as one unit with the unit that follows. Spacing, punctuation, and capitalization are ignored. Such prefixes include *d, da, de, de la, del, des, di, du, el, fitz, l, la, las, le, les, lu, m, mac, mc, o, saint, sainte, san, santa, sao, st, te, ten, ter, van, van de, van der,* and *von der* (*st, sainte,* and *saint* are indexed as written).

	Units Assigned		
	1	2	3
Gerald Steven St. Simon	Stsimon	Gerald	Steven
Carol Louise del Rio	Delrio	Carol	Louise

QUICK REFERENCE GUIDE

Filing Equipment and Supplies

TYPES OF FILING CABINETS

Vertical files (Figure 13-5)	Vertical files cabinets have pullout drawers where files are stored. Files are retrieved by lifting the appropriate file up and out. These are often used for business records and documents, and should include a locking device.
Open-shelf lateral files (Figure 13-6)	Records in open-shelf lateral file cabinets are retrieved by pulling them out laterally from the shelf. This type of cabinet is used most often with color-coded filing systems where visual inspection makes it possible to ensure files are kept in the proper order. Open-shelf lateral files are the most popular manual patient record system. It is necessary to be able to close and lock the open-shelf lateral files to protect confidentiality.
Movable file units	Movable file units allow easy access to large record systems and require less space than vertical or lateral files. These units may be electrically powered to move on floor tracks or may be physically moved with a handle mechanism. The movable shelving unit is electrically powered to open aisles for accessing files or to close aisles when those files do not need to be accessed. There are also movable file storage units that will automatically travel on a computer-controlled carousel track, moving files around until the required section reaches the operator.

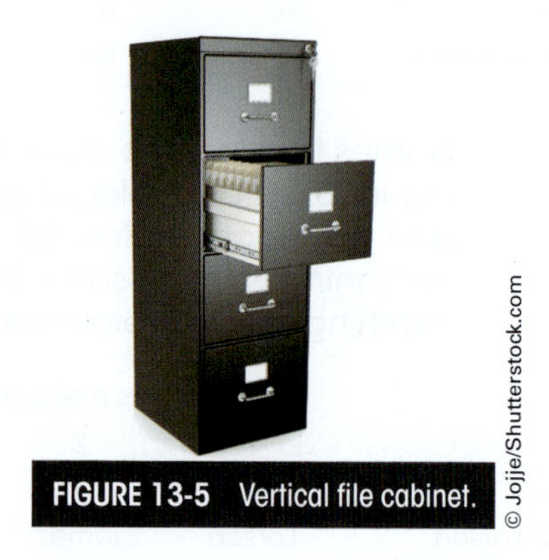

FIGURE 13-5 Vertical file cabinet.

© Jojje/Shutterstock.com

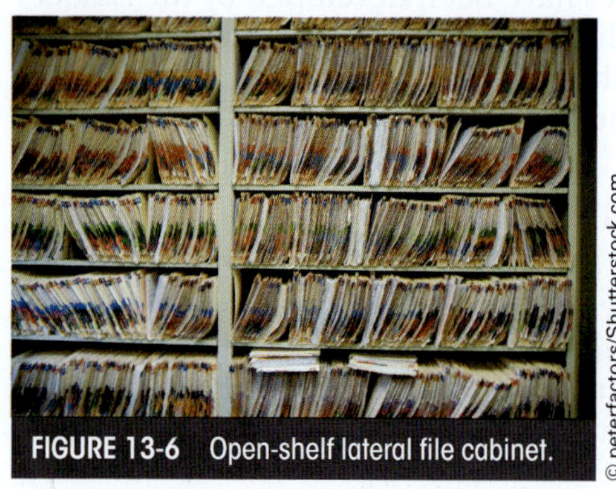

FIGURE 13-6 Open-shelf lateral file cabinet.

© peterfactors/Shutterstock.com

FILING SUPPLIES

File folders 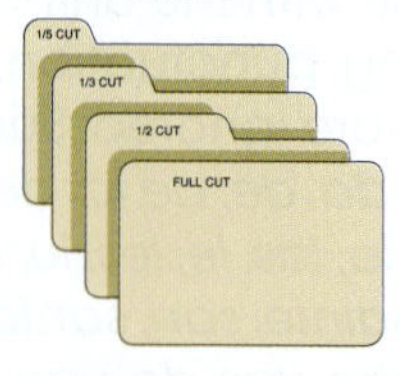	File folders are designed to use different types of labels. Extending along the top edge (the edge that will be visible when filing) are tabs that are cut in varying sizes and positions to allow for different methods of labeling. File folders should be constructed of good-quality card stock. If they are too light in weight, they will soon be bent, torn, and battered from use. They need to be sturdy enough for years of use.
Identification labels 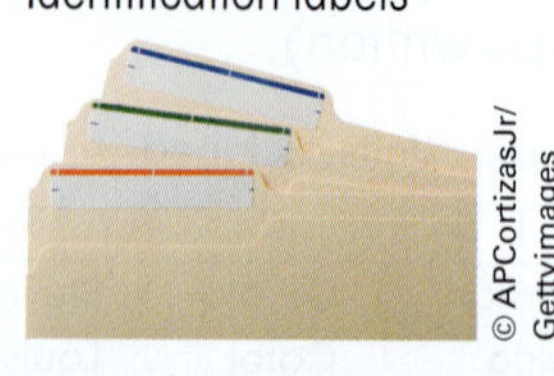 © APCortizasJr/ Gettyimages	A variety of labels are used to display the information required to select the correct name or number designation for a particular file. The identification label is adhered either along the top of the file folder (top tab) in vertical file cabinets or along the side of the file folder (side tab) in lateral file cabinets.

(continues)

Guides and captions 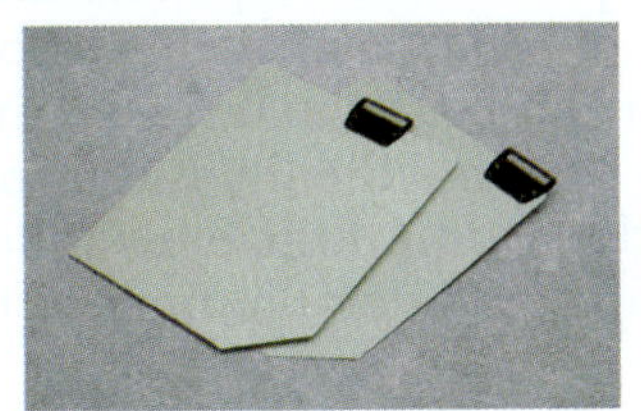	Guides are used to separate file folders. Guides are somewhat larger than file folders and are of heavier stock. Guides are described by the position of the tab, designated according to its location. For instance, a tab located at the far left would be in the first position, the next one to the right would be in the second position, and so forth. Guides are used in vertical and lateral systems.
	
	Captions are used to identify major sections of file folders by more manageable subunits (e.g., AA–AC, A, B, Office Supplies). Captions are marked on the tabs of the guides. These are denoted as single caption and double caption:
	• *Single captions* contain just one letter, number, or unit:
	  • A, B, C, D
	• *Double captions* contain a double notation to denote a range of files:
	  • Ab–Be, Co–Dy, Ho–Le

Out guides 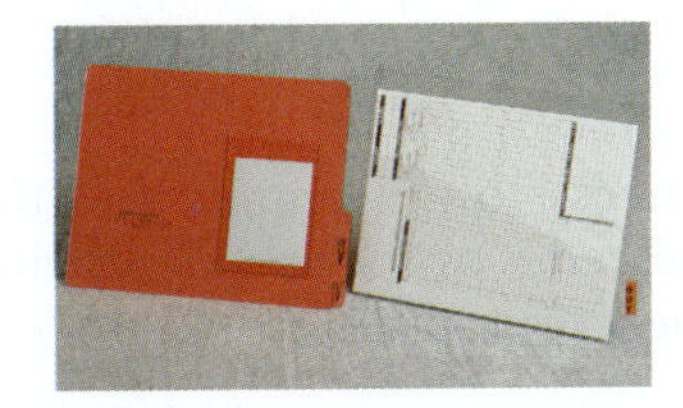	**Out guides**, or out sheets, are devices to help in tracking charts. An out guide is a piece of card stock or a plastic/paper sheet kept in place of the patient chart when the chart is removed from the filing storage.

Rule 4. When titles are used, they are considered as separate indexing units. If the title appears with first and last names, the title is considered to be the last indexing unit. When dealing with patient charts, the first name always accompanies the title and last name.

	Units Assigned			
	1	2	3	4
Dr. Marlene Elaine Smith	Smith	Marlene	Elaine	Dr
Prof. Marcia Tai Lewis	Lewis	Marcia	Tai	Prof

Rule 5. Names that are hyphenated are considered as one unit.

	Units Assigned		
	1	2	3
Adele Marie Johnson-Smith	Johnson-smith	Adele	Marie
Ray Steven Reynolds-Martin	Reynolds-martin	Ray	Steven

Rule 6. When indexing names of married women, the name is indexed by the legal name. Remember that patient charts are legal documents, making this practice necessary (use cross-referencing as necessary).

	Units Assigned			
	1	2	3	4
Amy Sue Sung (Mrs. John)	Sung	Amy	Sue	Mrs John
Tami Jo Strizver (Mrs. Todd)	Strizver	Tami	Jo	Mrs Todd

Rule 7. Seniority and professional or academic degrees are the last indexing unit and are used only to distinguish identical names.

	Units Assigned			
	1	2	3	4
James Edward Brown, Jr.	Brown	James	Edward	Jr
James Edward Brown, Sr.	Brown	James	Edward	Sr

Rule 8. Mac and Mc are filed in their regular place alphabetically. Some clinics will provide a special guide for both Mac and Mc for ease in filing.

Mabbott
MacDonald
Mazziotti
McAffe

Rule 9. Numeric units are broken down such that numeric seniority terms are filed before alphabetic terms.

	Edward Lee Kletka, IV
BEFORE	Edward Lee Kletka, Jr.
	George Lee Curtis, II
BEFORE	George Lee Curtis, Sr.

Filing Identical Names

When names are identical, the address may be used to order files. The address is indexed by:

First .... City
SECOND .... STATE
Third .... *Street Name*
FOURTH .... **ADDRESS #**

Therefore, the following Acme Drug Supply files would be arranged from first to last as follows:

1. Acme Drug Supply, **839** *Kentucky Boulevard,* Crawford, MISSOURI
2. Acme Drug Supply, **683** *Wildflower Avenue,* Fairbanks, ALASKA
3. Acme Drug Supply, **1539** *Wildflower Avenue,* Fairbanks, ALASKA
4. Acme Drug Supply, **742** *Terminal Street West,* Fairbanks, ARIZONA
5. Acme Drug Supply, **731** *Terminal Street East,* New York, NEW YORK

Although this is the official indexing rule, most medical facilities prefer alternative methods for filing identical charts. The primary consideration here is that patient addresses often change frequently. Therefore, preferred methods include date of birth or Social Security number.

STEPS FOR FILING MEDICAL DOCUMENTATION IN PATIENT FILES

Before a discussion of the common filing systems, it is helpful to review procedural steps that accurately and efficiently process data sheets, laboratory requests, dictation, and so forth from the time they are generated to the time the file is returned to the medical records section. Efficiently following these steps will save considerable time in the clinic.

Inspect

Carefully inspect the report to identify the patient, subject, or file to whom the information belongs. Remove clips and staples. Make certain the information is complete.

Index

Use the indexing process to determine how the chart would be located, properly identifying indexing units and their order.

Code

Coding in medical records is the process of marking data to indicate how information is to be filed. If using a system other than a strict alphabetic system, determine the proper coding for the chart so it can be retrieved. Otherwise, identify the indexed units by underlining or highlighting. This makes refiling more effective and ensures that the item will always be filed in the same place. If a cross-reference is required, identify the cross-reference by double underlining and placing an *X* nearby. This chapter includes detailed information on coding and cross-referencing.

Sort

If there are a number of reports/documents to be filed, sort them into units according to the captions on the charts. This will eliminate wasted time in working back and forth through the alphabet or numbers.

File

The papers are placed in the proper charts and the charts returned to their proper place in the medical records section. Be alert to the labels and refile any information or charts that have been misfiled.

FILING TECHNIQUES AND COMMON FILING SYSTEMS

Three major filing systems are commonly used in the clinic setting: alphabetic, numeric, and subject. The alphabet is intrinsic to all methods, and the basic rules for filing, covered previously, are used in all systems.

Color coding is used a high percentage of the time in all three systems to minimize filing errors. Another system, geographic, is seldom used in the clinic unless there are multiple clinics. Even then, a form of color coding may be used.

Color Coding

Color coding is a technique often used in the three major filing systems. Numerous color-coding systems are available. Patient charts most often use an alphabetic system of color coding, although color coding can be used in numeric filing as well. There are a number of large suppliers that offer color systems and records management systems. Color coding may seem complicated at first, but once medical assistants understand the principles behind it and practice its application a number of times, the task becomes much easier, and there is immediate recognition if a chart is misfiled.

Color coding makes retrieval of files more efficient with the use of visible color differences that facilitate easier maintenance of the files. Color-coding filing systems also use an alphabetic system; after they are coded by color, that designation is used to order the files alphabetically.

Tab-Alpha System. The various forms of the Tab-Alpha system are designed primarily for filing systems in small clinics that use vertical files where all individual charts are clearly visible in one unit.

Each alphabetic letter is assigned a different color. Each folder has a color-coded label. Only full-cut folders are used:

- Colored labels are applied over the edge of the full cut for the first two letters of the key indexing unit (Winston, Paul Lewis: WI).
- A third white label is placed over the tab edge, which contains all of the indexing units (Winston, Paul Lewis).
- In addition, some clinics use a color-coded label to indicate the last year the patient was seen. This makes an efficient method for easily identifying active and inactive files.
- Any additional labels (e.g., allergies, last year seen, or industrial claim) are attached to the chart according to the clinic procedure.

Alpha-Z System. Forms of the Alpha-Z system are designed for use with either open lateral files or vertical drawer files (Figure 13-7A). Alphabetic letters are used as the primary guides. Breakdowns of alphabetic combinations are added as determined by the needs of a particular facility.

A combination of 13 colors is used in the Alpha-Z system with white letters on a solid colored background for the first half of the alphabet and white letters on a colored background with white stripes for the second half of the alphabet (Figure 13-7B).

The 13 colors used are shown in Figure 13-8. Folders have three labels:

- The first label contains the typed name, a color block, and the letter of the alphabet for the first letter of the first indexing unit:

  Winston, Lewis Paul YELLOW *W*

- The second and third labels are color-coded to correspond to the second and third letters of the first unit:

  ***I* on pink background and *N* on red-striped background**

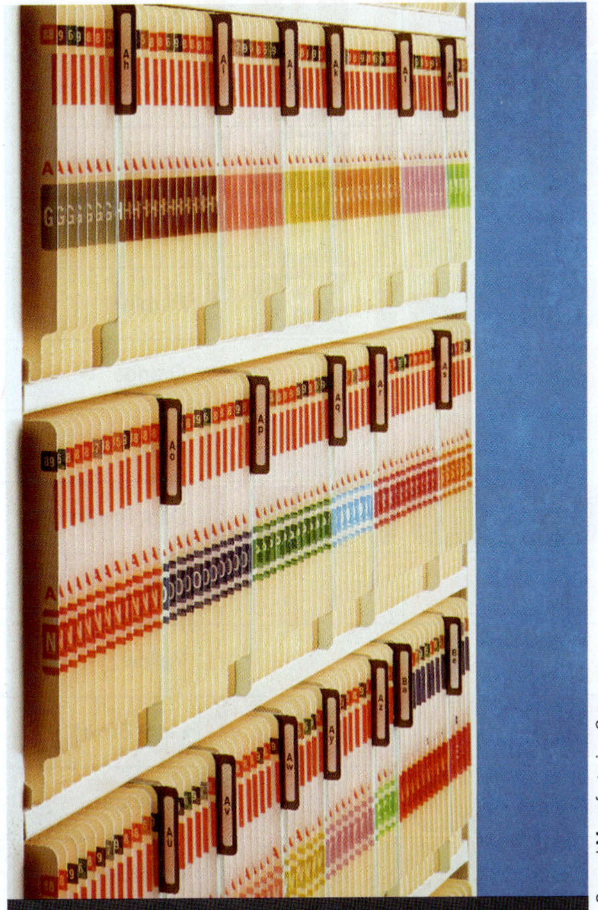

FIGURE 13-7A Color-coding filing system uses open-lateral shelving unit with color-coded files.

Courtesy Smead Manufacturing Company

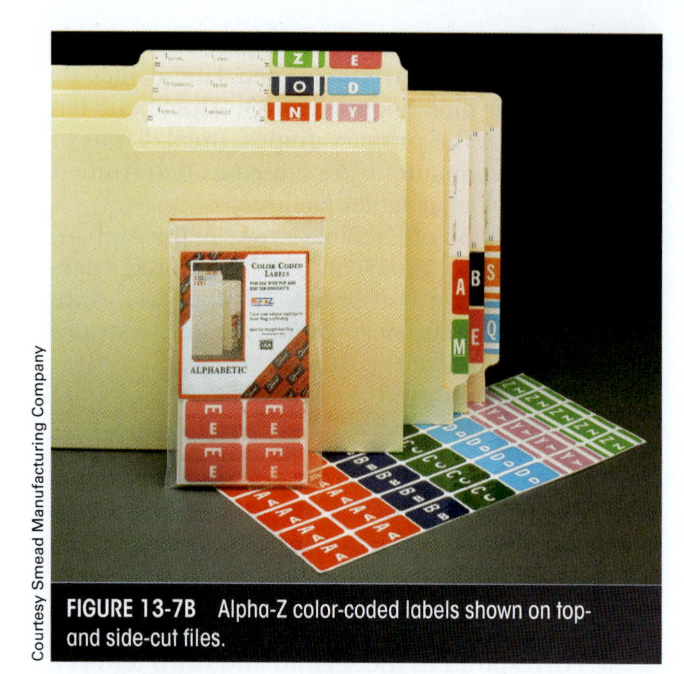

Courtesy Smead Manufacturing Company

FIGURE 13-7B Alpha-Z color-coded labels shown on top- and side-cut files.

White Letter Colored Background	White Letter Striped Colored Background	Color
A	N	Red
B	O	Dark Blue
C	P	Dark Green
D	Q	Light Blue
E	R	Purple
F	S	Orange
G	T	Gray
H	U	Dark Brown
I	V	Pink
J	W	Yellow
K	X	Light Brown
L	Y	Lavender
M	Z	Light Green

FIGURE 13-8 Thirteen colors are used in the Alpha-Z system.

Customized Color-Coding Systems. Many clinics use color systems to meet specific needs.

Colored File Folders by First Name. One method color codes the first letter of the first name. The folders then are filed alphabetically by last name.

Example: *A* is assigned red folders; *M* is assigned green folders; *S* is assigned blue folders

Annette Samuels	Red folder
Michael Taylor	Green folder
Susan Boyer	Blue folder

Many small medical clinics use this system and find it quite effective. In the multiprovider urgent care center, this would be quite time-consuming when locating files for patients of all providers.

Colored File Folders by Last Name. Another method using this system assigns colored folders according to the first letter of the last name. The folders are then filed alphabetically.

Example: *S* is assigned pink folders; *B* is assigned gray folders.

Bill Schwartz	Pink folder
Corey Boyer	Gray folder

This system makes it easy to spot folders that have been misfiled under an incorrect first letter, but it does not break it down further for misfiling within the first-letter guides.

Color-Coded Numbers. The color-coded number system is used in a numeric filing system and operates in the same way as alphabetic systems. Numbers from 0 to 9 are color coded. The appropriate colored numbers are then placed on the tabs of the patient's folder.

Alphabetic Filing

Procedure

Strict alphabetic filing is one of the simplest filing methods, as files are strictly maintained by assigning a label to each file. The first letter of that label (e.g., Jones, Invoices, or Pharmacies) is then used to alphabetize the files from A to Z. When a limited number of files are accessed, this is an acceptable method of maintaining records. Also note that every filing system will utilize the alphabet somewhere. Procedure 13-2 provides steps for manual filing with an alphabetic system.

PROCEDURE 13-2

Manual Filing with an Alphabetic System

PURPOSE:

To demonstrate an understanding of the principles of alphabetic filing.

EQUIPMENT/SUPPLIES:

- Documents to be filed
- Dividers with guides
- Miscellaneous number file section
- Alphabetic card file and cards
- Accession journal, if needed

PROCEDURE STEPS:

1. Inspect and index. **RATIONALE: Ensures that the chart is ready for filing and determines the order in which the chart will be filed.**
2. Sort the charts alphabetically. **RATIONALE: Determines the order and placement of the record; allows for a second assessment for placement.**
3. Create cross-reference files according to clinic policy.
4. File the charts appropriately.
5. Check the placement with the charts immediately before and after the chart being filed. **RATIONALE: Makes certain the chart is filed in the correct location.**

Numeric Filing

Numeric filing is organized by number rather than by letter. A key benefit of numeric filing is that it preserves patient confidentiality because the individual's name is not obviously apparent on the file folder. The numeric filing systems most often used in medical facilities are straight numeric and terminal digit.

Straight Numeric. Straight numeric filing places charts in exact chronological order according to assigned number. For example, records numbered 45023, 45024, and 45025 will be in consecutive order on a shelf. This is an easy system to learn and use; however, there are some disadvantages. The greater number of digits to recall, the greater the chance for error. Numbers transposition is common. Chart number 45024 can be misfiled as chart number 54024. The use of color with straight numeric can decrease misfiling.

Terminal Digit. In terminal digit filing, a six-digit number is most often used with a hyphen dividing three parts of two digits, for example, 85-32-07 and 86-32-07. Within these numbers, the primary units are the last two numbers; the middle digits are the secondary units; the first two numbers are the third and final units considered. In a terminal digit file, there are 100 primary sections from 00 to 99 to be considered. The medical assistant will consider the primary section first, match the record with the same group to the secondary set of digits next, and then file in numerical order by the third unit.

The advantage to this system is that files and numbers are equally distributed. Only every 100th new medical record will be filed in the same primary section. Filing using the straight numerical order of the first two numbers is simple to learn.

Middle Digit. In middle digit systems, the staff still files according to pairs of digits, but the pairs of digits are in different positions. The middle pair of digits is primary, the pair of digits to the left is secondary, and the pair of digits on the right is third.

The terminal digit and middle digit systems are most likely seen in hospitals and large multi-provider clinics.

Components of Numeric Filing. Four essential components are used with a numeric system, whether it is a manual or computerized system.

Serially Numbered Dividers with Guides. Consecutive numeric guides (5, 10, etc.; 50, 100, etc.) separate the individual file folders into smaller groups of files.

Miscellaneous (General) Numeric File Section. This is reserved for records that have not been assigned numbers. Patients should automatically be assigned a number on the first visit. However, on occasion patients cannot be assigned a number initially. The miscellaneous section is generally in front of all the numeric folders for ease of locating items. Files in the miscellaneous section are filed alphabetically by patient name. This is the best place for the miscellaneous file(s) for two reasons:

1. They do not have to be moved each time a numbered file is added to the back of the order.
2. In a large system of files, retrieval from the front is quick and easy.

Alphabetic Card File. This alphabetic file is necessary as a source to locate numeric files or records. A card contains name, address, and file number (or an ***M*** if located in the miscellaneous section); any **cross-reference** is here rather than in the numeric files.

The alphabetic card file in a manual system would be equivalent to the computerized record of the patient and whatever number is assigned to him or her in that computer record. If using a computerized system, the program generally will automatically cross-reference the number with the alphabetic list that was generated with the initial entry. If laboratory data on Leo M. McKay come into the clinic, there will need to be a method to know where to locate his chart to file the report, that is, the alphabetic listing.

With a manual system, the alphabetic file is kept in an index card fashion. This file will contain the complete name and address (and any other information denoted by the clinic policy, e.g., insurance and emergency numbers).

Noted with this information there needs to be either an ***M*** for miscellaneous (for those items not assigned a number) or an assigned number (Figures 13-9A and B).

If a cross-reference is required, prepare a cross-reference card and include an ***X*** next to the file number (or ***M***) to indicate this is the cross-reference card and not the primary location (Figure 13-9C).

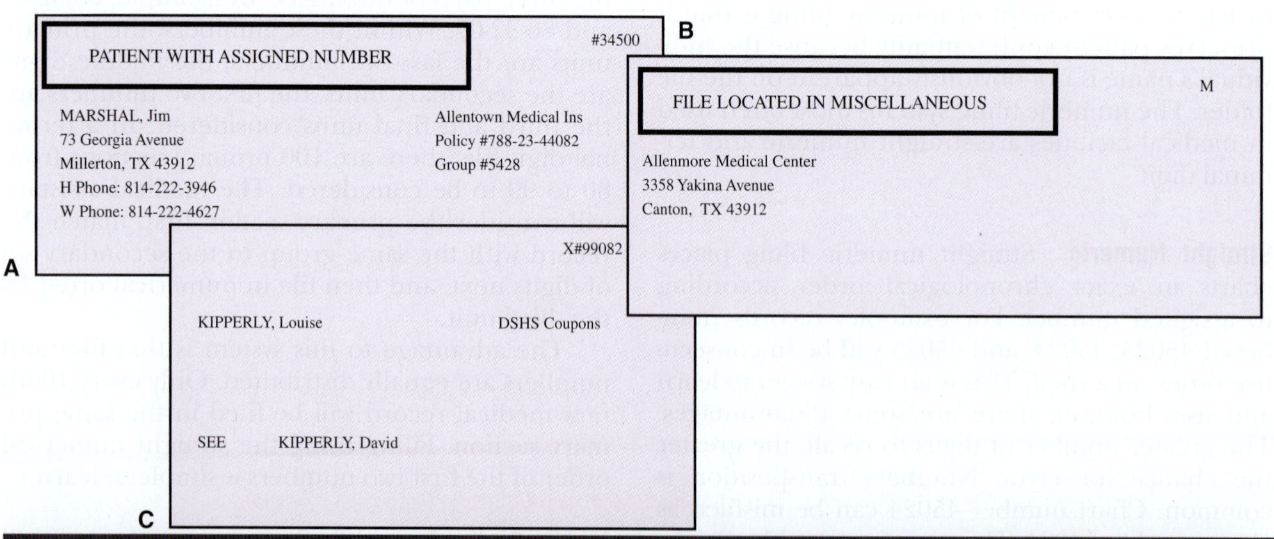

FIGURE 13-9 Card files used in a numeric filing system: (A) Patient with an assigned number. (B) Business record has not had a number assigned and is located in miscellaneous section. (C) Cross-reference card.

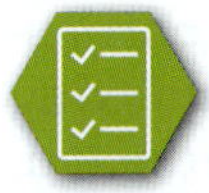

Accession Record. The **accession record** is a journal (or computer listing) where numbers are preassigned. Each new item to be assigned is written on the line next to the number (Figure 13-10). Each new entry for which a chart will be created must be assigned a number. A computerized system would have an accession record in its memory bank. Procedure 13-3 provides numeric filing steps.

Subject Filing

Procedure

There are many reasons why material would be filed using a system of subjects in a medical clinic. If providers are doing research, they might wish to index research according to diseases. Subject files are convenient for locating frequently used services or for filing reference materials for patient needs. Insurance company information also might be filed by subject.

When using a subject filing system, scan the material to determine the subject or theme. As with color-coding and numeric filing, an alphabetic file is necessary. This can be either a subject list or an index card file listing the subjects. Also, as with numeric filing, all cross-reference cards are done only with alphabetic file listings.

Within the folders, material can be arranged either alphabetically or chronologically; keep in

PROCEDURE 13-3

Manual Filing with a Numeric System

PURPOSE:

To demonstrate an understanding of the principles of the numeric filing system.

EQUIPMENT/SUPPLIES:

- Documents to be filed
- Dividers with guides
- Miscellaneous numeric file section
- Alphabetic card file and cards
- Accession journal, if needed

PROCEDURE STEPS:

1. Inspect and index. RATIONALE: Ensures that the information is ready for filing and determines how the chart will be located.
2. Code for filing units. Check the alphabetic card file for each piece to see if the card has already been prepared. RATIONALE: Determines the number under which the chart will be filed.
3. Write the number in the upper right-hand corner if the piece has been assigned a number. RATIONALE: Tells you the number to be used in filing.
4. If no number is assigned (i.e., it has an *M* for miscellaneous), check the miscellaneous file. If a miscellaneous item is ready to be assigned a number, make a card and note the number in the right-hand corner of the card file, cross out the *M*, and make a chart file. RATIONALE: Tells you if a number should be prepared because of numerous items in the miscellaneous file, or if the piece to be filed should stay in the miscellaneous file.
5. If there is no card, make up an alphabetic card including a complete name and address, and then write either *M* or assign a number. RATIONALE: Ensures that there is always an alphabetic card with necessary demographic information and an assigned number or *M* for each piece of information and chart.
6. Cross-reference if necessary and file the card properly. You are then ready to file the document in the appropriate file folder/chart. RATIONALE: Ensures less likelihood of misfiling if necessary cross-references are prepared.
7. File in ascending order. RATIONALE: Establishes a pattern for filing.

ACCESSION LOGBOOK	
#	File Name
800	CARRERA, Jaime
801	AU, Rhoda
802	TREMONT Drug Supply
803	
804	
805	
806	
807	

FIGURE 13-10 Accession record or log sequentially lists predetermined numbers to be used to assign to numeric records. The next number available in this system is 803.

mind the objective for maintaining the particular files. For instance, if using subject indexing for research projects providers have conducted, identify the subject category; then in the material, code an item for reference to that specific material. Procedure 13-4 provides subject filing steps.

Choosing a Filing System

To select a filing system, each facility must decide what the primary objectives are with respect to storage of patient files, business records, and research files. How will the charts be used primarily? Will information need to be tracked by others not familiar with the records? Often more than one filing system will be used, such as alphabetic filing for patient charts, a numeric system for research subjects, and a subject system for miscellaneous correspondence.

PROCEDURE 13-4

Procedure

Manual Filing with a Subject Filing System

PURPOSE:

To demonstrate an understanding of the principles of the subject filing system.

EQUIPMENT/SUPPLIES:

- Documents to be filed by subject
- Subject index list or index card file listing subjects
- Alphabetic card file and cards

PROCEDURE STEPS:

1. Review the item to find the subject. **RATIONALE: Checks the item for the main topic of information to determine where the piece will be filed.**
2. Match the subject of the item with an appropriate category on the subject index list. **RATIONALE: Saves you time so that you do not create an unnecessary subject index list.**
3. If the item contains information that may pertain to more than one subject, decide on the proper cross-reference. **RATIONALE: Ensures that any confusion will be checked with a cross-reference.**
4. If the subject title is written on the material, underline it. **RATIONALE: Readily identifies the subject used for filing.**
5. If the subject title is not written on the item, write it clearly in the upper right-hand corner and underline (______) it. **RATIONALE: Indicates the subject used for filing; consistently places the subject in the expected place.**
6. Use a wavy (~~~) line for cross-referencing and an *X* as with alphabetic and numeric filing. **RATIONALE: Clearly identifies any cross-referencing.**
7. Underline the first indexing unit of the coded units. **RATIONALE: Ensures the correct order for filing.**

The number of documents to be filed is one primary determinant in selecting an alphabetic or numeric system. Alphabetic filing is quite manageable for many clinics. However, when the number of patients is quite large, a numeric system becomes practical because an infinite set of numbers is available. With the numeric system, there is only one of each assigned designation. However, with an alphabetic system, there are a number of common names (e.g., Smith, Jones, Adams, and Johnson) that can have many multiples requiring additional sorting to narrow the search for the correct chart. In addition, with multiple charts of the same last name, the chance for misfiling increases.

Legal

Confidentiality is another reason to select a numeric filing system. Confidentiality of charts is maintained more easily with numeric files because no name is visible on the outside of the chart. In addition, numerically referenced records can be used in research activities where random sampling and anonymity are required.

To make the medical facility HIPAA compliant when traditional paper-based or manual charts are used, you need to ensure that no patient-identifiable information is located on the outside of the chart. This includes the patient address or any other information that might be used to determine the identity of the patient, including Social Security number, birth date, or phone number. Any information that reveals a health condition or payment status also must be removed from the outside of the chart. Recall the earlier example of locked storage cabinets for manual files. Note that all file cabinets are to be closed and locked when no one is immediately present in the clinic; that includes lunch time when the staff may be eating in the staff lounge.

FILING PROCEDURES

By adhering to some common principles in medical records management, any filing system will be more effective and will enable the medical assistant to store, identify, retrieve, and maintain medical records efficiently.

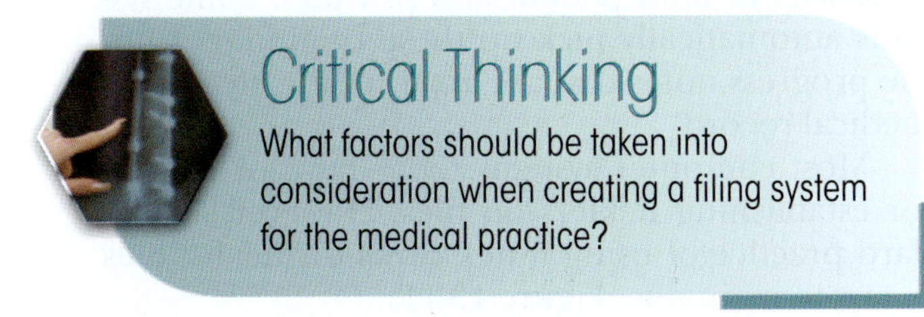

Critical Thinking

What factors should be taken into consideration when creating a filing system for the medical practice?

Cross-Referencing

In running an efficient medical facility, files must be stored for quick and accurate retrieval. If there is any doubt as to where a particular file would be located, cross-reference the file. Many clinics fail to take the extra time it requires to do this. However, with the growing number of foreign names, hyphenated names, and stepfamilies, it is well worth the effort. When the clinic receives a letter and a release of information form inquiring about medical facts on Mr. David Kipperly's four stepchildren who were involved in an accident, how will these files be located? If they are cross-referenced under the stepfather's name, this will be a relatively easy procedure. However, if the medical assistant is unfamiliar with the family (as in a larger urgent care center with a large volume of patients), this may become a time-consuming job. Another scenario might involve insurance information on Janet Morgan. A search of the records does not produce a file for any Janet Morgan. The reason for this is that Janet Morgan is married, and her chart has been filed under Janet Hill-Morgan. Time spent cross-referencing contributes to a more efficient method of retrieving information.

A cross-referencing system does not need to be elaborate. It is quite sufficient to use inserts with labels attached that are inserted in the appropriate place in the storage units. For instance, a plain piece of cardstock, rather than a file or chart, could be inserted for "Janet Morgan." This insert would simply have a label directing one to the location of the primary file.

The proper steps for cross-referencing, together with several examples where cross-referencing might be used, are discussed in the next section.

Steps for Cross-Referencing

1. Identify the primary filing label.
2. Make a proper file to be used as the primary location for all medical records.
3. Identify one (or more) alternatives where one might find the file.
4. For the alternative filings, make a cross-reference sheet, card, or dummy chart that lists the primary reference and refers back to the location of the primary file.

Example: The patient, Jaime Renae Carrera, has made it known to the clinic that most of his information received will refer to the name Renny Carrera, as this is his preference. The SEE reference will identify where the primary file is located.

PRIMARY FILE:	Carrera, Jaime Renae
X-REFERENCE FILE:	Carrera, Renny
	SEE Carrera, Jaime Renae

Rule 1. **Married Individuals.** When taking a spouse's name, the primary file would be the patient's legal name with the cross-reference listed under the spouse's.

PRIMARY FILE:	Au, Rhoda A. (Mrs.)
	Lee Au
X-REFERENCE FILE:	Au, Mrs. Lee
	SEE Au, Rhoda A. (Mrs.)

Rule 2. **Foreign Names.** The primary file would be located under the patient's legal name. It is important, therefore, that you identify the first, middle, and surname (last name) when the patient comes for the first visit. Unless people are familiar with a particular group of names, the first, middle, and surnames are often confused with one another. Again, your experience will teach you which cross-references should be set up.

PRIMARY FILE:	Sing, Yange Teah
X-REFERENCE FILE:	Yange, Sing Teah
	SEE Sing, Yange Teah
X-REFERENCE FILE:	Teah, Yange Sing
	SEE Sing, Yange Teah

Rule 3. **Hyphenated Names.** With the proliferation of hyphenated names, it is common for materials to be listed under different combinations of the hyphenated name. For instance, a married woman may have records under her maiden name, her husband's surname, and her hyphenated name. Therefore, it is necessary to make two cross-references.

PRIMARY FILE:	Krenshaw-Skiple, Rose Marie
X-REFERENCE FILE:	Skiple, Rose Marie
	SEE Krenshaw-Skiple, Rose Marie
X-REFERENCE FILE:	Krenshaw, Rose Marie
	SEE Krenshaw-Skiple, Rose Marie

Rule 4. **Multiple Listings.** A great deal of correspondence is received with multiple listings of names. At times, the medical clinic may receive correspondence from only one of the involved parties. Rather than keep a separate file for each, maintain a primary file as listed on the letter and then cross-reference file(s) for the individual names.

PRIMARY FILE:	Olsen, Piper, and Dillard Associates
X-REFERENCE FILE:	Piper, Richard C., M.D.
	SEE Olsen, Piper, and Dillard Associates
X-REFERENCE FILE:	Olsen, Francis William, M.D.
	SEE Olsen, Piper, and Dillard Associates
X-REFERENCE FILE:	Dillard, Thomas E., M.D.
	SEE Olsen, Piper, and Dillard Associates

Tickler Files

Sticky notes and writing notes on the calendar are popular methods of reminding clinic personnel to follow up with some required action. However, a well-organized, efficient clinic will maintain what is known as a **tickler file**, a method that serves as a reminder that some action needs to be taken at a date in the future.

Some systems have a calendar that pops up to allow reminders to be placed on the calendar. The computer system reminds you of the note when that particular day arrives. Some EMR systems have built-in reminders that automatically give a reminder for such things as annual physical examinations, monthly blood pressure checks, medication checks, and anything else that might be beneficial to both patient and provider. Some systems automatically pick up these reminders from the progress notes that are a part of the electronic medical record.

Most computer systems today have provisions for establishing ticklers on files. However, a standard practice of using index cards for tickler files is easy to maintain (Figure 13-11).

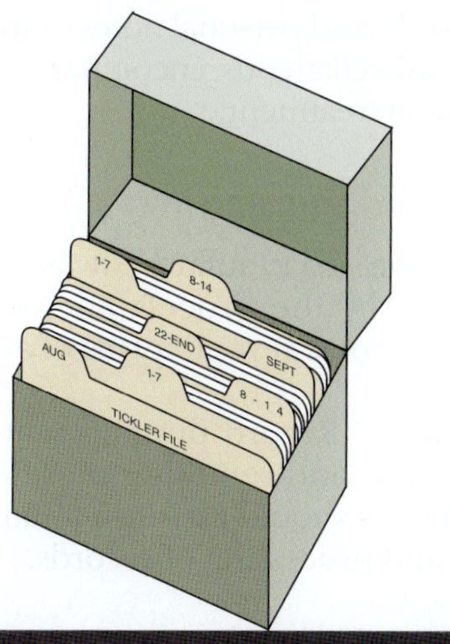

FIGURE 13-11 Tickler files should be reviewed daily or weekly to follow up on activities and actions that must be taken.

The tickler card should contain the following information:

- Patient name
- Tickler date (when action should be taken)
- Required action (e.g., schedule surgery or mail reminder)
- Additional relevant information (e.g., telephone number)

If action is to be taken with a patient or on behalf of the patient (e.g., scheduling a hospital admittance or sending a reminder of a checkup visit), place the information on the tickler card as soon as possible so this task is not forgotten.

When filing records, be sure to look for words such as *on ________ date we will, pending action,* or *follow-up,* indicating that some course of action needs to be taken.

It is important to remember that any tickler system, whether manual or computerized, is worthless if the reminder is not adhered to and appropriate action taken.

Release Marks

It is a good practice to use some type of release mark (date stamp, initials, check mark) on every item that is filed. Ideally, the provider should initial the document after it has been read. Then, if action is required by the medical assistant, a release mark is in a consistently identified place on every document. If no action is required after the provider has signed or initialed, place a release mark on the document. A release mark on every piece of information serves as an excellent quality-control measure.

Checkout System

Many clinics have developed dummy charts or files labeled "out sheets" or "out guides" for use when the chart is removed. Most of these guides are identified by an OUT label or metal holder, but they could be assigned a particular color; the key is that they stand out as different from the primary folders.

On the out guide, there should be a minimum of the following information:

- A record of when the chart was removed
- Where the chart can be located

Other information that is useful to note includes:

- Expected date of return
- Actual date the chart was returned
- Signature of the individual checking out the record
- Notation on what section of the chart file was borrowed, such as a laboratory report or specialty examination

Some clinics prefer to have *temporary folders* rather than just an out guide. There are also out guides with pockets to file data in the absence of a chart. This allows for data storage on a temporary basis until the primary file is returned. The data can then be filed permanently when the primary folder is returned. If these folders are of a different color or have a different type of tab/label, they can be spotted easily so the staff can track the temporary files to be sure they do not become permanent folders.

Locating Missing Files or Data

Misfiling can occur for a number of reasons. When this situation occurs, a specific procedure must be established to conduct a search for the missing information. By systematically searching, the missing data usually can be located. This systematic search can be aided by making a mental note of the particular items that commonly are misplaced, such as thin-paper laboratory reports, small laboratory slips, and look-alike names such as "Ward" filed under "Wart" or "Adam" filed under "Adams." Make a note of what was misfiled and where the information was located to more easily locate similar items in the future.

To locate missing pieces of information when the correct file is located but not the particular item within that file:

- Check all of the items within the file.
- Check other files with similar labels.

To locate missing files:

- Check the folders filed before and after the proper location of the misplaced file.
- Look at folders with similar labels.
- Check the provider's desk, the desk tray, and with other clinic personnel.
- If using a color-coding system, look for folders with the same coding as the misplaced file.
- If using a numeric system, look for possible transposition of combinations of numbers.
- Check for transposition of first and last names.
- Check for alternative spellings of names or look-alike names.

Misplaced files can be frustrating and time-consuming to locate. The best strategy is to check files for the proper filing order whenever returning or retrieving a file folder. When removing a file to answer a question, leave the file following it sticking out slightly to make its return easy and correct. Most importantly, when finished with a record, refile it immediately.

Filing Chart Data

Types of Reports. The patient's chart is the key source of information relating to treatment. A number of reports are kept in the chart, all serving to provide a total picture of patient care. Following are the most common documents that are part of the patient's medical record (see Chapter 15 for other documents).

Clinical Notes. Clinical notes include documentation such as the medical history, the physical examination, and the follow-up notes. They track the patient's course of treatment.

Correspondence. Filing of correspondence varies. Some file all types of correspondence together. Others file correspondence about the patient's treatment with the clinical notes.

Laboratory Reports. Included in laboratory reports are X-ray reports, CT scans, ultrasound reports, blood work, urinalysis, EEGs, ECGs, physical therapy–related reports, and pathology reports—information related to clinical data that assess the patient's condition.

Miscellaneous. The miscellaneous category includes insurance-related papers, requests for transfer of medical records, and personal notes from/to patients. In general, miscellaneous encompasses matters not related to direct treatment.

Retention and Purging

As information accumulates, it is necessary to maintain files by the process known as **purging**. Purging can involve several forms of action.

Record Purging. Record purging requires sorting through records and removing those not in active use. Each facility should establish a standard policy for control and processing of records.

States have different time requirements for retention of various types of records that will take into account the statute of limitations (see Chapter 6). Table 13-1 lists general guidelines. As a way of controlling risk and practicing responsible risk management, many facilities choose to maintain large numbers of inactive files rather than to destroy any records. Check with the Medical Practice Act in your state to determine record-keeping requirements.

Active Files. Active files include records that need to be readily accessible for retrieval of information.

Inactive Files. Inactive files consist of records that need to be retained for possible retrieval of information. Files not currently being accessed for information would thus become inactive. Often, the type of practice dictates the relevant time period when files are determined to be inactive (generally 2 to 3 years).

Closed Files. Closed files are those that are no longer required. Again, patient files are retained for significantly longer periods of time because of litigation and research considerations, usually 3 to 6 years beyond the statute of limitations.

CORRESPONDENCE

Most clinics process a considerable amount of correspondence not directly related to patient care. Such items include employment applications, letters from/to pharmaceutical representatives, advertisements for medical supplies, magazine subscription information, and letters to/from other providers on a variety of subjects. This correspondence is processed using alphabetic filing rules. However, an additional step is necessary to determine whether the correspondence is incoming

TABLE 13-1

RECORDS FOR RETENTION

PATIENT INDEX FILES These include appointment books or daily appointment sheets. They are kept for an indefinite period. They may be required for litigation or research.
CASE HISTORIES The length of storage depends on state requirements and individual practice requirements. Product liability cases have deemed long-term storage of these records necessary (20+ years). The records of minors must be retained at least until the age of majority. The statute of limitations is a deciding factor as well, usually 3 to 6 years. If records are to be destroyed because of the death of a provider or closure of a practice, the following procedure is required: Each patient should be notified of the circumstances and given the opportunity to have his or her records forwarded to another provider. After notification, the records must be retained for a "reasonable" period (determined by state regulations). A period of 3 to 6 months is generally determined to be a "reasonable" period. The records must be destroyed by burning or shredding to protect confidentiality.
LABORATORY AND X-RAY DATA Originals should be retained permanently with the patient's case history.
PERSONAL/PROFESSIONAL RECORDS Professional licenses should be stored permanently in a secure location.
OFFICE EQUIPMENT RECORDS These records are generally kept until the warranties and depreciation are no longer valid. They should be kept in an easily accessible location if under maintenance contract.
INSURANCE RECORDS Professional liability policies are kept permanently. Other policies are kept in active files while in force.
FINANCIAL RECORDS Bank records are kept in active files for up to 3 years and then placed in inactive storage. Tax records must be retained permanently.

or outgoing. The correspondence must be filed under some aspect that will be distinctly identifiable; that is, what idea, subject, or name would most likely be thought of if someone wanted to retrieve that correspondence or file additional relevant correspondence.

Even when scanning documents for importing to the EMR, how to determine the category or subject for a document needs to be established. The digital version of the document can then be archived in the appropriate place within the record.

Filing Procedures for Correspondence

Once it is determined whether correspondence is incoming or outgoing, follow the basic rules for filing. In addition:

- Remove paper clips and staple items together.
- Inspect to see if the item is ready to be filed; that is, if appropriate action has been taken. If not, take care of copies and enclosures, and then place notes in the tickler file for future action before proceeding with the indexing.
- On incoming correspondence, be sure the letterhead is in direct relation to the letter.

Example: A personal letter written by a patient on hotel stationery—index the signature on the letter.

Example: When both the company name and the signature are important, index the company name. A letter from Preston Industries written by the company president—index Preston Industries, not the president's name, which may change.

Example: If there is no letterhead and you have determined the material is not relevant to a patient, index the name on the signature line. A letter received from Carlton Fiske, RPT, advising your clinic of services his firm has to offer your patients—index Fiske.

- On outgoing correspondence, look at the inside address and the reference line.

Example: A letter to the District Court regarding Karen Ritter, an employee who is summoned to jury duty—index Karen Ritter rather than District Court.

Example: If the correspondence is relevant to a patient, index the patient's name. A letter RE: Wayne Elder—index under Elder.

Example: If the correspondence is not relevant to a patient, look to the inside address for the indexing information. A letter inquiring about cost estimates for redecorating the clinic reception room—index the firm in the inside address, and cross-reference to the subject (redecorating clinic).

Example: When the inside address is relevant and contains both a company name and a person's name, index the company name. (This avoids the problem of personnel changes.) Cross-referencing would be done under the individual name. A letter to Marvin Fairchild, President of Brandex Pharmaceuticals—index Brandex Pharmaceuticals with a cross-reference for "Marvin Fairchild, President, SEE Brandex Pharmaceuticals."

Example: If the letter is personal, the name of the person to whom the letter is written would be used for indexing purposes. Dr. Lewis writes a letter to Dr. Whitney, one of his colleagues, asking if he plans to attend an upcoming conference—index Dr. Whitney.

- On incoming or outgoing correspondence, code the indexing units of the designated label. If the correspondence is being cross-referenced, be sure to note the cross-referencing unit and place the *X* in a visible place. You may find that the body of the letter contains an important name or subject.
- Create a miscellaneous folder for items that do not have enough in number to warrant an individual folder. Items in the miscellaneous folder are filed alphabetically first, and then identical items are filed with the most recent piece on top. An individual folder is then created when enough pieces accumulate on a particular item.

ELECTRONIC MEDICAL RECORDS

Total electronic automation in any medical facility is a major undertaking. It can be both frightening and exhilarating. Careful study of systems available, impact on providers and staff, time necessary for moving from manual to electronic files, and costs involved are measured against the benefits incurred.

With the government's mandate to have EMRs for most patients and Congress pushing to make all Medicare-covered prescriptions transferred electronically, EMRs are here to stay and one day will replace all paper/manual medical records. Evidence shows that fewer errors are created in EMRs because the "human element" is decreased. If all the data are entered correctly, the computer software "does all the thinking" to find the chart, store information appropriately, create reminder notices, check all medications for any contraindications, and flag any warning to providers, such as high cholesterol or blood pressure readings moving into the "alert" zone. The EMR will keep a record of all patient appointments and any missed appointments as well as any piece of information that might be found in a manual patient record. EMR software creates, stores, edits, and retrieves patient data. It has the added advantage of allowing more than one person to access a chart at the same time.

EMR software can be purchased as a single-computer application or as part of a larger "practice management" software package. Often, medical facilities start with one aspect of a practice management software package (usually not EMRs) and then gradually add the other pieces. EMRs are capable of the following:

- Create and print customized encounter forms and superbills
- View patient records of all provider encounters and laboratory results, transcription notes, radiologic images, and so forth
- Utilize predefined templates to make examination notes, procedures, review of systems, and postoperative checks quicker and more efficient
- Indicate or choose medications (from a predetermined list of those most prescribed), with specific instructions that can be electronically admitted into the chart and to the pharmacy
- Flag any drug interactions, contraindications, or allergies related to the patient
- Give providers pen units or small computers in which to enter data with a simple touch of the pen
- Provide providers and necessary staff members with immediate access to the patient record

- Be easily retrieved and never lost or misplaced
- Eliminate the manual coding and filing of medical charts
- Reduce the amount of phone tag retrieving necessary information from a paper file
- Create reminders for follow-up as necessary
- Provide a more efficient method of signing charts
- Can be emailed to a referring provider or easily printed, whether part of or the whole chart

EMRs require that providers use computers to open and view charts and write prescriptions. Progress notes can be created using clinical templates and a point-and-click form of entry. Commonly used clinical phrases can be dropped into the progress note with a push of a button. If providers prefer to dictate and have their notes transcribed, that can also be done. The transcribed and entered note will automatically update relevant information such as problem lists, vital signs, laboratory results, and so on. As voice recognition improves, it will become possible for the provider to speak the entries normally keyed into the system.

Confidentiality is often mentioned as a concern in EMRs, but with the ability to limit network access, system administrators can identify access and privileges according to the desired policy of the clinic. The EMR is fully recognized as a legal document, is able to track any changes made, and can be presented to a court of law. Because a standard part of any EMR installation is a system backup, you should never be without a medical chart even if the system goes down for a brief period.

Most medical assistants working in facilities that are fully computerized say they hardly remember how they could function any differently. They also report that moving from the manual to the electronic system can be frustrating at times, but it is worth the effort in the long run.

Archival Storage

Most providers preserve patient medical records for at least the life of their practice. This obviously is a space-consuming prospect, particularly in today's large practices. Computers help to solve this dilemma through EMRs. This not only eliminates the bulky storage problems encountered with traditional records, but records can be retrieved and viewed almost instantaneously on a computer screen.

One of the advantages of the EMR is the small amount of storage needed for all the patient charts; but remember that computer files, including patient charts, should have a backup system that stores the information in a secure place should there be a computer problem. Some systems provide for automatic backup every 30 minutes or less. Some systems include a second hard drive that stores data as they are being created or as often as determined by facility policy. With an effective and efficient backup system, no one on the clinic staff will ever be without a patient chart when it is needed.

Transfer of Data

EMRs are easily emailed in whole or in part. Computers also streamline transfer of records from one medical facility to another. Faxing is an everyday part of the medical clinic. Gone is the time when it took a provider days to obtain information vital to treating a patient. Within minutes, a patient's entire medical record can be sent electronically from one clinic to another. Scanners (optical character recognition) are devices that allow information to be converted to an image on the computer screen. For instance, a patient's entire medical record can be scanned by the device and then recreated as a computer file exactly as it was in paper form.

Confidentiality

Legal

Maintaining confidentiality is a major issue in using the computer and online devices for storage and transfer of medical information. Not enough emphasis can be placed on the confidentiality issue. Medical assistants employed in a medical facility will hear and see information that is completely private. It is never appropriate to discuss any of that information outside the clinic with any individual unless it is a person who needs that information for medical reasons. It is also unwise to discuss private information within the facility if it is not your concern, and especially if your voice might be overheard by someone waiting in an examination room, a patient using the restroom, or individuals in the reception area. An appropriate situation in which information can be shared is when giving the name, address, and Social Security number or clinic number to the radiology department that will be performing the X-rays ordered by the provider.

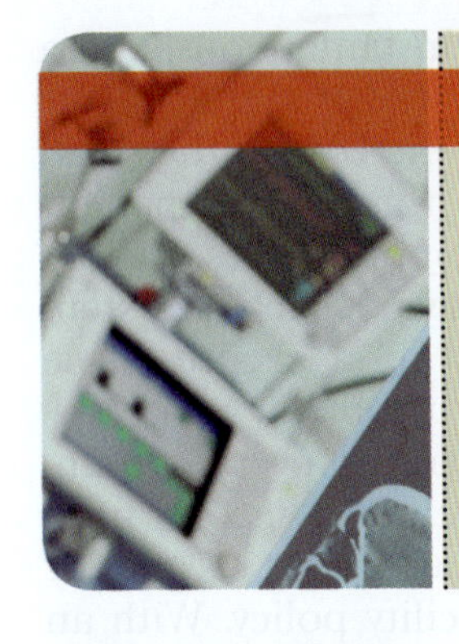

CASE STUDY 13-1

Refer to the scenario at the beginning of the chapter.

CASE STUDY REVIEW

1. Juanita Hansen is waiting in the clinic. Dr. Lewis and the staff are scrambling to find Juanita's test results. What can be done now to make certain Juanita has not made the trip unnecessarily?
2. Identify steps to be taken to prevent this situation from happening another time.

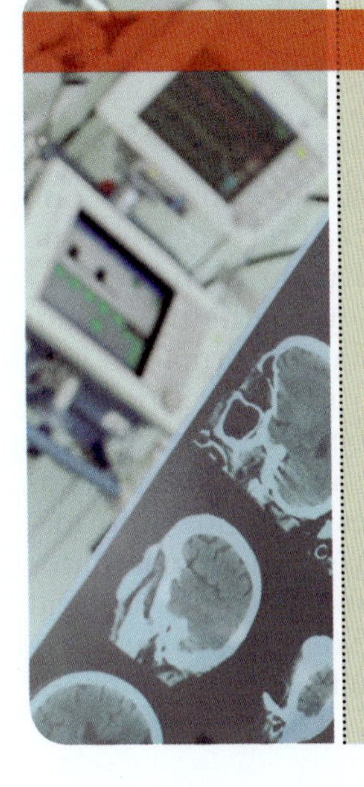

CASE STUDY 13-2

Ellen Armstrong, CMAS (AMT), administrative medical assistant at Inner City Health Care, has been chiefly responsible for managing this clinic's medical records. However, because Ellen is only a part-time employee, the clinic manager feels she needs to delegate some of the responsibility of maintaining all clinic files to Liz Corbin, CMA (AAMA), a medical assistant who also works part time. Ellen knows the system well and had a hand in designing an effective numeric filing method that both ensures patient confidentiality and satisfies the needs of Inner City and its large volume of patients. Now she is trying to orient Liz, who has little experience with the filing system, to the intricacies of medical records management.

CASE STUDY REVIEW

1. What is a good starting point for Liz Corbin's education in medical records management?
2. What are the basic procedures for filing any piece of documentation that Liz needs to learn?
3. Under the direction of the clinic manager, Inner City is gradually shifting to a computerized system for all operations. Eventually, patient files will be computerized. What can Ellen and Liz do to prepare for this eventuality?

Summary

- Records management plays an ever-increasing role in the clinic setting today. With the need for thorough and proper documentation, a majority of interactions on the patient's behalf are concerned with proper information processing.
- It is imperative that medical records be managed efficiently, and that the medical assistant possesses the skills required for sorting, filing, retrieving, and maintaining information effectively.
- Proper use of electronic medical records is necessary to ensure appropriate use of features to preserve documentation integrity and prevent fraud, waste, abuse, and improper payments.
- The medical assistant must understand the procedures for properly documenting, maintaining, updating, purging, correcting, and releasing medical information using both paper charts and EMR/PM systems.
- The medical assistant must be able to accurately create paper charts and electronic records for patient medical records.
- Types of medical records and information storage includes POMR and the SOAP note method, the SOMR method, and the chronological arrangement method.
- Basic rules for filing and applying the steps for filing medical documents include the procedural steps Inspect, Index, Code, Sort, and File.
- Medical assistants must be familiar with other filing techniques in addition to alphabetic, which can be used for patient or other types of organizational uses in a clinic setting. These include numeric filing, subject filing, cross-referencing, and tickler files.
- The medical assistant must be aware of proper archiving of medical records and backup systems for the EMR system.

Study for Success

To reinforce your knowledge and skills of information presented in this chapter:

- Review the *Key Terms* and *Learning Outcomes*
- Consider the *Critical Thinking* features and *Case Studies* and discuss your conclusions
- Answer the questions in the *Certification Review*

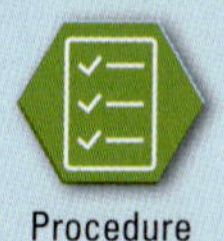

- Perform the *Procedures* using the *Competency Assessment Checklists* on the *Student Companion Website*

CERTIFICATION REVIEW

1. What is the name of the process for maintaining order in files by separating active from inactive files?
   a. Indexing
   b. Coding
   c. Purging
   d. Alphabetizing
2. What is the name of the system used as a reminder of action to be taken on a certain date?
   a. Accession log
   b. Tickler file or reminder note
   c. Release mark
   d. Purging system
   e. Outguide
3. What is the name of the tool used to ensure that records are tracked when borrowed in order to maintain an accurate filing system?
   a. Release mark
   b. Out guide
   c. Alphabetic card file
   d. Cross-reference file
4. What answer describes the correct indexing for units 1, 2, 3, 4 in the name John Porter O'Keefe II?
   a. O'Keefe John Porter II
   b. John Porter O'Keefe II
   c. II O'Keefe John Porter
   d. The "II" would be disregarded
   e. John Porter O'Keefe
5. Of the four systems of filing, what is the best for every ambulatory care setting?
   a. The numeric system
   b. The color-coding system
   c. One customized to the needs of the clinic
   d. The alphabetic system
6. Who owns the medical record?
   a. The patients for whom the record is about
   b. Insurance carriers who help to pay medical costs
   c. The providers who create the record
   d. The insurance carrier
   e. Both a and c
7. What is the process for making corrections to the medical record?
   a. They are made by erasing the error and replacing it with the correction.
   b. They are made by placing a single line through the error and replacing it with the correction.
   c. They are never made to charts because of the legal nature of the information.
   d. They are made only by the provider.
8. Which of the following statements about EMRs is false?
   a. They are initially more expensive than paper medical records.
   b. They should be available to most Americans by 2020.
   c. They eliminate coding and filing of medical charts.
   d. They create reminders for follow-up as necessary.
   e. Solo practitioners are least likely to use EMRs.
9. When identical names are being indexed, which indexing system is preferred in a medical system?
   a. The address
   b. The telephone number
   c. The birth date or Social Security number
   d. A preassigned clinic number
10. What are the preferred steps for filing medical documentation?
    a. Code, index, sort, inspect, file
    b. Inspect, code, index, sort, file
    c. Sort, inspect, index, code, file
    d. Inspect, index, code, purge
    e. Inspect, index, code, sort, file

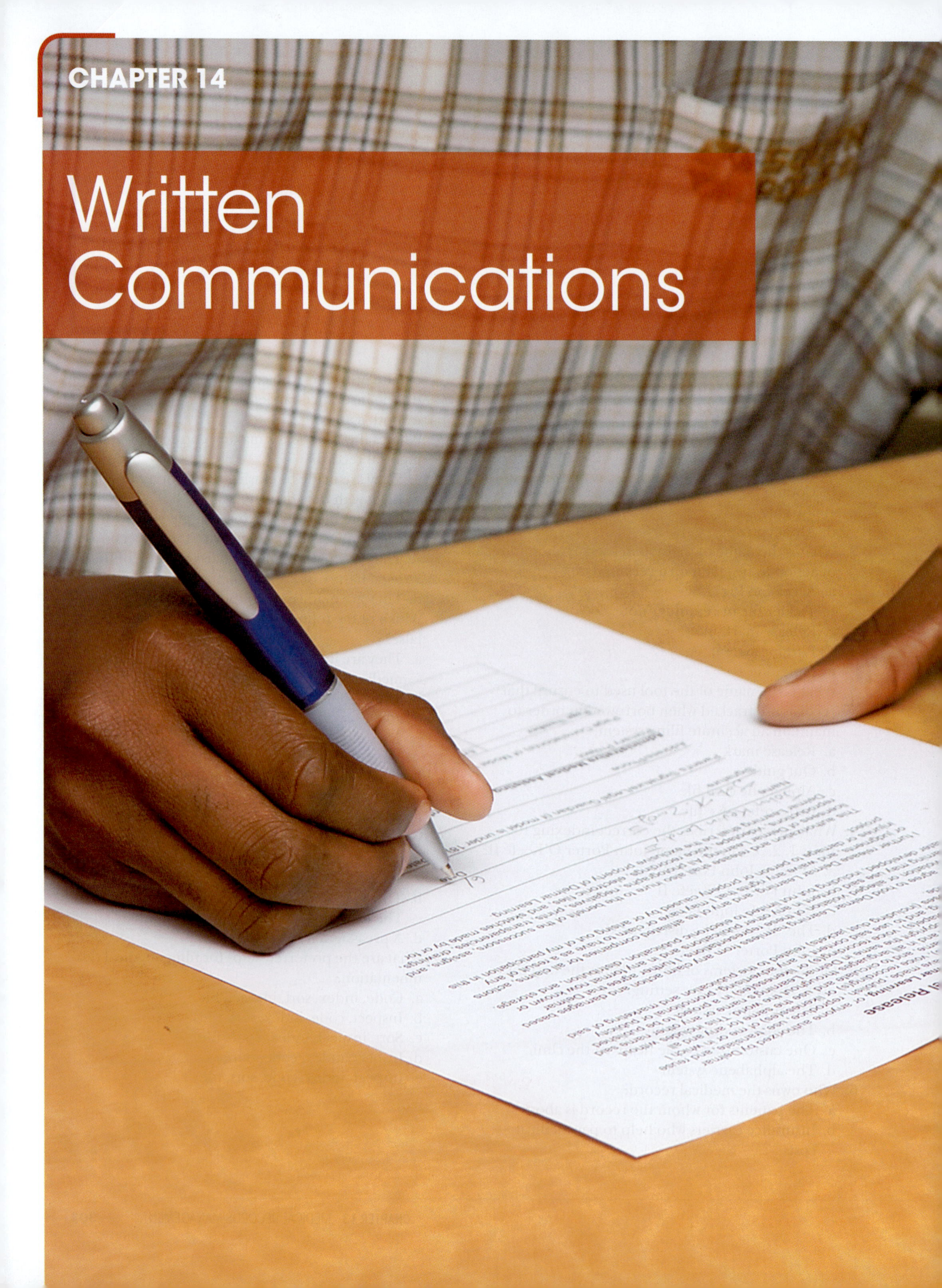

CHAPTER 14

Written Communications

LEARNING OUTCOMES

1. Define and spell the key terms as presented in the glossary.
2. Identify the role of the medical assistant in producing written communications.
3. List the four major letter styles.
4. Compose and key letters using appropriate components of a business letter.
5. Identify various types of form letters that may be written by the medical assistant.
6. Proofread a letter for grammar, spelling, and content.
7. Use proper proofreading marks to correct a document.
8. Describe the various classifications of mail and determine when each class should be used.
9. Address envelopes to satisfy postal regulations.
10. Discuss legal and ethical issues relating to written communications, as well as HIPAA regulations.

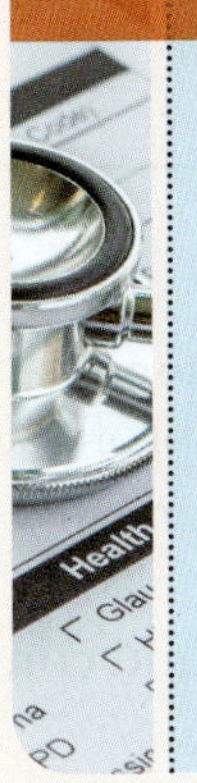

KEY TERMS

agenda
blind copy
bond paper
form letter
full block letter
keyed
memorandum (memo)
minutes
modified block letter, indented
modified block letter, standard
optical character recognition (OCR)
portfolio
proofread
simplified letter
watermark
ZIP+4

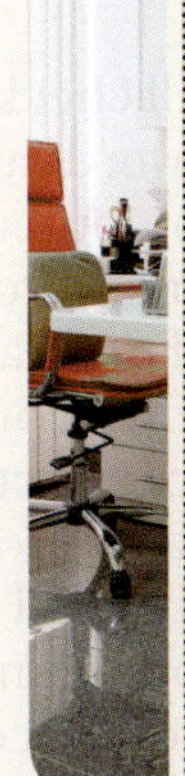

SCENARIO

When they are produced with care, written communications can be a time-consuming part of the administrative medical assistant's day. This is why Marilyn Johnson, CMA (AAMA), the clinic manager at Inner City Health Care, has compiled a style manual for the multiprovider practice. Marilyn is clearly aware that professional appearing and worded letters send a positive message to all recipients. Yet, she wants to make correspondence writing and producing as efficient as possible; her style manual provides an easy-to-use resource for anyone in the clinic responsible for composing or sending written documents.

In her style manual, Marilyn has included examples of the "house" letter format, which is block style; a list of commonly used medical terms for easy spelling reference; answers to common questions staff have in regard to word usage; proofreader's marks; proper addressing procedures for envelopes and packages, depending on whether they are being sent by U.S. mail or by an alternative delivery method; and a quick list of the best ways to send various types of correspondence. Marilyn has also included a list of "Do Nots" to help her staff avoid mistakes in their written communications.

Chapter Portal

One of the key responsibilities of the administrative medical assistant is written communication. Letters to patients, to referring providers, to other health care organizations, and even interoffice correspondence should be thoughtfully composed, carefully produced according to the style selected by the clinic manager, and mailed and delivered in a way that is both time and cost efficient.

Written correspondence is important in conveying a professional image of the clinic and impacts public relations either positively or negatively. It must also be remembered that written documents provide a permanent or legal record in the event of any litigation and thus must be carefully and accurately worded.

In most clinics, medical assistants are responsible for creating many forms of written communications. Examples of these forms of communications include:

- Various types of letters, such as letters to order supplies and equipment, letters replying to various types of inquirie, collection letters, and promotional letters
- Memoranda and interoffice communications
- Referrals, consultation, and surgical report letters
- Written instructions for patients
- Meeting agendas and minutes
- Promotional brochures
- Policy and procedure documents

COMPOSING CORRESPONDENCE

The medical assistant must always remember that the quality of the correspondence reflects the standards of the medical clinic. It is important to also remember that there is a difference between social correspondence and business correspondence. Social correspondence tends to be lengthy and personal in nature, whereas business correspondence should be clear, concise, courteous, and accurate. It is best to keep business letters to one page in length whenever possible.

Writing Tips

Rosemary Fruehling, a writer and lecturer, states, "Business writing is good when it achieves the purpose the author intended." Practice and careful attention to detail are required to write effective business letters. Writing tips for consideration include:

- Follow the style and format determined by your provider-employer. Providers often prefer a professional, formal style of letter composition.
- Think about key points to be addressed in the letter and organize them before beginning composition. The first paragraph should identify what the letter is about and focus the reader's attention.
- Establish a tone of voice. Be personable and cordial in tone while remaining professional.
- Use only language that the reader will understand.
- Most sentences should be short and contain only one idea or thought.

Spelling

It is important that all correspondence contain no misspelled or incorrectly used words. When in doubt, always look the word up in a dictionary (Table 14-1). When checking spelling in a dictionary, develop the habit of reading the definition as well. This will help imprint the correct spelling and meaning of the word.

Be careful about relying on the spell check function of your computer; many medical words are not formatted into the computer. The computer does not recognize if you have used the wrong word, only that the word is spelled incorrectly. For example, the words *to, too,* and *two* may all be spelled correctly but may be misused within the sentence structure.

It may be helpful to develop a list of frequently misused words in an alphabetized notebook, card index, or special file on your computer (Table 14-2). Several computer word processing software packages contain English/medical spell check features. A new word that is not currently identified in the spell check or medical check package may be added to the program.

TABLE 14-1

FREQUENTLY MISSPELLED MEDICAL TERMS

abscess	malaise
aneurysm	ophthalmology
arrhythmia	palliative
calcaneus	parenteral
cirrhosis	pharynx
clavicle	pneumonia
curettage	pruritus
diarrhea	psychiatrist
hemorrhage	pyrexia
hemorrhoids	rheumatic
homeostasis	rhythm
humerus	roentgenology
ileum	sphygmomanometer
ilium	staphylococcus
ischemia	vesical
ischium	vesicle
larynx	

Proofreading

Before presenting any correspondence to the provider for signature or mailing, the document should be **proofread**. Proofreading is the process of reading the document and checking for accuracy. Accuracy involves checking to be sure that the correct grammar, spelling, punctuation, and capitalization have been used and that the message is clear and concise and presented in a logical organization.

Proofreading marks most commonly used are shown in Figure 14-1. Standard proofreading marks are symbols and short notations that are used to mark up documents indicating corrections and solutions to errors. Some proofreading tips that may be useful include:

- Proofread each document twice, once on the screen checking for obvious errors and then on a hard copy to be sure everything is accurate and makes sense.
- Prepare the document, set it aside, and proofread a third time later. Inaccuracies or errors may "jump" out in a later review.
- Do not proofread when tired.
- If the document is long, proofread in several short intervals.
- Read a long document to another person and have him or her check sentence structure and content accuracy.
- Use a card or ruler as a guide to maintain your place within the document.
- Use a piece of colored clear plastic over the document to rest your eyes. This is especially helpful when proofing a long document.

TABLE 14-2

FREQUENTLY MISUSED WORDS

advice	advise		hear	here	
affect	effect		hole	whole	
capital	capitol		knew	new	
coarse	course		know	no	
coma	comma		lean	lien	
command	commend		patience	patients	
complement	compliment		personal	personnel	
comprehensible	comprehensive		plain	plane	
council	counsel		precede	proceed	
conscience	conscious		principal	principle	
deposition	disposition		right	write	
device	devise		stationary	stationery	
elicit	illicit		taught	taut	
eligible	illegible		their	there	they are
elude	allude		to	too	two
ensure	insure	assure	vain	vein	
explicit	implicit		weak	week	
farther	further		weather	whether	
heal	heel		you	your	you are

Mark	Example	Mark	Example
∧	Insert	⊏	Move left
	Delete	⊐	Move right
#	Insert space	⊓	Move up
⌣	Close up space	⊔	Move down
	Delete and close up	⊐⊏	Center
#	Close up, but leave normal space		Insert comma
eq.#	Equal space between words		Insert apostrophe
‖	Align type vertically	:/	Insert colon
=	Align type horizontally	⊙	Insert period
Sp	Spell out (Wd or 5)	?/	Insert question mark
TR	Transpose letters (words or)		Insert quotation marks
BF	Boldface type		Insert semicolon
ROM	Roman type		Insert hyphen
ITAL	Italic type		Insert em dash
CAP	Capital letter		Insert en dash
LC	Lower case letter		Subscript
SC	Small caps		Superscript
STET	Let it stand	¶	Paragraph indent
WF	Wrong font	no ¶	No indent; run in
			Break; start new line

FIGURE 14-1 Common proofreader's marks.

Proofreading in the Cloud

When several persons are involved in preparing a complex document, proofreading involves one person reviewing and making changes and then sending it to the other author for their concurrence. If changes are made the cycle is repeated. The Cloud has changed the need for the back and forth transferring of a document from one author to another or between the author and an assistant. As of 2012, both Google apps and Microsoft Office 365 apps are available on the Cloud allowing composition of documents on a server that is available to multiple users having access via a password. The Microsoft Office 365 App allows sharing of documents by several users for modification and review, but not interactively. The Google documents sharing feature allows multiple users to change a document interactively during the same session. This makes the proofreading process much simpler and if combined with a conference call, simplifies obtaining agreement on changes to text.

COMPONENTS OF A BUSINESS LETTER

Procedure

The following sections describe the components of most business letters. Procedure 14-1 provides steps for preparing and composing business correspondence. Figure 14-2 graphically illustrates the placement of business letter components, Table 14-3 provides guidelines for preventing errors in letter placement, and Figure 14-3 illustrates how placement can be altered to suit letter size.

PROCEDURE 14-1

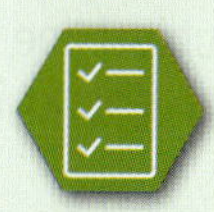
Procedure

Preparing and Composing Business Correspondence Using All Components (Computerized Approach)

PURPOSE:

Prepare and compose a rough draft and final-copy letter using appropriate language and letter style to convey a clear and accurate message to the recipient.

EQUIPMENT/SUPPLIES:

- Computer, word processor and printer
- Printed letterhead and plain second sheet
- Dictionary
- Thesaurus
- Medical dictionary
- Style manual

PROCEDURE STEPS:

1. Organize key points to be addressed in a logical sequence. RATIONALE: To assist in writing an effective letter.
2. Go to Page Setup and set document margins, paper size and source, and layout. ***Paying attention to detail***, set the fonts to be used and paragraph parameters. Name and save the document. RATIONALE: Saves time and loss of formatting.
3. Compose a rough draft of the letter. With time and experience, these outlining steps may be eliminated before drafting the letter. RATIONALE: Business correspondence should be clear, concise, courteous, and accurate. A draft letter aids in checking that the letter is logical and achieves the intended purpose.
4. Use language that is easily understood. State the reason for the letter in the first paragraph and encourage action in the last paragraph. RATIONALE: For communication to take place, both parties must understand the message. The letter must be written so that the recipient understands the language and responds appropriately.
5. Read the draft for obvious errors in grammar, spelling, and punctuation. Use the appropriate reference material (dictionary, style manual, spell check, and so on) to check any inaccuracies. Read again for content. Is the message accurate, logical, and organized appropriately? Save the document again if any changes were made. Lay the letter aside and read it once more at a later time. RATIONALE: Reading several times allows you to concentrate on different elements of the letter. Errors may jump out when reading for the third time.
6. Choose the letter format that is customary to your clinic. Established templates saved on the computer or provided on computer software are time savers. RATIONALE: The letter style should be efficient to prepare and professional in appearance and content to represent the provider-employer in a professional manner.
7. Key in the date or use the computer's auto date feature on line 15 or two to three lines below the letterhead. RATIONALE: Using the component parts of a business letter ensures that the letter is professional in appearance and represents the provider-employer in a professional manner.
8. Key the recipient's name and address flush with the left margin beginning on line 20. RATIONALE: Using the component parts of a business letter ensures that the letter is professional in appearance and represents the provider-employer in a professional manner.
9. On the second line below the recipient's address, key the salutation flush with the left margin. Follow the salutation with a colon. RATIONALE: Using the component parts of a business letter ensures that the letter is professional in appearance and represents the provider-employer in a professional manner.

(continues)

10. Key the subject of the letter on the second line below the salutation flush with the left margin, if the subject line is being used. RATIONALE: Using the component parts of a business letter ensures that the letter is professional in appearance and represents the provider-employer in a professional manner.
11. Begin the body of the letter on the second line below the salutation or subject line. The body format will depend on the style of letter used. For example, if the full block format is used, paragraphs will begin flush with the left margin. Single space within paragraphs; double space between paragraphs. RATIONALE: Using the component parts of a business letter ensures that the letter is professional in appearance and represents the provider–employer in a professional manner.
12. Key the complimentary closure on the second line below the body of the letter. Capitalize only the first letter of the first word of the complimentary closure (e.g., Respectfully yours). RATIONALE: Using the component parts of a business letter ensures that the letter is professional in appearance and represents the provider-employer in a professional manner.
13. Key the signature four to six lines below the complimentary closing. RATIONALE: This ensures that the recipient will be able to determine who sent the letter.
14. If reference initials are used, key the initials two lines below the keyed signature (e.g., WL:jg). RATIONALE: Using the component parts of a business letter ensures that the letter is professional in appearance and represents the provider-employer in a professional manner.
15. Key the enclosure or copy notation one or two lines below the reference initials. RATIONALE: Using the component parts of a business letter ensures that the letter is professional in appearance and represents the provider-employer in a professional manner.
16. ***Paying attention to detail,*** proofread the document and make corrections as necessary. RATIONALE: All information contained in the letter must be accurate and written in a clear and concise manner with logical organization. The grammar, spelling, punctuation, and capitalization must be correct to ensure a professional appearance and represent the provider-employer in a positive manner.
17. Save the document again and print two copies. RATIONALE: The document is saved on the computer, and a copy for signature and mailing is produced. A hard copy for the file is also established.
18. Prepare the envelope. Place the envelope flap over the letter and attach it with a paper clip. RATIONALE: Prepare the envelope using U.S. postal regulations to ensure delivery in a timely manner. Proofread to be sure the address is accurate to ensure deliverability. By placing the envelope flap over the letter and attaching it with a paper clip, the two will not become separated.
19. Place the letter on the provider's desk for review and signature. RATIONALE: The provider's signature signifies the letter is accurate, sends the intended message, and represents the clinic in a professional manner.
20. File a copy of the letter in an appropriate filing system. RATIONALE: May be needed in the future for reference or as documentation.

Date Line

The date is usually **keyed** on line 15 or two to three lines below the letterhead. In keying, data are input by keystrokes on a computer. The date should be completely written out as January 15, 20XX, rather than 1/15/20XX. (If military style is used, the format would be 01 January 20XX.)

Inside Address

The inside address is keyed flush with the left margin. This address may be two, three, or four lines. Some rural areas only require two lines. If the letter is addressed to a provider, the credentials appear after the name. Do not type Dr. John Jones, M.D. (Both Dr. and M.D. are titles; use one or the other.)

Salutation

The salutation is keyed flush with the left margin on the second line below the inside address. A colon follows the salutation. The formal salutation should refer to the receiver of the letter using

1, 1.5, or 2" Margin

Your Name
Street Address
City, State ZIP+4
Area Code and Phone
Email address

1 line

Date

4 lines

SPECIAL NOTATIONS (e.g., **PERSONAL, CONFIDENTIAL, CERTIFIED MAIL**)

1 line

Recipient's Name
Company Name
Company Address

1 line

SUBJECT: (Subject of Letter, e.g., **RESIGNATION, PATIENT NAME ...**)

1 line

Dear (Recipient's Name):

1 line

SUBJECT: (Alternate location for SUBJECT LINE)

1 line

When using block format to write a business letter, all of the information is typed flush with the left margin. When using modified block or indented formats as shown here, your address block and date are five spaces to the right of the page center. The first line of each paragraph is indented 0.5 inch.

1 line

When more than three or four paragraphs are required, headings may be used for each paragraph to help the reader. The headings should be short and capture the key topic of that section of the letter. Headings should be **Boldfaced** or Underlined with the first letter of each word capitalized. Letters that have more than one page should have a heading on each continuation page that gives the name of the addressee, page number, and date.

1 line

After the body of the letter comes the closing, signature block, reference initials, enclosure information, and carbon copy information.

1 line

Sincerely yours,

4 lines

Your Name
Your Title

1 line

YN/TN (Initials of writer and typist)

1 line

cc: (Names receiving copy)

FIGURE 14-2 Placement of business letter components.

title and last name (e.g., "Dear Mr. Marshal:"). If the receiver and sender know each other well, the receiver's first name may be used (e.g., "Dear Jim:").

TABLE 14-3

GUIDELINES FOR LETTER PLACEMENT

The following guidelines are helpful in preventing errors in placement:

1. An imaginary picture frame should surround the letter. Margins may be 1, 1.5, or 2 inches (see Figure 14-3).
2. The last line of the letter should end no less than 1 inch from the bottom of the page.
3. Do not divide the last word on a page.
4. A minimum of three lines should be keyed on the second page of a letter. When dividing a paragraph at the bottom of a page, keep a minimum of two lines on the bottom of the page and two lines at the top of the next page.
5. If using a computer to prepare letters, it is easy to make adjustments to create a professional letter.
6. Use single space within paragraphs.
7. Use double space between paragraphs.

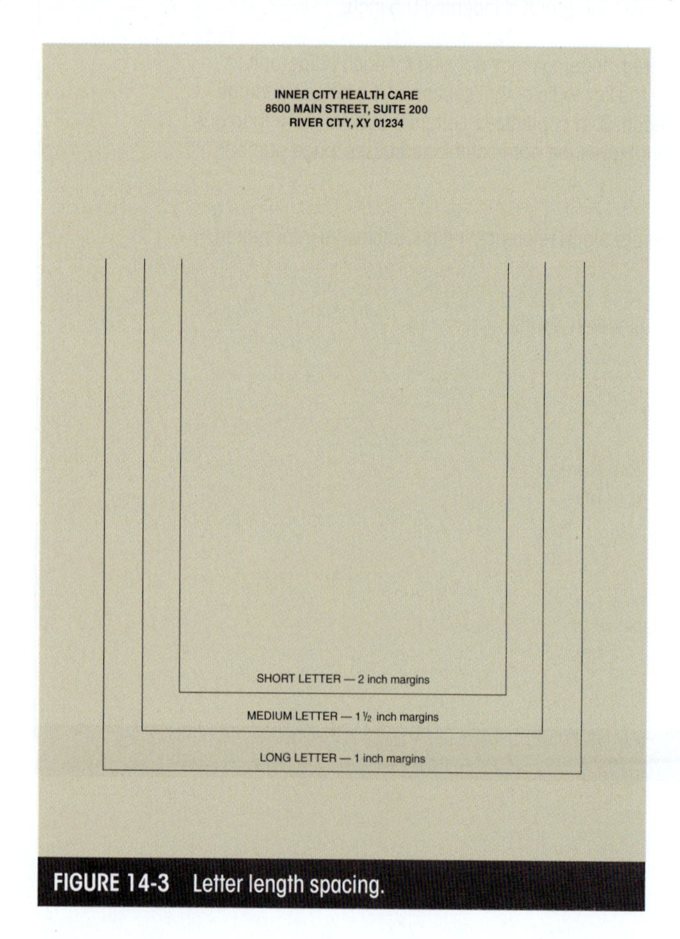

FIGURE 14-3 Letter length spacing.

Subject Line

If used, the subject line is keyed on the second line below the salutation starting at the left margin. This may begin flush with the left margin, indented five spaces, or centered. The patient's name or subject (meeting or topic) may be used on the subject line.

Body of Letter

The body of the letter should begin on the second line below the salutation unless a subject line is used that precedes two lines above the body. The body format will depend on the style of letter used. Paragraphs will begin flush with the left margin in full block letter style, or they may be indented five spaces when using the modified block letter style.

Complimentary Closing

The complimentary closure begins on the second line below the body of the letter. The closure depends on the formality of the letter. Only the first letter of the first word of the complimentary closure is uppercase.

The style used in the complimentary closure should correspond with the salutation (Table 14-4).

Keyed Signature

A keyed signature is a professional courtesy to the reader. Often, a letter is received in which the signature of the sender is not legible. The keyed signature should be at least four lines below the complimentary closing. This space may be lengthened to six lines if you are keying a short letter.

TABLE 14-4

RECOMMENDED COMPLIMENTARY CLOSINGS

LETTER STYLE	COMPLIMENTARY CLOSING
Formal	Respectfully yours or Respectfully
General	Very truly yours or Yours truly or Sincerely or Sincerely yours
Informal (used when reader and writer are on first-name basis)	Regards or Best wishes

Reference Initials

The reference initials used may only be those of the person named in the keyed signature if the same person composed and signed the letter. If reference initials are used, the name of the individual composing the letter should be in uppercase letters with the medical assistant's initials keyed in lowercase letters.

Example:

WL:jg or WL/jg

Enclosure Notation

The enclosure indication can be either one or two lines below the keyed reference initials.

The number of enclosures may be indicated using one of several methods:

- Enclosures
- Enc.
- 1 Enc.
- 2 Enclosures
- Enclosures (2)

Some enclosures should be identified specifically, for example, a check for $84. Enclosures also may be sent under separate cover. If this method is used, state that the enclosure is under separate cover. It may be written as: Enclosure under separate cover: Sarah Jones's medical record.

Copy Notation

If copies of the letter are to be sent to other parties, the copy notation should be one or two lines below the reference initials. The notation *c* (copy) or *pc* (photocopy) should be followed by the name of the person receiving the copy. When more than one person is to receive a copy of the original letter, key *c*: by the first name. Align the other names under the first person identified alphabetically or by rank.

Example:

c: Joseph Brown, MD
John Smith, MD

A **blind copy** notation *bcc*: may be used to send copies of the letter to individuals without the recipient's knowledge. This message is only keyed on the copy of the individual receiving the blind copy. The use of blind copies has decreased and in some practices is no longer used.

Postscripts

Postscripts (abbreviated as P.S.) may be used to:

1. Express an afterthought
2. Identify a thought that has been intentionally deleted from the body of the letter
3. Make a strong significant point

Postscripts are keyed two spaces below reference initials and enclosures.

Continuation Page Heading

There are two methods used to begin the continuation page heading. There should be at least a 1-inch space at the top of each continuing page of the letter. Plain paper matching the color, weight, size, and quality of the letterhead should be used. The following are examples of appropriate continuation page headings.

Example:

(1 inch from top of page)

Jeremy Brown, MD -2- May 4, 20XX

or

Jeremy Brown, MD
Page 2
May 4, 20XX

LETTER STYLES

The administrative medical assistant may be responsible for creating a variety of letters that support the needs of the clinic. Word processing software has business letter and memo templates that are useful in creating these documents.

Communication

One efficient approach to letter composition is to create a **portfolio** or database of frequently used **form letters**. Individualize letters by using the current date and the receiver's name and mailing address. When a form letter is carefully composed and produced, it may not be perceived as a form letter by the recipient.

With the provider-employer's permission, the medical assistant may sign certain letters, including most form letters. Form letters that may be written by the medical assistant include:

- Letters to thank referring providers
- Letters emphasizing to patients criteria for care as directed by the provider
- Letters announcing new insurance or HMOs accepted

- Letters to order supplies or subscriptions
- Letters acknowledging speaking engagements
- Letters to announce vacation schedules or other clinic closures
- Letters to announce new staff
- Letters to remind patients of payment due or notification of collection procedures

Letters prepared for the provider's signature should be placed with an addressed envelope on the provider's desk for review and signature. Place the envelope flap over the letter and attach with a paper clip. Also include with the letter any enclosures for the provider's approval, as well as the patient file (if applicable for paper charts) if it will be needed for reference.

Four major styles of letters are used by medical and professional clinics:

1. Full block
2. Modified block, standard
3. Modified block, indented
4. Simplified

Full Block

The **full block letter** is the most time efficient for the clinic because the medical assistant does not have to use excessive motion to tab indentions or to place address, complimentary close, or keyed signature. When using the full block style, all lines begin flush with the left margin, and mixed punctuation is used (a colon is placed after the salutation and a comma after the complimentary closing). This style is suggested when desiring a contemporary-looking efficient letter.

Modified Block

In the **standard modified block** style letter, all lines begin at the left margin with the exception of the date line, complimentary closure, and keyed signature, which usually begin at the center position or five spaces to the right of center. Figure 14-4 illustrates a modified block style letter without indention.

The assistant may choose to use the **indented modified block** style letter. In this format, the first line of each paragraph may be indented five spaces. Figure 14-5 illustrates a modified block style letter with indented paragraphs.

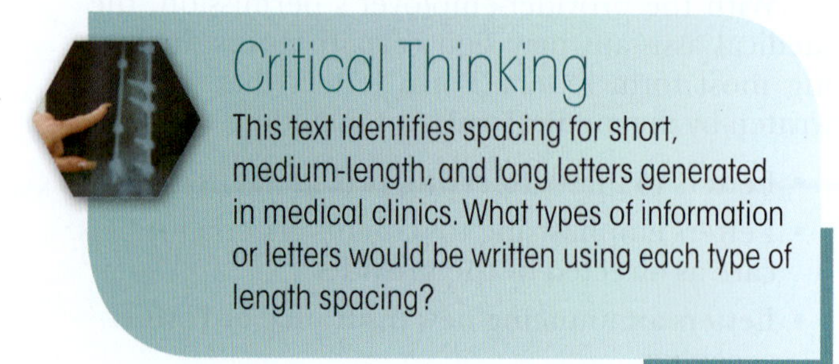

Critical Thinking

This text identifies spacing for short, medium-length, and long letters generated in medical clinics. What types of information or letters would be written using each type of length spacing?

Simplified

The **simplified letter** style omits the salutation and complimentary closure. All lines are keyed (input by keystroke) flush with the left margin. The subject line is keyed in capital letters three lines below the inside address. The body of the letter begins three lines below the subject line. The signature line is keyed in all capital letters four lines below the body of the letter. The Administrative Management Society recommends this style of letter. However, in medical clinics, this style is most often used when sending a form letter. Figure 14-6 illustrates a simplified style letter.

SUPPLIES FOR WRITTEN COMMUNICATION

Begin written communication at the computer workstation by checking to see that all supplies required to prepare the document are at hand. Check the computer settings and turn the printer on. Load the correct letter stock paper into the printer when the document is ready to be printed. The paper should be **bond**, of good quality, and at least 20 to 24 pound stock with a watermark. A **watermark** is legible when paper is held to the light. Choose a shade of white, cream, or gray bond paper.

Although colored paper may be more eye-catching, it does not display a professional image. Also, be sure that the paper stock is compatible with printers used in the clinic.

Letterhead

The letterhead style and design is usually chosen by the provider(s) and may include a specially designed logo for the practice. The provider/practice name, street address or post office box number, city, state, ZIP code, and telephone number with area code are usually printed on the letterhead. Many clinics also add their fax number and email address. Letterhead information may be placed at either side or in the center of the paper.

Second Sheets

When an order is placed for letterhead, the medical assistant should order additional plain paper

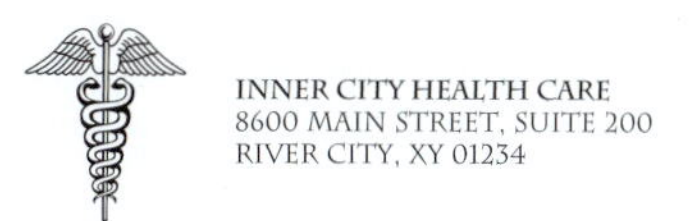

January 12, 20XX (approximately 15th line)

Jeremy Brown, MD (approximately 20th line)
111 S Main
Blossom, UT 10283-1120

Dear Dr. Brown:

SUBJECT: Blossom Medical Society Meeting

Thank you for inviting me to speak at the Blossom Medical Society Meeting June 15, 20XX. As requested, my topic will describe the use of MRI in assisting physicians to make a more accurate diagnosis without resorting to invasive procedures. The exact title of my speech will be sent by next Friday.

Please have your clinic manager send information regarding the number of participants expected, time of meeting, location, and any other details that will assist me in preparing my speech.

I will write or call if I have any additional questions.

Yours truly,

Winston Lewis, MD

Winston Lewis, MD

WL:ea

Enclosure: Handout on MRI

FIGURE 14-4 Sample standard modified block style letter; all elements start at left margin, except date, complimentary closing, and keyed signature.

of the same stock as the letterhead to be used for second page sheets. The number of sheets will vary from clinic to clinic. If providers normally dictate long letters, this must be taken into consideration when ordering quantities.

Printing Multipage Business Letters

Printing multipage business letters on letterhead stationery requires use of more than one tray in the printer, unless you want to collate the letterhead or hand feed it into the printer. The simplest procedure is to place the letterhead stationery into a tray other than the default tray. Then go to File, Page Setup, Paper Source, and from the menu that appears, specify the tray containing the letterhead stationery. The menu lets you choose the tray for the first page and the tray for the rest of the document. Make sure that the Apply To box is set for Whole Document.

Envelopes

The stock and quality of the envelopes should match the stationery used in the clinic. The address should be standardized so that it contains all delivery address elements. The correct name, city, state, and ZIP+4 codes must be used so that mail is processed efficiently and effectively.

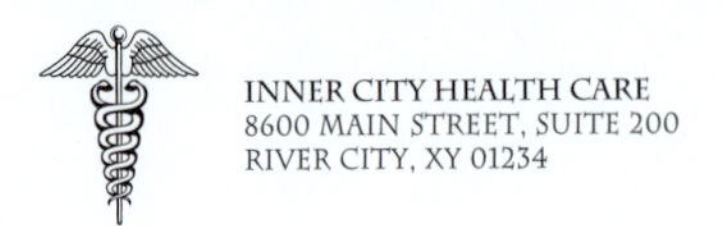
INNER CITY HEALTH CARE
8600 MAIN STREET, SUITE 200
RIVER CITY, XY 01234

January 12, 20XX (approximately 15th line)

Jeremy Brown, MD (approximately 20th line)
111 S Main
Blossom, UT 10283-1120

Dear Dr. Brown:

Blossom Medical Society Meeting

Thank you for inviting me to speak at the Blossom Medical Society Meeting June 15, 20XX. As requested, my topic will describe the use of MRI in assisting physicians to make a more accurate diagnosis without resorting to invasive procedures. The exact title of my speech will be sent by next Friday.

Please have your clinic manager send information regarding the number of participants expected, time of meeting, location, and any other details that will assist me in preparing my speech.

I will write or call if I have any additional questions.

Yours truly,

Winston Lewis, MD

Winston Lewis, MD

WL:ea

Enclosure: Handout on MRI

FIGURE 14-5 Sample modified block style letter with indented paragraphs. This format is the same as the standard modified except that the subject line and paragraphs are not left-justified.

Example:

JEREMY BROWN MD
111 S MAIN
BLOSSOM UT 10283-1120

If Dr. Brown uses a post office box for the delivery of his mail, that address should be used. The postal service delivers to the last line before the city, state, and ZIP+4 code.

Example:

JEREMY BROWN MD
PO BOX 1453
BLOSSOM UT 10283-1120

Place the intended delivery address on the line immediately above the city, state, and ZIP+4 code. The other address may be placed on a separate line above the delivery line.

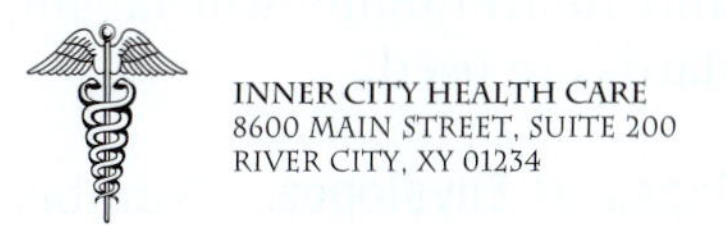

INNER CITY HEALTH CARE
8600 MAIN STREET, SUITE 200
RIVER CITY, XY 01234

January 12, 20XX (approximately 15th line)

Jeremy Brown, MD (approximately 20th line)
111 S Main
Blossom, UT 10283-1120

(triple-space)

SUBJECT: BLOSSOM MEDICAL SOCIETY MEETING

(triple-space)

Thank you for inviting me to speak at the Blossom Medical Society Meeting June 15, 20XX. As requested, my topic will describe the use of MRI in assisting physicians to make a more accurate diagnosis without resorting to invasive procedures. The exact title of my speech will be sent by next Friday.

Please have your clinic manager send information regarding the number of participants expected, time of meeting, location, and any other details that will assist me in preparing my speech.

I will write or call if I have any additional questions.

Winston Lewis, MD (4 line spaces)

WINSTON LEWIS, MD

WL:ea

Enclosure: Handout on MRI

FIGURE 14-6 The simplified style letter has no salutation or complimentary closing. The subject line and keyed signature are all upper case.

Example:

JEREMY BROWN MD
111 S MAIN
PO BOX 1453
BLOSSOM UT 10283-1120

This letter would be received at the post office box, not the street address.

General Standards for Addressing Envelopes. **Optical character recognition (OCR)** is a type of software that recognizes and decodes characters written on envelopes. The U.S. Postal Service uses OCR that recognizes various types of machine print, hand-print, and cursive styles. This automates the reading of most addresses on envelopes, although the Postal Service estimates that 30 million pieces of hand-written envelopes must still be decoded and delivered every day. The U.S. Postal Service suggests that the address on letter mail be machine-printed with a uniform left margin. It should be formatted in a manner that allows an OCR to recognize the information and find a match in its address files.

A scanner reads the ZIP code on the bottom line and prints a bar code in the lower right corner of the envelope. Envelopes that are handwritten cannot be read by the OCR. These letters must wait for more costly and slower manual sorting.

To conform to standards, eliminate all punctuation in the envelope address with the exception of a hyphen in the ZIP+4 code. Leave a minimum of one space between the city name and two-character state abbreviations and the ZIP+4 code. The OCR can read a combination of uppercase and lowercase characters in addresses but prefers all uppercase characters (see Procedure 14-2).

Dark ink on a light background using uppercase letters is the suggested method in preparing a keyed address. There should be a uniform left margin on all lines of the address. An imaginary rectangle that extends ⅝ to 2¾ inches from the bottom of the envelope with 1 inch on each side should contain the address. The lower right edge should be kept free of any marks. This area will contain the bar code, whether it is preapplied or printed by an OCR. The bar code area is ⅝ inch from the bottom and 4½ inches from the right side of the envelope.

The U.S. Postal Service publishes several pamphlets and booklets that describe the format to be used when sending any mail. Check with the postal service regarding the latest publications. Service and deliverability will be improved if these standards are used.

Types of Envelopes. Number 6¾ and number 10 are the envelopes most often used. A window envelope may also be used, especially when mailing statements.

Number	Size
6¾	6½" long × 3" wide
10	9½" long × 4" wide
7	7½" long × 3" wide

See Figure 14-7 for an example of an envelope with the suggested zone sizes for OCR reading. The address on the statement need only be keyed once. The entire address is capitalized with no punctuation. Only one space should be used between the state abbreviation and the ZIP code. When this statement is folded with the address in view, it may be inserted into a window envelope. Make certain that the entire address is visible through the window.

PROCEDURE 14-2

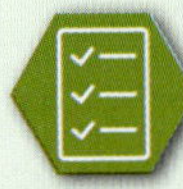

Addressing Envelopes According to U.S. Postal Regulations

PURPOSE:

To address envelopes according to U.S. Postal Service regulations to ensure timely delivery.

EQUIPMENT/SUPPLIES:

- Computer or word processor and printer with envelope tray
- Envelopes
- Address labels
- U.S. Postal Service Publication 221, *Addressing for Success*

PROCEDURE STEPS:

1. Insert the envelope in the printer and select the envelope format from the software program. When using a word processor or computer, labels may be used rather than printing directly on the envelope. The label is then adhered to the envelope. Many printers have an envelope tray and software that will transfer the address from the letter to the envelope. This feature is a time saver because you key the address only once. RATIONALE: U.S. postal regulations suggest that the address on letter mail should be machine printed, with a uniform left margin.
2. Visualize an imaginary rectangle on the envelope. The rectangle extends 5/8 inch to 2¾ inches from the bottom of the envelope, with 1 inch on each side. The address is placed within this rectangle (Figure 14-7). RATIONALE: U.S. postal regulations suggest that the address on letter mail should be machine printed, with a uniform left margin.

(continues)

3. Key the address in uppercase letters. Be sure to maintain a uniform left margin on all lines. Eliminate all punctuation in the address except the hyphen in the ZIP+4 code. RATIONALE: Leave a minimum of one space between the city name and the two-character state abbreviation and the ZIP+4 code. A scanner reads the ZIP+4 code on the bottom line and prints a bar code in the lower right corner of the envelope. The OCR prefers all uppercase characters.
4. If you are not using preprinted envelopes, key the return address in uppercase letters in the upper left corner of the envelope. Include the name on the first line; address on the second line; and city, state, and ZIP+4 code on the third line. RATIONALE: The return address should be printed in the upper left corner of the envelope should the letter need to be returned to the sender for any reason.
5. ***Paying attention to detail***, proofread the envelope and make corrections as necessary. RATIONALE: When all information is correct, processing will take place efficiently and correctly.

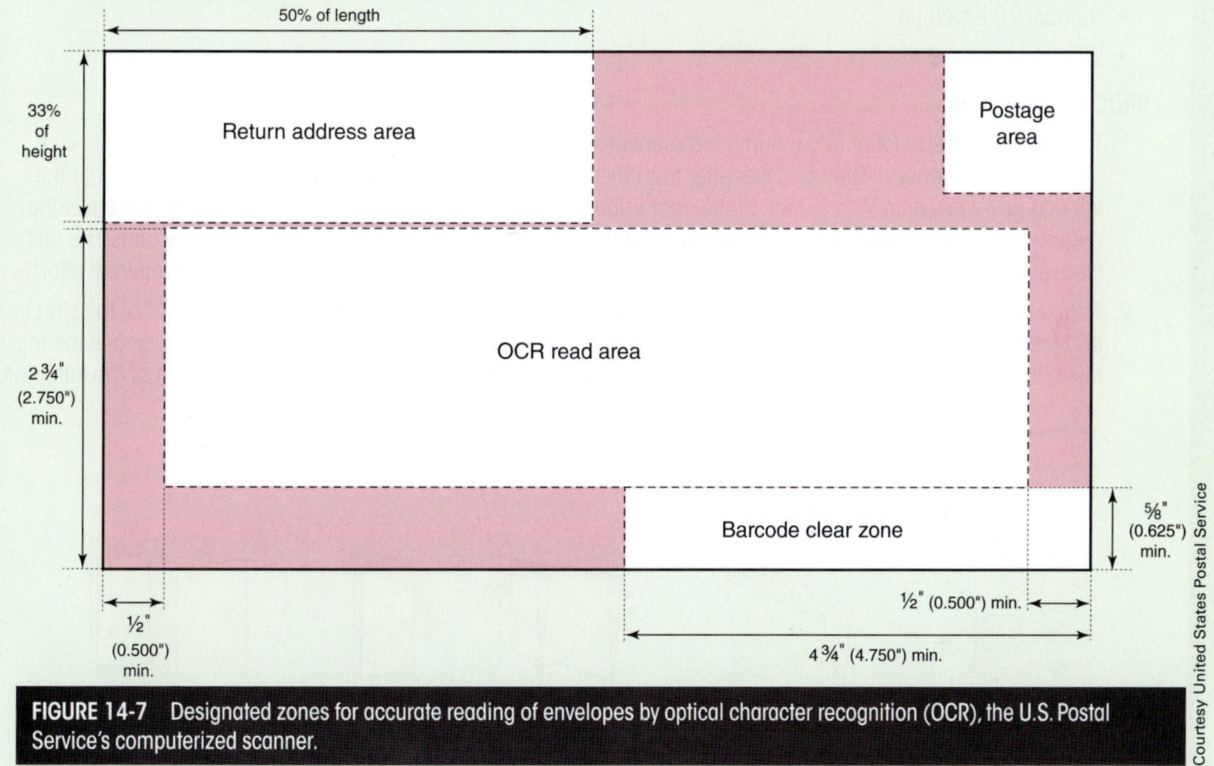

FIGURE 14-7 Designated zones for accurate reading of envelopes by optical character recognition (OCR), the U.S. Postal Service's computerized scanner.

To prepare envelopes for mailing, lay all envelopes facing upward in a row with the flaps displayed. Moisten all the envelopes with a sponge. With the dominant hand, seal the flap; with the nondominant hand, push the envelope aside while the next flap is closed. Procedure 14-3 illustrates letter folding and placement of envelopes for closure. The use of premoistened or peel-off strips helps speed up the process.

Mail Merge

Mail Merge lets you create form letters, envelopes, or mailing labels using data from a data source. You would use this feature to send mailings to your client base or to a list of prospects, among others. Mail Merge permits sending a form letter with envelopes to hundreds of recipients in a matter of minutes.

The client names and addresses are first stored in a Mail Merge data source, which can be a table or database such as Microsoft Excel. For Microsoft Word, a Mail Merge data source can be created by selecting Mail Merge in the Tools menu, selecting Mail Merge Helper, and following the instructions given in Helper. Almost all word processor programs let you carry out a Mail Merge with an external database. You will need to consult the program manual for details.

PROCEDURE 14-3

Folding Letters for Standard Envelopes

PURPOSE:

To fold and insert letters into envelopes so that the letters fit properly in the envelopes.

EQUIPMENT/SUPPLIES:

- Letters to be mailed
- Number 6¾ envelope
- Number 10 envelope
- Window envelope

PROCEDURE STEPS:

1. To fit a standard-size letter into a number 6¾ envelope, fold the letter up from the bottom, leaving ¼ to ½ inch at the top, and crease it. Then fold the letter from the right edge about one third the width of the letter. Fold the left edge over to within ¼ to ½ inch of the right-edge crease. Insert the left creased edge first into the envelope (Figure 14-8A). RATIONALE: Ensures a proper fit of the letter into the envelope with a minimum of folds. The last crease made enters the envelope first. This enables the recipient to begin to read the letter with minimal effort.
2. To fit a standard-size letter into a number 10 envelope, fold the letter up about one third the length of the sheet and crease it. Then fold the top of the letter down to within ¼ to ½ inch of the bottom crease, and crease the top. Insert the top creased edge first into the envelope (Figure 14-8B). RATIONALE: Ensures a proper fit of the letter into

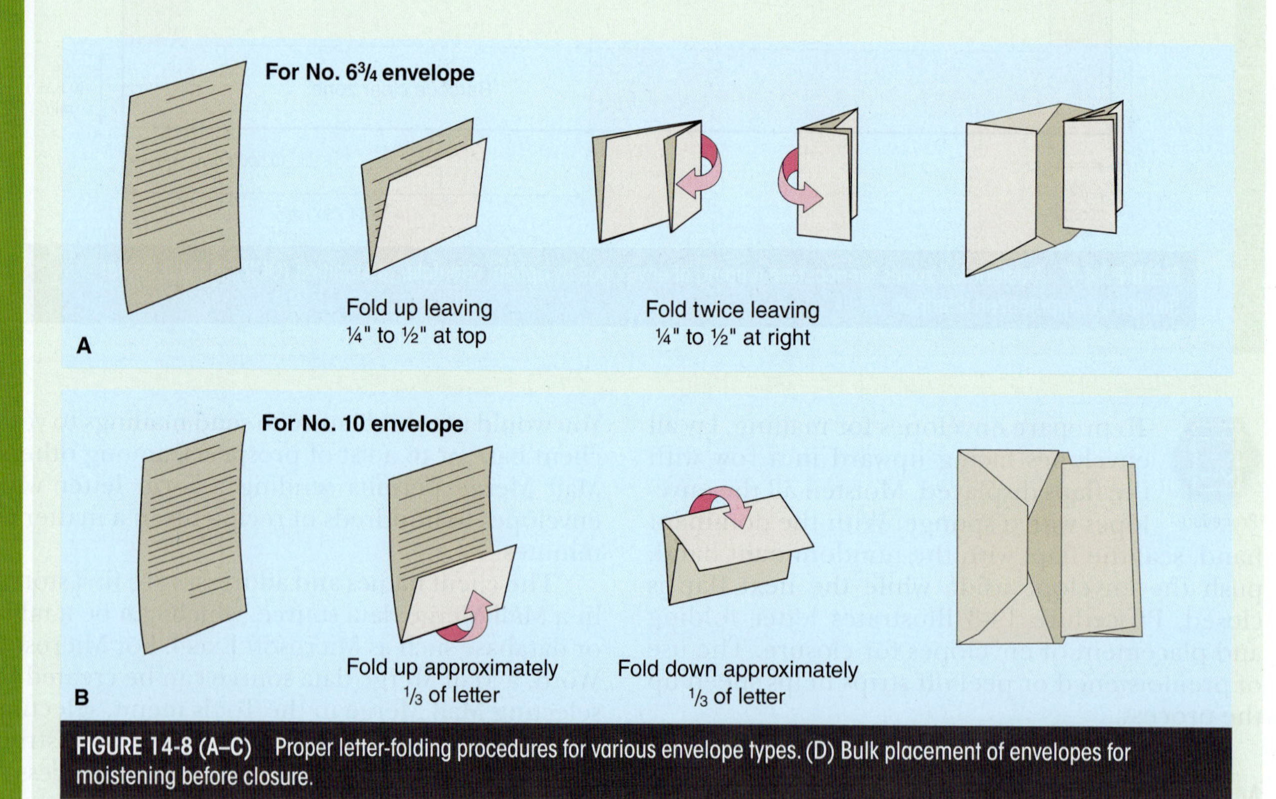

FIGURE 14-8 (A–C) Proper letter-folding procedures for various envelope types. (D) Bulk placement of envelopes for moistening before closure.

(continues)

the envelope with a minimum of folds. The last crease made enters the envelope first. This enables the recipient to begin to read the letter with minimal effort.

3. To fit a standard-size letter into a window envelope, turn the letter over and fold the top of the letter up about one third the length of the page so that the address is facing you. Then fold the bottom of the letter back to the first crease. Insert the letter into the envelope bottom first (Figure 14-8C). ***Paying attention to detail,*** you should be able to read the entire address through the window. RATIONALE: Ensures that the entire address can be read through the window envelope and be delivered correctly.
4. Place envelopes as shown in Figure 14-8D to moisten before sealing. RATIONALE: Provides efficient method of sealing multiple letters for mailing.

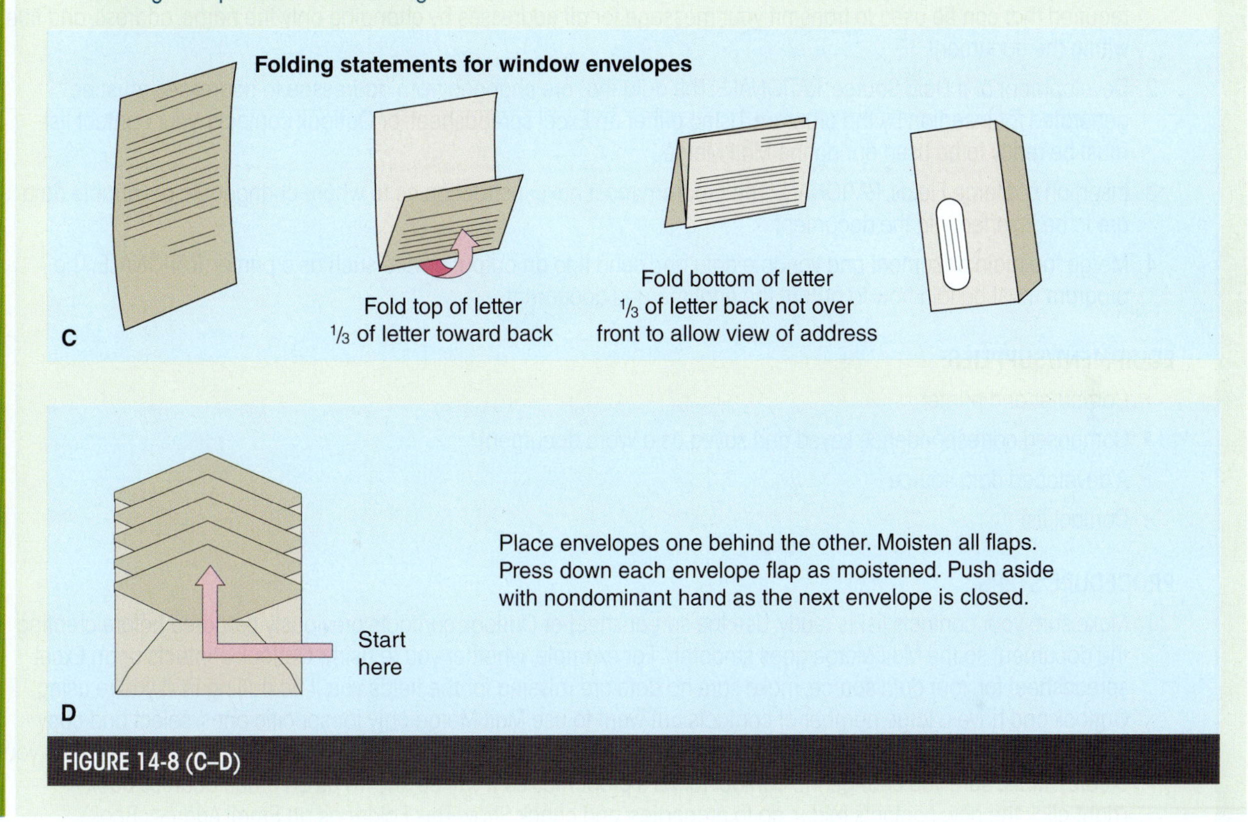

FIGURE 14-8 (C–D)

Separate fields are suggested in the database for first name, last name, title, address, city, state, and postal code. To preclude time-consuming changes, three fields should be used for address, to accommodate clients with complex addresses. If a field is not required, leave it blank.

The Mail Merge Helper will give you the choice of editing the main document. Compose the document you want to send, and for each field where you want a new name or address, select Insert Merge Field, and then select the name of the field you want to insert. You are now ready to print the form letters. Select Mail > Merge-Mail > Mail Merge Helper from the Tools menu and select Printer from the Merge To box. Your printer should show the documents in the queue. Procedure 14-4 gives step-by-step instructions for using Mail Merge.

OTHER TYPES OF CORRESPONDENCE

Other specialized types of correspondence the medical assistant may be involved in preparing include memoranda, meeting agendas, and meeting minutes.

Memoranda

A type of interoffice correspondence is the **memorandum**, or **memo** for short. The use of memos permits messages to be sent quickly and without

PROCEDURE 14-4

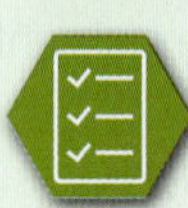
Procedure

Creating a Mass Mailing Using Mail Merge

PURPOSE:

To create a mass mailing using the computer's Mail Merge Helper feature contained within Microsoft Word. The procedure consists of four steps:

1. Create a generic main document to be sent to different addressees. RATIONALE: A clear and concise document is required that can be used to transmit your message for all addresses by changing only the name, address, and title within the document.
2. Development of a Data Source. RATIONALE: The data that are changed from addressee to addressee must be generated for insertion by the program. Using either an Excel spreadsheet, or Outlook contacts, your contact list must be ready to be used during the Mail Merge.
3. Insertion of Merge Fields. RATIONALE: The program must have instruction as to where changeable or variable data are to be inserted into the document.
4. Merge the main document and variable data and send it to an output device such as a printer. RATIONALE: The program must be told how to output the final merged document.

EQUIPMENT/SUPPLIES:

- Computer and printer
- Composed correspondence keyed and saved as a Word document
- A developed data source
- Contact list

PROCEDURE STEPS:

1. Make sure your contacts list is ready. Use the spreadsheet or Outlook contacts previously prepared before creating the document so the Mail Merge goes smoothly. For example, whether you're using Outlook contacts or an Excel spreadsheet for your data source, make sure no data are missing for the fields you'll be pulling in. If you're using Outlook and have a large number of contacts but want to use Mail Merge only for specific ones, select and copy those contacts to a new folder. (To do this, select the contacts, right-click, choose Move and then Copy to Folder you create). Make sure you change the contact folder's properties so it will be shown as an email address book (right-click the new contacts folder, go to properties, and check Show This Folder as an Email Address Book).
2. Create a new blank document in Word.
3. Navigate to the Mailings tab.
4. Click Start Mail Merge and select your document type by selecting Letters.
5. Click Select Recipients and choose to create a new list, use an existing list, or choose from Outlook contacts.
   a. If you select Use an Existing List, you will be asked to browse to the file on your computer and then confirm the data table.
   b. If you select Choose from Outlook Contacts, you'll be asked to choose the Outlook contact folder and then add or remove recipients from the merge. Therefore, it is advised in step 1 to create a new contacts folder for your Mail Merge, so you will not have to scroll through all of your contacts in this small box.
6. Create the content for your document and insert the placeholders. When you get to the part where information is obtained and needs to be personalized from your data source, insert a placeholder with either the Insert Merge Field button or one of the two shortcuts Word offers for common fields: Address Block and Greeting Line.

(continues)

7. Use the Address Block shortcut. As the name suggests, Address Block creates a placeholder for a name and address, which is useful when creating letters, mailing labels, or envelopes. With both the Address Block and Greeting Line shortcuts, you'll be able to specify what gets inserted and preview what it will look like.
8. If the preview seems to be missing information, click Match Fields to tell Word where the data are for the missing fields. When the preview looks good, click OK, and Word will insert the address placeholder.
9. If applicable, insert other fields into your document. For other placeholders you might need, click on Insert Merge Field and select the field you want to insert at that point in the document.
10. Click Preview Results to preview the merge results after the document is finished and all fields are inserted.
11. If all looks good, click Finish & Merge and you can print individual documents, send them as email messages, or edit each individual document as needed.
12. Repeat this for other types of documents using Mail Merge. In addition to letters (which can be any sort of document), emails, envelopes, labels, or directories may be selected as the document type. Word also has a Step-by-Step Mail Merge Wizard (click the Mailings tab and then Start Mail Merge), which walks you through the process above.

labor-intensive preparation. The memo format may already be preformatted on your computer software. If not, it is easy to design your own memo format.

The side margins should be set for 1 inch. Begin to key the memo heading 2 inches from the top of the page (line 13). The heading includes the words *date, to, from,* and *subject,* which should be boldfaced and capitalized. The words should each be keyed on a separate line with a double space between each line. By setting a tab stop 10 spaces in from the left margin, you will be able to tab to each entry and clear the headings to add the appropriate information. Triple space after the entry for the subject heading.

The body of the memo may begin at the left margin or may be set 10 spaces in so that the text starts directly beneath the typed headings. No salutation is required in a memo. Figure 14-9 provides a sample memo.

DATE: August 25, 20XX (key heading 2 inches from top of page, line 13)

TO: Staff of Inner City Health Care (embolden and capitalize headings and double space between them)

FROM: Marilyn Johnson, Clinic Manager

SUBJECT: Vacation Schedule (triple space after the subject)

Doctors Lewis & King will be on vacation January 1–15. Please do not schedule appointments during that time for either doctor. Clinic personnel should report to work as usual. During this two-week period, we will be preparing for the annual audit.

FIGURE 14-9 Sample memorandum.

Meeting Agendas

Most meetings operate by following *Robert's Rules of Order, Newly Revised* as their parliamentary authority. The outlined order of business is as follows:

- Reading and approval of the minutes
- Reports of officers, boards, and standing committees
- Reports of special committees (ad hoc)
- Special orders
- Unfinished business and general orders
- New business
- Date and time of next scheduled meeting

The **agenda** lists the specific items that the group plans to discuss at the meeting under each of the above-mentioned divisions. The medical assistant preparing the agenda must determine the topics that are to be discussed. Copies of the agenda should be sent to each group member before the meeting date, and extra copies should be taken to the meeting for those who may have misplaced or forgotten to bring the agenda with them to the meeting. Figure 14-10 provides a sample meeting agenda.

Meeting Minutes

A written record of what transpired during a meeting is called the **minutes**. The minutes should record what business actions were taken during

AGENDA
STAFF MEETING
Tuesday, September 1, 20XX
Location–Conference Room

Reading and approval of last months' minutes
Reports
  Risk Management Committee
  Personnel
Unfinished business
  Purchase of new X-ray machine
New business
  Doctors Lewis & King vacation January 1–15
  Annual audit
Date and time for next meeting
Adjournment

FIGURE 14-10 Sample meeting agenda.

the meeting, who made each motion and what it was, who seconded the motion, any pertinent discussion, and whether the motion was passed. In the medical clinic, a designated person will take the minutes during a meeting, and then prepare the data for approval and documentation. In some cases, the clinic may rotate the responsibility of taking of minutes among staff members.

The first paragraph of the minutes should contain the following information:

- Kind of meeting (regular, special, emergency)
- Name of the group or association
- Date, time, and place of the meeting
- Who officiated at the meeting and names of members present and absent
- Whether the previous meeting minutes were read and approved

The body of the minutes should include a paragraph discussing each subject matter or each item listed on the agenda. All motions should be recorded including the exact wording of the motion, the name of the person making the motion, the person seconding the motion, and whether the motion passed or failed. If the meeting had a guest speaker, the speaker's name and title and the subject of the presentation may be included in the minutes.

The last paragraph should contain the next meeting date, time, and place and the time of adjournment for this meeting. The person recording the minutes should sign them, and a copy of all minutes should be maintained in a notebook designated for that purpose. The minutes can also be scanned and saved to a hard drive or backup location. It is important that reliable backup is maintained, in two separate places, of all important documentation, especially if the originals are destroyed. Corporations are required to have regular meetings with recorded minutes for legal purposes. Figure 14-11 provides a sample of recorded minutes.

PROCESSING INCOMING AND OUTGOING MAIL

The management of written communications also involves developing procedures for sorting, distributing, and otherwise processing incoming mail. It also includes posting and shipping outgoing items by the most cost- and time-effective method.

Incoming Mail and Shipments

All mail should be sorted by type before opening. Incoming mail includes telegrams, faxes, certified or registered letters, personal letters, emails, checks from patients, insurance forms, invoices, medical journals, newspapers, magazines for the reception area, and advertisements regarding equipment and supplies.

Once it is categorized, incoming mail is directed to the appropriate personnel in the clinic. Checks from patients and invoices may be distributed to the bookkeeper, insurance forms to the insurance clerk, medical journals and advertisements can be placed on the provider's desk, and magazines and newspapers can be placed in the reception area.

Integrity

Personal or confidential letters should not be opened unless the medical assistant has been given this responsibility by the provider or clinic manager.

Use a letter opener to open all mail before taking out the contents and reading the document. After removing the contents:

- Stamp or write the date it was received in the clinic in the area of the document designated for this notation.
- If the address is not included on the letter, write the address on the letter, as identified on the envelope or on the bank check (if a patient is making a payment).
- When a colored reply envelope is sent with the statement to the patient, payments returned in these envelopes can speed up the sorting process.

STAFF MEETING MINUTES

The monthly staff meeting of Inner City Health Care was held Tuesday, September 1, 20XX, in the conference room. The meeting was called to order by Marilyn Johnson, Clinic Manager. Those members present included: Dr. Lewis, Dr. King, Walter Seals, Nancy McFarland, Ellen Armstrong, Joe Guerrero, Gwen Carr, and Thomas Myers.

The previous meeting's minutes were read and approved as published.

Gwen Carr, CMA (AAMA), heading the Risk Management Committee, reported that a thorough walk-through of the clinic had taken place to assess safety issues. It was determined that the pull cords on the blinds could pose a potential hazard to small children. Gwen made a motion that the blinds be upgraded with new vinyl louvered blinds with the plastic rod-type louver adjuster. Nancy McFarland seconded the motion. After discussion, a unanimous vote was cast to replace the blinds at the earliest time possible.

Walter Seals, Human Resource Manager, announced that he would be posting an opening for a CMA (AAMA) to work in the lab. All staff personnel were asked to share information about this opening with professionals who might be interested in working at Inner City Health Care.

Discussion was presented by Doctors Lewis & King regarding the purchase of a new X-ray machine. A committee consisting of Nancy McFarland, Joe Guerrero, and Thomas Myers was appointed to investigate the specific needs of the clinic and to locate appropriate vendors. They will present their findings at the next scheduled staff meeting.

New business items include the fact that Doctors Lewis & King will be on vacation January 1–15, 20XX. We are asked to not schedule appointments for them during that time.

Marilyn Johnson discussed preparations for the annual audit during the vacation period of Doctors Lewis & King. She will provide a schedule and timeline at the next staff meeting.

The next scheduled meeting will be October 3 at 12:30 PM in the conference room.

The meeting adjourned at 1:45 PM.

Ellen Armstrong

FIGURE 14-11 Sample meeting minutes.

- Look into the envelope to make certain that all contents have been removed.
- Attach the letter to the envelope with a paper clip, preferably on the left side.

Reply promptly to all requests, answering letters according to date of arrival; emergency situations need to be managed immediately.

Outgoing Mail and Shipments

Before placing postage on outgoing mail, weigh the item to be mailed, using a manual or electronic scale. A manual scale will read ounces. The assistant will then affix the appropriate postage, either stamps or postal meter. An electronic scale will automatically display the correct postage. If your clinic has a postal meter, this should be used to expedite mail. Metered mail does not have to be canceled or postmarked at the post office.

Procedure

A postage meter is leased or purchased from a manufacturing company recommended by the postal service. However, the postage meter must be taken to the

Critical Thinking

For the next week, practice sorting and prioritizing your personal incoming mail. If you live with others, ask permission to sort their mail and deliver it to them. Follow procedures outlined in this chapter. Write a paragraph about what you have learned by completing this exercise and how this experience might translate to a medical facility.

post office to purchase postage. The meter is locked for the amount of postage purchased. Clinics that send a large volume of mail may purchase a postage meter. Procedure 14-5 provides steps for preparing outgoing mail.

Postal Classes

The Postal Service provides a range of mail classes and pricing to accommodate most user needs. Visit http://www.usps.com and use the Calculate a Price tool to find prices for mailing various mailing pieces (envelopes, boxes, etc.) from one ZIP code to another.

Formats for Efficient Mail Processing

Certified and registered markings should be placed below the stamp or approximately nine lines from the right top edge of the envelope. *Personal* or *confidential* notation should be keyed in all caps three lines below the return address. Adherence to other regulations will ensure accurate, timely delivery.

ZIP+4. ZIP+4 consists of the basic five ZIP code digits followed by a hyphen and four additional digits. The use of ZIP+4 will expedite the delivery of mail. If the envelope has been prepared properly to be read through OCR, the digits will be converted to a bar code. This piece of mail then goes to the bar code sorter, which rapidly sorts for the final destination.

Abbreviations. When addressing mail, use the abbreviations for states and U.S. possessions (Figure 14-12) and use official postal service abbreviations for street suffixes, directionals, and locators (Figure 14-13).

International Mail

Classes of international mail include letters and letter packages, postcards and postal cards,

PROCEDURE 14-5

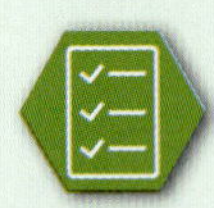

Procedure

Preparing Outgoing Mail According to U.S. Postal Regulations

PURPOSE:

To prepare outgoing mail for expeditious delivery.

EQUIPMENT/SUPPLIES:

- Manual or electronic scale
- Postage meter or stamps
- Envelope or package to be mailed

PROCEDURE STEPS:

1. Sort the mail according to postal class. For example, all single-piece letters that weigh less than 11 ounces are included in first-class mail. Correspondence and statements are sent in this classification. RATIONALE: Sorting by postal class expedites processing at the post office.
2. Using the manual or electronic scale, weigh the item to be mailed. ***Paying attention to detail***, if you are using a manual scale, read the weight in ounces and compute the amount of postage due. If you are using an electronic scale, the correct postage will be displayed on the scale. RATIONALE: Correct postage on each postal item is essential to ensure faster delivery service.
3. Using a postal meter or stamps, affix the appropriate postage to the piece to be mailed. Use of a postal meter expedites delivery of mail because metered mail does not have to be canceled or postmarked at the post office. RATIONALE: Correct postage on each postal item is essential to ensure faster delivery service.
4. Place the prepared mail in the area of the clinic designated for outgoing mail or deliver the mail to the post office according to clinic policy. RATIONALE: Ensures that all mail going out is centrally located and that the postal worker can pick up outgoing mail and deliver incoming mail efficiently.

AL	Alabama	NE	Nebraska
AK	Alaska	NV	Nevada
AS	American Samoa	NH	New Hampshire
AZ	Arizona	NJ	New Jersey
AR	Arkansas	NM	New Mexico
CA	California	NY	New York
CO	Colorado	NC	North Carolina
CT	Connecticut	ND	North Dakota
DE	Delaware	MP	No. Mariana Islands
DC	Dist. of Columbia	OH	Ohio
FL	Florida	OK	Oklahoma
GA	Georgia	OR	Oregon
GU	Guam	PA	Pennsylvania
HI	Hawaii	PR	Puerto Rico
ID	Idaho	RI	Rhode Island
IL	Illinois	SC	South Carolina
IN	Indiana	SD	South Dakota
IA	Iowa	TN	Tennessee
KS	Kansas	TX	Texas
KY	Kentucky	TT	Trust Territory
LA	Louisiana	UT	Utah
ME	Maine	VT	Vermont
MD	Maryland	VI	Virgin Islands, U.S.
MA	Massachusetts	VA	Virginia
MI	Michigan	WA	Washington
MN	Minnesota	WV	West Virginia
MS	Mississippi	WI	Wisconsin
MO	Missouri	WY	Wyoming
MT	Montana		

FIGURE 14-12 Abbreviations for states, territories, and the District of Columbia.

aerograms (airmail letters), printed matter, direct sacks of printed matter, matter for people who are blind, small packets, and parcel post. Special services such as insurance, recorded delivery, registered mail, restricted delivery, return receipt, special delivery, cash on delivery mail, and certified mail are also available. For the most current information on rates and services, inquire at the local postal service.

AVE	Avenue	PL	Place
BLVD	Boulevard	RD	Road
CT	Court	STA	Station
CTR	Center	ST	Street
CIR	Circle	TPKE	Turnpike
DR	Drive	VLY	Valley
EXPY	Expressway		
HTS	Heights	APT	Apartment
HWY	Highway	RM	Room
IS	Island	STE	Suite
JCT	Junction	PLZ	Plaza
LK	Lake	N	North
LN	Lane	E	East
MTN	Mountain	S	South
PKY	Parkway	W	West

FIGURE 14-13 Abbreviations for street suffixes, directionals, and locators.

LEGAL AND ETHICAL ISSUES

Written communication, no matter what form is used, must take into consideration legal and ethical issues. A copy of all written communication should be maintained in the patient medical record or in clinic files should it be needed at a later date.

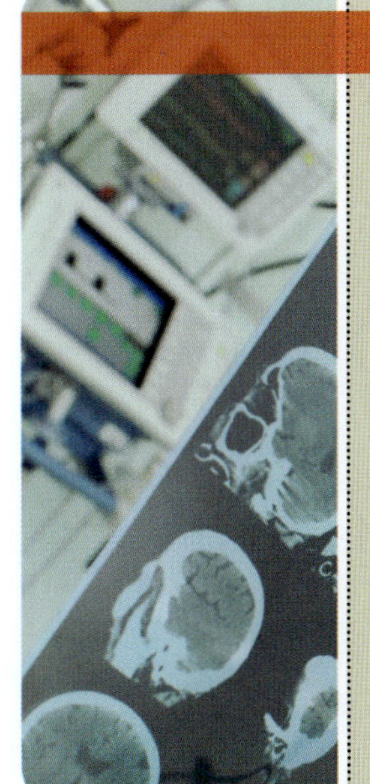

CASE STUDY 14-1

Refer to the scenario at the beginning of the chapter.

When she was assembling the style manual for all written communications generated by Inner City Health Care, clinic manager Marilyn Johnson wanted it to be as comprehensive as possible. Therefore, she gathered research over a period of months, noting problems the clinic had experienced in written communications, such as letters going out without the provider's signature. She became familiar with proofreading devices that would ensure letter-perfect correspondence. She also developed source materials on the different classes of mail and the services of the U.S. Postal Service.

CASE STUDY REVIEW

1. Marilyn is ready to outline the manual. Review the chapter information and create an outline indicating major topic headings for the Inner City Health Care style manual.
2. Because a few of the medical assistants are not comfortable with composing, what writing tips can Marilyn include to make them more confident?
3. Marilyn wants all letters to look alike. What information should she include to educate the manual users about the components of a standard letter?

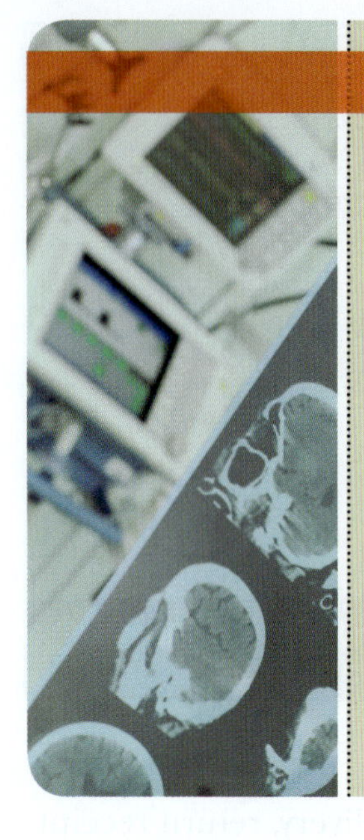

CASE STUDY 14-2

Inner City Health Care is considering adopting the use of clinical email because many of their patients have home computers and use email in their day-to-day communications. Clinic manager Marilyn Johnson is concerned about maintaining patient confidentiality and appropriate use of clinical email. She has decided to develop a written agreement of understanding and plans to ask each patient to sign the agreement before transmission of any clinical email is instituted. Marilyn also believes a privacy disclaimer could be of legal value to the clinic. Review Chapter 11's section on email etiquette for a sample disclaimer.

CASE STUDY REVIEW

1. Marilyn is developing the agreement of understanding. What are some key elements that should be included in the agreement?
2. Responding to patients using email correspondence is different than social communication. What are some guidelines for email correspondence that will be helpful to remember?
3. List several advantages and disadvantages to using email in the ambulatory health care setting.

Summary

- Written correspondence is important in conveying a professional image of the clinic and impacts the practice either positively or negatively.
- Written documents provide a permanent or legal record in the event of any litigation and thus must be carefully and accurately worded.
- The medical assistant must understand the components of a business letter and organizing the placement of these components in the proper order and spacing on a page.
- The medical assistant must be familiar with the various letter styles and properly setting up the components of each style.
- Medical assistants must know how to use Mail Merge for the creation of envelopes and mailing lists.
- Other types of correspondence include memoranda, meeting agendas, and taking meeting minutes.
- The medical assistant must know how to process incoming and outgoing mail, including types of postal mail classes.

Study for Success

To reinforce your knowledge and skills of information presented in this chapter:

- Review the *Key Terms* and *Learning Outcomes*
- Consider the *Critical Thinking* features and *Case Studies* and discuss your conclusions
- Answer the questions in the *Certification Review*

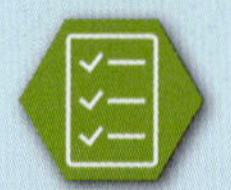
Procedure

- Perform the *Procedures* using the *Competency Assessment Checklists* on the *Student Companion Website*

CERTIFICATION REVIEW

1. How should you proofread a letter?
   a. Never read it against the document
   b. Always proof it only on the computer screen
   c. Read long documents a section at a time
   d. Always finish the job no matter how tired you may be
2. How can form letters be individualized?
   a. Form letters are never individualized
   b. By using the current date, receiver's name, and mailing address
   c. By limiting form letters to a select number of uses
   d. By using a letter style other than Simplified
   e. Form letters will be individualized if mailed first class only
3. Of the four major letter styles, which is the most contemporary?
   a. Full block
   b. Modified block, standard
   c. Modified block, indented
   d. Simplified
4. What form letters can the medical assistant sign for the provider?
   a. Letters to thank referring providers
   b. Letters to order supplies
   c. Letters to announce new staff
   d. None of these
   e. All of these
5. On what line is the subject line keyed?
   a. On line 15 or two to three lines below the letterhead
   b. On the second line below the inside address
   c. Four lines below the complimentary closing
   d. On the second line below the salutation
6. Which of the following is a guideline for letter placement?
   a. Use single line space within paragraphs.
   b. When dividing a paragraph at the bottom of a page, keep two lines on the bottom of the page and two lines at the top of the next page.
   c. A minimum of three lines should be keyed on the second page of a letter.
   d. None of these
   e. All of these
7. After removing the contents from incoming mail, what should you do?
   a. Stamp the date it was received in the clinic.
   b. Look in the envelope to make certain that all contents have been removed.
   c. If the address is not included on the letter, write it on the letter as it appeared on the envelope.
   d. All of these
8. Computer disks, film, video tapes, and books are sent in which postal class?
   a. Express
   b. First class
   c. Bulk rate
   d. Second class
   e. Media class
9. First-class mail is divided into which two subclasses?
   a. Automation and nonautomation
   b. Periodical and standard mail
   c. Standard A and standard B
   d. Bulk and parcel post mail
10. What is the most time efficient letter style for creating a variety of letters?
    a. Watermark
    b. Standard modified block
    c. Full block letter
    d. Indented modified block
    e. Simplified letter

CHAPTER 15

Medical Documents

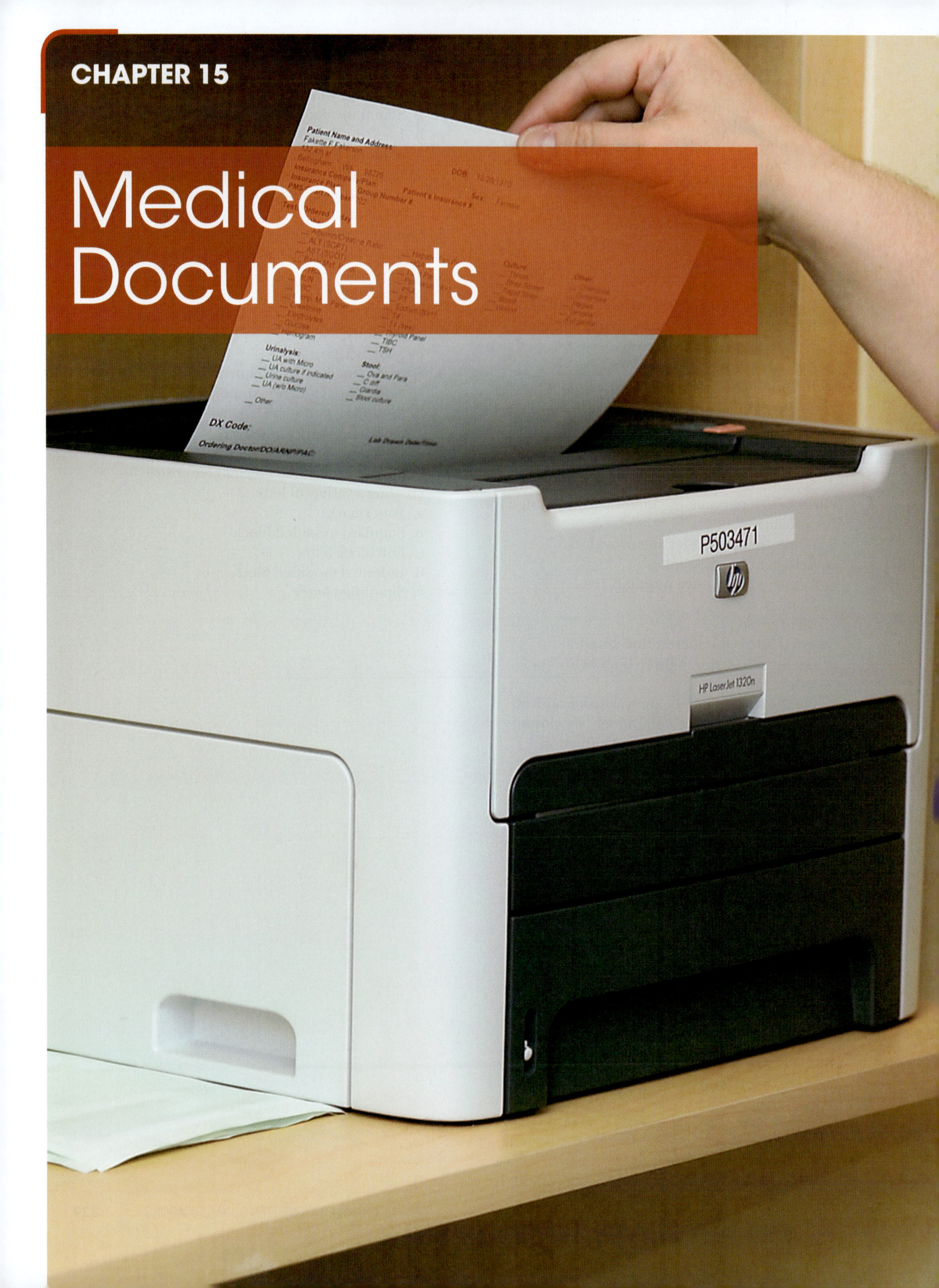

LEARNING OUTCOMES

1. Define and spell the key terms as presented in the glossary.
2. Discuss the changing role of medical transcription.
3. Discuss the impact of electronic health records on medical transcription.
4. List a minimum of three reasons for justifying outsourcing medical transcription.
5. Discuss voice recognition software and its impact upon medical transcription.
6. List responsibilities of the medical transcriptionist serving as editor of medical documents.
7. Review the importance of quality assurance and risk management.
8. Describe the process of flagging and its significance.
9. Discuss what is meant by the term *authentication* and identify three ways it may be done related to medical reports.
10. State what is meant by *privileged* information.
11. Identify four ways the medical transcriptionist can be compliant with the Health Insurance Portability and Accountability Act (HIPAA).
12. Differentiate among chart notes, history and physical examination reports, radiology and imaging reports, operative reports, pathology reports, consultations, discharge summaries, autopsy reports, and correspondence.
13. Discuss turnaround time and its importance to medical records.

KEY TERMS

- Association for Healthcare Documentation Integrity (AHDI)
- auditor
- autopsy report
- certified medical transcriptionist (CMT)
- chart notes
- chief complaint (CC)
- confidentiality agreement
- consultation report
- current reports
- discharge summary (DS)
- editor
- electronic medical record (EMR)
- flag
- gross examination
- Health Insurance Portability and Accountability Act (HIPAA)
- history and physical examination (H&P) report
- history of the present illness (HPI)
- medical transcriptionist (MT)
- microscopic examination
- old report or aged report
- operative report (OR)
- outsourcing
- pathology report
- present problem (PP)
- privileged
- progress notes
- quality assurance (QA)
- radiology report
- registered medical transcriptionist (RMT)
- review of systems (ROS)
- risk management
- STAT report
- turnaround time (TAT)
- voice recognition software (VRS)

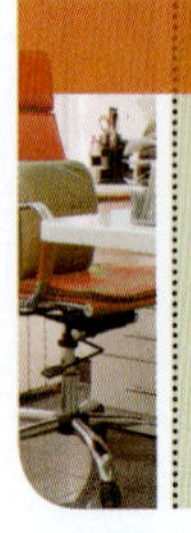

SCENARIO

Inner City Health Care, a multispecialty clinic, employs two full-time medical transcriptionists. Marilyn Johnson, CMA (AAMA), is the clinic manager and has former training and experience as a medical transcriptionist. This experience provides her with the basic understanding necessary to manage the medical transcription and medical records department of the clinic. Marilyn is very cost conscious and is exploring outsourcing all medical transcription.

Chapter Portal

The development of new technology over the last few years is impacting medical facilities in a variety of ways. Computerized medical facilities have implemented electronic medical records (EMR), may use voice recognition software (VRS) and electronic signatures, or may outsource transcription to other areas of the United States or to foreign countries. These changes have a direct impact on the position medical transcriptionists (MT) once held in the medical environment. Today, the MT may be more involved with quality assurance (QA), risk management, and editing the completed document rather than transcribing written or dictated medical information.

THE CHANGING ROLE OF MEDICAL TRANSCRIPTION

Medical transcriptionists (MT), sometimes referred to as health care documentation specialists, listen to voice recordings dictated by health care providers and create medical records in the proper format for the type of document and according to the standards of the facility. MT may also review and edit medical documents created by speech recognition technology, to ensure accuracy between what was dictated and the document produced. An MT that does not actually type the document, but rather compares dictation to the text produced by the voice recognition software, and then edits the text where needed, may sometimes be called a dictation editor or a medical transcription editor.

Today's cost-conscious and rapidly changing economy along with new technology has brought about many changes to the MT profession. The following paragraphs discuss major changes impacting medical transcription today.

Electronic Medical Records

Clinics using **electronic medical records (EMR)** rather than paper-based medical records may delegate much of the MT's responsibility to other medical personnel. For example, the MA may record directly into the EMR the reason for the visit, medications the patient is currently taking, including over-the-counter and herbal products; height and weight; vital signs; and any observations. The provider, using the computer, has access to the entire patient medical record and may call up test results, various images, diagnoses, and treatment plans for verification or comparison. The provider may add to the EMR document by directly keying in chart notes or by dictating to a digital recording system or may use voice recognition software. The provider may complete and transmit prescriptions directly to a pharmacy or forward all or part of the medical record to a referring provider.

Each entry into the EMR is automatically date and time stamped, which facilitates documentation and tracking of patient care and outcomes. The EMR provides easy access to quickly locate accurate and readily usable information about the patient at the point of care. EMR are much more efficient in the clinical decision-making process than the old cumbersome paper-based patient records. EMR may be sent to all medical personnel involved in the care of a patient in a matter of seconds.

We have covered the process of changeover to a computerized system in the medical clinic in Chapter 10, but we have not covered the process of the physical transition from existing paper medical records to electronic health records. Two issues must be resolved: How much of the paper chart do we convert to a digital format and how do we make the majority of the existing clinical history available to the physician? Several options are available:

- *All patient charts are scanned into the EMR system.* This choice is the most attractive option, but it is also the most costly. Although the basic scanning can be performed by a relatively unskilled worker, a trained medical professional must file the data in the appropriate category of the new medical record so that it can be readily located by the medical provider.

- *Partial scanning of patient charts.* Charts are pulled for existing patients scheduled for the coming week and only the clinically pertinent information from the past three to six visits as identified by the medical provider are scanned and filed in the new system. This process is repeated until partial paper records for all patients are included in the EHR system. This approach requires that paper records be actively retained for a period before they are archived.
- *Do not scan any old information.* Develop an EHR record for all patients from a given date and have the old paper record for existing patients available for the medical provider for as long as the provider feels necessary. At some point the provider will no longer have a need for the paper record and it can be archived.

Some practices receive a lot of calls regarding patient questions or pharmacy requests. The summary page of the paper record can be scanned for all patients to establish an EHR that is useful in fulfilling these types of requests. One of the options for transitioning paper records can then be used to develop a more complete EHR for each patient.

The conversion of paper records to electronic records is most readily accomplished by scanning. It could be done using practice personnel; however, it is more cost effective for an outside firm that will come onsite to do the work. Care must be exercised to follow all HIPAA regulations. A trained medical professional will still be required to ensure that the records are filed appropriately in the EHR system.

The file system used in establishing an EHR system must be carefully thought out to ensure that the medical provider can easily retrieve data. The EHR program being used is a good place to begin in planning the details of the file system while tailoring it to the specific type of medical practice. Documentation of the file system and the conversion procedure is a first step to maintaining consistent nomenclature and data format throughout the conversion.

Outsourcing

Transcription is a task that is presently outsourced by many large clinics and hospitals. **Outsourcing** is the practice of contracting with a service outside the clinic or hospital to a company where the task can be accomplished at a lower cost and with a faster turnaround time. Outsourcing companies usually are located in countries where a source of English-speaking educated labor is present, the pay rate is low, and a stable business climate exists. Currently, outsourcing organizations are located in areas of the United States and Canada as well as offshore at companies primarily located in the United Kingdom, India, and the Philippines.

Today's medical clinics must keep a keen eye on the bottom line—cost. Some advantages given to support outsourcing of medical transcription include the following:

- Outsourcing transcription frees administrative and support personnel to complete tasks that often are delayed because of time crunch factors.
- Outsourcing companies are on the job 24/7 and 365 days of the year, so the medical clinic need not be concerned about vacation periods or sick leave. Someone is always on the job.
- Outsourcing companies focus on transcription without having to answer telephones, schedule appointments, or deal with any number of interruptions encountered in the medical clinic. Therefore, documents are more accurate, standardized, and completed with less turnaround time.
- Outsourcing transcription frees floor space (real estate) previously used to support a line item expense and converts it to a source of revenue.
- Outsourcing saves on costly employee benefits packages.

Digital dictation by the provider can be readily sent to the outsource organization that performs the transcription using the Internet, with the completed document returned in similar fashion. Some important considerations before outsourcing transcription include the following:

- Be sure the medical clinic and the transcription service are using compatible hardware and software.
- Investigate quality assurance, security, HIPAA, and confidentiality measures.
- Be cost conscious. Most transcription fees are calculated by the line, but it may be more cost effective to pay by the minute of recorded dictation time. A digital dictation system allows one to measure to the 10th or 100th of a minute.
- A transcription service that uses a digital dictation system should have a user-friendly method of tracking transcribed documents. The work should be able to be located in less than 3 minutes.

- When using a digital dictation system, a provider's dictation is available to the transcriptionist as soon as the provider hangs up the phone, allowing for no lost time, which equates to cost containment.

Outsourcing is rapidly eliminating the need for the traditional transcriptionist in medical facilities. This practice is in turn being replaced by the use of voice recognition software.

Voice Recognition Software

Voice recognition software (VRS), also known as speech recognition, automatic speech recognition (ASR), or natural language recognition software, converts voice to text using a computer. In essence, the software "translates" the sounds spoken into written words. This type of program has improved greatly in recent years, translating with little error. Specialized programs are capable of translating highly technical medical terminology.

The latest generation of VRS uses continuous speech technology, which allows the speaker to speak more naturally. All VRS systems require an enrollment process, during which a person sits at the computer and reads sample text out loud to help train the speech recognition software to understand the particular voice pattern. VRS integrates easily with Windows applications, including Microsoft Word, Outlook Express, Internet Explorer, and AOL Instant Messenger. Some VRS products are marketed that work with personal digital assistants (PDAs) and smartphones.

Medical Transcriptionist as Editor

With the use of EHR, outsourcing, or VRS methods of transcription, the MT professional is now serving as the **quality assurance (QA)** manager, responsible for **risk management**, and the **editor** or **auditor** of transcribed documents. A QA manager establishes a process that provides accurate, complete, consistent health care documentation in a timely manner. Figure 15-1 shows data flow for transcribed medical records produced using outsourcing and speech recognition software.

Editing is the process of reviewing the transcribed document for accuracy and clarity. It is important to remember that one must not change the dictator's style or meaning when editing. Common errors are

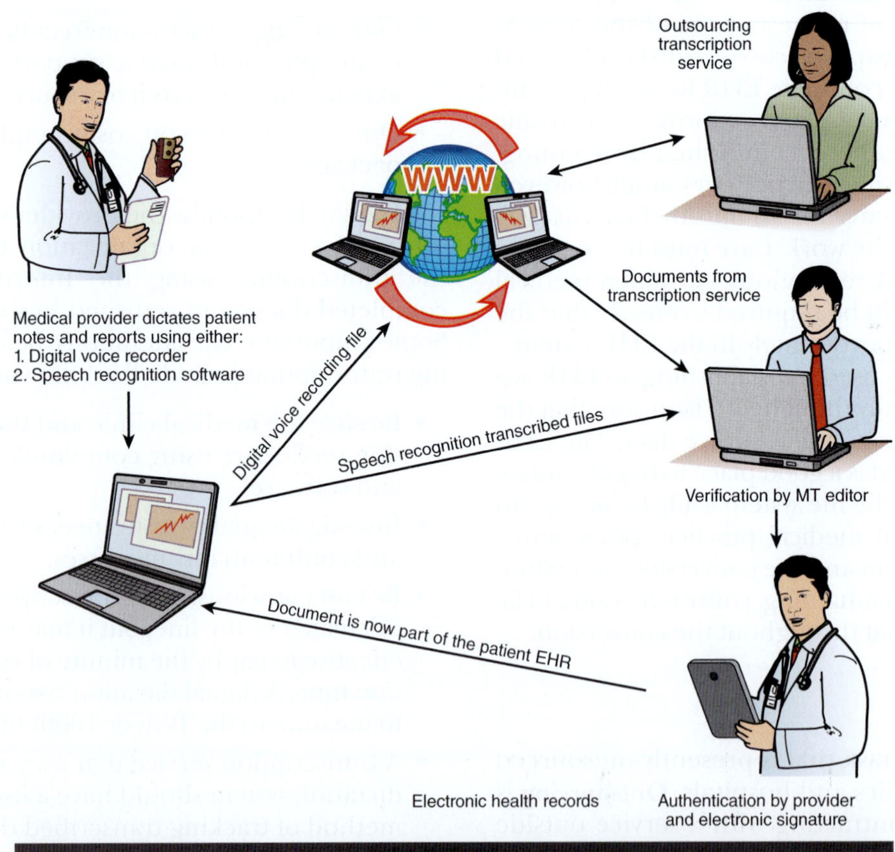

FIGURE 15-1 Data flow for transcribed medical records produced using outsourcing and speech recognition software.

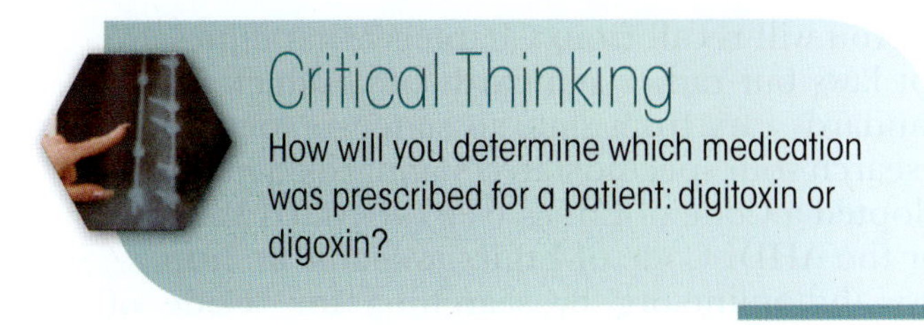

usually in sentence structure, punctuation, and spelling. They are easily changed without altering the dictator's style or meaning. Sound-alike words are another area where errors occur.

The **Association for Healthcare Documentation Integrity (AHDI)** recommends the following principles when reviewing a document:

- Compare the transcribed report against dictation. Do not just read the document.
- Use industry-specific standards for style, punctuation, and grammar (e.g., *The Book of Style for Medical Transcription*).
- Consider risk management issues.
- Third parties, such as the QA person, proofing a document should provide feedback to the transcriptionist. Although 100% accuracy is desired, accuracy of audited documents should not be less than 98%. Accuracy less than this figure requires corrective action.

If the MT encounters a term that cannot be interpreted or something new that cannot be referenced, the MT should **flag** that section of the document to alert the dictator that something needs to be corrected or resolved. The flagged message may indicate the provider is cut off, what the term sounds like, or the message is incomprehensible. Provide as much information as you can to assist the dictator in recalling the dictated area in question.

Flagging procedures vary from one facility to another and may depend upon the method used to transcribe documents. In large facilities using EHR, VRS, or outsourcing, the flagged documents may be referred directly to QA personnel. The notation may be incorporated into the computerized document using a color-code approach with a flag message. The correct information then can be added to the document and the color coding removed. In-house flagging may simply consist of a sticky note or a preprinted flag attachment.

Authentication

In most cases, the provider dictating the information will sign or authenticate the document. At times an attending provider or physician assistant will be responsible for dictating the material. The provider's signature on the document indicates that the information was accurate and complete at the time of dictation and as transcribed.

In today's technological world, electronic signatures have become common practice. The words *electronically signed by [provider's name]* underneath the signature are keyed to indicate an electronic signature. Electronic signatures may also be accomplished through:

- Use of alphanumeric computer key entries as identification
- Use of an electronic writing device
- Use of a biometric system

Medicare and the Joint Commission guidelines require that the signature on medical reports, electronic or handwritten, be completed by the provider dictating the information and not delegated to anyone else. Federal law, state law, and Joint Commission accreditation standards all address the issue of electronic signatures.

CONFIDENTIALITY AND LEGAL ISSUES

Confidentiality means treating the patient's medical information as private and not for publication. The patient has a right to privacy; therefore, medical information is **privileged**. Privileged information may only be communicated with the patient's permission or by court order. The MT must learn to follow the motto: *What you see here and what you hear here must stay here when you leave here.*

Health Insurance Portability and Accountability Act Regulations

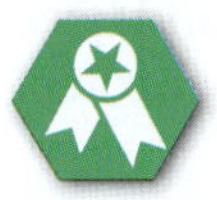

Health Insurance Portability and Accountability Act (HIPAA) regulations are government rules and procedures that have resulted from legislation designed to protect the confidentiality of patient information ranging from medical records to personal identification numbers that, if divulged, could result in identity theft.

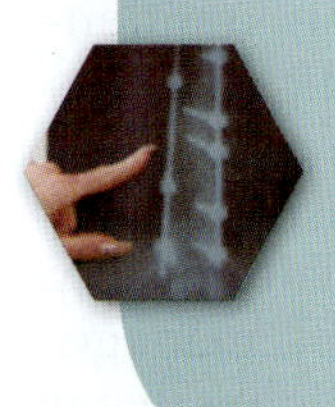

Critical Thinking

How would you go about designing a medical transcription workstation that was ergonomic and compliant with HIPAA regulations? Review Chapter 10.

The MT can meet most HIPAA regulations by adhering to the following simple rules:

- Do not divulge medical records you transcribe to anyone other than the dictator, your supervisor, or an authorized QA person. Files should not be discussed with the patient. Do not divulge files to an attorney or insurance representative without consulting with risk management personnel.
- Safeguard files in your possession. Take reasonable steps to keep files secure, such as keeping tapes and hard copy of reports in a locked file cabinet, using passwords for computer files, installing virus protection software, and using a firewall if appropriate. Do not carelessly carry files around on your person or in your car.
- Transmit files electronically only with the permission of your client or the dictating provider, and then agree on the proper procedures and protocols for transmission.
- Have a signed business associate agreement or similar document that defines the protocols you are expected to follow to protect patient confidentiality.

These general rules do not constitute legal advice; consult with appropriate legal counsel for specific questions.

Protocols

Protocols are the procedures your clinic has in place to ensure patient confidentiality. You are usually required to sign a **confidentiality agreement** stating that you will comply with the established procedures. Your contracts, together with the protocols, become a part of the institution's documentation demonstrating compliance with HIPAA regulations. The purpose of your signing a contract is to substantiate that you have received training and have been instructed in proper procedures to protect medical records.

From the MT's viewpoint, risk management involves protecting the confidentiality of the medical records and ensuring the accuracy of those records.

MTs are in an excellent position to assist the risk management officer, through their commitment to quality and their awareness of confidentiality procedures and possible medical errors indicated in the dictated data. Should a problem or error be detected that could be a risk management problem, the MT should immediately notify his or her superior, clinic manager, risk management officer, or the employer's or client's legal staff according to clinic policy.

You will recall from Chapter 7 that ethics are not laws but rather standards of conduct. These standards vary from state to state, so you should research your specific state's standards. The AHDI adopted a Code of Ethics (see the AHDI Web site for the AHDI Code of Ethics available at: http://www.ahdionline.org by searching for "Code of Ethics") for professional MTs.

Although, in certain cases, the MT can be held financially responsible for errors and omissions, the MT usually is under the jurisdiction of *respondeat superior*, meaning that the provider-director or clinic manager is responsible for the wrongful acts of the MT working under his or her supervision. This is not meant to imply that MTs should not protect themselves by instituting some personal risk management, such as carrying errors and omissions insurance. Insurance should be considered particularly if the MT is operating a home business and contracting transcription work.

Medical records are documents governed by laws and may be subpoenaed for review by various courts. The medical report may play a major role in substantiating injury or malpractice claims.

TYPES OF MEDICAL DOCUMENTS

Medical reports become part of the patient's permanent medical record and are vital to continued patient care. Other providers, attorneys, insurance companies, or the court may review the medical reports in part or in their entirety. Therefore, the medical report must be neat, accurate, and complete. *Neat* refers to a medical report that is legible and assembled to permit easy access to information as needed. *Accurate* means that the dictation has been transcribed as dictated, and *complete* indicates that the document has been dated correctly and signed or initialed by the dictator.

Complete documentation of medical reports is also important for payment or reimbursement of services for which the provider expects to be paid. The billing and diagnosis codes reported on the health insurance claim form must be supported by the documentation contained within the medical report.

A new trend in transcription is the integration of digital images directly into the transcribed record. The response to inputting digital images (photographs, scans, and radiographs) has been positive from both the local health care community and patients themselves. This is attributed to easier understanding of a picture by patients and more precise presentation using both pictures and written text to medical professionals.

The tools required for integrating digital images into word processing programs is already available to most MTs in their current Microsoft Word software packages. They only have to obtain the digital images from their provider-employer. If the transcribed record is included in the EHR, digital images can be attached, allowing other providers to view, enlarge, and manipulate the images at will.

The transcribed medical report may be formatted in a variety of styles similar to business correspondence. Common transcribed reports include:

1. Chart notes and progress notes
2. History and physical examination reports
3. Radiology reports
4. Operative reports
5. Pathology reports
6. Consultations
7. Discharge summaries
8. Autopsy reports
9. Correspondence

Hospitals and practices may require a specific format for reports different from those described in the following examples. A few helpful formatting rules are:

- Use section headings that clarify the report.
- Do not add sections left out by the dictator.
- Do not include unnecessary confidential information unless specifically instructed to do so.
- Note who dictated the report, if not the attending provider, and provide space for both to sign. The initials of the transcriptionist should be on the signature page.
- Use 1-inch margins all around, unless the document is to be filed in a chart that has a top opening, then use a 1.25-inch margin at the top only. If using sticky paper for chart notes, use 0.5-inch margins.
- Use paragraph format.

Chart Notes and Progress Notes

Chart notes, sometimes referred to as **progress notes**, are a concise description of the patient's encounter with the medical clinic. They are chronologically listed and may include in-person visits to the clinic and telephone and electronic mail (email) inquiries. Chart notes should be filed in the chart within 24 hours of the encounter. The present problem, the provider's physical findings, and the treatment plan should be identified within the chart note. Laboratory test results also may be included. The provider or clinic personnel may enter chart note information as informal handwritten notes, or keyed notes affixed to the appropriate space. All notes documented must include the date, time, and signature of the person entering the data along with his or her credential. This information is pertinent for follow-up questions or for litigation purposes. Figure 15-2 shows a sample chart/progress note in an EHR.

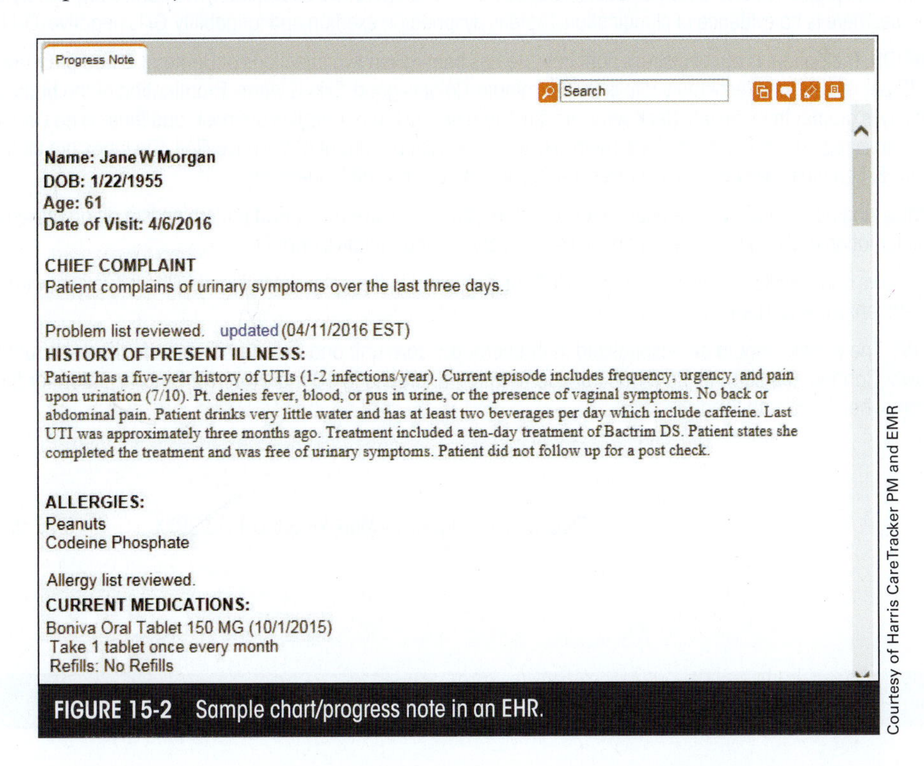
Progress Note

Search

Name: Jane W Morgan
DOB: 1/22/1955
Age: 61
Date of Visit: 4/6/2016

CHIEF COMPLAINT
Patient complains of urinary symptoms over the last three days.

Problem list reviewed. updated (04/11/2016 EST)
HISTORY OF PRESENT ILLNESS:
Patient has a five-year history of UTIs (1-2 infections/year). Current episode includes frequency, urgency, and pain upon urination (7/10). Pt. denies fever, blood, or pus in urine, or the presence of vaginal symptoms. No back or abdominal pain. Patient drinks very little water and has at least two beverages per day which include caffeine. Last UTI was approximately three months ago. Treatment included a ten-day treatment of Bactrim DS. Patient states she completed the treatment and was free of urinary symptoms. Patient did not follow up for a post check.

ALLERGIES:
Peanuts
Codeine Phosphate

Allergy list reviewed.
CURRENT MEDICATIONS:
Boniva Oral Tablet 150 MG (10/1/2015)
Take 1 tablet once every month
Refills: No Refills

FIGURE 15-2 Sample chart/progress note in an EHR.

Courtesy of Harris CareTracker PM and EMR

History and Physical Examination Reports

The **history and physical examination (H&P) report** documents information relating to the patient's main reason for treatment. The report is divided into two sections. The first is the history, which includes the **chief complaint (CC)** or **present problem (PP)**, a description of symptoms, problems, or conditions that brought the patient to the clinic; **history of the present illness (HPI)**, a chronological description of the development of the patient's illness; past medical and surgical history; family history; and social history.

The second section is the **review of systems (ROS)** and inquiry about the system directly related to the problems identified in the HPI. The provider determines the extent of the examination performed and documented based on the problems presented. The findings of the actual physical examination make up the documentation for the physical examination section of the report.

The Joint Commission accredits and regulates all policies and procedures of hospitals and provider's clinics owned by hospital organizations. The Joint Commission requires that hospitals provide H&P reports to be filed in patient charts within 24 hours of admission. Occasionally, the patient is seen in the provider's clinic and a decision is made to admit the patient to the hospital. In this case, the examination is performed in the clinic, but the report is dictated to the hospital that transcribes the document and files it within the patient's chart. The H&P format may also be used to document a patient's annual physical examination in the clinic. Figure 15-3 shows a sample H&P Report.

HISTORY AND PHYSICAL EXAMINATION

PATIENT: Donald Waite
CHART #: 97223

HISTORY: The patient is a 72-year-old male who was admitted because of intermittent, moderately severe chest pain starting from the substernal region radiating to the back and to the left arm and associated with a choking sensation. The pain lasted from minutes to half an hour and was relieved by two nitroglycerin tablets.

This condition has been going on for the last two weeks. The patient has known arteriosclerotic heart disease and since his discharge in July 20XX, has been doing reasonably well on Procardia, nitrates, Persantine, and digoxin.

PAST HISTORY: The patient had a pacemaker implantation for sick sinus syndrome four years ago. He has a history of angina and myocardial infarction. He also has essential hypertension.

His past surgical history includes an appendectomy and bilateral herniorrhaphies. He has no allergies.

The patient still works as a projectionist in a movie house. He does not smoke but drinks occasionally. He denies any history of diabetes, liver, or kidney disease. There is no evidence of claudication. There is dyspnea on exertion and fatigability. GI is negative; GU is negative.

PHYSICAL EXAMINATION: The patient is out of distress right now. He has been given two injections of Demerol. Blood pressure is 120/68, ventricular rate is 72 per minute, and respiratory rate is 20 per minute. Color is good. Skin is warm. Examination of the head shows that right lenticular opacity is greater than the left. Neck veins are flat. There are no bruits. Carotids are brisk, and there is no evidence of thyroid enlargement. The heart is regular with no S3 gallops. There is a systolic ejection murmur at the base III/VI. The lungs are clear. The abdomen shows surgical scars. Extremities have no edema. Pulses are 2+, and there is no calf tenderness.

IMPRESSION: Unstable angina secondary to coronary artery disease with obstructive and mixed pattern spasm on an affixed lesion. Status postpacemaker implantation and degenerative joint disease with cervical degenerative arthritis.

Review of the EKG shows nonspecific ST-T wave changes in II, III, and aVF and in the anterolateral leads. Chest X-ray showed cardiomegaly, and the enzymes are pending.

RECOMMENDATIONS: The patient should be hospitalized in the coronary care unit and monitored. The nifedipine should be increased up to 60 mg—slowly. Continue Persantine. Continue transderm nitro—increase to 10 mg/24 hr (0.4 mg/hr). Monitor the blood level. Consider angiogram when he is stabilized.

Electronically signed by Mark King, MD 11/3/20XX 5:37 PM

MK/jg

d: 11/2/XX
t: 11/2/XX

FIGURE 15-3 Sample history and physical examination report.

Radiology and Imaging Reports

A **radiology report** is a description of the findings and interpretations of the radiologist who studies the diagnostic procedure. Examples of radiology reports are X-ray studies, computed tomography (CT) scans, magnetic resonance image (MRI) scans, nuclear medicine procedures, and fluoroscopic studies. In some cases, a contrast medium is administered either orally or by injection before the procedure is performed. A scan is a procedure that requires the use of radioactive isotopes.

When dictating, the radiologist may switch from present to past tense; that is, the procedure was performed in the past tense, and the findings are given in the present tense.

Stereoscopy and tomography are technologies that view structures within the body in dimensions or layers. Computed tomography uses radiography with computers to visualize a slice of the body part. Sonograms and echograms are another imaging technology that uses high-frequency sound waves to compose a picture of an area of the body. Magnetic resonance imaging produces sectional images of the body without the use of radiology. New technologies create the need for understanding the imaging process and appropriate documentation of patient information.

When transcribing radiology or imaging reports, the date of service should be used rather than the date of dictation. Other details to be included within the report may include:

- Number and type of views taken
- Any special circumstances that could affect the examination
- Quality of the study (clear or blurry)
- Abnormal findings
- Normal findings
- Radiologist's impression, interpretation, diagnosis, and recommendations
- Signature of the radiologist

The report should be filed in the patient's chart within 4 to 8 hours of the procedure. Sufficient documentation must be in the report for the provider to use if he or she must prove that the study was medically necessary or if justification for reimbursement is required. Figure 15-4 shows an example of a radiology report.

MERCY MEDICAL CENTER
300 Main Street
Denver, CO 80201

RADIOLOGY #: 23445

PA & LATERAL CHEST Date 10/07/XX

The pulmonary vessels are clearly outlined and are not distended. There are not any typical signs of redistribution. A few increased interstitial markings persist, but there are no typical acute Kerley B-lines. There may be a little residual pleural effusion at the costophrenic sinus and posterior gutters. Most of the pulmonary edema and effusion has otherwise cleared. The chest is not hyperexpanded. The thoracic vertebrae show spurring but no compression.

IMPRESSION:

1. No signs of elevated pulmonary venous pressure or frank failure at this time.
2. Residual pleural effusion is seen in the costophrenic sinus and posterior gutters, either residual or recent congestive failure.

BILATERAL MAMMOGRAMS Date: 10/07/XX

Bilateral xeromammograms were obtained in both the mediolateral and craniocaudal projections. There is no previous exam for comparison. There is slight asymmetry of the ductal tissue in the lower outer quadrant of the right breast. There are no dominant masses, clusters of microcalcifications or pathologic skin changes identified.

IMPRESSION: Normal bilateral mammogram.

Electronically signed by
Renny Genray, MD 10/08/20XX 11:21 AM

JOHN DOE, M.D. SMITH, HARRIET #123456-7
Dictated by: Renny Genray, M.D.
D&T: 10/07/XX | 10/07/XX | RG/mt

RADIOLOGY REPORT

FIGURE 15-4 Sample radiology report.

Operative Reports

The **operative report (OR)** chronicles the details of a surgical procedure performed in a hospital, outpatient surgical center, or clinic. The surgeon or assistant dictates the OR immediately after the operation. The OR describes the surgical procedure, preoperative and postoperative diagnoses, and specimens removed. It sometimes includes a sponge count and instrument inventory, an estimate of blood loss, and the condition of the patient on leaving the operating room. The report should also include the name of the primary surgeon and any assistants. The type of anesthesia and name of the anesthesiologist should also be included in the report. Often the report will end with disposition or where the patient was transferred when he or she left the operating room and the condition of

PATIENT: Joseph Oritz

DATE: 6/25/XX

SURGEON: Raja Rao, MD

PREOPERATIVE DIAGNOSIS: Crohn's disease requiring central venous access for hyperalimentation.

POSTOPERATIVE DIAGNOSIS: Crohn's disease requiring central venous access for hyperalimentation.

OPERATION: Insertion of left-sided subclavian double-lumen central venous catheter.

ANESTHESIA: 1% lidocaine.

PROCEDURE: The patient was placed in the supine position with the neck extended to the right side. The left side of the chest was prepared and draped in the usual manner using Betadine solution. The subclavian vein on the left side was percutaneously and easily entered, and the guide wire was advanced into the superior vena cava. The double-lumen central venous catheter with VitaCuff was placed through the guide wire into the superior vena cava. Good blood flow was obtained. The catheter was sutured to the skin using 2-0 silk sutures and connected to IV solution.

A dry sterile dressing was applied.

The patient tolerated the procedure well.

Electronically signed by
Juan Esposito, MD 06/25/20XX
4:15 PM

JE/urs

d: 6/25/XX
t: 6/27/XX

FIGURE 15-5 Sample operative report.

the patient at the time of transfer. The authenticated report should be filed in the chart as soon as possible after surgery so that other staff members caring for the patient will have needed information. Figure 15-5 shows a sample OR.

Pathology Reports

A **pathology report** is generated to describe the **gross** and **microscopic examinations** performed on organs, lesions, tissue samples, or body fluid removed during a surgical procedure. In some cases, the pathologist examines the specimen before the patient is sutured to determine if a more extensive surgical procedure is required (e.g., in the case of malignant tumors).

Pathologists generally dictate the report in the present tense because they interpret the pathologic findings as they view the specimens. The report must be completed within 24 hours of receipt with

PATHOLOGY REPORT

PATHOLOGY NO.:	792 304	
DATE:	12/20/XX	
CHART NO.:	56 84 20	
NAME:	Lee Allen Au	AGE: 15 Female
DEPARTMENT:	Surgery	MD: Dr. Raja Rao
TISSUE:	Appendix	
HISTORY:	Right Lower Quadrant Pain	

CLINICAL DIAGNOSIS: RLQ Pain

PATHOLOGICAL REPORT: The specimen is labeled appendix and is received in formalin. The specimen consists of an appendix that measures 6 × 1 × 0.5 cm in greatest dimension. The serosa surface has some white fibrinoid material attached to it and on a cross section. Some purulent fibrinous material can also be seen. Representative sections are submitted in 1 cassette.

DIAGNOSIS: Acute suppurative appendicitis with periappendicitis and mesoappendicitis.

Electronically signed by
Mark King, MD 12/20/20XX
2:22 PM

MK/gc

d: 12/20/XX
t: 12/20/XX

FIGURE 15-6 Sample pathology report.

a copy maintained by the laboratory and copies sent to each provider involved in the case. The original is maintained in the patient's chart. Figure 15-6 shows a sample pathology report.

Consultation

When one provider requests the services of another provider in the care and treatment of a patient, a **consultation report** is generated. The information may be disseminated in the form of a report or within the body of a letter. The contents of the consultation report/letter usually consist of all of the elements of an H&P with a focused history of the patient's illness and the body system directly related to the consultant's area of specialty. The consultant also includes within the report/letter the findings, supporting laboratory data, diagnosis, and suggested course of treatment. The report/letter usually ends with a comment from the consulting provider thanking the admitting provider for the referral. It should be filed in the patient's medical record within 24 hours of receipt. Figure 15-7 shows a sample consultation report.

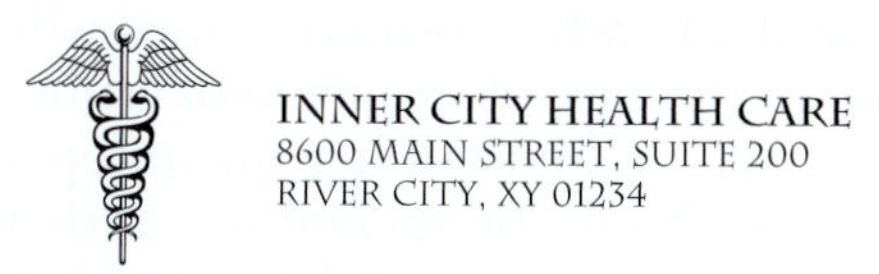

January 4, 20XX

Margaret Holly, MD
Metroma Medical Center
900 Union Street, Suite 208
Metroma, MI 11666

RE: MARY O'KEEFE

Dear Dr. Holly:

Thank you for referring Mary O'Keefe to our clinic. She presented today stating that she recently relocated to Clinton with her husband and children to be closer to her parents. Mary has been experiencing symptoms suggestive of pregnancy and is here for evaluation. Over the past three weeks, she has noticed increased tenderness of her breasts, fatigue, and a feeling of being bloated. A home pregnancy test was positive.

Her past medical history is positive for the usual childhood diseases and the births of two children, following normal pregnancies. She has a negative past surgical history.

She has no allergies to medications and takes Tylenol for occasional headaches. She is married and has two children, ages 3 years and 12 months. She is employed part-time in an insurance office. She does not smoke or drink.

The family history is noncontributory.

On review of systems, her complaints are limited to those described above. She has had no nausea or vomiting, and no change in bowel habits. She has no dizziness, no fevers, and no urinary symptoms.

Physical examination revealed a 32-year-old white female in no acute distress. HEENT normocephalic, atraumatic. PERRLA, EOMI. The thyroid was not enlarged, and there was no cervical adenopathy. The lungs were clear. The heart had a regular rate and rhythm. The abdomen was soft and nontender. Bowel sounds were normal. The extremities revealed trace ankle edema. The neurological examination was within normal limits. Pelvic examination confirmed a gravid uterus, compatible with a very early pregnancy.

An abdominal ultrasound has been ordered and a beta HCG was drawn.

I believe Mary is pregnant and I will put her on our OB regimen starting with monthly visits. Thank you for your kind referral.

Sincerely,

Mark King, MD

Mark King, MD

MK/nf

FIGURE 15-7 Sample consultation report.

Discharge Summaries

The **discharge summary (DS)** documents the patient's history of hospital admissions. The DS includes the reason for hospital admission, a description of what transpired while the patient was in the hospital, the final diagnosis, follow-up instructions, discharge medications, patient's condition at discharge, and prognosis for recovery. If the patient is transferred to another facility such as a skilled nursing facility, the report is changed from DS to transfer summary. If the patient has expired during the stay, the report is usually called a death summary. The Joint Commission requires that the completed DS be filed in the patient's chart within 48 to 72 hours of discharge from the hospital. Figure 15-8 shows a sample DS.

Autopsy Reports

An **autopsy report** may also be called an autopsy protocol, a necropsy report, or a medical examiner report. Autopsies are performed to determine the cause of death or to ascertain and confirm presence of disease. It is important to understand that state law requires that autopsies be performed in certain situations. For example, an autopsy report is required when someone dies suddenly, when someone dies while unattended, or in the case of suspicion of crime.

When transcribing an autopsy report, more words should be spelled out and abbreviation use kept to a minimum because these records may be entered into a court of law and must be accurate and clearly understood. Many states require that military time be used when documenting the time a body arrives at the coroner's office. Temporary anatomic diagnoses should be placed in the medical report within 72 hours and in the completed report within 60 days. Figure 15-9 shows a sample autopsy report.

Correspondence

It is important for the MT to remember that all forms of medical correspondence also are considered medical documents and must be transcribed with the same care as any other medical

PATIENT: Kelly Cohen
CHART #: 29324

ADMITTED: 9/26/XX
DISCHARGED: 11/19/XX

HISTORY/LAB: This infant was born on 09/26/XX to a 30-year-old, gravida II, para 1 female, with a last menstrual period of 3/22/XX estimated date of confinement 2/29/XX. The mother had been observed regularly during her pregnancy. However, she did develop preterm labor necessitating early hospitalization. At that time, the mother was placed on antibiotics and dexamethasone and delivered at approximately 26 weeks' gestation. At the time of delivery, the membranes ruptured spontaneously and fluid was clear. The infant had an Apgar score of 5 and 8 at 1 and 5 minutes, respectively. The infant required intubation in the delivery room and was then transferred to the NICU. On admission, weight was 1,159 grams, length 38.5 cm, head circumference 25.5 cm, chest circumference 26 cm. Assessment was 26 weeks' gestation.

COURSE/CONDITION ON DISCHARGE/DISPOSITION: At the time of admission the infant had respiratory distress, was intubated, and required Survanta. The infant was placed on IV fluid and antibiotics, and appropriate blood work was done. During the hospitalization, the infant improved with regard to the respiratory distress. However, the infant developed bronchopulmonary dysplasia, hyperbilirubinemia, and apnea of prematurity. The infant was placed on the appropriate medications and improved steadily. Her weight increased gradually. During the hospitalization, the infant was evaluated by Dr. Lally of Ophthalmology who will follow up on an outpatient basis.

The infant was discharged home on 11/20/XX. She had a hearing test, eye examination as stated, and was going to receive home physical therapy three times a week. She was on Fer In Sol drops and was feeding on Neosure and breast milk. The overall prognosis was guarded to good.

FINAL DIAGNOSIS: Preterm, 26-week female infant, appropriate for gestational age, apnea of prematurity, anemia, respiratory distress syndrome, bronchopulmonary dysplasia, hyperbilirubinemia, and presumed sepsis.

Electronically signed by Amy M. Cox, MD 09/27/20XX 8:15 AM

AMC/nf

d:11/20/XX
t: 11/20/XX

FIGURE 15-8 Sample discharge summary report.

AUTOPSY REPORT

Patient Name:	George Matthews
Hospital No.:	11509
Necropsy No.:	98-A-19
Admitting Physician:	Joe Abbott, M.C.
Pathologist:	Loraine Muir, M.D.
Date of Death:	04/05/20XX, 9 PM
Date of Autopsy:	04/06/20XX, 8 AM
Admitting Diagnosis:	Adenocarcinoma, maxilla.
Prosector:	Keith Johnson, P.A.

FINAL ANATOMIC DIAGNOSIS

1. Old fibrotic myocardial infarction of the anterior and septal walls of the left ventricle with anterior ventricular aneurysm, 4.5×3.0 cm.
2. Patchy old fibrotic myocardial infarction of the lateral and posterior septal walls of the left ventricle.
3. Probable recent ischemic changes, especially of the anterior and septal walls of the left ventricle.
4. Severe calcified atherosclerotic coronary vascular disease with up to 95% stenosis of the right coronary artery (RCA), up to 70% stenosis of the left anterior descending (LAD) coronary artery, and greater than 95% stenosis of the left circumflex coronary artery (LCCA).
5. Bilateral arterionephrosclerosis.
6. Atherosclerotic vascular disease, aorta, moderate to severe; circle of Willis, moderate.
7. Old infarct of right inner and inferior occipital lobe; small lacunar infarct, right caudate nucleus.
8. Bilateral pulmonary congestion, moderate.
9. Chronic passive congestion, liver, mild.
10. Simple cysts, right and left kidneys, up to 5.5 cm.
11. Diverticulum, 2.5 cm, duodenum.
12. Diverticulosis, sigmoid colon.
13. Status post partial left maxillectomy for adenocarcinoma, recent.

Electronically signed by Elizabeth M. Jones, MD 04/26/20XX 6:17 PM

EMJ:xx

D:04/26/XX
T: 04/26/XX

FIGURE 15-9 Sample autopsy report.

report would. Review Chapter 14 for information regarding various styles and formats for business correspondence. Figure 15-10 shows a sample of medical correspondence.

TURNAROUND TIME AND PRODUCTIVITY

Specific time limits are often established for completion of medical reports. **Turnaround time (TAT)** indicates the specific time period in which a document is expected to be completed from the time it is received by the transcriptionist until it is returned to the provider to sign and made a part of the permanent medical record.

Turnaround times for hospital reports fall into three categories:

1. ***STAT reports.*** Should be completed within 2 to 4 hours.
2. ***Current reports.*** Should be completed within 24 hours or less.
3. ***Old reports or aged reports.*** DS reports are an example, except when the patient is being transferred to another facility. Old reports should be completed within 48 to 72 hours or less.
4. *When requesting copies of a medical record* the usual TAT is 7 to 10 business days.

Different facilities have different requirements; however, the transcriptionist or clinic personnel responsible for medical records should be aware that failure to meet deadlines could result in disciplinary or legal action. The reason for this stringent adherence to turnaround time is that STAT and current reports can influence timely treatment of the patient.

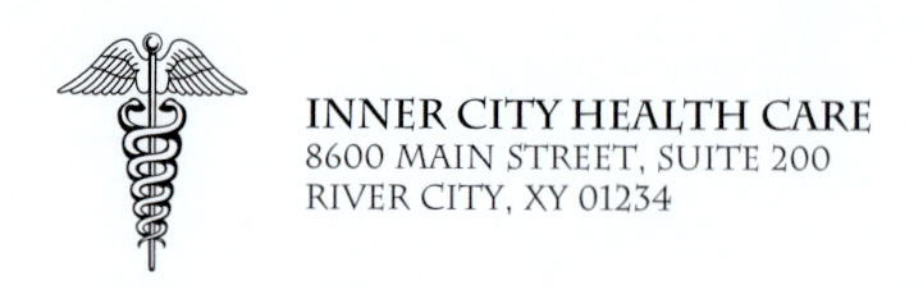

January 4, 20XX

Susan Smith, Coordinator
Special Project Division
American Drug Company
90058 Northover Road
Welfond, PA 44578

Dear Ms. Smith:

It is my understanding that your department oversees the Aid for Patients program, which provides Glucogenasin for indigent patients. I am interested in learning more about this.

I have a 74-year-old female patient who would be greatly helped by this medication. She suffers with hypertension, adult onset diabetes mellitus, and moderate angina. Medication compliance has been a problem; however, we feel that this new drug, with its q.d. dosage, will be easy for her to deal with.

Any information you could forward would be appreciated.

Yours truly,

Winston Lewis, MD

Winston Lewis, MD

WL/tm

FIGURE 15-10 Sample medical correspondence.

DOCUMENTATION

8/28/XX Removed cast from right wrist and instructed patient to make an appointment with PT. Radiology, BQL/ CMA (AAMA) 9/12/XX________________________

Workload, as well as productivity of the transcriptionist, affects turnaround time. When workload is too great to meet turnaround times, the medical records administrator must be notified immediately. Once a job has been accepted, the transcriptionist or transcription service is legally bound to meet the schedule short of a major catastrophe of the type legally considered to be an "act of nature."

MEDICAL TRANSCRIPTION AS A CAREER

The medical transcription career has changed significantly in the United States. The career continues to evolve with the introduction of new technology and outsourcing. Most healthcare providers use either digital or analog dictating equipment to transmit dictation to medical transcriptionists. The Internet has grown to be a popular mode for transmitting documentation and allows for faster turnaround time. Speech recognition technology electronically translates sound into text and creates drafts of reports. The MT serve as QA managers, oversee risk management, and function as editors or auditors of medical documents. Medical transcriptionists are invisible, and yet invaluable, members of the patient care team.

MTs serving as editors enjoy detective work and are curious; if terminology is new to them, they use references to research and learn more. MTs must be self-disciplined, detail oriented, and independent, and usually they are perfectionists. They are dedicated to professional development and enthusiastically committed to learning. MTs possess integrity and understand the importance and legal implications of medical confidentiality.

Professionalism Related to Medical Transcription

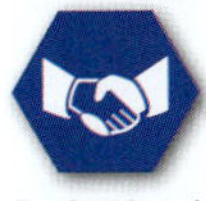

Professionalism as related to medical transcription has many requirements. Following is advice on how to maintain a professional attitude.

- *Display a professional manner and image.* Working as an MT requires good hygiene practices and dress attire appropriate to the surroundings. The MT should always respect others and use good communication skills.
- *Demonstrate initiative and responsibility.* Demonstrating initiative means being to work early enough to organize and begin the workday at the appointed time. All deadlines must be met or changes approved.
- *Work as a member of the health care team.* The MT is a member of the health care team and as such must sign a business associate agreement and a confidentiality agreement. The MT should report incidents of confidentiality discrepancies and any perceived medical procedural errors to appropriate risk management personnel.
- *Prioritize and perform multiple tasks.* The MT must prioritize the documents to be edited to satisfy turnaround time and maintain productivity standards.
- *Adapt to change.* The MT must be flexible and willing to change. Technological advances require being open to new ways of handling medical documents. The MT's role and job description are changing to meet today's new demands.
- *Enhance skills through continuing education.* New technology, breakthroughs in medicine, and new medications are recognized daily as researchers explore ways in which to treat disease and increase longevity. The MT must remain current with new medical developments to maintain professionalism.

A qualified MT, described as one with a minimum of 2 years' experience in performing medical transcription in a variety of medical and surgical specialties, may wish to become a **certified medical transcriptionist (CMT)**, through a voluntary examination from the AHDI. Recent graduates, or MTs with less than 2 years' experience, may apply to become **registered medical transcriptionists (RMT)**. For additional information regarding AHDI credentialing, visit AHDI's Web site at: http://www.ahdionline.org.

PROCEDURE 15-1

Transcribing Medical Referral Letters

Procedure

PURPOSE:

To transcribe (type) medical referral letters using word processing software based on physician dictation.

EQUIPMENT/SUPPLIES:

- Computer and word processing software
- Source documents

PROCEDURE STEPS:

1. After setting up the transcription equipment and inserting the tape, open the word processing software.
2. Using the general formats for each document type, prepare and transcribe (type) the physician's dictation as shown on the source document. Use proper punctuation and grammar.
3. When complete, save the document.
4. Print the letter so the physician may sign it and turn in a copy to your instructor. Prepare a mailing envelope(s).
5. Close the word processor when done.

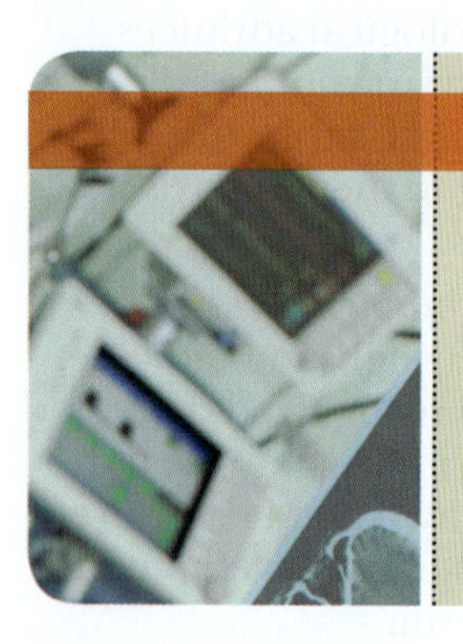

CASE STUDY 15-1

Refer to the scenario at the beginning of the chapter.

CASE STUDY REVIEW

1. List important issues Marilyn will want to consider before outsourcing medical transcription.
2. Using your favorite search engine, research outsourcing as well as VRS options. Write a summary of your findings and state your rationale for supporting either outsourcing, VRS, or keeping the transcription in-house.

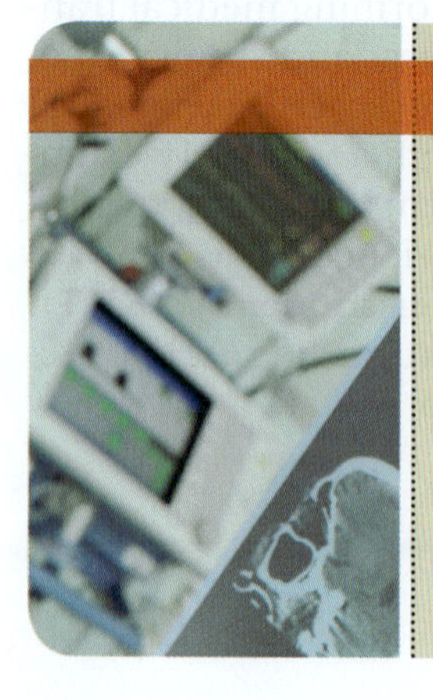

CASE STUDY 15-2

At Inner City Health Care, the MT has just transcribed the following content in a document: "This patient developed a persistent lesion on the inner aspect of the left upper lip. This lesion was at the junction of the vermilion and mucous membrane. A punch biopsy was obtained of this 1-cm lesion and was read as a probable verrucous squamous cell carcinoma of the lower lip."

CASE STUDY REVIEW

1. What inconsistencies, if any, do you find within this content?
2. What should the MT do to verify inconsistencies and inaccuracies?
3. How should these inconsistencies and inaccuracies be corrected?

Summary

- Medical documentation is a vital part of patient health care; without it, it is impossible to provide quality health care, to bill insurance carriers properly to ensure providers are reimbursed for services rendered, and to support and protect the provider should records be subpoenaed.
- The medical transcriptionist must keep all patient information strictly confidential and may be asked to sign a confidentiality agreement.
- Medical transcriptionists will continue to be medical language specialists, and are increasingly becoming editors as the use of voice recognition software becomes more prevalent.
- The medical assistant must understand the methods of accurately and confidentially converting paper records into digital documents in the EMR by scanning and then selecting the most useful information for use by the providers and staff.
- Medical document types include chart notes and progress notes, history and physical examination reports, radiology reports, operative reports, pathology reports, consultations, discharge summaries, autopsy reports, and correspondence.
- Proper formatting must be used for each medical document.
- Medical transcriptionists must have basic skills in transcribing or editing frequently used documents in a clinic.

Study for Success

To reinforce your knowledge and skills of information presented in this chapter:

- Review the *Key Terms* and *Learning Outcomes*
- Consider the *Critical Thinking* features and *Case Studies* and discuss your conclusions
- Answer the questions in the *Certification Review*

Procedure

- Perform the *Procedure* using the *Competency Assessment Checklists* on the *Student Companion Website*

CERTIFICATION REVIEW

1. What three factors influence the changing role of medical transcription?
   a. Cost
   b. Changing economy
   c. New technology
   d. All of these
2. What are examples of new technology used in medical transcription?
   a. EHR
   b. Outsourcing
   c. VRS
   d. Authentication
   e. All of these
3. Why does a medical transcriptionist place a flag within a medical document?
   a. The dictator made a mistake.
   b. The dictator could not be understood.
   c. The transcriptionist made an error.
   d. None of these.
4. What is the definition of authentication?
   a. Use of an electronic signature
   b. The information was accurate and complete at the time of dictation and as transcribed, and has been signed and dated by the dictating provider
   c. Use of a biometric system
   d. Use of an alphanumeric computer key entry as identification
   e. The typing was done by a medical transcriptionist
5. What would the medical transcriptionist do when there is a question that cannot be resolved?
   a. Guess at what is being dictated
   b. Edit the document and exclude what cannot be understood
   c. Flag the document
   d. Refuse to transcribe documents for that provider

6. What is the turnaround time for most STAT reports?
   a. Same as aged reports
   b. Current
   c. Within 2–4 hours
   d. Within 24 hours
   e. Both a and b
7. What is the definition of an H&P report?
   a. It is divided into a history section and the ROS section.
   b. It is sometimes referred to as a progress note.
   c. It describes gross and microscopic examinations.
   d. It documents the patient's history of hospital admission.
8. Which of the following is true of autopsy reports?
   a. They are also called narcolepsy reports.
   b. They determine cause of death, ascertain and confirm presence of disease.
   c. They should be brief and contain many abbreviations.
   d. They are always required to use military time.
   e. Temporary diagnoses should be placed within 24 hours.
9. In what time frame should chart notes be filed?
   a. 12 hours
   b. 24 hours
   c. 4–8 hours
   d. 48–72 hours
10. Which of the following statements is true regarding the CMT?
   a. It is a requirement.
   b. It is voluntary.
   c. It requires a minimum of 2 years' experience in a variety of specialties.
   d. Both b and c are correct.
   e. None of these

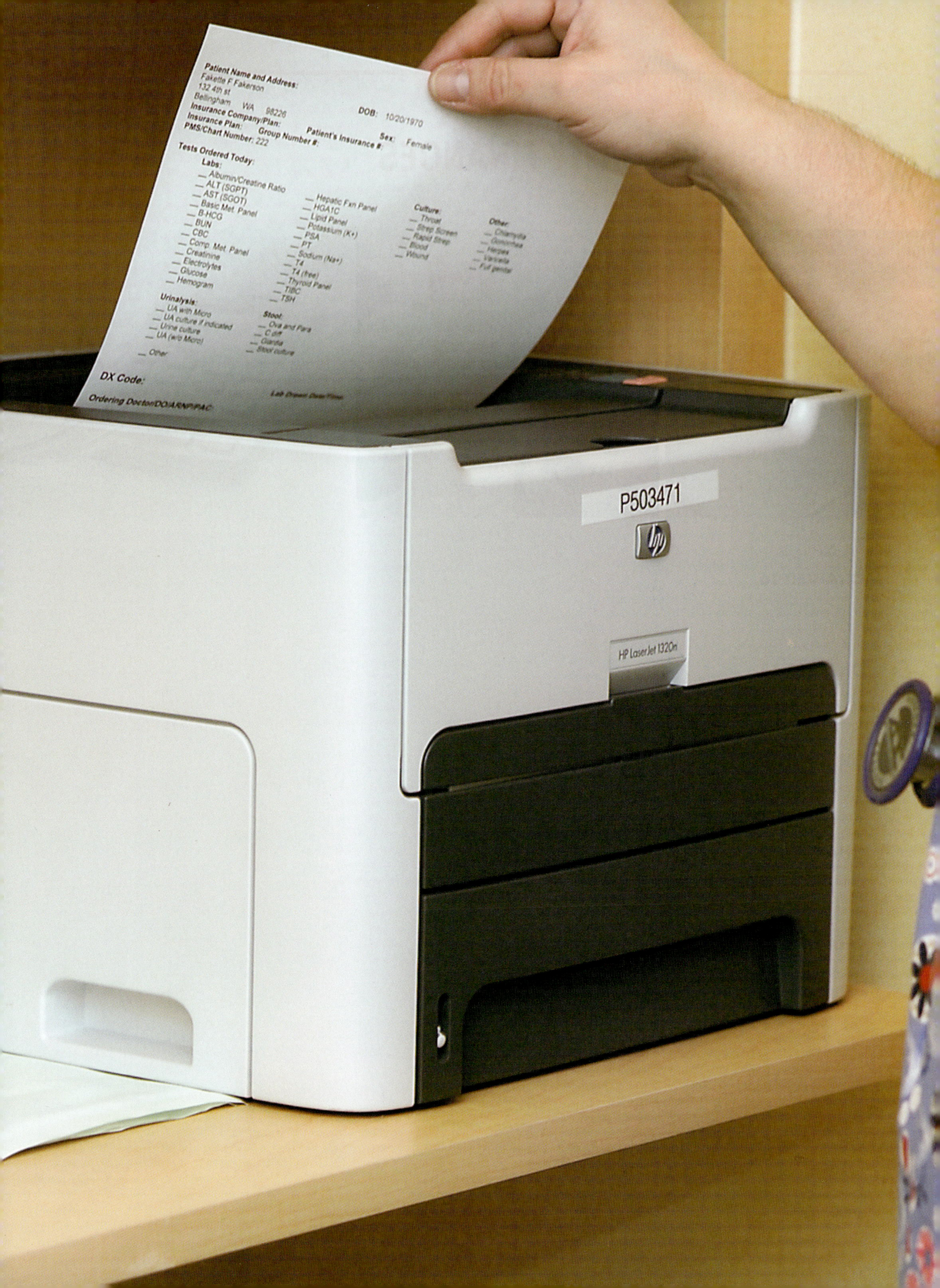

Patient Name and Address:
Fakette F Fakerson
132 4th st
Bellingham WA 98226
DOB: 10/20/1970
Insurance Company/Plan:
Patient's Insurance #:
Sex: Female
Insurance Plan: Group Number #:
PMS/Chart Number: 222
Tests Ordered Today:
Labs:
— Albumin/Creatine Ratio
— ALT (SGPT)
— AST (SGOT)
— Basic Met. Panel
— B-HCG
— BUN
— CBC
— Comp. Met. Panel
— Creatinine
— Electrolytes
— Glucose
— Hemogram
— Hepatic Fxn Panel
— HGA1C
— Lipid Panel
— Potassium (K+)
— PSA
— PT
— Sodium (Na+)
— T4
— T4 (free)
— Thyroid Panel
— TIBC
— TSH
Culture:
— Throat
— Strep Screen
— Rapid Strep
— Blood
— Wound
Urinalysis:
— UA with Micro
— UA culture if indicated
— Urine culture
— UA (w/o Micro)
— Other
Stool:
— Ova and Para
— C diff
— Giardia
— Stool culture
DX Code:
Lab Drawn Date/Time:
Ordering Doctor/DO/ARNP/PAC:
P503471
HP LaserJet 1320n

UNIT V
MANAGING FACILITY FINANCES

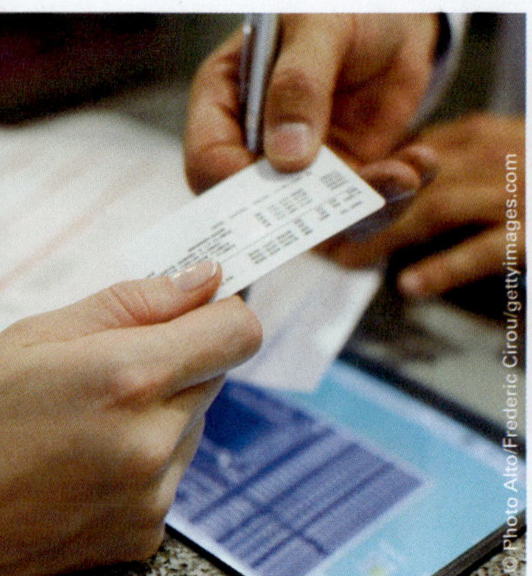

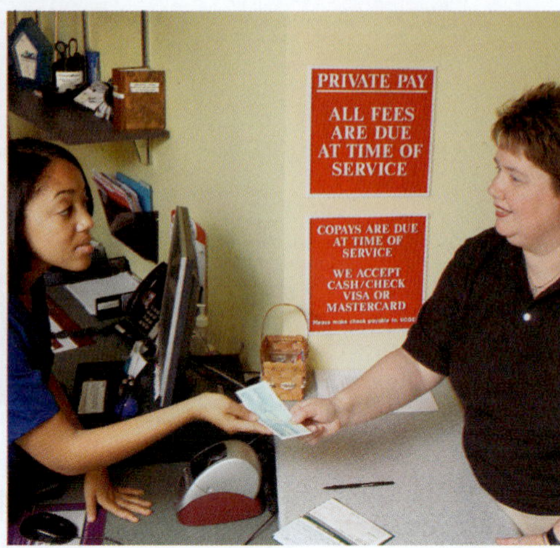

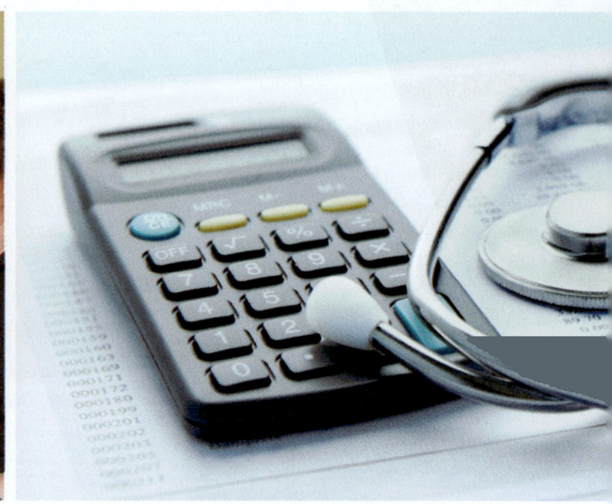

© Photo Alto/Frederic Cirou/gettyimages.com

ATTRIBUTES OF PROFESSIONALISM

The administrative medical assistant often handles medical insurance billing and bookkeeping, especially when recording transactions from both patients and insurance plans. The medical assistant must be comfortable with handling money and following up for collections when necessary. Each patient must be respected, and not be stereotyped due to their type of insurance coverage, lack of coverage, or ability to pay.

It is not unusual for medical services to be provided at a discount, through negotiated contracts with insurance plans, courtesy adjustments for patients that need them, and other situations where collecting the full fee for service is not possible. The medical assistant must navigate patient questions regarding their insurance and accounts while maintaining a positive, professional, and respectful attitude. This promotes dignity for the patient and an atmosphere conducive to healing, which allows the patient to feel comfortable returning for follow-up care and health maintenance.

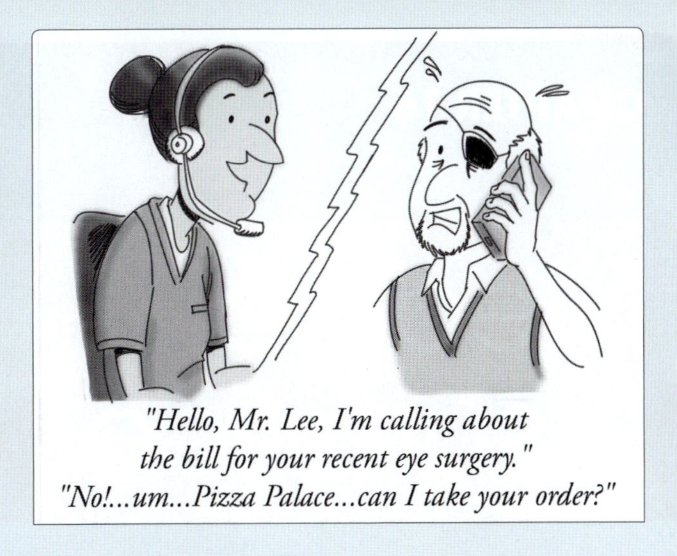

"Hello, Mr. Lee, I'm calling about the bill for your recent eye surgery."
"No!...um...Pizza Palace...can I take your order?"

Listed below are a series of questions for you to ask yourself, to serve as a professionalism checklist. As you interact with patients and colleagues, these questions will help to guide you in the professional behavior that is expected every day from medical assistants.

Ask Yourself

COMMUNICATION

- ☐ Do I display professionalism through written and verbal communication?
- ☐ Do I speak at each patient's level of understanding?
- ☐ Do I display appropriate body language?
- ☐ Do I respond honestly and diplomatically to my patients' concerns?
- ☐ Do I show sensitivity when communicating with patients regarding third party requirements?
- ☐ Does my knowledge allow me to speak easily with all members of the health care team?
- ☐ Do I utilize tactful communication skills with medical providers to ensure accurate code selection?

PRESENTATION

- ☐ Am I courteous, patient, and respectful to patients?
- ☐ Do I display a positive attitude?
- ☐ Do I display a calm, professional, and caring manner?
- ☐ Do I demonstrate empathy to the patient?
- ☐ Do I display sensitivity when managing appointments?

COMPETENCY

- ☐ Do I pay attention to detail?
- ☐ Do I ask questions if I am out of my comfort zone or do not have the experience to carry out tasks?
- ☐ Do I display sound judgment?
- ☐ Am I knowledgeable and accountable?
- ☐ Do I demonstrate professionalism when discussing the patient's billing record?
- ☐ Do I display sensitivity when requesting payment for services rendered?
- ☐ Do I interact professionally with third party representatives?

INITIATIVE

- ☐ Do I show initiative?
- ☐ Am I flexible and dependable?
- ☐ Do I direct the patient to other resources when necessary or helpful, with the approval of the provider?
- ☐ Do I implement time management principles to maintain effective office function?
- ☐ Do I assist co-workers when appropriate?

INTEGRITY

- ☐ Do I work within my scope of practice?
- ☐ Do I demonstrate sensitivity to patient rights?
- ☐ Do I protect the integrity of the medical record?
- ☐ Do I protect and maintain confidentiality?
- ☐ Do I immediately report any error I made?
- ☐ Do I do the "right thing" even when no one is observing?

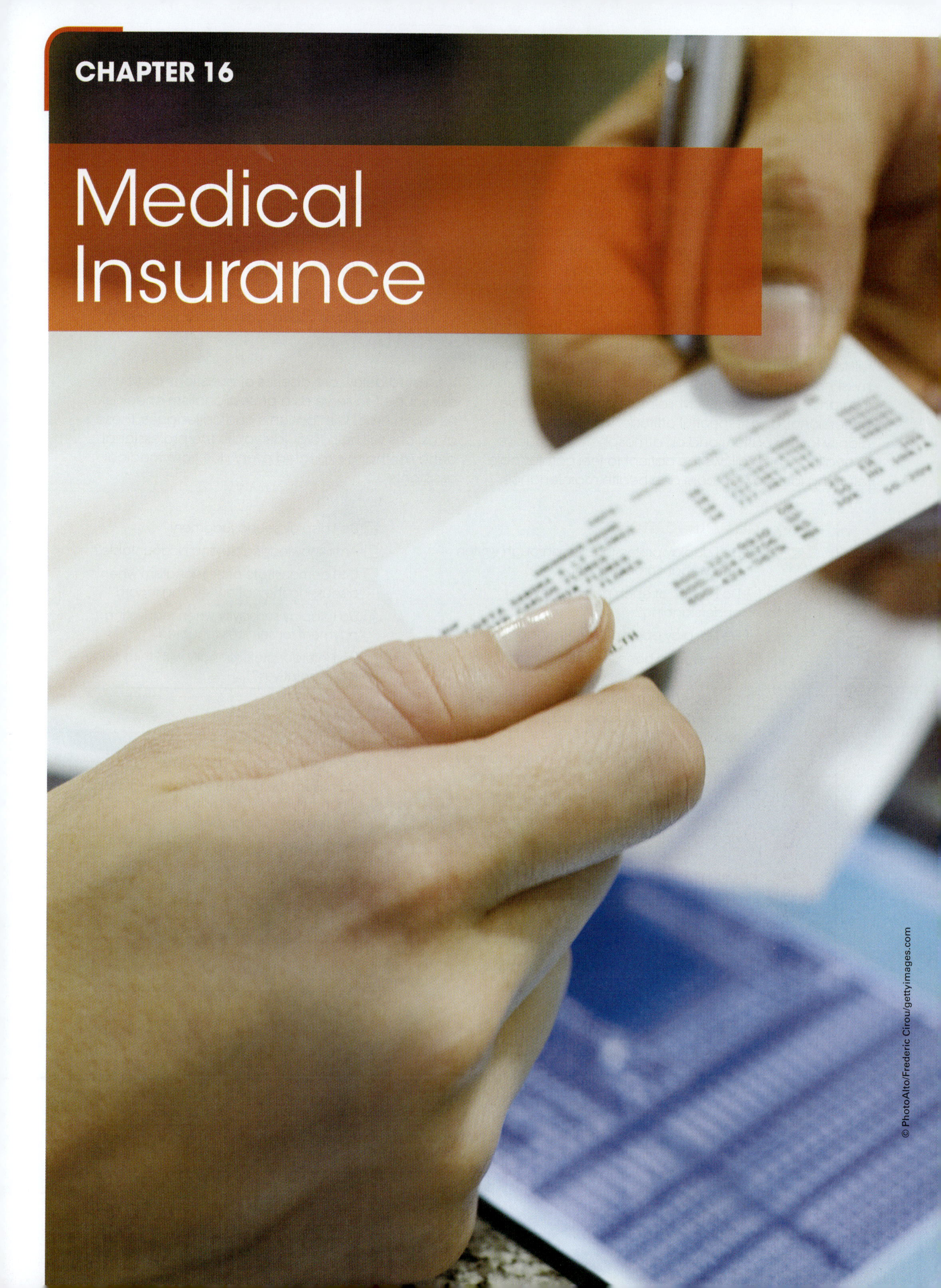

CHAPTER 16

Medical Insurance

LEARNING OUTCOMES

1. Define and spell the key terms as presented in the glossary.
2. Define the terminology necessary to understand and submit medical insurance claims.
3. List at least five examples of medical insurance coverage and discuss their differences.
4. Identify models of managed care.
5. Screen patients for insurance, verifying eligibility for managed care services.
6. Obtain managed care referrals, precertification, and preauthorization, including documentation.
7. Discuss workers' compensation as it applies to patients.
8. Discuss types of provider fee schedules.
9. Define diagnosis-related groups.
10. Discuss legal and ethical issues related to medical insurance and the provider's office.
11. Explore career opportunities in the insurance profession.
12. Describe procedures for implementing managed care and insurance plans.

KEY TERMS

abuse
adjustment
assignment of benefits
beneficiary
benefit period
birthday rule
capitation
Centers for Medicare and Medicaid Services (CMS)
co-insurance
coordination of benefits (COB)
co-payment
crossover claim
deductible
Defense Enrollment Eligible Reporting System (DEERS)
diagnosis-related groups (DRGs)
donut hole
exclusion
exclusive provider organization (EPO)
explanation of benefits (EOB)
fraud
health maintenance organization (HMO)
HIC number (HICN)
hospital outpatient prospective payment system (OPPS)
independent provider association (IPA)
integrated delivery system (IDS)
limiting charge
major medical insurance
managed care organization (MCO)
Medicare Part A
Medicare Part B
Medicare Part C
Medicare Part D
Medigap policy
personal injury protection (PIP)
point-of-service (POS) plan
preauthorization
preferred provider organization (PPO)
primary care provider (PCP)
referral
remittance advice (remit, RA)
resource-based relative value scale (RBRVS)
Self funded health care
subscriber
traditional indemnity insurance (FFS)
TRICARE
triple option plan
usual, customary, and reasonable (UCR)
Workers' Compensation insurance

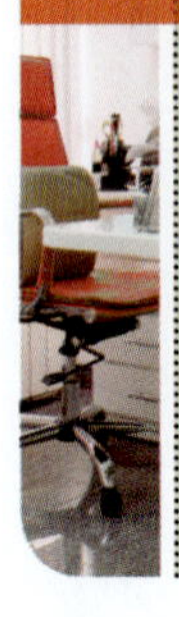

SCENARIO

At Inner City Health Care, a multi provider clinic in a large city, medical assistant Ellen Armstrong, CMAS (AMT), is responsible for all patient billing procedures. Inner City participates in a number of insurance plans, so Ellen must stay abreast of policy changes regarding reimbursement, preauthorizations, and claims filing. She also tries to become acquainted with the conditions of each patient's insurance coverage and helps patients understand their responsibility, if any, for payment. Finally, Ellen holds periodic meetings with her assistants to update them; she continually stresses to them the importance of timeliness in filing claims and the need for absolute accuracy in diagnosis and procedure codes, which must always reflect services actually performed.

Chapter Portal

An understanding of medical insurance and proper coding techniques is absolutely critical to the survival of the medical clinic. In recent years, much has changed in medical insurance coverage: more patients are choosing health maintenance organizations (HMOs) and other managed care options, and even traditional insurance carriers such as Blue Cross and Blue Shield are modifying their insurance plans to include some aspect of managed benefits.

In some ways, managed care coverage has simplified the patient's responsibility for payment, but it is more important than ever for the medical assistant to be accurate, timely, and conscientious in both filing insurance claim forms and understanding—and helping the patient to understand—the conditions of individual insurance policies.

The increasing complexity of health insurance today means that medical assistants must continually update their base of information. This chapter provides the groundwork for understanding the role of insurance, its terminology, and its various forms, and it gives the medical assistant the confidence to take responsibility for claim filing in the ambulatory care setting.

UNDERSTANDING THE ROLE OF HEALTH INSURANCE

Health insurance was designed to help individuals and families compensate for the high costs of medical care. Medical care consists of the diagnosis of diseases/disorders and the care and treatment provided by the health care team of professionals to individuals who are ill or injured. Medical care, which also includes preventive services, is designed to help individuals avoid health or injury problems and is termed *health care.*

Health care insurance is a contract between an individual policyholder and a third-party or government program that reimburses the medical provider or the policyholder for medically necessary treatment or preventive care covered by that specific health care provider.

There is much discussion today about changes in the health care insurance industry. Foremost is the goal that health care insurance should be available to all citizens of the United States. In the past, health insurance was usually tied to the employment package that covers the employee, and possibly the spouse and dependent children. One problem with work-related coverage is that some part-time employees are not eligible for health insurance and thus often go uninsured. Another problem is if an employee takes a position elsewhere, medical benefits may not transfer equally. If a family member is ill with a preexisting condition such as cancer or diabetes mellitus, the new insurance policy may not cover that disease or condition for a fixed time period. This time-dependent limitation of coverage is known as an **exclusion**. If health insurance has previously been in effect for at least 18 months and any lapse in coverage between policies did not exceed 63 days, a preexisting condition cannot be given as a reason for exclusion. Some states have laws limiting the length of an exclusion period; otherwise it is at the discretion of the carrier. An exclusion also may include illnesses or conditions for injury specifically not covered by the policy.

The Patient Protection and Affordable Care Act (PPACA), signed into law by President Barack Obama in 2010, is intended to help resolve many of these concerns. The Act requires that all individuals who do not already have medical insurance coverage through a group plan with their employer or coverage through Medicare or Medicaid to purchase health coverage. There are many parts to the PPACA, which all together will be making many changes to our health insurance industry over the next 10 years. For example, as of January 2014, insurance companies were longer permitted to charge policyholders a preexisting condition a higher premium. It is also stated in the PPACA that by 2018, insurance plans are not to charge a co-payment if the office visit is for preventive medicine, such as well-women and well-child visits.

Another controversial aspect of health insurance is refusal to provide coverage for certain procedures because they have not been sufficiently proved to be effective. Although more insurance companies are beginning to cover procedures such as in vitro fertilization, there remain many other plans that do not agree. Because most insurance carriers will not extend coverage to experimental treatment, family and friends of patients often gather for fund-raising drives to ensure that medical costs are covered.

Not all insurance carriers cover the same exposures equally, and few carriers pay at the same rate. Similarly, carriers do not charge the same premiums to policyholders. Some insurance companies cover individuals, families, or employee groups through work or through groups such as the American Association of Retired Persons (AARP). Some premiums reflect the insured person's past medical history and the company's exposure in covering the person. Premiums may be less if the insured person selects a higher annual deductible. Other premiums represent the rate that a group is able to obtain based on the group's claim history.

MEDICAL INSURANCE TERMINOLOGY

Before discussing the types of insurance coverage, one must understand the language used by the insurance industry. The terminology is specific in meaning and has been tested in courts of law to further define its meanings.

Terminology Specific to Insurance Policies

A policy is an agreement between an insurance company or government program and the insured, or **beneficiary,** that is, the person covered under the terms of the policy. The insured may also be referred to as the **subscriber**. The insured person may include as beneficiaries a spouse and dependent minor children; others may be included if related by blood and dependent on the insured for more than 50% of their support. The insurance carrier pays a percentage **(co-insurance)** of the cost of the services covered under the policy in exchange for a monthly premium or charge. This premium is paid by the insured or the employer, or it is shared by both.

At the inception or beginning of the policy, the insured is given an identification card, which must be presented before receiving medical treatment. This card contains the insured person's name, identification number, group number, and any co-payment amount or restrictions for treatment. The back of the insurance card contains an address where claims should be submitted and telephone numbers needed to receive prior authorization for treatment when required.

Deductible. The language of the policy spells out the terms of the coverage. Usually there is an annual **deductible**, or an amount of money that the insured must pay out-of-pocket for medical services before the policy begins to pay. This deductible can range from $100 to $5,000, or an even greater amount, depending on the language of the policy. The deductible must be met each calendar year by medical charges that are incurred after the inception or anniversary date of the policy, usually at the beginning of each year.

For instance, if Boris Bolski went to the provider on January 22 and incurred $258 in charges but his policy did not go into effect until February 1, none of these charges would apply toward his deductible. If, however, he returned to the doctor on February 3 and incurred another $85 charge, that amount could be applied against his deductible.

Co-insurance. After application of the deductible to the submitted bills, the insurance policy pays a percentage of the remaining amount. This percentage or co-insurance can vary from 50% to 100% depending on the language in a specific policy. Most traditional plans pay 70% to 80%.

Co-payment. Some insurance policies, especially **health maintenance organizations (HMOs)** and other managed care policies, require the patient to make a payment of a specified amount, for instance, $20 or $50, at the time of treatment. This payment must be collected at the time of the office visit. Some policies have both a **co-payment** and a co-insurance clause. In addition, co-payment amounts may differ between a primary physician and a specialist. For example, the co-payment to the primary physician may be only $20 per office visit. However, when a patient visits a specialist, the co-payment may increase to $35. Co-payments may also be applied in the emergency room (ER) setting. Often, the ER co-payment is waived if the patient is admitted to the hospital. The co-payment may be possibly waived in other situations, such as when a patient is coming in for a follow-up visit after surgery for suture removal.

Preexisting Condition. Under the Affordable Care Act, health insurance companies cannot refuse to offer coverage or charge higher premiums because of a pre-existing condition. A pre-existing condition is a diagnosis the patient had before the date new health coverage begins. In addition, premiums cannot be higher based on gender. These rules went into effect for plans beginning on or after January 1, 2014.

The only exception to this rule is for any "grandfathered" individual health insurance plan that was purchased on or before March 23, 2010 that was not changed to reduce benefits or increase costs to the policyholder. If a patient has a grandfathered plan, they may not have some of the rights and protections other plans offer under the Affordable Care Act. The insurer must notify the patient if they have a grandfathered plan.

If a patient has a grandfathered plan, they may opt to switch to a plan that offers protections under the ACA during the annual open enrollment period. If the plan ends at any time during the year, a patient may switch at that time and purchase a plan outside of the open enrollment period.

As a medical assistant that works with insurance in the clinic, it is important to be aware of the protections that do not apply to grandfathered plans. These include coverage of preventative care, guarantee to appeal coverage decisions, protection of choice of doctors and access to emergency care, yearly limits on coverage, and coverage of a pre-existing condition. Protections that apply to all plans, including grandfathered individual plans do include no lifetime limits on coverage, and coverage for adult children up to age 26. As with any insurance plan, eligibility should be verified and plan details obtained as applicable to the clinic before services are rendered to the patient. In this manner, any non-covered services or out of pocket expenses can be discussed with the patient ahead of time.

Exclusions. Exclusions are noncovered services and are an important part of a policy. Some policies exclude services that are not medically necessary, such as cosmetic surgery, whereas other policies may allow these procedures with certain criteria that makes them medically necessary. An example might be repair of a deviated septum of the nose, due to frequent infections, snoring, and breathing problems. Other examples of exclusions or non-covered services might be preexisting conditions, dental services, chiropractic services, or routine eye examinations. Not every policy has the same exclusions.

Coordination of Benefits. Most health insurance policies have a clause that coordinates the benefits of one policy with those of another when a patient has dual coverage. Dual coverage, or having more than one policy, will put into effect this clause, named **coordination of benefits (COB)**.

Coordination of benefits rules follow a set of guidelines as put forth by the National Association of Health Insurance Commissioners (NAIC). The purpose of these guidelines is to avoid duplicate payment for medical services when there are two policies.

It is important to understand that COB is further determined by type of plan, whether the covered person is the insured or a dependent on the plan, and if there is Medicare and/or Medicaid, the rules are different.

Insurance carriers will use the following general guidelines:

- Group plans are those provided by an employer or other entity that are primary for the insured or subscriber. Group plans that do not have a COB clause will always be primary.
- Individual insurance, or those policies that are purchased by the insured and are not through an employer, normally pay benefits without regard to group policies. These policies might provide their own guidelines for dual insurance, and each needs to be verified.
- When dependent children have dual coverage (one policy per parent), determining the primary is done using the **birthday rule**. The plan of the parent whose birthday falls earliest in the year is the primary policy. Thus, if the father's birthday is October 17 and the mother's birthday is May 12, the mother's policy is primary. The year of the birth date is not relevant. If the parents have the same birthday, the policy in effect the longest is primary. For children of divorced parents who are covered under both parents' policies, the policy of the custodial parent usually is primary.

- Medicare and Medicaid have different guidelines which can be affected by the beneficiary being employed or retired, the size of the employer, and if the insured has certain diseases. These include end-stage renal disease and amyotrophic lateral sclerosis (ALS).

Whichever insurance is primary pays for covered services up to the maximum allowed under the plan, less the deductible and co-payment. The secondary insurance will coordinate the benefits and pay as appropriate, but the amount is never to exceed the total amount of the services. If the secondary insurance offers a COB, it will only consider the percentage paid as if it were primary.

Explanation of Benefits. The insurance carrier generates an **explanation of benefits (EOB)**, which is mailed to each patient (or may be obtained online). The EOB is a statement summarizing how the insurance carrier determined the reimbursement for services received by the patient. The backside of the EOB addresses questions frequently asked and defines the terms used within the EOB. The EOB is not to be considered a bill; it simply details information as to how the claim was processed by the insurance carrier. Figure 16-1 shows an example of an EOB.

Remittance Advice. The provider's office receives a **remittance advice** (**remit**, or **RA**) from the insurance carrier. The provider's RA summarizes all of the benefits paid to the provider within a particular period of time. The RA includes all of the patients covered by a specific insurance for that time period. The difference between the provider's charges and the amount paid by the insurance carrier may be billed to the patient. Figure 16-2 shows an example of a remittance advice.

Terminology Specific to Billing Insurance Carriers

There is specific terminology that one must understand when submitting insurance claims for medical benefits. Most clinics bill all appropriate insurance carriers to ascertain that the claim is made and the provider receives payment.

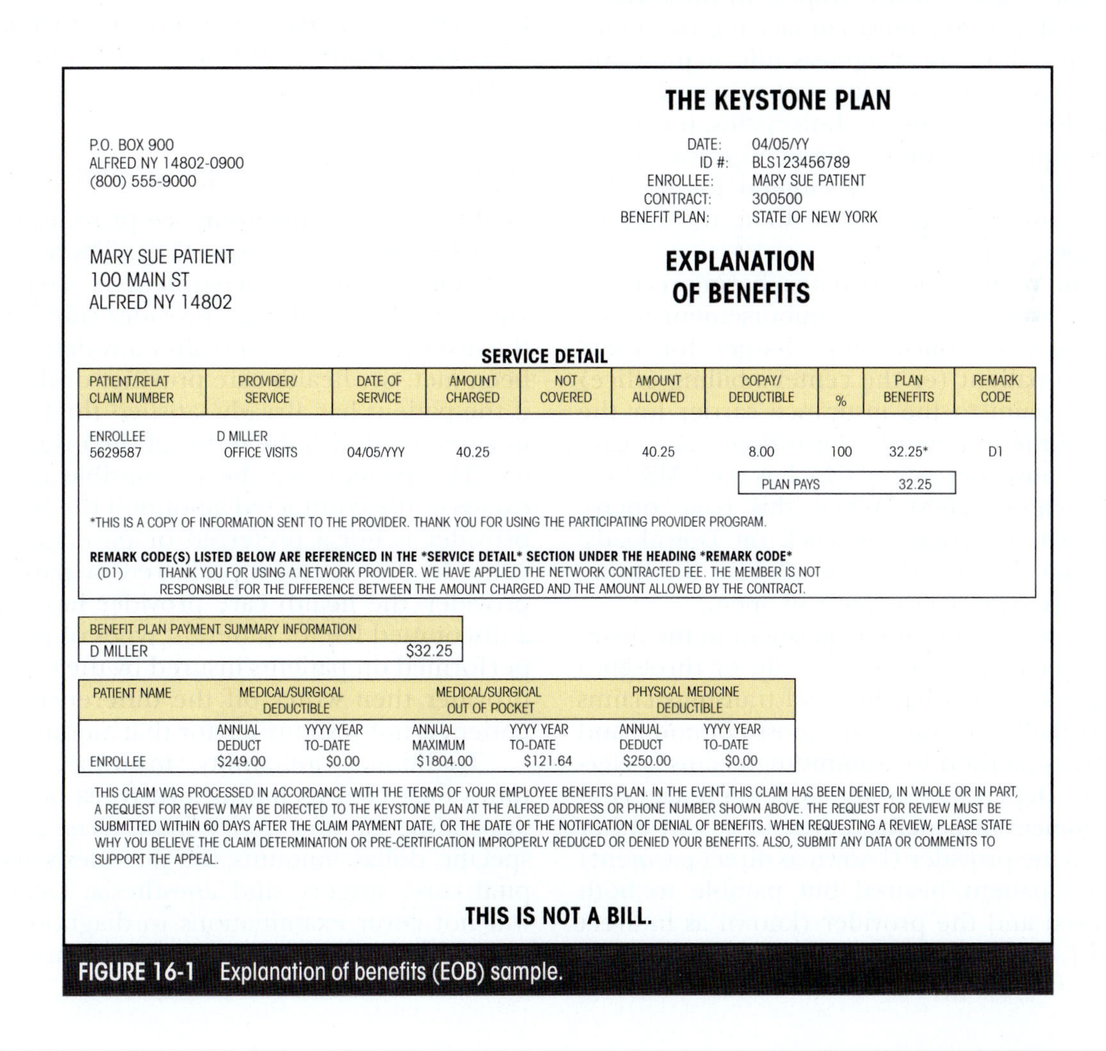

THE KEYSTONE PLAN

P.O. BOX 900
ALFRED NY 14802-0900
(800) 555-9000

DATE: 04/05/YY
ID #: BLS123456789
ENROLLEE: MARY SUE PATIENT
CONTRACT: 300500
BENEFIT PLAN: STATE OF NEW YORK

MARY SUE PATIENT
100 MAIN ST
ALFRED NY 14802

EXPLANATION OF BENEFITS

SERVICE DETAIL

PATIENT/RELAT CLAIM NUMBER	PROVIDER/ SERVICE	DATE OF SERVICE	AMOUNT CHARGED	NOT COVERED	AMOUNT ALLOWED	COPAY/ DEDUCTIBLE	%	PLAN BENEFITS	REMARK CODE
ENROLLEE 5629587	D MILLER OFFICE VISITS	04/05/YYY	40.25		40.25	8.00	100	32.25*	D1
						PLAN PAYS		32.25	

*THIS IS A COPY OF INFORMATION SENT TO THE PROVIDER. THANK YOU FOR USING THE PARTICIPATING PROVIDER PROGRAM.

REMARK CODE(S) LISTED BELOW ARE REFERENCED IN THE *SERVICE DETAIL* SECTION UNDER THE HEADING *REMARK CODE*
(D1) THANK YOU FOR USING A NETWORK PROVIDER. WE HAVE APPLIED THE NETWORK CONTRACTED FEE. THE MEMBER IS NOT RESPONSIBLE FOR THE DIFFERENCE BETWEEN THE AMOUNT CHARGED AND THE AMOUNT ALLOWED BY THE CONTRACT.

BENEFIT PLAN PAYMENT SUMMARY INFORMATION	
D MILLER	$32.25

PATIENT NAME	MEDICAL/SURGICAL DEDUCTIBLE		MEDICAL/SURGICAL OUT OF POCKET		PHYSICAL MEDICINE DEDUCTIBLE	
	ANNUAL DEDUCT	YYYY YEAR TO-DATE	ANNUAL MAXIMUM	YYYY YEAR TO-DATE	ANNUAL DEDUCT	YYYY YEAR TO-DATE
ENROLLEE	$249.00	$0.00	$1804.00	$121.64	$250.00	$0.00

THIS CLAIM WAS PROCESSED IN ACCORDANCE WITH THE TERMS OF YOUR EMPLOYEE BENEFITS PLAN. IN THE EVENT THIS CLAIM HAS BEEN DENIED, IN WHOLE OR IN PART, A REQUEST FOR REVIEW MAY BE DIRECTED TO THE KEYSTONE PLAN AT THE ALFRED ADDRESS OR PHONE NUMBER SHOWN ABOVE. THE REQUEST FOR REVIEW MUST BE SUBMITTED WITHIN 60 DAYS AFTER THE CLAIM PAYMENT DATE, OR THE DATE OF THE NOTIFICATION OF DENIAL OF BENEFITS. WHEN REQUESTING A REVIEW, PLEASE STATE WHY YOU BELIEVE THE CLAIM DETERMINATION OR PRE-CERTIFICATION IMPROPERLY REDUCED OR DENIED YOUR BENEFITS. ALSO, SUBMIT ANY DATA OR COMMENTS TO SUPPORT THE APPEAL.

THIS IS NOT A BILL.

FIGURE 16-1 Explanation of benefits (EOB) sample.

ABC INSURANCE COMPANY
100 MAIN STREET
ALFRED NY 14802
1-800-555-1234

REMITTANCE ADVICE

DAVID MILLER, M.D.
101 NORTH STREET

ALFRED, NY 14802

PROVIDER #: 123456
PAGE #: 1 OF 1
DATE: 04/05/YY
CHECK/EFT #: 000235698

PERF PROV SERV DATE POS NOS PROC MODS BILLED ALLOWED DEDUCT COINS GRP/RC AMT PROV PD

NAME BAKER, JENNY HIC 235962541 ACNT BAKE1234567-01 ICN 1235626589651 ASG Y MOA MA01
236592ABC 0405 0405YY 11 1 99213 75.00 50.00 0.25 0.00 CO-42 15.00 50.00
PT RESP 10.31 CLAIM TOTALS 75.00 50.00 0.25 0.00 15.00

NET 50.00

TOTALS	# OF CLAIMS	BILLED AMT	ALLOWED AMT	DEDUCT AMT	COINS RC AMT	TOTAL AMT	PROV PD ADJ AMT	PROV AMT	CHECK AMT
	1	75.00	50.00	0.25	15.00	65.25	50.00	0.00	50.00

FIGURE 16-2 Remittance advice (single claim) sample.

Many policies require **preauthorization** before certain procedures or before a visit can be made to a specialist or a physical therapist. In these cases, the medical assistant must contact the insurance carrier with all of the diagnosis information and the proposed course of treatment. For instance, if a patient has a diagnosis of cholecystitis, preauthorization requires notification and approval before referring that patient to a surgeon for possible cholecystectomy. If this is not done, the surgery may not be covered.

A claim occurs when patients, having received treatment, wish to receive reimbursement under their insurance policies for charges for treatment. The patient (or the center's billing office) sends the claim to the insurance carrier for the amount of the treatment. This is done via a claim form, the most common of which is the CMS-1500 (02-12) (Figure 16-3). When this page opens, scroll down the page and click on Downloads: Intermediary-Carrier Directory. A PDF file listing all Medicare regional carriers will open.

The completed claim form is sent to the insurance carrier by mail, electronically, or through a holding system that batches and transmits claims at timed daily intervals. The most common and expeditious method for submitting claims is electronically. Depending on the policy language and the **assignment of benefits**, payment is sent either directly to the provider (known as direct payment) or to the patient/insured but payable to both the insured and the provider (known as indirect payment).

TYPES OF MEDICAL INSURANCE COVERAGE

In today's health care environment, medical assistants need to be aware of the different types of medical insurance policies.

Traditional Indemnity Insurance

Traditional indemnity insurance provides coverage on a fee-for-service basis (FFS). There is usually a deductible and a co-payment or co-insurance amount. The health care provider submits bills to the insurance carrier, and after any deductible has been met, the health care provider or the patient, if the patient has already satisfied the bill, is paid in agreement with the terms of the insurance policy. The patient may be responsible for fees in excess of the contracted amount if the health care provider is not a preferred or participating provider. In the case of a preferred or participating provider, the health care provider has agreed to a discounted fee for different types of procedures performed on patients insured by the carrier. The provider then writes off the difference, and the patient is not responsible for that amount.

Traditional indemnity insurance is sometimes marketed as having two types of coverage, depending on the policy. *Basic insurance* covers specific dollar amounts for provider's fees, hospital care, surgery, and anesthesia. Generally, it will not cover examinations to diagnose or treat fertility problems, but more carriers are covering

HEALTH INSURANCE CLAIM FORM

APPROVED BY NATIONAL UNIFORM CLAIM COMMITTEE (NUCC) 02/12

PICA | PICA

CARRIER

PATIENT AND INSURED INFORMATION

1. MEDICARE (Medicare#) | MEDICAID (Medicaid#) | TRICARE (ID#/DoD#) | CHAMPVA (Member ID#) | GROUP HEALTH PLAN (ID#) | FECA BLK LUNG (ID#) | OTHER (ID#)

1a. INSURED'S I.D. NUMBER (For Program in Item 1)

2. PATIENT'S NAME (Last Name, First Name, Middle Initial)

3. PATIENT'S BIRTH DATE MM DD YY SEX M F

4. INSURED'S NAME (Last Name, First Name, Middle Initial)

5. PATIENT'S ADDRESS (No., Street)

6. PATIENT RELATIONSHIP TO INSURED Self Spouse Child Other

7. INSURED'S ADDRESS (No., Street)

CITY STATE

8. RESERVED FOR NUCC USE

CITY STATE

ZIP CODE TELEPHONE (Include Area Code) ( )

ZIP CODE TELEPHONE (Include Area Code) ( )

9. OTHER INSURED'S NAME (Last Name, First Name, Middle Initial)

10. IS PATIENT'S CONDITION RELATED TO:

11. INSURED'S POLICY GROUP OR FECA NUMBER

a. OTHER INSURED'S POLICY OR GROUP NUMBER

a. EMPLOYMENT? (Current or Previous) YES NO

a. INSURED'S DATE OF BIRTH MM DD YY SEX M F

b. RESERVED FOR NUCC USE

b. AUTO ACCIDENT? YES NO PLACE (State)

b. OTHER CLAIM ID (Designated by NUCC)

c. RESERVED FOR NUCC USE

c. OTHER ACCIDENT? YES NO

c. INSURANCE PLAN NAME OR PROGRAM NAME

d. INSURANCE PLAN NAME OR PROGRAM NAME

10d. CLAIM CODES (Designated by NUCC)

d. IS THERE ANOTHER HEALTH BENEFIT PLAN? YES NO *If yes*, complete items 9, 9a, and 9d.

READ BACK OF FORM BEFORE COMPLETING & SIGNING THIS FORM.

12. PATIENT'S OR AUTHORIZED PERSON'S SIGNATURE I authorize the release of any medical or other information necessary to process this claim. I also request payment of government benefits either to myself or to the party who accepts assignment below.

SIGNED ____ DATE ____

13. INSURED'S OR AUTHORIZED PERSON'S SIGNATURE I authorize payment of medical benefits to the undersigned physician or supplier for services described below.

SIGNED ____

PHYSICIAN OR SUPPLIER INFORMATION

14. DATE OF CURRENT ILLNESS, INJURY, or PREGNANCY (LMP) MM DD YY QUAL.

15. OTHER DATE QUAL. MM DD YY

16. DATES PATIENT UNABLE TO WORK IN CURRENT OCCUPATION FROM MM DD YY TO MM DD YY

17. NAME OF REFERRING PROVIDER OR OTHER SOURCE | 17a. | 17b. NPI

18. HOSPITALIZATION DATES RELATED TO CURRENT SERVICES FROM MM DD YY TO MM DD YY

19. ADDITIONAL CLAIM INFORMATION (Designated by NUCC)

20. OUTSIDE LAB? YES NO $ CHARGES

21. DIAGNOSIS OR NATURE OF ILLNESS OR INJURY Relate A-L to service line below (24E) ICD Ind.

A. B. C. D.
E. F. G. H.
I. J. K. L.

22. RESUBMISSION CODE ORIGINAL REF. NO.

23. PRIOR AUTHORIZATION NUMBER

24. A. DATE(S) OF SERVICE From MM DD YY To MM DD YY	B. PLACE OF SERVICE	C. EMG	D. PROCEDURES, SERVICES, OR SUPPLIES (Explain Unusual Circumstances) CPT/HCPCS MODIFIER	E. DIAGNOSIS POINTER	F. $ CHARGES	G. DAYS OR UNITS	H. EPSDT Family Plan	I. ID. QUAL.	J. RENDERING PROVIDER ID. #
1								NPI	
2								NPI	
3								NPI	
4								NPI	
5								NPI	
6								NPI	

25. FEDERAL TAX I.D. NUMBER SSN EIN

26. PATIENT'S ACCOUNT NO.

27. ACCEPT ASSIGNMENT? (For govt. claims, see back) YES NO

28. TOTAL CHARGE $

29. AMOUNT PAID $

30. Rsvd for NUCC Use

31. SIGNATURE OF PHYSICIAN OR SUPPLIER INCLUDING DEGREES OR CREDENTIALS (I certify that the statements on the reverse apply to this bill and are made a part thereof.)

SIGNED DATE

32. SERVICE FACILITY LOCATION INFORMATION

a. NPI b.

33. BILLING PROVIDER INFO & PH # ( )

a. NPI b.

NUCC Instruction Manual available at: www.nucc.org

FIGURE 16-3 CMS-1500 (02/12) claim form.

routine physical and preventive care. **Major medical insurance** covers catastrophic expenses resulting from illness or injury.

Some traditional indemnity insurance plans and most managed care insurance carriers require the patient to select a **primary care provider**, or **PCP**. The PCP becomes the first medical practitioner caring for the patient, is also known as the gatekeeper, and is responsible for making referrals for further treatment by specialists or for hospital admission. The insurance carrier frequently will refuse payment for treatments not referred by the PCP.

Blue Cross and Blue Shield (BCBS). Whereas many traditional policies are offered by commercial carriers, the "Blues" are the largest payer groups in the United States, with 36 independent and locally operated franchises. Originally, Blue Cross started as a prepaid hospital plan, and Blue Shield later was added to cover physician provider services. In the early 1980s, the two merged to become the BCBS Association. Independent franchises may be organized as not-for-profit or for-profit.

Today, BCBS offers coverage for large employer groups, small businesses, and individual plans. Additionally, BCBS also serves as a Medicare fiscal intermediary (FI), administrating the Medicare program regionally throughout the United States, District of Columbia, Canada, Puerto Rico, and Jamaica. In the United States, a Medicare fiscal intermediary acts on behalf of the government to review reimbursement and coverage, and pays on approved claims.

A BCBS participating provider (PAR) chooses to sign a member contract and receives an incentive. PARs agree to accept the BCBS reimbursement as payment in full for covered services. BCBS agrees to reimburse providers directly and in a shorter turnaround time.

Each policyholder is given a card with the subscriber's name and a three-character letter prefix identification number. The letter prefix is important because it indicates under which BCBS plan the person is insured. This identification number must be included on each claim form submitted to BCBS; if it is not included, the claim will be denied.

Managed Care Insurance

Managed care insurance involves a **managed care organization (MCO)** that assumes the responsibility for the health care needs of a group of enrollees. The MCO can be a health care plan, hospital, provider group, or health system. The MCO contracts with an insurance carrier, or is itself the carrier, to take care of the medical needs of the enrolled group for a fixed fee per enrollee for a fixed period, usually a calendar year. This payment system is called capitation. If the medical costs exceed the fixed fee, the MCO/provider loses income; conversely, if the costs are less than the fixed fee, the MCO/provider makes a profit. An MCO relies on as large an enrollee base as possible to average the cost of medical care.

MCOs were established in an attempt to curb medical costs and provide for more efficient use of medical resources. Almost all MCOs use PCPs as case managers or utilization management services to control what medical resources are used for each patient and to strictly control treatment plans and discharge planning. This policy has led to disputes over quality of care, and many states have enacted laws requiring external quality reviews by independent organizations. The quality-control programs include government oversight, patient satisfaction surveys, review of grievances, measurement of the health status of the enrolled group, and reviews by accreditation agencies. Medicare has established measurable standards for MCOs through its Quality Improvement System for Managed Care (QISMC) program. The federal government requires providers to disclose incentive packages with MCOs to avoid conflicts of interest resulting in reduced level of care solely for the purpose of reducing costs or treatment, thus recognizing a profit at the expense of patient care.

Six models exist for managed care organizations:

1. ***Exclusive provider organization (EPO).*** Enrollees must obtain their medical services from a network of providers or health care facilities that are under exclusive contract to the EPO. The state insurance commissioner regulates EPOs.
2. ***Integrated delivery system (IDS).*** Enrollees obtain medical services from an affiliated group of service providers. The service providers consist of private practices and hospitals that share practice management and services to reduce overhead. An IDS may also be called one of the following: integrated service network, delivery system, horizontally integrated system, vertically integrated system or plan, health delivery network, or accountable health plan.
3. ***Health maintenance organization (HMO).*** Enrollees obtain medical services from a network of providers who agree to fixed fees for services but are not under exclusive contract to the insurance carrier.

4. ***Point-of-service (POS) plan.*** The enrollee has the freedom of obtaining medical services from an HMO provider or by self-referral to non-HMO providers. In the case of self-referral, the enrollee will have to pay greater deductibles and co-insurance charges.
5. ***Preferred provider organization (PPO).*** Enrollees obtain services from a network of providers and hospitals that have contracted their services at a discounted fee to an insurance company on a nonexclusive basis.
6. ***Independent practice association (IPA).*** Enrollees obtain medical services from an association of independent physician providers and other medical entities. Services are provided to MCOs either by capitation, flat fee, or a negotiated FFS schedule.
7. ***Triple option plan.*** Enrollees have the option of using the coverage as a traditional, HMO, or PPO health plan. This is also called a 3-in-1 plan.

Table 16-1 lists differences between traditional and managed care policies.

Health maintenance organizations, or HMOs, are probably the most familiar managed care organizations. Originally, HMOs were designed to provide a full range of health care services and preventative care. Some HMOs are referred to as "one-stop" medical care, as the providers, diagnostic imaging, laboratory, pharmacy, and other services are located under one roof. More recently, the HMO without walls has become more commonplace, which is typically a network of participating providers within a defined geographic area.

TABLE 16-1

DIFFERENCES BETWEEN TRADITIONAL AND MANAGED CARE POLICIES

TRADITIONAL PLANS	MANAGED CARE
Usually can go outside provider network	Usually must stay inside provider network
Co-insurance	Co-pay each visit
Annual deductible	No annual deductible
Illness or injury only	Preventive treatment, as well as illness and injury
Premium paid monthly to company by employer or subscriber	Premium paid monthly to company by employer or subscriber
Provider paid by fee for service	Provider paid by capitation

The Impact of Managed Care. The emergence of managed care in today's society provides new administrative and clinical challenges to members of the health care team as they struggle to provide the best health care while working within limitations often imposed by insurance carriers. Virtually all health care settings, whether they are individual or group practices, or urgent care centers, are experiencing the impact of managed care. Providers network and compete to serve patients better and more cost-efficiently.

Under managed care, critics charge, health care dollars have grown scarce, providers must strive to provide the same quality for reduced reimbursement, preapprovals must be obtained for many services, and some services may be denied because they are not considered cost-effective.

Clinically, managed care may set limits on services or length of services. Second opinions are encouraged and sometimes required. In some systems, the patient's PCP is considered the *gatekeeper*, approving and providing referrals to specialists and more costly procedures, surgery, and tests. Critics of managed care point out that restricting or denying services may lead to an increase in professional liability.

Administratively, paperwork and documentation have become increasingly important to ensure proper reimbursement. Although it is the patient's responsibility to understand the conditions of the insurance policy, these are often difficult to understand or interpret. The medical staff must be fully aware of when a preapproval or treatment plan is required, when a second opinion is necessary for reimbursement, and other clauses and restrictions that affect care and reimbursement for care.

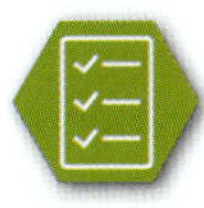
Procedure

At the same time, although managed care is challenging even the most resilient of providers, the very real need to keep costs down has also generated considerable creativity and energy among the health care profession as providers seek to use technology more efficiently; as they collaborate on new, cost-effective delivery methods; and as everyone involved in health care—insurers, providers, and patients—works together to contain costs by emphasizing prevention and lifestyle changes. Procedure 16-1 provides the steps involved in applying managed care policies and procedures.

PROCEDURE 16-1

Applying Managed Care Policies and Procedures

PURPOSE:

To apply managed care policies and procedures that the provider or medical facility has partnership agreements with.

EQUIPMENT/SUPPLIES:

- Managed care contracts
- Managed care policies and procedures manuals
- Patient record
- Authorized forms from managed care organizations
- Clerical supplies

PROCEDURE STEPS:

1. Determine which managed care organization the patient has contracted with. RATIONALE: To ensure that the correct policies and procedures are applied to the correct organization.
2. Contact the insurance carrier(s) via telephone to:
   a. Verify the patient has insurance in effect and is eligible for benefits.
   b. Confirm any exclusions or noncovered services.
   c. Determine deductibles, co-payments, or any other out-of-pocket expenses that the patient is responsible for paying.
   d. Ask if preauthorization is required for referrals to specialists or for any procedures and/or services. RATIONALE: Ascertains that insurance is viable and what benefits and patient expenses are established within the contract.
3. Record the name, title, and telephone number and extension of the insurance person contacted. RATIONALE: Documents the name of the individual providing the information. If questions arise at a later date, a contact is readily available.
4. Collect any forms necessary to process the patient claims. RATIONALE: Submitting correct forms to the managed care organization expedites the process.
5. ***Paying attention to detail***, document the information collected in the patient's medical record and on the Verification of Eligibility and Benefits form. RATIONALE: Provides a record of what has taken place.
6. ***Show initiative*** by attending seminars and workshops offered by managed care organizations or in-service training sessions. RATIONALE: Promotes obtaining up-to-date information regarding managed care policies and procedures.

Original Medicare

Medicare, also referred to as Original Medicare, was established in 1966, and is the largest medical insurance program in the United States. Most individuals 65 years and older, individuals with a disability that keeps them from working, and individuals with chronic kidney disease and amyotropic lateral sclerosis (ALS, also known as Lou Gehrig's disease) are eligible for Medicare.

Medicare coverage consists of Parts A, B, C, and D. Part A is the Medicare program for hospitalization and requires no monthly premiums. Parts B, C, and D require monthly premiums to be paid by the patient, with the amount depending upon income and specific plans selected. Medicare and Medicaid are administered by the **Centers for Medicare and Medicaid Services (CMS)** which is an agency within the U.S. Department of Health and Human Services.

An **HIC number (HICN)** is the identification number of a Medical beneficiary. Both CMS and the Railroad Retirement Board (RRB) issue

Medicare HIC numbers. The format of an HIC number issued by CMS is a Social Security number followed by an alpha or alphanumeric suffix. For patients with Railroad Retirement benefits, an alpha prefix precedes the Social Security number.

Medicare Part A. **Medicare Part A** covers hospital admission and stay, home health care, and hospice care. It has a substantial deductible and a limit to the number of hospital days per stay and the total number of hospitalizations per year. Medicare Part A pays only a portion of a patient's hospital expenses, which are calculated on a **benefit period** basis. A benefit period begins with the first day of hospital stay and ends when the patient has been out of the hospital for 60 consecutive days. Many individuals subscribe to supplemental insurance (called Medigap policies) to cover the substantial deductible.

Individuals not yet 65 years old who already receive retirement benefits from Social Security, the Railroad Retirement Board, or disability are automatically enrolled in Part A and Part B. For all other qualified individuals, Medicare becomes effective the month of their 65th birthday. Three months before their 65th birthday, or the 24th month of disability, individuals are sent an initial enrollment package containing information about Medicare and a Medicare card. If both Medicare Parts A and B are desired, they simply sign the Medicare card and keep it in a safe place for use when needed. Figure 16-4 shows a sample Medicare card. Figure 16-5 is an example of the Railroad Retirement Board (RRB) card.

Medicare Part B. **Medicare Part B** covers outpatient expenses that include providers' fees, physical therapy, laboratory tests, radiologic studies, ambulance services, and charges for durable medical equipment. Durable medical equipment (DME) charges are for items that can withstand repeated use, and are meant to serve only a medical purpose (meaning they are not needed in the absence of illness or injury). Such equipment includes such items as canes, crutches, walkers, commode chairs, and blood glucose monitors. Part B does not cover medications *except* certain diabetic testing supplies. Medicare Part B requires a monthly premium, which is adjusted annually and can be dependent on income level.

In 2016, the patient must pay an annual deductible of $166 before Medicare Part B will begin to pay its share of the bills. Medicare then reimburses 80% of the Medicare fee schedule for medical care and 100% for laboratory fees. Medicare's fee schedule was adopted in 1992 and is based on the **resource-based relative value scale (RBRVS).** The RBRVS was developed using values for each medical and surgical procedure based on work, practice, and malpractice expenses and is factored for regional differences.

Figure 16-6 shows how the Medicare worksheet would look if there were no exclusions or deductions.

Medical service providers can elect to accept Medicare fee schedules and become a participating provider (PAR), or they may accept assignment on a case-by-case basis as a nonparticipating provider (non-PAR). Medical providers, whether PAR or

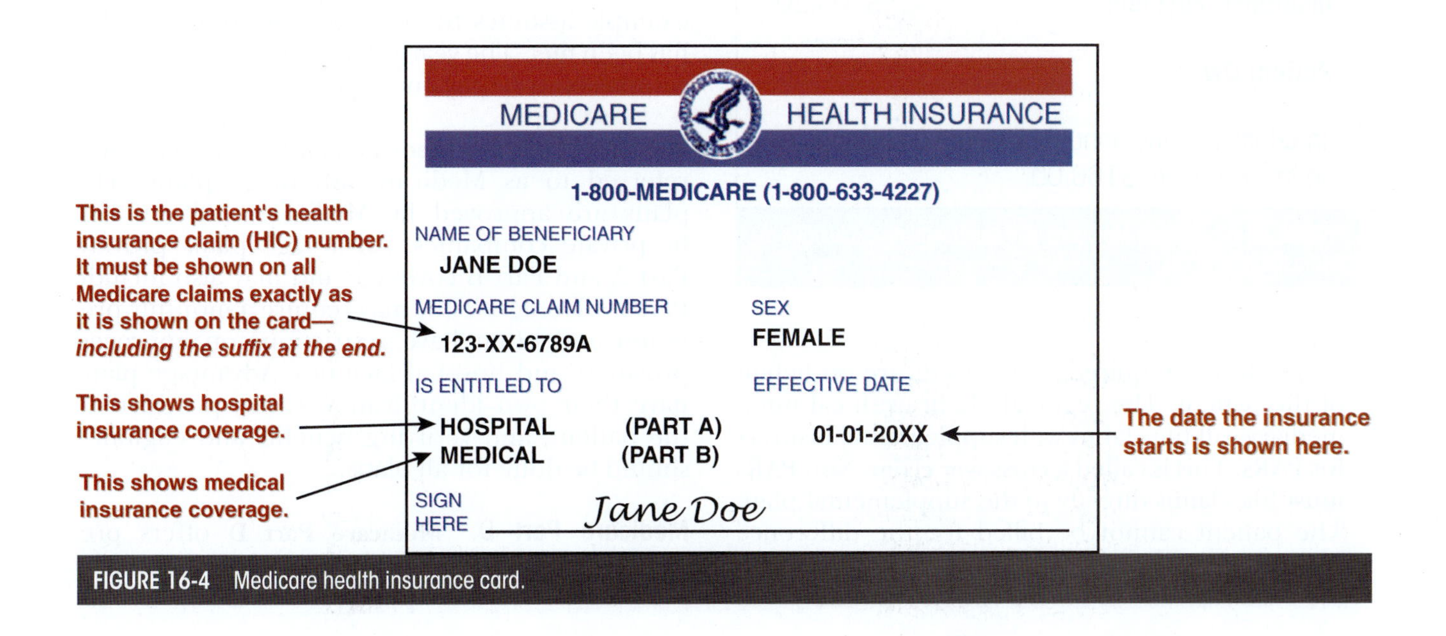

FIGURE 16-4 Medicare health insurance card.

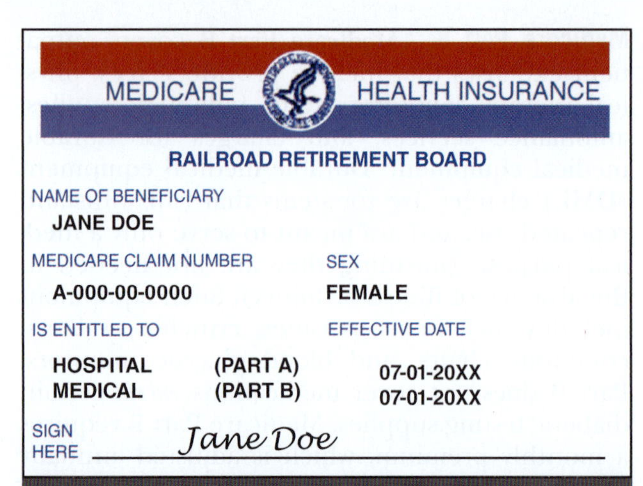
MEDICARE HEALTH INSURANCE

RAILROAD RETIREMENT BOARD

NAME OF BENEFICIARY
JANE DOE

MEDICARE CLAIM NUMBER: A-000-00-0000
SEX: FEMALE

IS ENTITLED TO / EFFECTIVE DATE
HOSPITAL (PART A) 07-01-20XX
MEDICAL (PART B) 07-01-20XX

SIGN HERE *Jane Doe*

FIGURE 16-5 Railroad Retirement Board (RRB) Medicare health insurance card.

Allowed Charges	
Office visit	$205.00
Return visit	+ 90.00
Total Charges	$295.00
Less deductible	–166.00
Subtotal	$129.00
Apply 80% co-insurance	x 80%
Insurance Payment	$103.20
Patient Owes	$25.80*

*In addition to the annual Medicare deductible, in this example, $166.00.

FIGURE 16-6 Sample Medicare worksheet with no exclusions or deductions.

non-PAR, are required to bill Medicare on behalf of the patient. The regional Medicare fiscal intermediary will file claims with supplemental insurers for PARs. This is called a **crossover claim**. Non-PARs must file claims directly to the supplemental plan. The patient cannot be billed for the difference between the participating provider's charges and the Medicare allowed fee. Providers can drop out

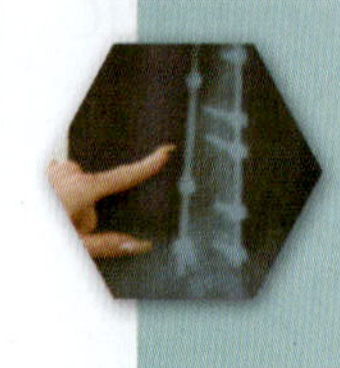

Critical Thinking

A Medicare patient has an office visit and is seen by a PAR provider. The allowed charge for the visit is $150. An insurance claim form is submitted to the local Medicare fiscal intermediary to apply against the deductible. At the next visit, the allowed charge is $125.00. This bill also is submitted to Medicare. How much of the bill will insurance pay after the deductible has been subtracted? How much does the patient owe?

of Medicare and enter into a contract with their Medicare patients that allows them to charge what they wish for services, but they must not bill Medicare for any services for the next 2 years, except in cases of emergency or urgent care.

In the example shown in Figure 16-7 the RBRVS allowed charge is applicable to both the participating and nonparticipating provider in computing the benefits Medicare pays to the provider. However, the non-PAR provider is limited to 95% of the RBRVS allowed charge in computing the amount of co-insurance. In addition, the non-PAR provider may only charge the patient up to 115% of the Medicare allowed amount. This is called the **limiting charge**. The difference between the limiting charge and the actual charge cannot be collected from the patient. The PAR provider must write off the difference between what the provider charges for the procedure and the Medicare allowed charge as a courtesy adjustment. This example assumes the yearly Medicare deductible has been met. The yearly deductible is the patient's responsibility to pay out of pocket.

Medicare Part C. **Medicare Part C** is commonly referred to as Medicare advantage plans. The plans are approved by Medicare and are run by private companies. Advantage plans provide Part A and Part B coverage and may also include Part D coverage. They may require a monthly premium and often have restrictions on approved providers and hospital facilities. Advantage plans have their own identification cards, provided to the patient, and verifying benefits and eligibility should be done for all plans.

Medicare Part D. **Medicare Part D** offers prescription drug coverage for everyone covered by Medicare. Part D requires a monthly premium

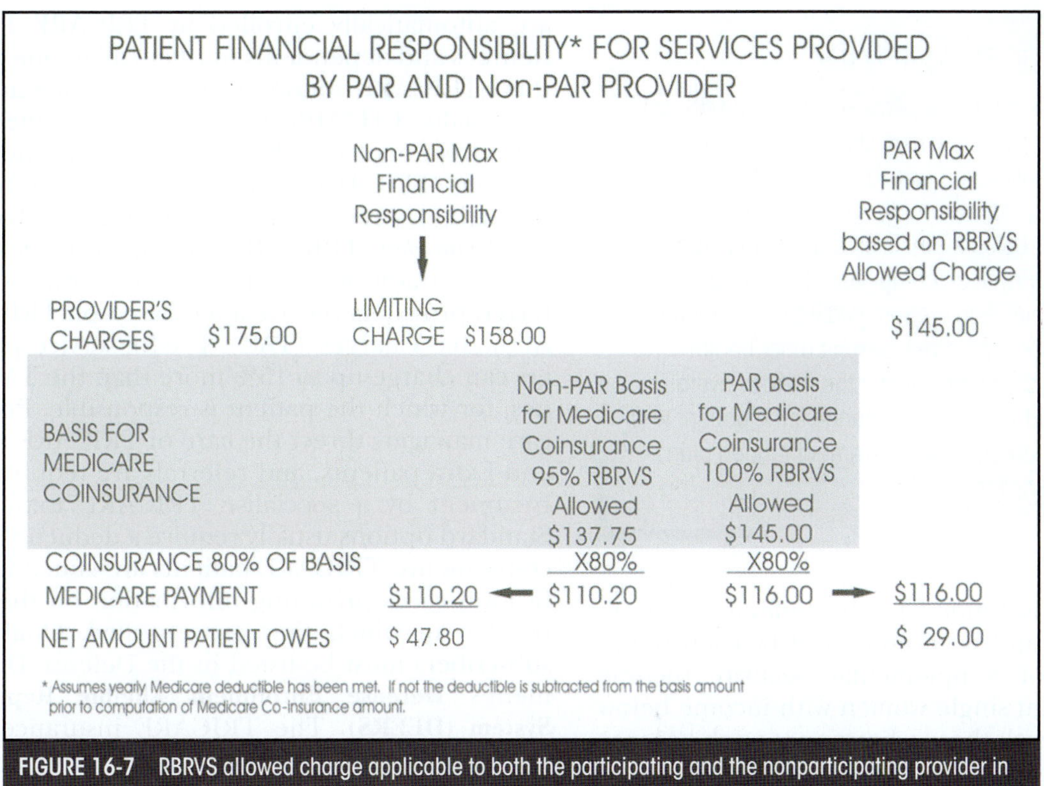

FIGURE 16-7 RBRVS allowed charge applicable to both the participating and the nonparticipating provider in computing the benefits Medicare pays to the provider.

that varies depending on the plan selected. In the case of advantage plans, the cost of Part D may be administered by private companies.

Part D prescription drug coverage plans have a unique feature called the **donut hole** or coverage gap. As of 2016, all plans provide coverage until the total drug costs reach $3310, then the patient is totally responsible for the next $3752 of drug costs. After that, the patient only pays a small co-payment for each prescription until the end of the calendar year. Drug coverage plans vary greatly. Selection should be based on convenience, cost, and drugs covered by the plan.

Medicare Supplemental Insurance

Medicare supplemental insurance is a secondary insurance that may cover Medicare deductibles, co-insurance requirements, and additional procedures not covered by Medicare. It is purchased by the patient through an insurance carrier or is provided as part of an employee retirement package. Supplemental **Medigap policies** are filed with the carrier by the Medicare regional carrier. The regional carrier is not required to file claims for employee retirement plan supplemental packages on behalf of the patient. Supplemental insurance frequently requires the patient to seek treatment with specific providers and hospitals. Different programs have different coverage, which is dependent on the carrier and state requirements and should be determined when scheduling an appointment.

Medicaid Insurance

Medicaid insurance, also known as Title 19, or XIX, and Medi-Cal in California, was designed to assist those on public assistance, low income persons over the age of 65, the people with disabilities between the ages of 18 and 65, and those that

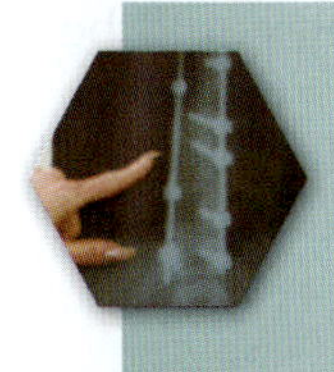

Critical Thinking

A patient has an office visit and is seen by a non-PAR provider whose office does not accept Medicare assignment. The charges are $175; however, the Medicare allowable amount is $125. A return office visit is charged at $100, with a Medicare allowable amount of $80. The $166 deductible has not yet been satisfied for the year. How much does the patient owe?

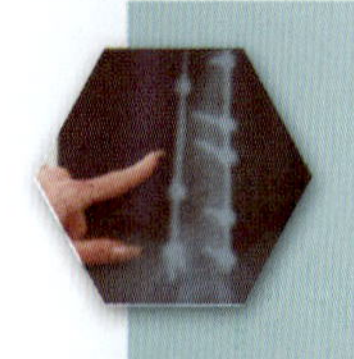

Critical Thinking

Some insurance plans set limits on services or length of services. Do you agree with this policy, and give rationale as to why or why not? Example: A patient with a knee replacement is on a managed care plan. Physical therapy benefits during rehabilitation are reduced if the patient does not show progress, despite other health issues that may hinder the therapy overall. Would your answer change if the patient was covered under a government funded plan, such as Medicaid?

are blind. It is funded by the federal and state governments and is administered by each state's department of Supplemental Security Income (SSI). Pregnant single women with income below the poverty level; those who cannot work because of emotional, mental, or physical difficulties; and people who are on Aid to Families with Dependent Children may qualify for this program. Recipients have an identification card for the program. Not all providers accept Medicaid patients. When referring a patient to a specialist or another provider, it is wise to ascertain whether that provider accepts patients with Medicaid. A referral form prepared by the PCP or referring provider usually is required.

Because Medicaid is always secondary to any supplemental insurance, claims to Medicaid are considered only after all other insurance payments have been made. When a person has both Medicare and Medicaid, charges are submitted first to Medicare and last to Medicaid.

Legal

Because Medicare and Medicaid are federal programs, errors in billing could be construed as fraud, for which there are criminal penalties. It is therefore imperative that all billing practices conform to the legal requirements of these programs.

TRICARE

TRICARE, formerly the Civilian Health and Medical Program for Uniformed Services (CHAMPUS), is medical insurance for active duty, activated guard, reserves, and retired members of the military, and their families and survivors. Active duty, guard, and reserve service members are automatically enrolled in TRICARE Prime. Retirees and dependents must enroll in one of the three TRICARE options: Prime, Extra, or Standard (originally CHAMPUS). TRICARE Prime provides treatment mainly through military hospital facilities. TRICARE Extra provides care primarily through contracted civilian providers called *preferred providers*. TRICARE Standard provides care through traditional fee-for-service providers. Preferred providers receive a fee based on TRICARE Allowable Charges (TAC). Fee-for-service providers can charge up to 15% more than the TAC values, for which the patient is responsible. Primary care managers direct the care of TRICARE Prime and Extra patients, and referrals are required for treatment by a specialist. TRICARE Extra and Standard options usually require a deductible and co-payments. TRICARE patients are issued identification cards providing information on the type of plan in which they are enrolled. Qualifying subscribers must be listed in the Defense Department's **Defense Enrollment Eligible Reporting System (DEERS).** The TRICARE insurance program is managed by three regional centers in the United States and by a TRICARE overseas center.

Civilian Health and Medical Program of the Veterans Administration

Civilian Health and Medical Program of the Veterans Administration (CHAMPVA) is medical insurance for spouses and unmarried dependent children of a veteran with permanent total disability resulting from a service-related injury and for the surviving spouse and children of a veteran who died of a service-related disability. The patient has an identification card for the program. The program is administered by the Health Administration Center in Denver, Colorado.

Workers' Compensation Insurance

Workers' Compensation insurance is medical and paycheck insurance for workers who sustain injuries associated with their employment. In some instances, the insurance covers family members in the case of death of the worker. The employer usually pays the premium to the state or an insurance carrier designated by the state. Some large employers assume the insurance risk and are self-insured. Federal and state laws define minimum standards for Workers' Compensation programs. Workers' Compensation covers 100% of associated medical expenses. Claims are filed with the insurance carrier. Although most workers are insured under state programs, federal programs exist for the following specific groups:

- Office Workers' Compensation Programs (OWCP)
- Energy Workers' Occupational Illness Compensation Program
- Federal Black Lung Program
- Federal Employees' Compensation Act Program (FECA)
- Longshore and Harbor Workers' Compensation Program
- Mine Safety and Health Administration (MSHA)

Personal Injury Protection (PIP) Insurance

Personal injury protection (PIP) insurance is a component of automobile insurance that covers medical and hospital expenses due to a motor vehicle accident (MVA). It is often referred to as no-fault insurance because it pays out claims regardless of who is at fault in an accident. Other common terms are auto medical payment (AMP), Med Pay, and medical payments coverage. These terms are interchangeable and refer to the same no-fault insurance. Payments are based on the limits of the policy, and may pay for as much as 80% of expenses. PIP insurance covers the policyholder, but in some cases, may also extend to passengers and pedestrians involved in a car accident.

In addition to hospital and medical expenses, PIP may also cover lost wages as a result of a car accident, help pay costs of services, such as having someone take children to school, child care, or grocery shopping, and funeral expenses.

Coverage requirements vary by state; some require that drivers carry it, in others, it is optional. If a state requires PIP, there will be minimum coverage requirements. If not, the limits can be adjusted by what the policyholder chooses and can afford. Currently, the states that require PIP include Delaware, Florida, Hawaii, Kansas, Kentucky, Massachusetts, Michigan, Minnesota, New Jersey, New York, North Dakota, Oregon, Pennsylvania, and Utah.

PIP coverage is also required in Maryland, Texas, and Washington; however, a driver can sign a waiver and opt not to purchase the coverage. In this case, an exclusion agreement is signed, where the driver agrees to forego coverage, and affirms understanding that there is no personal injury protection and they will be liable for expenses sustained in a MVA as applicable.

Because PIP insurance regulations and requirements change, staying up to date on the topic and what is required in the state where you are located is a good idea.

Self-Funded Health Care

With **self-funded health care**, also known as **self-insurance**, the employer operates its own health plan, instead of purchasing a plan from an insurance carrier to cover employees. When operating a self-funded plan, the employer pays for the services of the insurance carrier to administrate the plan. Each self-insured plan differs in coverage and claim filing requirements. The plan administrator should be contacted before scheduling a patient appointment.

Medical Tourism Insurance

Medical tourism is an unusual option being added to conventional insurance plans in an effort to control rising health care costs. It consists of health-provider networks paying the insured client to go abroad for treatment at internationally accredited hospitals. This insurance option has several potential disadvantages that may outweigh the reduced costs. Safety of blood supplies for transfusions and tissue for bone grafts is questionable in some countries, long distance travel may be dangerous for some patients, and returning patients may find it difficult to obtain follow-up care due to providers' concerns about exposure to possible malpractice lawsuits. Medical tourism options are quite new to the industry. At this time, whether this will become the new wave in insurance or will disappear from the future of insurance is uncertain.

SCREENING FOR INSURANCE

It is the responsibility of the medical assistant to screen all new patients for their insurance. New patients should be asked to arrive 15 to 20 minutes earlier than their appointment time to complete a patient registration form. The form requests vital information that enables the medical office to contact the patient, process his or her billing and insurance claims, know who to contact in case of emergency, authorize payment of insurance benefits, and record method of payment. Commercial forms are available for purchase or can be designed by office management personnel for this purpose.

The medical assistant should review each section of the patient registration form to verify that all information is complete and legible. Many offices make a photocopy of the patient's driver's license and attach it to the registration form. This procedure helps in identifying the correct person through photo identification should it be necessary. It is important to verify the spelling of all patient names: first, middle, and last.

Ask the patient to show his or her health insurance card and verify the effective date and pertinent information. All medical offices should make a photocopy of both sides of the card to maintain in the patient's chart, or scan both sides of the card and upload to the patient's electronic medical record. In most cases, the back of the card contains information about any deductible, co-payment, and preapproval requirements, as well as the insurance company's name, address, and telephone number. It also shows any special claim submission instructions.

Each time a patient checks in, the medical assistant should ask questions to verify the following insurance information:

- Request DOB (date of birth) to establish correct patient.
- Confirm the patient's current address.
- Confirm the patient's insurance carrier and plan.
- Ask for the patient's insurance card and verify information and effective dates.
- Determine whether the insurance carrier covers the procedure.
- Determine that the patient's PCP is performing the procedure.
- Confirm whether a referral is required and whether an authorization number or authorization code is required. Confirm evidence of qualifying has been secured.
- Establish proof of eligibility (see Figure 16-8).

When screening patients for insurance, it is important to understand the philosophy of the medical office. Some see patients regardless of ability to pay; responsible medical assistants will investigate all avenues for reimbursement first. Some situations include the patient who is eligible for Medicaid but has not yet applied, or the patient who has applied for Medicaid but has not yet received notification of qualification. Procedure 16-2 provides the steps for screening for insurance.

The medical assistant should investigate and verify that all avenues have been taken to achieve the proof of eligibility that the office needs to receive reimbursement from Medicaid. This may include calling the Medicaid office to verify eligibility or going online and printing a proof of eligibility directly from the Medicaid system. This electronic data exchange system is called an *envoy*. Proof of eligibility cards are distributed to recipients and are in effect for at least a year. However, the most common avenue to ensure that services will be reimbursed is not to see any patient who does not have proof of Medicaid coverage. Medicaid sends an eligibility Medical Assistance Identification (MAID) (medical coupon) to the patient the first day of each month. This coupon guarantees the ambulatory care center payment for the services provided. Unless it is an emergency, some offices will not schedule

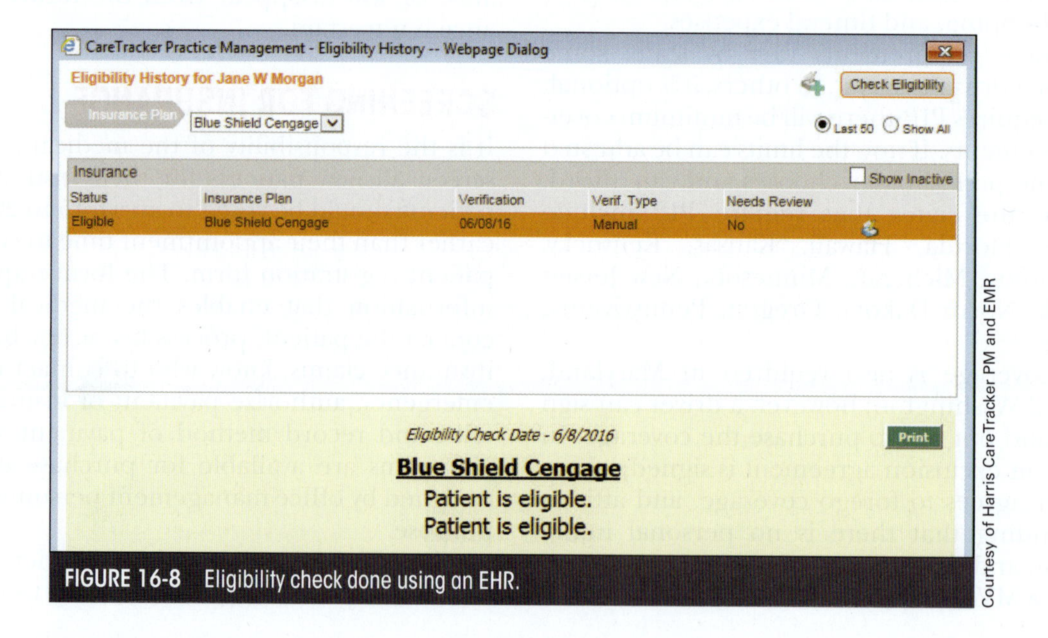

FIGURE 16-8 Eligibility check done using an EHR.

Courtesy of Harris CareTracker PM and EMR

PROCEDURE 16-2

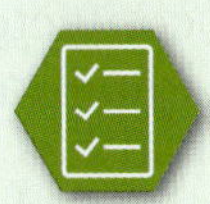

Procedure

Screening for Insurance

PURPOSE:

To verify insurance coverage and obtain vital information required for processing and billing insurance claim forms.

EQUIPMENT/SUPPLIES:

- Patient registration forms
- Clipboard and black ink pen
- Patient's chart

PROCEDURE STEPS:

1. When scheduling the first appointment, ask the patient to bring his or her insurance card and to arrive 15 to 20 minutes before the appointment time to complete the patient registration form. RATIONALE: The insurance card is required to verify effective dates and pertinent information relative to insurance coverage. The registration form also requests vital information necessary for patient care and insurance billing.
2. When the patient turns in the completed registration form, review it immediately, ***paying attention to detail,*** to be sure that all information has been collected and is legible. RATIONALE: It is important that all requested information is included on the registration form and that the medical assistant can read it clearly when processing the insurance claim forms. If information is not provided on the claim form or is incorrect, the insurance carrier may deny the claim.
3. Ask the patient for his or her insurance card. Make a photocopy of both sides of the card to be maintained in the patient's chart, or scan the insurance card and upload to the patient's electronic medical record. RATIONALE: The insurance card provides vital information, including correct spelling of patient's name, insurance plan numbers, effective dates, telephone numbers to call regarding referrals and preauthorizations, and information about any deductible and co-payment.
4. Verify proof of eligibility for Medicaid patients. The patient should have his or her proof of eligibility card with him or her, or you may need to make a telephone call directly to Medicaid or use the online electronic data exchange system to determine proof of eligibility. RATIONALE: This information is required for Medicaid reimbursement.
5. Each time a patient checks in, whether established or new, the following information should be verified:
   - Address. Confirm the patient's current address and telephone number. RATIONALE: Patients may have moved and may not realize they had not reported the new address and telephone number to the office.
   - Verify insurance coverage. RATIONALE: This information is required for correct claims processing and billing procedures.
   - Using the copy of the insurance card, verify the information and effective dates. Also be sure that a photocopy of the card is maintained in the patient's chart. RATIONALE: This is a means of keeping insurance records current for billing purposes.
   - Determine whether the insurance carrier covers the procedure. RATIONALE: If the carrier does not cover the procedure, reimbursement will need to come from a third party or the patient.
   - Determine that the correct provider is performing the procedure. RATIONALE: This information is needed for reimbursement purposes.
   - Determine whether a referral is required and whether an authorization number or code is needed. RATIONALE: Reimbursement by the carrier cannot take place without the proper documentation and authorization number.
   - Confirm that evidence of qualifying has been secured. RATIONALE: Proof of eligibility must be verified for reimbursement from Medicaid.

Medicaid patients before the fifth of each month. This allows ample time for the beneficiary to receive the medical coupon. If the patient presents for an appointment without a medical coupon, and proof of eligibility cannot be determined elsewhere, it is common practice to have that patient reschedule the appointment. The exception is an emergency.

Medical assistants with responsibility for billing are vital to the success of a clinic. Billing the insurance carriers promptly, completing claim forms properly, billing patients as needed, and keeping track of aging accounts will do much to ensure a flow of adequate income. In all insurance matters, be available to patients with questions regarding their insurance or accounts because a friendly attitude helps patients feel positive about the care they receive and establishes a long-term relationship.

REFERRALS AND AUTHORIZATIONS

When a PCP refers a patient to a specialist, the term **referral** is used by managed care facilities. Referrals may be denied because of incomplete information contained on the referral form or because a medical necessity was not established. Referrals are generally categorized as one of three types:

- *Regular.* Usually takes 3 to 10 working days to review procedures and approve
- *Urgent.* Usually takes about 24 hours for approval
- *Stat.* May be approved via telephone after faxing the information to the utilization review department

The most common referral used by managed care plans is the regular referral. The member services department must be contacted to check the status of a referral. It is important to never tell the patient that the referral has been approved until you have obtained a hard copy of the *authorization* (a managed care term for approved referrals). Be sure to review the content of the referral carefully. The typical referral will contain important information regarding its limitations, such as:

- Number of authorized visits to the provider
- The type of services authorized
- Expiration date (i.e., most will last for only 90 days)

Preauthorizations and *precertifications* are terms used to determine whether a service or procedure is covered and if the insurance plan approves it as medically necessary. Preauthorization is required for some services, hospital admissions, inpatient and outpatient surgeries, and most elective procedures (Procedure 16-3). Once approved, an authorization number will be provided. The patient also receives a letter containing the authorization number and the approved services. The patient must present this letter to the specialist's office on the day the service is provided.

When questions arise regarding preauthorization, precertification, or referral procedures, the medical assistant should call the plan's contact number for specific information. Many offices

PROCEDURE 16-3

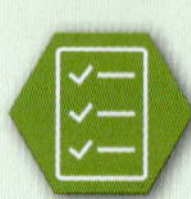

Obtaining Referrals and Authorizations

PURPOSE:

To ascertain coverage by the insurance carrier for specific medical services, hospital admissions, inpatient or outpatient surgeries, elective procedures, or when the PCP elects to refer the patient to another provider.

EQUIPMENT/SUPPLIES:

- Patient's medical chart and copy of his or her insurance card
- Name and telephone number of the contact person for the carrier
- Referral form
- Telephone/fax machine
- Pen/pencil

(continues)

PROCEDURE STEPS:

1. Collect all necessary documents and equipment (patient's chart/record, insurance carrier's information and telephone number). RATIONALE: Allows for efficient use of time in acquiring the referral or authorization.
2. Determine the service or procedure requiring preauthorization. You will also need to know the name and telephone number of the specialist involved and the reason the request is being sought. RATIONALE: This information is required to complete the referral form to obtain authorization from the patient's insurance carrier.
3. Complete the referral form, being sure to include all pertinent information. RATIONALE: The request may be denied if all information has not been included.
4. Proofread the completed form, ***paying attention to detail.*** RATIONALE: Because of the importance of this step, accuracy is critical.
5. Fax or electronically send the completed form to the insurance carrier. RATIONALE: The completed form apprises the carrier of the patient's medical condition, requests preauthorization for treatment, requests a verification or authorization number, and confirms the treatment plan.
6. Maintain a completed copy of the referral form in the patient's chart. RATIONALE: The form can be accessed in the future should questions arise.

find it helpful to maintain a reference log regarding these requirements. Information to maintain includes:

- Name of the insurance plan
- Address and telephone number
- Name and telephone number of contact person or the person with whom you spoke
- Co-payment amount and deductible information
- Inpatient and outpatient surgery benefits
- Preauthorization requirements, second-opinion options
- Participating hospitals, radiology service providers, laboratories, and physicians

The authorization number and referral numbers are entered in Box 23 of the CMS-1500 form when billing for services.

DETERMINING FEE SCHEDULES

A provider charges for services using a variety of means for computing a fee schedule. Although all of the fee computation plans vary and give somewhat different results, they all have common elements. Note the following examples:

- *The overhead or practice expenses for the clinic or office.* This category includes rental of the physical building or office space and equipment; utilities; cost of medical supplies inventory; and salaries of nurses, medical assistants, bookkeepers, and other personnel who are paid on a salary or contract basis. It also includes cost of employee benefits such as retirement plans, sick leave, and vacation time.
- *The cost of medical malpractice insurance.* This cost is separated from the charge for general insurance, which is included in the preceding category, because of the significant portion of the fee attributed to this item and because it varies greatly for different types of services. Obstetric/gynecologic procedures are probably the greatest for the entire medical community, including surgical procedures.
- *Hourly rate for the services provided by the provider.* This rate varies depending on the skill and training required for the procedure, the cost of living in the area, and the rate charged by other providers in the area. (The law of supply and demand applies here as in any other economic arena.) Surgeons charge a greater rate than providers in general practice, rates are greater in a metropolitan area than in a rural area, and experience level commands greater rates.

All of these cost elements are derived on an hourly basis. The sum of the above elements combined with the time required is used to arrive at the fee schedule for a procedure or service.

The advent of insurance plans, Medicare, and managed care plans has resulted in specific formulas being developed and accepted by the different plans to establish a fee schedule acceptable to the carrier. Several of the fee schedule systems in common usage are discussed in the following sections.

All of them, however, incorporate the preceding three elements (practice expenses, malpractice expenses, and provider's experience).

Usual, Customary, and Reasonable Fees

The **usual, customary, and reasonable (UCR)** fee schedule is a fee system that defines allowable charges that will be accepted by insurance carriers. The actual rate may vary from one carrier to another, but the process is the same.

- Usual fee is the provider's average fee for a service or procedure. This fee is based on the economic analysis of the practice described earlier in this section.
- Customary fee is the average or range of fees within the geographic area that an insurance carrier will accept. It is frequently tied to a national average for a similar metropolitan or rural setting.
- Reasonable fee is the generally accepted fee for services or procedures that are extraordinarily difficult or complicated and require more time and effort by the provider.

An example of the operation of the UCR system is as follows. An insurance carrier operating on the UCR fee schedule may have determined a customary fee range for a new patient office visit with history taking and physical examination to be $140 to $225 for that region. If the amount billed by the provider were $160, the provider would be reimbursed for the service in full. Had the provider billed $250, the reimbursement would be $225, and the provider would have to write off the $25 nonallowed charge. The amount the provider would have to write off is often referred to as an **adjustment**. Providers who participate in UCR systems cannot bill the patient for the nonallowable charge.

Resource-Based Relative Value Scale (RBRVS)

Medicare has used the RBRVS since 1992. Under this system, a provider's services are reimbursed based on relative value units (RVUs). Each service, procedure, and medication is assigned a code compiled from the *Current Procedural Terminology* (CPT) manual issued by the American Medical Association for procedures and the *International Classification of Diseases, 10th Revision, Clinical Modification* (ICD-10-CM) manual for diagnoses issued by the World Health Organization. Medicare then issues three RVUs for each code in the *Medicare Fee Schedule* (MFS) manual issued each year. The RVUs are for provider's work, practice expenses, and malpractice expenses. The practice expense is further differentiated based on location, that is, whether the work was done in a hospital (facility) or in a clinic or office (nonfacility). The nonfacility practice expense further differentiates between whether the nonfacility is transitioned or fully implemented. A geographic practice cost index (GPCI) related to the geographic area where the provider is located is issued for each RVU category. The GPCI is based on the ZIP code for the address of the practice or wherever the service is performed. The payment for service is then established from the sum of the geographically adjusted RVUs multiplied by a nationally uniform conversion factor for services.

The Formula for Calculating Payment Schedules

The American Medical Association provides a simplified table to assist with calculating the Medicare payment schedule. The Omnibus Budget Reconciliation Act of 1989 (OBRA 89) geographic adjustment provision requires all three components of the relative value for a service—physician work relative value units (RVUs), practice expense RVUs, and professional liability insurance (PLI) RVUs—to be adjusted by the corresponding GPCI for the locality. In effect, this provision increases the number of components in the payment schedule from three to the following six:

- Physician work RVUs
- Physician work GPCI
- Practice expense RVUs
- Practice expense GPCI
- PLI RVUs
- PLI GPCI

The general formula for calculating Medicare payment amounts for 2016 is shown in Table 16-2. The data to place into the formula changes annually, and can be obtained through the American Medical Association website (www.ama-assn.org) in the "Physician Resources" area.

The Medicare conversion factor is a scaling factor that converts the geographically adjusted

TABLE 16-2

MEDICARE FORMULA FOR PAYMENT OF SERVICES

	Work RVU1 × Work (GPCI)[2]
+	Practice Expense (PE) RVU × PE GPCI
+	Malpractice (PLI) RVU × PLI GPCI
	= Total RVU
×	CY 2016 Conversion Factor of $35.8043 (Jan 1.-Dec. 31, 2016)
	= Medicare Payment

number of relative value units (RVUs) for each service in the Medicare physician payment schedule into a dollar payment amount. The initial Medicare conversion factor was set at $31.001 in 1992.

Budget Neutrality Adjustment (BNA) in the Medicare Fee Schedule

In 2009, Medicare changed its payment calculation in the Physician Fee Schedule. It moved the Budget Neutrality Factor from the Work RVU to the Conversion Factor.

The conversion factor decreased, but fees increased. This provided a 4-6% increase in E/M services. In previous years, applying the budget neutrality factor to the work RVU had the effect of decreasing payments more for services with high work RVU values.

Clinics should review their third party contracts to be sure the BNA is not included in the calculation of fees. Contract amounts that are based on the Resource Based Relative Value Scale should be determined as a conversion factor multiplied by the total RVUs. If the fee is a percentage of Medicare, then the payer is including the BNA in the calculation and being paid less. Procedure 16-4

PROCEDURE 16-4

Computing the Medicare Fee Schedule

PURPOSE:

To compute the Medicare allowable (MA) payment for services.

EQUIPMENT/SUPPLIES:

- CPT book
- Computer
- Calculator

PROCEDURE STEPS:

1. Using the *Current Procedural Terminology* (CPT) book, obtain the CPT code for the exact procedure or service for which a fee schedule is being computed. **RATIONALE: Accurate code must be obtained to ensure correct billing.**
2. Using the Medicare Fee Schedule, which is issued each year, determine the relative value units for (a) provider's time (work), (b) practice expense (PE), and (c) costs of malpractice insurance (MP) listed for the CPT code in step 1. These factors represent the relative amount of a fee allocated to each item.
3. Using the Medicare fee schedule, determine the geographic practice cost index (GPCI). This factor accounts for different cost of living values for urban versus rural and geographic locations in the United States.
4. Using the Medicare Fee Schedule, determine the relative value unit (RVU) conversion factor (CF). This factor converts RVU units to dollars based on an average for the entire United States.
5. Compute the Medicare allowable fee for the procedure or service using the equation supplied in Table 16-2.

provides steps for computing the Medicare allowable fee schedule.

Diagnosis-Related Groups

In order to consider a claim for accepted reimbursement, Medicare will carefully examine the **Diagnosis-Related Groups (DRGs)**. These designations are part of a reimbursement strategy that is designed to focus upon the diagnoses of the patient instead of the services rendered. They ensure that all given diagnoses are as specific as possible and also justify the length of a patient's stay in the hospital. This concept also brings together conditions that were known to be related to one another and could prove medical necessity, as well as validate the treatments given.

Hospital Inpatient Prospective Payment System

The inpatient prospective payment system (IPPS) is a reimbursement system for hospitals based on similar diagnosis-related groups (DRGs) of inpatients discharged. Rather than the traditional method of payment based on actual costs incurred in providing care, DRGs are based on an average cost for treatment of a patient's condition. The hospital is reimbursed for each discharge according to a predetermined rate for each DRG.

Hospital Outpatient Prospective Payment System

The **hospital outpatient prospective payment system (OPPS)** is a reimbursement system for hospital outpatients, certain Part B services furnished to hospital inpatients who have no Part A coverage, and partial hospitalization services furnished by community mental health centers. All services are classified into groups called Ambulatory Payment Classifications (APCs). Payments are established for each APC, and the hospital is reimbursed for each patient. Depending on the services provided, hospitals may be paid for more than one APC for an encounter.

Capitation

Capitation is a payment system used primarily by managed care organizations. A fixed dollar amount is reimbursed to the provider for patients enrolled during a specific period. The payment per patient is independent of services or procedures provided to a patient. To be financially responsible, this system requires enrollment of a large number of patients so that a few patients do not unduly skew an average cost. This type of system requires extensive practice of preventive medicine to be cost-effective.

LEGAL AND ETHICAL ISSUES

Most Medicare claims are now required to be submitted electronically, and private payers in growing numbers are also using electronic claims submission. In a computerized system, everything related to billing and reimbursement is computerized and transmitted electronically. If the office is participating in CMS's Electronic Data Interchange (EDI), it will be assigned a unique identifier number that constitutes its legal electronic signature. Be cautious with this electronic signature, because the office is responsible for any and all claims made with it. The Health Insurance Portability and Accountability Act (HIPAA) of 1996 (specifically title II, subtitle F) regulates the security and privacy of transmitted health care information. Review HIPAA's regulations in Chapters 11 and 15.

Integrity

The medical assistant faces legal and ethical issues related to insurance issues on a daily basis; therefore, it is important that each patient be treated equally and fairly. As mentioned in Chapter 4, it is critical that patients not be stereotyped, regardless of whether they have multiple insurance plans or are not covered by any insurance plan at all. Every patient must be cared for objectively, with respect, and in a professional manner.

Legal

Medical personnel are bound by law to maintain the confidentiality of all medical information and must be able to recognize information that is protected by privacy rules and understand how it is to be handled. Protected health information (PHI) may be considered individually identifiable health information. This includes information that describes the health status of an individual, including basic demographics and the use of medical services, as well as information that either identifies or can be used to identify an individual. Medical personnel must remember that informed consent is not consent to use and disclose personal information.

Insurance Fraud and Abuse

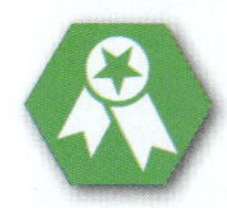

Insurance **fraud** and **abuse** may be involved in more than 10% of submitted medical claims according to the Insurance Information Institute. These estimates include both intentional as well as accidental coding and billing irregularities and, if detected and proved, such irregularities can result in legal action against the practice or clinic and personnel responsible for or having knowledge of the irregularities. Personnel involved in coding and billing should be alert for both accidental and intentional coding and billing irregularities and bring them to the attention of responsible managers. If no corrective action is taken, all personnel involved, including managers, are legally responsible to report the irregularities to the insurance carrier. Examples of fraudulent insurance activities include but are not limited to:

- Coding to a higher level of service to increase revenue (upcoding)
- Misrepresenting the diagnosis to justify payment
- Billing for services, equipment, or procedures that were never provided
- Unbundling service procedure codes
- Charging uninsured patients less than insured patients
- Receiving rebates or any type of compensation for referrals (kickbacks)

Insurance abuse involves activities that are inconsistent with accepted business practices. Some examples of abuse include but are not limited to:

- Charging for services that are not medically necessary
- Overcharging for services, equipment, or procedures
- Improper billing practices
- Violating participating provider agreements with insurance companies

Heavy penalties, including a $10,000 fine per claim form plus three times the fraudulent claim amount, may be sanctioned on individuals who knowingly and willfully misrepresent information submitted on insurance claim forms to gain greater payments or benefits.

To protect yourself and the medical practice from committing insurance fraud and abuse, you should begin by identifying risk areas based on errors in the past history of billing and insurance claims processing. Practice internal audits to monitor compliance with written protocols. Participate in seminars and in-service programs to keep current with coding and billing practices. Be sure to use only the current year's coding manuals to ensure accuracy. Code only what is documented in the medical record, and ask for clarification when needed.

An auditor should check claim forms, whether submitted electronically or by hard copy, to see that they are completed correctly. Include all pertinent dates and diagnostic and procedural coding information necessary for insurance payers to generate reimbursement. Auditors look specifically for any indicators of insurance fraud and abuse.

PROFESSIONAL CAREERS IN INSURANCE

To be successful in the health insurance specialist field, training and entry-level requirements are essential. An opportunity for employment in these specialties is greater for those with a college degree that includes course-work in medical terminology, anatomy and physiology, pharmacology, insurance and coding procedures, and communication skills.

Personal attributes that enhance employment possibilities as health insurance specialists include, but are not limited to, the following descriptions: self-motivated, works well independently, detail oriented, a critical thinker, ethical, maintains confidentiality, cooperative, reliable, and adaptable.

The following Internet links will help you explore a variety of health insurance specialist career opportunities.

- American Academy of Professional Coders (AAPC) at http://www.aapc.com
- American Health Information Management Association (AHIMA) at http://www.ahima.org
- American Medical Billing Association (AMBA) at http://www.ambanet.net
- Alliance of Claims Assistance Professionals (ACAP) at http://www.claims.org
- National Electronic Billers Alliance (NEBA) at http://www.nebazone.com

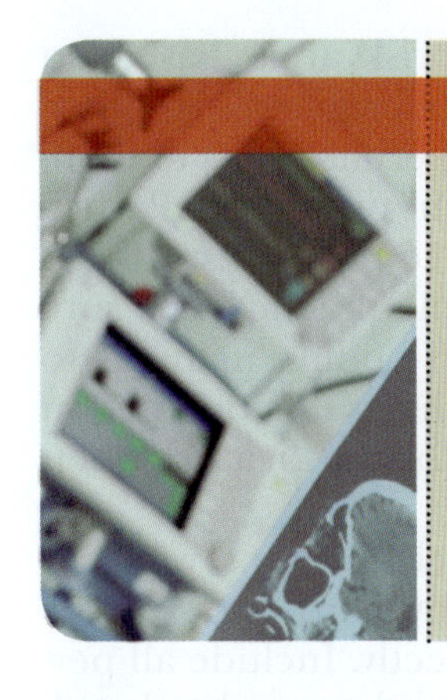

CASE STUDY 16-1

Refer to the scenario at the beginning of the chapter.

CASE STUDY REVIEW

1. Identify ways that Ellen Armstrong, CMAS (AMT), can stay abreast of policy changes regarding reimbursement.
2. List options for Ellen to take in order to be up to date with insurance coverage so that she can help patients understand their responsibility, if any, for payment.
3. Recall steps for screening patients for insurance. Why is this so important?

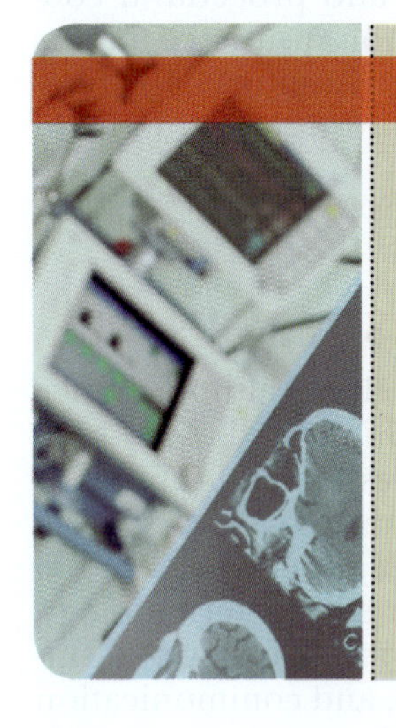

CASE STUDY 16-2

Ellen Armstrong, CMAS (AMT), is responsible for all patient insurance billing procedures. Ellen has the following information:

	Total Charges	Allowed Charges
Office visit	$150.00	$100.00
Return visit	$80.00	$75.00

Deductible has not been satisfied.

CASE STUDY REVIEW

1. Calculate the patient's correct billing if the provider accepts assignment.
2. Calculate the patient's correct billing if the provider does not accept assignment.

Summary

- An understanding of medical insurance terminology and various types of coverage is vital to a thriving clinic.
- The increasing complexity of health insurance today means that medical assistants must continually update their base of information.
- The Affordable Care Act has introduced a number of challenges, and as the number of Americans with coverage continues to grow, so will the need for a good understanding of medical billing and coding principles for medical assistants.
- Medical assistants must develop strong communication skills to explain insurance procedures to patients, and make contact with representatives to determine eligibility and verification of benefits.
- The medical assistant will need to be familiar with medical insurance terms and how these terms apply to the clinic, the policyholder, and impact on proper reimbursement. These terms include *beneficiary; policyholder; subscriber of a plan; deductibles; co-insurance and co-payments; exclusions and preexisting condition exclusions for grandfathered individual plans; coordination of benefits (COB), explanation of benefits (EOB), and remittance advice (RA) notices, preauthorization,* and *assignment of benefits.*
- Insurance plan types include traditional insurance, managed care insurance models (EPO, IDS, HMO, POS, PPO), Medicare (Parts A, B, C, and D) and Medicaid/Medi-Cal, Tricare, Workers' Compensation, and personal injury protection (PIP) insurance.
- Medical assistants must know screening techniques for insurance data and how to obtain referrals and precertifications as required by insurance plans.
- The medical assistant must be aware of legal and ethical issues as they relate to medical insurance in order for PHI to be protected, and minimize or eliminate unintentional insurance fraud and abuse.

Study for Success

To reinforce your knowledge and skills of information presented in this chapter:

- Review the *Key Terms* and *Learning Outcomes*
- Consider the *Critical Thinking* features and *Case Studies* and discuss your conclusions
- Answer the questions in the *Certification Review*

Procedure

- Perform the *Procedures* using the *Competency Assessment Checklists* on the *Student Companion Website*

CERTIFICATION REVIEW

1. Which of the following is the most common avenue to ensure that services will be reimbursed?
   a. Do not see any patient who does not have proof of Medicaid coverage.
   b. Complete an envoy.
   c. Go online and print a proof of eligibility directly from the system.
   d. Ask patients if they are covered.
2. What is the most common insurance claim form?
   a. UB04 form
   b. ICD-9-CM
   c. CMS-1500 (02-12) form
   d. Assignment of benefits
   e. ICD-10-CM
3. Which of the following statements is an accurate description of Medicare?
   a. It was created by Title 19 of the Social Security Act.
   b. It covers most persons age 65 years and older.
   c. It is designed to cover prescriptions.
   d. It is handled separately by each state.
4. If the RBRVS allowable is $150 and the deductible has not been met, Medicare will pay how much?
   a. $20
   b. $40
   c. $120
   d. 80% of RBRVS allowable after $166.00 deductible
   e. None of these
5. How many primary MCO models are in operation across the U.S.?
   a. Four
   b. Three
   c. Six
   d. Eight
6. Which of the following statements is an accurate description of Medicaid insurance?
   a. It is funded by the federal government and administered by each state's department of SSI.
   b. It requires a Medigap policy.
   c. It consists of Part A, Part B, Part C, and Part D.
   d. It requires PARs to accept assignment.
   e. All of these
7. Which of the following statements is an accurate description of BCBS?
   a. They are locally based in all 50 states in the United States.
   b. They operate like MCOs.
   c. They recognize Medicare Part B.
   d. They are part of CHAMPVA.
8. Which of the following statements is an accurate description of TRICARE?
   a. It is part of CHAMPVA.
   b. It is part of OWCP, MSHA, and FECA programs.
   c. It is a self funded plan.
   d. It was formerly the Civilian Health and Medical Program for Uniformed Services.
   e. It no longer exists.
9. All of the following are examples of insurance fraud EXCEPT for what?
   a. Charging uninsured patients less than insured patients
   b. Charging for services that are not medically necessary
   c. Coding to a higher level of service to increase revenue
   d. Receiving rebates or any type of compensation for referrals
10. According to the birthday rule, which of the following is true?
   a. The father's insurance policy will always be the primary insurance plan.
   b. The policy with the later effective date will be the primary plan.
   c. The mother's policy will always be the primary insurance plan.
   d. The parent with the earlier DOB will carry the primary plan.
   e. The parent with the later DOB will carry the primary plan.

CHAPTER 17

Medical Coding

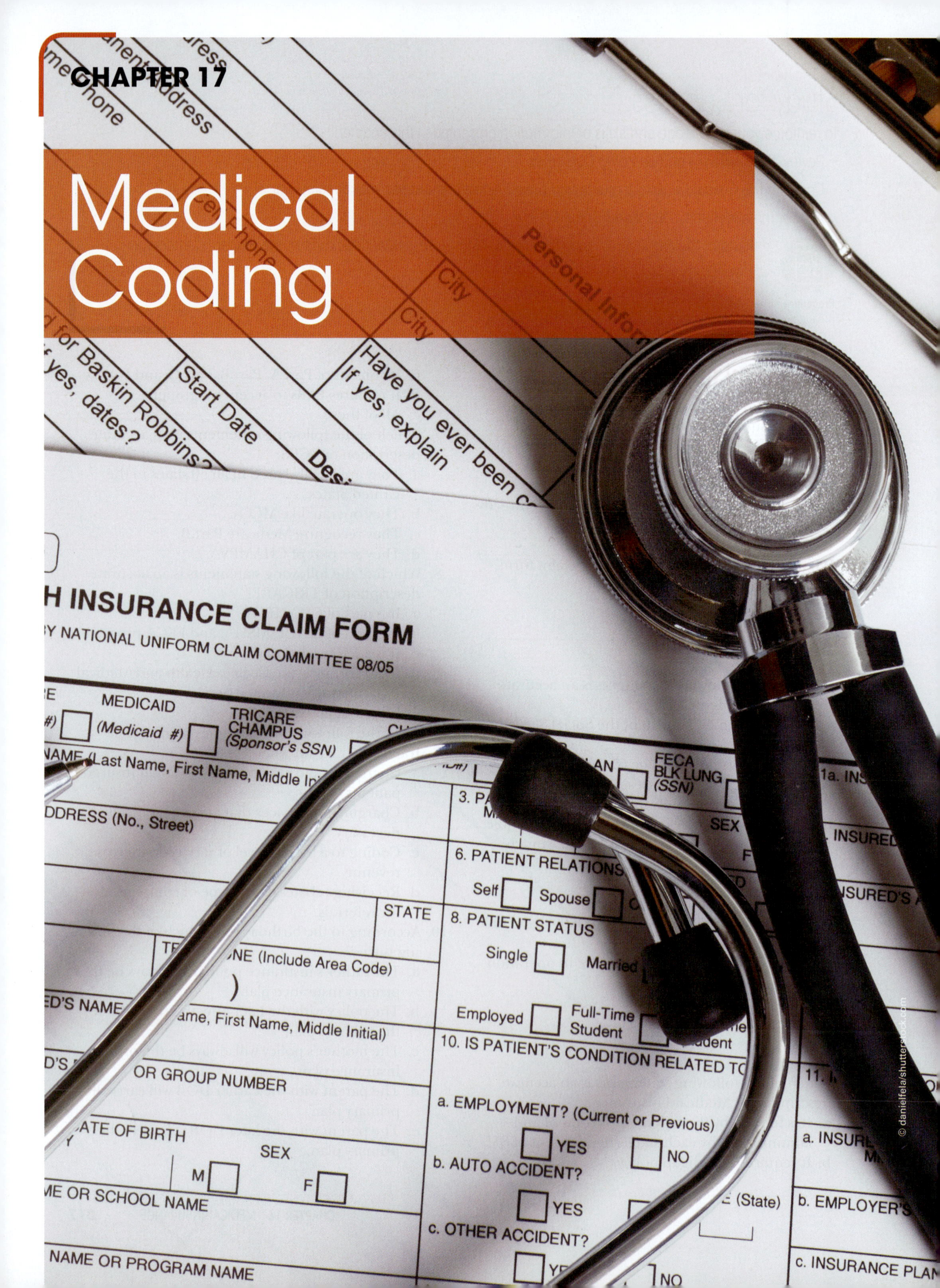

LEARNING OUTCOMES

1. Define and spell the key terms as presented in the glossary.
2. Define terminology necessary to understand and code medical insurance claim forms.
3. Describe how to use the most current procedural and diagnostic coding systems.
4. Code a sample claim form.
5. Apply third-party guidelines.
6. Recognize common errors in completing insurance claim forms.
7. Explain the difference between the CMS-1500 (02-12) and the UB-04 forms.
8. Compare processes for filing insurance claims both manually and electronically.
9. Discuss why claims follow-up is important to the ambulatory care setting.
10. Discuss legal and ethical issues related to coding and insurance claims processing.

KEY TERMS

- assumptive coding
- bundled codes
- claim register
- CMS-1500 (02-12)
- Current Procedural Terminology (CPT®)
- diagnosis
- down-code
- encounter form (superbill)
- explanation of benefits (EOB)
- Healthcare Common Procedure Coding System (HCPCS)
- ICD-10-PCS
- International Classification of Diseases, 9th Revision, Clinical Modification (ICD-9-CM)
- International Classification of Diseases, 10th Revision, Clinical Modification (ICD-10-CM)
- International Classification of Diseases, 10th Revision, Procedure Coding System (ICD-10-PCS)
- medical necessity
- modifiers
- morbidity
- mortality
- nomenclature systems
- point-of-service (POS) device
- symbols
- unbundling
- Uniform Bill 04 (UB-04)
- up-coding

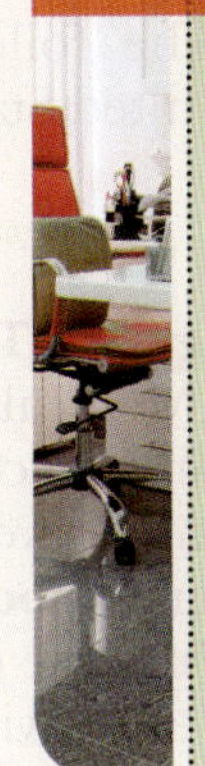

SCENARIO

At Inner City Health Care, a multiprovider clinic in a large city, medical assistant Ellen Armstrong, CMAS (AMT), is responsible for all patient billing procedures, including insurance claim forms. Ellen stresses with her colleagues the fact that coding is the basis for information exchanged between the health care providers and various agencies that compile health care statistics as well as third-party payers for health care services rendered to patients. Understanding medical terminology, anatomy, physiology, and how to code medical procedures and diagnoses accurately is a must. Using the computer to complete insurance forms, while considering common errors that may lead to denial of a claim, and transmitting the claims electronically are reviewed during in-service meetings. Ellen emphasizes that accurate coding must always reflect services actually performed and documented within the patient's chart.

Chapter Portal

Coding is the basis for the information on the claim form. Medical coding is mandatory for the accurate transmission of procedures and diagnosis information between health care providers and various agencies that compile health care statistics and the insurance companies that act as third-party payers for health care services rendered to patients. To code accurately, the medical assistant must have a good understanding of medical terminology, especially of those medical specialties found in the ambulatory care setting.

The use of computers to generate the insurance claim form and to transmit the form to the third-party payer is commonplace today. Computers are able to compute and compare numbers only. Letters that are in a sequence, such as the alphabet, are able to be compared as to their relativity to each other. For instance, *A* comes before *B* in the alphabet, and thus, a computer can compare those two values. For that reason, all charges, patient accounts, insurances, diagnoses and procedures, and even various categories are assigned letters or numbers (alphanumeric). The letters/numbers assigned to diagnoses and procedures (services) are called insurance codes. People whose jobs are to check accuracy of insurance codes and assign billing parameters (such as code modifiers) are called medical coders. (See the "Professional Careers in Insurance" section at the end of Chapter 16 for more information.)

INSURANCE CODING SYSTEMS OVERVIEW

Coding is the application of alphanumeric characters selected from standard terms used to describe a condition, disease, or service in health care. Medical codes come from complex **nomenclature systems** comprised of a detailed organization of information based on body systems. Health care staff need to use their knowledge about medical terminology, anatomy and physiology, pathophysiology, and pharmacology when performing medical coding tasks.

Purpose of Coding

Coding is done in order to process demographic, insurance, and coded medical diagnoses and procedures in order to request reimbursement for services and supplies used in health care. The coded information is analyzed to improve quality of medical care through the development and use of quality indicators, which provides information for public health and safety. This includes processes to decrease outbreaks of contagious diseases.

Another use of coded information includes the identification of risk factors used to develop standards for treatment and prevention of diseases. In addition, the purpose of coding includes the improvement and development of new treatments, supplies, and medications and technology. Payers use coded data to determine that the appropriate level of services are provided for specific conditions in order to make payment determinations. Health care costs are controlled through the combination of medical codes and documentation guidelines which are necessary to justify medical necessity for the services provided to the patient.

Medical necessity is required to ensure that services or procedures for a specific diagnosis or specified frequency are in order for consideration for reimbursement by the patient's insurance covered benefits. This is directed by 42 CFR 405.500 1995. The provider of services is responsible for documenting that the service is necessary and is covered by the insurance plan.

The HIPAA Administrative Simplification Act provision of 1996 ruled that electronic transmission of health care data complies with legal standards. It mandated the use of standardized code sets for submission of health care data.

CODE SETS

The process of translating written or spoken description of diseases, injuries, medical procedures, services, and supplies into numeric or alphanumeric format is called *coding*. The following coding systems are used within the United States.

Current Procedural Terminology (CPT®)

The **Current Procedural Terminology (CPT)** system was developed by the American Medical Association (AMA) to convert commonly accepted descriptions of medical procedures into a five-digit numeric code with two-digit numeric **modifiers** when required. CPT guidelines instruct the coder to add more codes. **Symbols** are used to visually represent instructions. Modifiers are important because they can impact the charge that is associated with the code. This system is used to code medical procedures such as clinic visits, X-rays, laboratory tests, and professional fees for providers who have performed surgery. Each CPT code has a fee schedule which is used to request reimbursement.

The American Medical Association publishes the CPT manual annually. The first edition was published in 1966. The six sections of the CPT coding system include:

Evaluation and Management	99201 to 99499
Anesthesiology	00100 to 01999, 99100 to 99140
Surgery	10021 to 69990
Radiology (Including Nuclear Medicine and Diagnostic Ultrasound)	70010 to 79999
Pathology and Laboratory	80047 to 89398
Medicine (Except Anesthesiology)	90281 to 99199, 99500 to 99607

To determine the CPT code, turn to the Category I section of the CPT code book and select one of the sections that constitutes the general classification of the procedure being coded (e.g., Surgery, Radiology). Then select the name of the procedure or service that accurately identifies what you are looking for. Read all of the codes that are indented below the main code. Indented codes provide greater specificity. Do not select a CPT code that only approximately defines the service performed. If you cannot find a name that exactly defines the service provided, report the service using the appropriate unlisted code. Unlisted codes are found at the end of each subsection in the CPT code book, and are also listed within the guidelines that precede each of the main sections. Most unlisted CPT codes end in 99. When using an unlisted code, a special report must be submitted with an insurance claim form to avoid denial or rejection. A special report will contain the nature, extent, and need of the procedure performed. An example of a special report would be the provider's operative note. Unlisted codes should not be used if a Category III code is available. This section is found in the back of the code book and gives temporary codes for emerging technologies, services, and procedures.

Evaluation and Management. The Evaluation and Management section takes every possible combination of visits into consideration and assigns each its own number. For instance, Mary O'Keefe, a new patient, is seen for a period of 45 minutes during which the provider takes a detailed history, examines the patient, and makes a medical decision of moderate complexity. The CPT code for this visit (99204) is found by looking under Office and Other Outpatient Services, New Patient. In another instance, Abigail Johnson, an established patient, is seen in the hospital for several days. These visits (99231, 99232, or 99233) would be found under Hospital Services, Subsequent Hospital Care. Codes for any type of evaluation and management are found in this section. In many clinics, the provider determines the level or charge for visits; however, the medical assistant must be familiar with all of the codes to make certain that billings are correct and that codes match the provider's documentation.

Anesthesiology. The Anesthesiology section includes all codes for anesthesia required for any procedure (with the exception of local anesthesia). The codes listed begin with the head and continue down the body to the legs and feet, concluding with anesthesia for radiologic procedures. If you want to find the correct code for anesthesia during a total hip replacement (arthroplasty), you will find Anesthesia in the index, look for the subterm *hip*, and refer to the range of codes listed: 01200 to 01215. When you refer back to the Anesthesia section, you find:

01200 Anesthesia for all closed procedures involving hip joint

01202 Anesthesia for arthroscopic procedures of hip joint

01210 Anesthesia for open procedures involving hip joint; not otherwise specified

01212 hip disarticulation

01214 total hip arthroplasty

01215 revision of total hip arthroplasty

As you read through the codes, you see that the correct code is 01214. Please note that this CPT code represents only the services provided by the anesthesiologist, not the surgical procedure itself.

Surgery. The section on surgery divides the codes according to body system. It begins with the integumentary system, and continues through subsequent systems ending with the ocular and auditory systems. The codes are very specific in this section, and care must be taken at all times to ensure the selection of the correct code. For example, a simple laceration repair of the neck is found as:

12001 Simple repair of superficial wounds of scalp, neck, axillae, external genitalia, trunk and/or extremities (including hands and feet): 2.5 cm or less

12002 2.6 cm to 7.5 cm

12004 7.6 cm to 12.5 cm

12005 12.6 cm to 20.0 cm

12006 20.1 cm to 30.0 cm

12007 over 30.0 cm

Thus, the exact length of the laceration and complexity of the repair can be found and coded correctly on the claim form. However, the aforementioned code description illustrates three important points. First, the code selected must represent the site of the laceration. Second, the code must represent the correct level of complexity for the repair. Third, the code must specify the correct length of the repair. If the medical assistant selects a code that is off by even just one digit, there would be a delay in reimbursement. The insurance claim would have to be corrected and resubmitted to the insurance company.

Radiology. Coding in the Radiology section covers each procedure done and each specific alteration to the procedure. For instance:

75889 Hepatic venography, wedged or free, *with* hemodynamic evaluation, radiological supervision, and interpretation

75891 Hepatic venography, wedged or free, *without* hemodynamic evaluation, radiological supervision, and interpretation

Radiologic procedures are not often done in the provider's clinic, although they may be in larger urgent care centers. Occasionally, chest X-rays are done or, in an orthopedic specialty, many skeletal X-rays may be done. More often, though, radiologic studies are ordered by the provider through a local facility that bills the insurance company directly, using the **diagnosis** the provider has provided.

Pathology and Laboratory. The Pathology and Laboratory section includes every test and combination of laboratory tests that can be ordered, as well as a section on surgical pathologic evaluation. This latter section includes specimens sent for examination, such as Pap smears, analysis of biopsy tissue from surgical sites, and tissue typing. Following is an example of a laboratory procedure code for hepatitis B that illustrates the complete selection of tests that may be ordered:

87340 Hepatitis B surface antigen (HBsAg)

86704 Hepatitis B core antibody (HBcAb); total

86705 IgM antibody

86706 Hepatitis B surface antibody (HBsAb)

87350 Hepatitis Be antigen (HBeAg)

86707 Hepatitis Be antibody (HBeAb)

Once again, it is very important that the code for the exact service be selected. The medical assistant should be aware of laboratory codes because when a laboratory test is ordered, the laboratory may call to clarify the order. If the coding is correct, the laboratory should have no questions.

For surgical pathologic evaluation, the codes are different. The level of examination (gross and microscopic) for the item determines the code. The provider usually determines these levels or the charge for these services based on the type of tissue obtained, and the reason for the service.

Medicine. The section of the CPT entitled Medicine includes codes for immunizations, injections, dialysis, allergen immunotherapy, and chemotherapy, as well as ophthalmologic, cardiovascular, pulmonary, and neurologic procedures, to name a few. Some of the procedures are considered invasive, although others are not. As in the earlier sections, there is a comprehensive breakdown of each procedure. For example:

Cardiography

93000 Electrocardiogram, routine ECG with at least 12 leads; with interpretation and report

93005 tracing only, without interpretation and report

93010 interpretation and report only

Chemotherapy Administration

96409 intravenous, push technique, single or initial substance/drug

96413 Chemotherapy administration, intravenous infusion technique; up to 1 hour, single or initial substance/drug

+96415 each additional hour (List separately in addition to code for primary procedure)

96416 initiation of prolonged chemotherapy infusion (more than 8 hours), requiring use of a portable or implantable pump

The plus symbol (+) before the CPT code indicates that the procedure is an add-on to a previously described procedure. For example, 96413 would be used to describe the service and the time administered up to 1 hour. Use +96415 for each additional 1 hour of administration.

Index. The final portion of the CPT code book is a comprehensive index listing every procedure alphabetically. The proper use of the CPT code book involves looking for the procedure in the index by its main term and then checking the number given to determine the precise code.

Category I codes found in the CPT have five numeric digits. This is the level of codes that are used the most to describe procedures and other professional services. Category II and Category III codes are made of four numeric digits and are followed by an alpha character. These codes would be used when no specific Category I code is available. Note that there are no decimal points in any of the codes. Each five-digit code stands for a specific procedure not duplicated elsewhere.

Modifiers. Occasionally, a service or procedure needs to be modified or altered in a certain way. In that case, there are two-digit numeric modifiers that can be applied to the five-digit CPT code. These modifiers can indicate unusual procedural services (–22), bilateral procedures (–50), multiple procedures (–51), two surgeons (–62), surgical team (–66), or repeat procedure by same provider (–76). The modifiers are listed in the inside front cover of each of the CPT code books as well as Appendix A of the book to alert the coder to use modifiers available for that code. In addition, there are other modifiers of an alpha or alphanumeric nature that are also listed in the front of the CPT code book. These modifiers come from the HCPCS code book, and are commonly used with CPT codes. Review the following examples that illustrate the use of modifiers:

- Surgical arthroscopy of the right shoulder with rotator cuff repair: 29827-RT
- Bilateral otoplasty, protruding ear, with or without size reduction: 69300-50
- Blepharoplasty of the lower right eyelid; extensive herniated fat pad: 15821-E4

Procedure

See Procedure 17-1 for instructions on CPT coding.

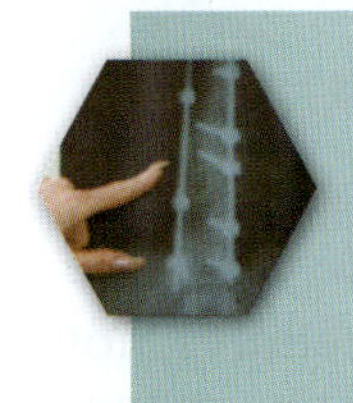

Critical Thinking

In which code book would you look to find the code for upper gastrointestinal endoscopy, simple primary examination (e.g., with small-diameter flexible endoscope) (separate procedure)? Which code did you select?

PROCEDURE 17–1

Procedure

Coding with Current Procedural Terminology

PURPOSE:

To convert commonly accepted descriptions of medical procedures (services) and visits of all types—clinic, hospital, nursing facility, home services—into a five-digit numeric code with two-digit numeric modifiers when required.

EQUIPMENT/SUPPLIES:

- CPT code book for the current year
- Copy of the encounter form and access to the patient's chart
- Pencil and paper

CASE SCENARIO:

Jane Smith, a new patient, is seen for 10 minutes, during which the provider takes a focused history and completes a problem-focused examination. A routine urinalysis, non-automated and without microscopy, is performed and a

(continues)

straightforward medical decision is made. Mary's preliminary diagnosis is painful urination. The urinalysis confirms a urinary tract infection. The provider writes her a prescription for an antibiotic and asks her to make an appointment in 10 days for another urinalysis to confirm the infection has cleared.

PROCEDURE STEPS:

1. Using the CPT code book, look in the Evaluation and Management section, Office or Other Outpatient Services, New Patient. Carefully read through the options until the code matching the described scenario has been found. RATIONALE: This section of the CPT code book provides codes used to report evaluation and management services provided in the provider's clinic or in an outpatient or other ambulatory care facility. You should have selected 99201.
2. Continue with the CPT code book, turn to the Index again, and look up Urinalysis, Routine. The code given is 81002. RATIONALE: This provides you with a code to investigate and determine its appropriateness.
3. Continue in the CPT code book and turn to the Pathology and Laboratory section. Follow the codes until you locate code 81002. When verifying the code, 81002 is an indented code and specifically states that the test is nonautomated, without microscopy. Be sure the description provided there matches what the provider has documented in the patient's chart. RATIONALE: To verify that the code is correct and matches documentation.

Healthcare Common Procedure Coding System (HCPCS)

Healthcare Common Procedure Coding System (HCPCS) was developed by Medicare as a supplement to the CPT system for procedures not defined with sufficient specificity. This system uses a five-digit alphanumeric code (one letter followed by four numbers) with an additional two-digit alphanumeric modifier if required. This code set includes supplies, durable medical equipment, and other medical services. Table 17-1 depicts the organization of the HCPCS codes.

Finding an HCPCS Code. Codes can be located by finding the main term or subterm in the alphabetical index. The name of the item, the type of service, the anatomical site, or abbreviation can also be used to look up the code. Modifiers are used to provide addition information about a service, item, or procedure. The code consists of a letter followed by four numbers. The Table of Drugs provides codes for the generic and brand names of drugs. Verify the code in the tabular list. You can also locate the code range and search the code that is needed.

International Classification of Diseases, Ninth Revision, Clinical Modification (ICD-9-CM)

The **International Classification of Diseases, 9th Revision, Clinical Modification (ICD-9-CM)** system was developed by the World Health Organization (WHO) in 1979 to classify all known diseases and disorders to assist in maintaining statistical records of **morbidity** (sickness) and **mortality** (death). Until October 2015, this system was used for both diagnostic coding (for all health care settings) and procedure coding (for inpatient services only). The ICD-9-CM code consists of a three-digit code (called a *category*) with one or two numeric digits following a decimal point. The ICD-9-CM coding manual was revised periodically and was updated yearly.

International Classification of Diseases, 10th Revision, Clinical Modification (ICD-10-CM)

The **International Classification of Diseases, 10th Revision, Clinical Modification (ICD-10-CM)** was developed by the World Health Organization in 1992. The official version is called the International Classification of Diseases (ICD-10). The WHO is responsible for revisions every 10 years. The United States implemented ICD-10-CM in October 2015 to replace ICD-9-CM. The National Center for Health Statistics is responsible for maintaining the diagnostic codes. The Centers for Medicare and Medicaid Services is responsible for maintaining the procedure codes for ICD-10-CM.

Revisions in ICD-10-CM from ICD-9-CM include the use of six and seven characters. In

TABLE 17-1

ORGANIZATION OF HCPCS CODES

CODE RANGE	DESCRIPTION
A0000 to A9999	Transportation services such as ambulance; medical and surgical supplies, including supplies for urinary incontinence, ostomy, respiratory, and dialysis; and radiopharmaceuticals
B4000 to B9999	Supplies, equipment, and nutritional products for enteral and parenteral nutrition
C1300 to C9899	New technology procedures, drugs, biologicals, radiopharmaceuticals, magnetic resonance angiography (MRA), and devices for outpatient hospitals to report
D Codes	Dental services—the ADA holds the copyright to D codes; they usually do not appear in the HCPCS manual
E0100 to C8002	Durable medical equipment (DME) for patient's activities of daily living, including crutches and oxygen equipment
G0008 to G9360	Procedures and services that may or may not have equivalent CPT codes, such as screening exams
H0001 to H2037	Mental health services, including treatment for alcohol and drug use
J0120 to J9999	Drugs that the patient does not self-administer
K00014 to K0900	DME for which there are no other HCPCS codes available, such as power wheelchairs
L0112 to L9900	Orthotics (devices that help to regain function) and prosthetics (replacement body parts), including cervical collars, lumbar support, artificial limbs, and male vacuum erection systems
M0064 to M0301	Codes represent an office visit for prescription drugs and miscellaneous therapies
P2028 to P9615	Pathology and laboratory services and blood products
Q0035 to Q9968	Temporary codes for drugs and supplies
R0070 to R0076	Transportation of portable diagnostic radiology equipment to provider locations
S0012 to S9999	Drugs, services, and supplies for Medicaid and other non-Medicare payers
T1000 to T5999	Medicaid services and supplies
V2020 to V564	Vision supplies, such as eyeglasses; hearing services and supplies; and speech language pathology services

Source: Centers for Medicare and Medicaid Services, www.cms.gov

addition, the codes have laterality and greater specificity. There were thousands of codes added from version ICD-9-CM. There are 1,943 new codes; 351 revised codes; and 313 deleted codes for the 2017 ICD-10-CM as published by CMS.

Revisions to the ICD-10-CM include codes that specify laterality such as the right arm or the left arm. Chapter 19, "Injury, Poisoning and Certain Other Consequences of External Causes (S00-T88)," has been expanded to include additional codes. There has been an increase of combination codes in which the code defines both a diagnoses and symptoms, reducing the need to record additional codes. The use of a sixth and seventh character contributes to greater specificity and validity for diseases, injuries, conditions, procedures, and so on. The official coding guidelines appear at the front of the coding manual as well as at the beginning of each chapter. In addition, there are two types of Excludes notes.

Tools used to convert ICD-9 to ICD-10 codes are called gem maps. These maps are published on the CMS Web site. It is important for many reasons to know how to convert the codes. One reason is to research and compare statistical data from the codes. Another reason is for claims resolution and processing of older claims. Because there are more codes in ICD-10, many of the codes do not directly convert from ICD-9.

The intent of the International Classification Disease system is to record morbidity and mortality. Morbidity is defined as conditions, injuries, or diseases that are not considered normal health. The physician documents changes in morbidity in the health record for each patient encounter. HIPAA mandates the recording of the various ICD-10-CM classifications as a standard in the electronic health care transactions for reporting purposes. Data generated from the reporting process are used to track diseases, injuries, and impairments in the population. Mortality means death.

There are 21 chapters in ICD-10-CM. Table 17-2 lists the code range and the description of each chapter.

ICD-10-CM uses conventions, instructional notes, punctuation marks, and abbreviations to help the coder select the appropriate code. Selecting the correct code is necessary in order for the code to be complete, correct, and accurate. The coding guidelines define the use of each convention. Examples include code also, code first, excludes 1, excludes 2, in diseases classified elsewhere, includes, not elsewhere classified (NEC), not otherwise specified (NOS), see, see also, and use additional codes. Examples of symbols include brackets, colon, parentheses, and a-point dash.

The coding guidelines are located at the beginning of the ICD-10-CM book as well as at the beginning of each chapter. The guidelines reference the appendices and sections. The coder must be familiar with these coding guidelines.

Procedure

See Procedure 17-2 for instructions on ICD-10-CM coding.

How to Find an ICD-10-CM Code. Using the main term, subterm, or synonym, search in the alphabetic index at the beginning of the code book. Find the code in the tabular section of the code book making sure to follow any instructions or directions described by symbols or coding guidelines.

ICD-10-PCS

ICD-10-PCS codes have seven alphanumeric characters. Each character has a specific meaning and/or value. The 16 sections of ICD-10-PCS include Medical and Surgical, Obstetrics, Placement, Administration, Measurement and Monitoring, Extracorporeal Assistance and Performance, Extracorporeal Therapies, Osteopathic, Other Procedures, Chiropractic, Imaging, Nuclear Medicine, Radiation Oncology, Physical Rehabilitation and Diagnostic Audiology, Mental Health, and Substance Abuse Treatment. These sections each have a number, which represents the first character of the PCS code. The remaining characters represent the following:

- The second place character represents the body system. There are 31 body systems that range from the central nervous system to the anatomical regions, lower extremities.
- The third place character represents the root operations. There are 31 root operations for the Medical Surgical section. Additional root operations are assigned for the other sections.
- The fourth place character represents the specific part of the body system on which the procedure is performed.
- The fifth place character for the Medical and Surgical codes is the approach used in the procedure. For example, an open approach means a cutting through of the skin or mucous membrane and any other body layers necessary to expose the site of the procedure.
- The sixth character indicates a device and specifies the device that remains after the procedure is completed. An example of one of the four types of devices is a cardiac pacemaker.
- The seventh character in the Medical Surgical section is a qualifier that has a unique value for an individual procedure.

TABLE 17-2

ICD-10-CM CODE RANGES AND DESCRIPTIONS

CODE RANGE	DESCRIPTION
A00 to B99	Certain infectious and parasitic diseases
C00 to D49	Neoplasms
D50 to D89	Diseases of the blood and blood-forming organs and certain disorders involving the immune mechanism
E00 to E89	Endocrine, nutritional, and metabolic diseases
F01 to F99	Mental, behavioral, and neurodevelopmental disorders
G00 to G99	Disease of the nervous system
H00 to H59	Diseases of the eye and adnexa
H60 to H95	Diseases of the ear and mastoid process
I00 to I99	Diseases of the circulatory system
J00 to J99	Diseases of the respiratory system
K00 to K95	Diseases of the digestive system
L00 to L99	Diseases of the skin and subcutaneous tissue
M00 to M99	Disease of the musculoskeletal system and connective tissue
N00 to N99	Diseases of the genitourinary system
O00 to O9A	Pregnancy, childbirth, and the puerperium
P00 to P96	Certain conditions originating in the perinatal period
Q00 to Q99	Congenital malformations, deformations, and chromosomal abnormalities
R00 to R99	Symptoms, signs, and abnormal clinical and laboratory findings, not elsewhere classified
S00 to T88	Injury and poisoning and certain other consequences of external causes
V00 to V99	External causes of morbidity
Z00 to Z99	Factors influencing health status and contact with health services

Source: Centers for Medicare and Medicaid Services, www.cms.gov

How to Use the ICD-10-PCS Code Book. Use the index at the beginning of the book. Using terms or general types of procedures, locate the correct PCS table which identifies the seven characters of the PCS code. Each code has a row that identifies the details of the procedure.

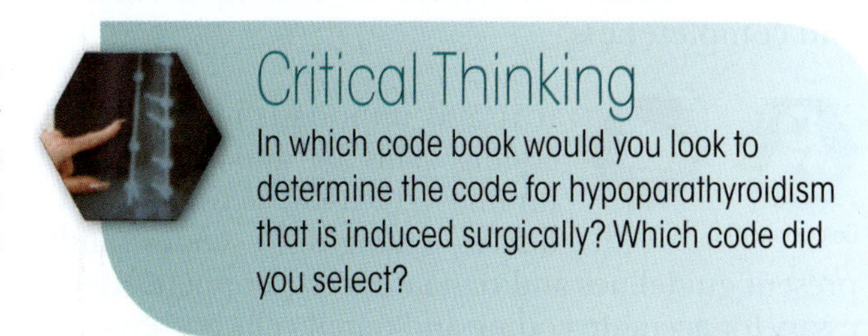

PROCEDURE 17–2

Coding with International Classification of Diseases, 10th Revision, Clinical Modification

PURPOSE:

The ICD-10-CM code books provide a diagnostic coding system for the compilation and reporting of morbidity and mortality statistics for reimbursement purposes.

EQUIPMENT/SUPPLIES:

- ICD-10-CM code books for the current year
- Copy of the encounter form and access to the patient's chart
- Pencil and paper

CASE SCENARIO:

Mary O'Keefe, a new patient, presents at the clinic today reporting painful, frequent urination. She is seen for 10 minutes, during which time the provider takes a focused history and completes a problem-focused examination. A routine urinalysis, nonautomated and without microscopy, is performed and a straightforward medical decision is made. Mary's preliminary diagnosis is painful urination. The urinalysis confirms a urinary tract infection. The provider writes her a prescription for an antibiotic and asks her to make an appointment in 10 days for another urinalysis to confirm the infection has cleared.

PROCEDURE STEPS:

1. Using the ICD-10-CM code book, the alphanumeric Index to Diseases, look up the main symptom or condition that brought the patient to the facility or the specific diagnosis confirmed by test results. In this case, the laboratory results confirmed a urinary tract infection. Code N39.0. RATIONALE: Uses alphanumeric index choosing urinary tract infection.
2. Using the tabular section, look up code N39.0. Read through all of the N39 listings to determine the appropriate code having the highest level of specificity. RATIONALE: Establishes the most accurate code: urinary tract infection, site not specified.

MEDICAL CODING

When performing billing procedures, medical assistants and medical administrative staff are expected to adhere to ethical standards and legal practices. All diagnostic and procedural codes reported must be supported by documentation in the patient's chart. Understanding medical terminology, anatomy, pathology, pharmacology, and information about procedures is critical to coding accuracy and completeness.

It is also important to maintain coding skills by attending continuing education activities that discuss changes in codes and present guidelines and regulatory requirements necessary for accurate coding and timely reimbursement for services and supplies. Networking with other medical coders is another valuable method of staying current with what is happening in this profession. Organizations such as the American Health Information Management Association (AHIMA) and the American Academy of Professional Coders (AAPC) offer webinars, seminars, and online training sessions.

CODING ACCURACY

Accuracy and completeness in coding is vitally important. Imprecise coding affects how quickly the provider is reimbursed and the correct amount of the reimbursement. Codes must be appropriate to the documentation. Insurance carriers always **down-code** if documentation or codes are ambiguous and reimburse the provider for the lowest possible fee. Following are the three primary reasons why down-coding happens:

- The coding system used on the claim form does not match the coding system used by the insurance carrier. Failure to routinely update the charge master contributes to this problem. The carrier's computer will convert the submitted claim code to the closest recognized code. In most cases, the reimbursement amount will be less because each CPT code is assigned a fee schedule.
- If a Workers' Compensation claims examiner has to convert a CPT code to a relative value scale (RVS) code, the examiner will select the lowest-paying code. When billing Workers' Compensation, always use the RVS system used by that carrier and match the code to the best description of the CPT code.
- When attached documentation does not match the written description of the procedure, the reimbursement will always be the lowest-paying code that fits the written description. Denial of payment may occur due to a lack of documentation for medical necessity. As stated earlier, medical necessity is required to ensure that services or procedures for a specific diagnosis or specified frequency are in order for consideration for reimbursement by the patient's insurance covered benefits.

Up-coding, also known as *code creep*, *overcoding*, or *overbilling*, occurs when—to obtain greater reimbursements—the insurance carrier is deliberately billed for a higher rate service than what was performed. Computer software programs have been developed to detect this practice easily and are called scrubbers. Often, complete audits are performed to assess the extent of up-coding practices. Sanctions and penalties are imposed on offenders due to fraud and abuse allegations.

Assumptive coding is assigning a code before the diagnostic code is confirmed.

The Medicare program, in particular, uses CPT codes, which are **bundled codes**. A bundled code is a grouping of several services that are directly related to a specific procedure and are paid as one. For example, surgical dressings and reading test results may be bundled into evaluation and management codes. **Unbundling** refers to separating the components of a procedure and reporting them as billable codes with charges to increase reimbursement rates. This procedure may also be termed *fragmentation*, *exploding*, or *à la carte medicine*. This practice is considered fraud and may lead to audit, sanctions, and penalties.

The more accurate the coding on the claim form, the less chance there is for error, the more quickly the provider is reimbursed, and the better the chance that the provider's reimbursement will reflect the actual charge. Many insurance carriers keep a fee profile of each provider's charges. This profile reflects the amount of each charge for each service and can affect the provider's reimbursement for those services.

Do not guess when coding. The code becomes a permanent part of the patient's-health record with the insurance carrier. If an incorrect code is used, that coded diagnosis will stay with that patient. This can be a difficult problem for insured persons if they change insurance carriers or if other health problems occur. Examples of protected diagnosis of health condition include HIV, AIDS, substance abuse, mental health conditions, and sickle cell anemia.

Consider a patient with hip pain. She has a history of ovarian cancer for which she has had radiology treatments. The hip pain is thought to be possible metastases from the original cancer site. When ruling out this possibility, the provider indicates the following code for the claim:

C79.89 Secondary malignant neoplasm of other specified sites: hip

When the pain is finally discovered to be arthritis and it is determined that the patient needs a hip replacement, the insurance carrier denies coverage for this operation for the following reason: The patient's condition is terminal, and the company does not want her to spend her last months having surgery and recovering from surgery when she is already in poor health. And, of course, there is the cost factor to consider in the eyes of the insurance carrier.

Incorrect coding can be a problem with ruling out a diagnosis. For instance, a patient presents many symptoms of peptic ulcer disease. Do not immediately code that patient as having that disease (which would be assumptive coding) until the diagnosis is confirmed. Instead, code the symptoms. When the tests come back and a specific diagnosis of peptic ulcer can be made, then code the disease as:

K27.7 chronic peptic ulcer, site unspecified, without hemorrhage or perforation

National Correct Coding Initiative (NCCI)

The Centers for Medicare and Medicaid Services (CMS) developed the National Correct Coding Initiative (NCCI) to promote national correct coding methodologies and to control improper coding leading to inappropriate payment in Part B claims. CMS developed its coding policies based on coding conventions defined in the AMA's CPT Manual, national and local policies and edits, coding guidelines developed by national societies, analysis of standard medical and surgical practices, and review of current coding practices.

CODING THE CLAIM FORM

For the insurance company to understand what is being billed, the claim form is completed by the medical assistant, administrative office staff, or billing clerk in the ambulatory care setting. The provider completes an **encounter form**, also known as a **superbill**, at the time of the visit. This encounter form (Figure 17-1) includes the date of service, the visit or consultation code, diagnoses for this visit, procedures done and laboratory tests ordered, and if necessary, the date the patient is to return. This information is then translated onto the claim form.

The **CMS-1500 (02-12)** is the claim form accepted by all insurance carriers (see Figure 16-3). This form is prepared using words and CPT codes

PLEASE RETURN THIS FORM TO RECEPTIONIST

NAME
Receipt No:

PLACE OF SERVICE: ( ) OFFICE ( ) COUNTY HOSPITAL ( ) COMMUNITY GENERAL HOSPITAL ( ) RETIREMENT INN NURSING HOME ( ) ______

DATE OF SERVICE ______

A. OFFICE VISITS - New Patient

	Code	History	Exam	Dec.	Time	
____	99201	Prob. Foc.	Prob. Foc.	Straight	10 min.	____
____	99202	Ex. Prob. Foc.	Ex. Prob. Foc.	Straight	20 min.	____
____	99203	Detail	Detail	Low	30 min.	____
____	99204	Comp.	Comp.	Mod.	45 min.	____
____	99205	Comp.	Comp.	High	60 min.	____

B. OFFICE VISIT - Established Patient

	Code	History	Exam	Dec.	Time	
____	99211	Minimal	Minimal	Minimal	5 min.	____
____	99212	Prob. Foc.	Prob. Foc.	Straight	10 min.	____
____	99213	Ex. Prob. Foc.	Ex. Prob. Foc.	Low	15 min.	____
____	99214	Detail	Detail	Mod.	25 min.	____
____	99215	Comp.	Comp.	High	40 min.	____

C. HOSPITAL CARE

	Dx	Units	Code	
1. Initial Hospital Care (30 min)	____	____	99221	____
2. Subsequent Care	____	____	99231	____
3. Critical Care (30-74 min)	____	____	99291	____
4. Each additional 30 min.	____	____	99292	____
5. Discharge Services	____	____	99238	____
6. Emergency Room	____	____	99282	____

D. NURSING HOME CARE

	Dx	Units	Code	
Initial Care - New Pt.				
1 Expanded	____	____	99322	____
2 Detailed	____	____	99323	____
Subsequent Care - Estab. Pt.				
3 Problem Focused	____	____	99307	____
4 Expanded	____	____	99308	____
5 Detailed	____	____	99309	____
6 Comprehensive	____	____	99310	____

E. PROCEDURES

		Code	
1 Arthrocentesis, Small Jt.	____	20600	____
2 Colonoscopy	____	45378	____
3 EKG w/interpretation	____	93000	____
4 X-Ray Chest, PA/LAT	____	71020	____

F. LAB

		Code	
1 Blood Sugar	____	82947	____
2 CDC w/differential	____	85031	____
3 Cholesterol	____	82465	____
4 Comp. Metabolic Panel	____	80053	____
5 ESR	____	85651	____
6 Hematocrit	____	85014	____
7 Mono Screen	____	86308	____
8 Pap Smear	____	88150	____
9 Potassium	____	84132	____
10 Preg. Test, Quantitative	____	84702	____
11 Routine Venipuncture	____	36415	____

F. Cont'd

	Dx	Units	
12 Strep Screen	____	87081	____
13 UA, Routine w/Micro	____	81000	____
14 UA, Routine w/o Micro	____	81002	____
15 Uric Acid	____	84550	____
16 VDRL	____	86592	____
17 Wet Prep	____	82710	____
18 ______	____	____	____

G. INJECTIONS

1 Influenza Virus Vaccine	____	90658	____
2 Pneumoccocal Vaccine	____	90772	____
3 Tetanus Toxoids	____	90703	____
4 Therapeutic Subcut/IM	____	90732	____
5 Vaccine Administration	____	90471	____
6 Vaccine - each additional	____	90472	____

H. MISCELLANEOUS

1 ______ ____ ____
2 ______ ____ ____

Mark diagnosis with (1=Primary, 2=Secondary, 3=Tertiary)

DIAGNOSIS NOT LISTED BELOW ______

DIAGNOSIS	ICD-10-CM 1, 2, 3	
Allergic rhinitis, unsp	J30.9	____
Anemia, unsp	D64.9	____
Anemia, iron deficiency, unsp	D50.9	____
Anemia, Vit. B12 deficiency, intrinsic factor	D51.0	____
Angina pectoris, other forms	I20.8	____
Abdominal pain, unsp	R10.9	____
Asthma, unsp, w/acute exacerbation	J45.901	____
Asthma, unsp, uncomplicated	J45.909	____
Atrial fibrillation, unsp	I48.91	____
Chest pain, other	R07.89	____
Bronchiolitis, acute, due to RSV	J21.0	____
Bronchitis, acute, unsp	J20.9	____
Bronchitis, NOS	J40	____
Cardiac arrest, cause unsp	I46.9	____
Cellulitis, unsp	L03.90	____
CI D/T, unsp occl/sten, unsp cereb art	I63.50	____
Contact dermatitis, NOS	L25.9	____
Contact dermatitis, irritant, due to solvents	L24.2	____
Convulsions, unsp	R56.9	____
COPD, unsp	J44.9	____
CVD, unsp, w/unsp sequelae	I69.90	____
Dehydration	E86.0	____

DIAGNOSIS	ICD-10-CM 1, 2, 3	
Depress dis, mjr, sing ep, unsp	F32.9	____
Diab mell, Type 2, w/o comp	E11.9	____
Diab mell, Type 2, w/ hyperglycemia	E11.65	____
Dizziness and giddiness	R42	____
Drug rx, adv, meds bio sub, init enc	T50.995A	____
Dysuria	R30.0	____
Edema, unsp	R60.9	____
Fatigue, other	R53.83	____
Fever, unsp	R50.9	____
Gastritis, acute, w/o bleeding	K29.00	____
Gastroenteritis, other spec, noninf	K52.89	____
GERD, w/o esophagitis	K21.9	____
Heart failure, unsp	I50.9	____
Hepatitis A, w/o hepatic coma	B15.9	____
Hypercholesterolemia, pure	E78.0	____
Hypertension, essential (primary)	I10	____
Hypoglycemia, unsp	E16.2	____
Hypokalemia	E87.6	____
Impetigo, unsp	L01.00	____
Lymphadenitis, nonspec, unspec	I88.9	____
Mental d/o, uns, D/T kwn phys cond	F09	____
Mono, inf, unsp, w/o comp	B27.90	____

DIAGNOSIS	ICD-10-CM 1, 2, 3	
Myocardial infarction, STE, unsp site	I21.3	____
Osteoarthritis, NOS	M19.90	____
Otitis externa, other infective, unsp ear	H60.399	____
Otitis media, NOS	H66.90	____
Peripheral vascular disease, unsp	I73.9	____
Pharyngitis, acute, unsp	J02.9	____
Pneumonia, unsp organism	J18.9	____
Prostate inflammatory disease, unsp	N41.9	____
Pulmonary heart disease, unsp	I27.9	____
Rash and other nonsp skin eruption	R21	____
Serous otitis media, chronic, unsp ear	H65.20	____
Sinusitis, acute, unsp	J01.90	____
Stomach and duodenum disease, unsp	K31.9	____
Tonsillitis, acute, unsp	J03.90	____
Upper respiratory infection, acute, unsp	J06.9	____
Urinary tract infection, unsp	N39.0	____
Urticaria, unsp	L50.9	____
Ventricular premature depolarization	I49.3	____
Viral agent, other, cause dis class elsew	B97.89	____
Weight loss, abnormal	R63.4	____

ABN: I UNDERSTAND THAT MEDICARE PROBABLY WILL NOT COVER THE SERVICES LISTED BELOW

A. ______ B. ______ C. ______

Date ______ Patient Signature ______

Doctor's Signature ______

RETURN: ______ Days ______ Weeks ______ Months ______

INNER CITY HEALTH CARE
8600 MAIN STREET, SUITE 200
RIVER CITY, XY 01234
PHONE No. (123) 456-7890
EIN# 00-1234560

□ W. LEWIS, M.D. NPI# 9995010111
□ M. KING, M.D. NPI# 9995020212
□ R. REYNOLDS, M.D. NPI# 9995030313

FIGURE 17-1 Encounter form.

for procedures performed and ICD-10-CM codes for diagnoses. Keep in mind that the codes must correlate; for instance, if a person had an ICD-10-CM diagnosis code of earache, otitis media, or H66.90, and the CPT procedure code indicated was 69090, ear piercing, the insurance company would question the claim and reject it for payment. The person completing the claim form must be *as precise as possible*. If the coding is wrong, the claim will be denied and the provider will not receive payment. Claims tracking investigates all coding errors and potential denial or delays in payment. Coding must correlate with the documentation note in the chart; otherwise, fraud is committed.

Coding the claim form is a precise way to communicate with the insurance carrier. Coding indicates the complexity of the visit using an evaluation and management CPT code, the diagnosis for the visit, and the specific procedures such as injections performed during the visit. This results in little confusion, and a minimum of additional communication is needed between the carrier and the provider's clinic because all information is contained in the codes.

For instance, Leo McKay, an established patient, is seen for an extended visit to determine the cause of his abdominal pain. Symptoms include diarrhea, fever, nausea, and anorexia. An abdominal ultrasound is ordered, as well as laboratory tests, and the results are unknown at the time of the insurance billing. The visit lasts 30 minutes and includes a full physical examination and a history of the present illness.

The CPT procedure coding for this visit is 99214, which reflects the examination and time spent with the patient, the history taken of this illness, and a medical decision of moderate complexity.

The ICD-10-CM diagnosis coding for abdominal pain is R10.9, for diarrhea R19.7, for nausea R11.0, and for anorexia R63.0. The claim form is submitted to the insurance carrier with these codes, and even though they are all symptoms, the claim will be paid because the visit and the tests ordered interrelate.

When the test results are known, they show a positive diagnosis of *Giardia lamblia*. The diagnosis code is changed to A07.1. Any further charges sent to the insurance carrier while Leo McKay is being treated for this problem are coded A07.1. The symptom codes from the first submission are dropped. *The Official ICD-10-CM Guidelines for Coding and Reporting* state that when signs and symptoms are integral to a definitive diagnosis, you are to code only for the definitive diagnosis.

Many electronic health records (EHR) use encoder programs (Figure 17-2), which are available online. Encoder programs are coding software programs that allow the user to locate CPT, ICD-10-CM, and HCPCS codes quickly using the computer. Many of the encoder programs permit the placement of bookmarks or notes for quick reference.

THIRD-PARTY PRIVACY, SECURITY, AND COMPLIANCE GUIDELINES

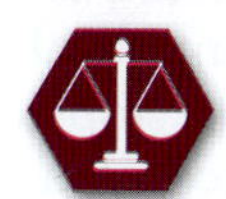
Legal

Integrity

Because patient information is easily accessed through medical charts, EHR, and the human factor, security and confidentiality measures must be in place in medical clinics. When patients schedule an appointment and are seen by the provider, they enter into a contract for specific services. The first party is the person receiving the contracted service. The second party

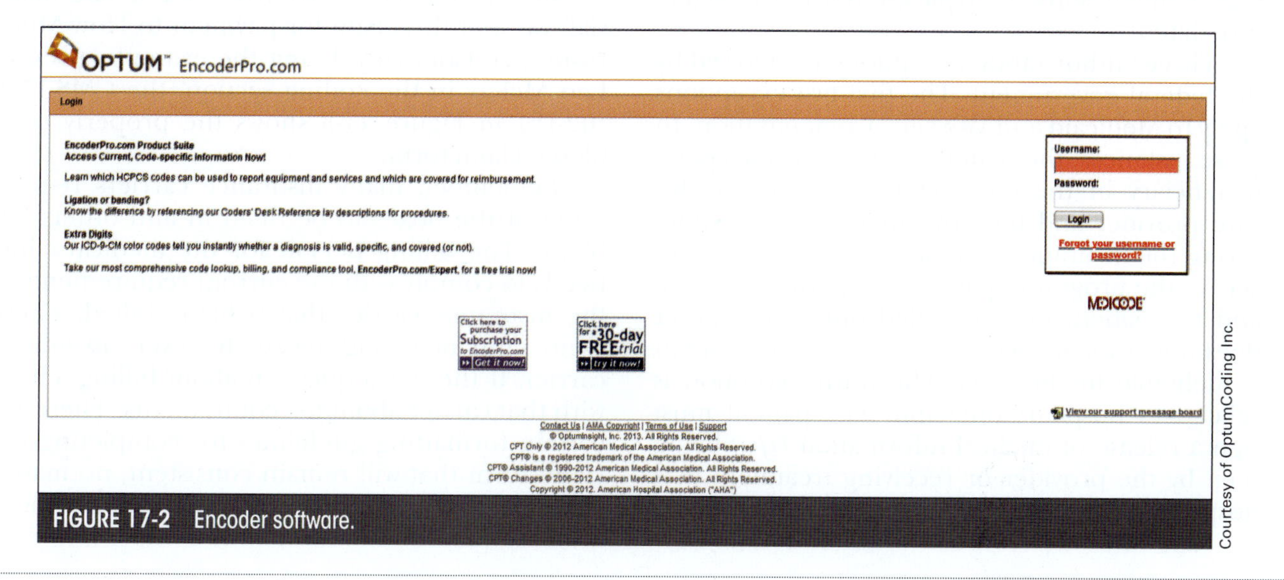

FIGURE 17-2 Encoder software.

Courtesy of OptumCoding Inc.

is the person or organization providing the service. A third party is one that is not involved in the patient–provider relationship but rather with reimbursement procedures.

The patient has a right to expect that his or her health information will not be disseminated to others without written permission to do so. Confidentiality issues involve restricting the health information to only those individuals who need to know. Compliance with Health Insurance Portability and Accountability Act (HIPAA) of 1996 regulations is one way to safeguard protected health information (PHI). Chapters 11, 12, 13, 14, 15, and 17 of the HIPAA regulations all place emphasis on HIPAA as it relates to PHI.

Authorization to release necessary medical information to payers, such as insurance carriers, must be obtained from the patient, the parent, or the guardian *before* any information is released. A *breach of confidentiality* is the release of unauthorized PHI to a third party. One way to prevent this when processing insurance claims forms is to ask the patient, parent, or guardian to sign an authorization to release medical information statement *before* the claim form is completed. The CMS-1500 (02-12) form provides space for this signature in block 12.

Some medical clinics, especially those that send claim forms electronically, develop their own specialized authorization for release of medical information form. The customized form must contain the specific name of the insurance company and must be signed by the patient, parent, or guardian. This form is generally valid for 1 year. The insurance company may request a copy of the signed form. When completing the CMS-1500 (02-12), block 12 may contain the words *SIGNATURE ON FILE* or the abbreviation *SOF*. Practice management software typically tracks the signature dates.

Three authorization exceptions are allowed by the federal government. The first two exceptions apply to Medicaid and Workers' Compensation. In these instances, the patient becomes a third-party beneficiary in the contract between the health care provider and the government agency sponsoring the insurance program. Providers agree to accept the program's payment as payment in full, and the patient may be billed only if the payer does not cover services rendered or if the patient is ineligible for benefits. The third exception is related to hospital admission. The patient must sign a release of medical information *before* being seen by the provider or receiving treatment in a hospital.

Procedure

Most states have specific laws related to release of protected medical information regarding mental health services and federally assisted alcohol and drug abuse programs. Patients being screened for HIV infection or AIDS must sign an additional authorization statement *before* information may be released regarding their status. See Procedure 17-3 for specific steps involved in authorization to release PHI to third-party payers.

COMPLETING THE CMS-1500 (02-12)

In most clinics today, the CMS-1500 (02-12) form is completed using data from the patient's EHR. In the few cases in which the clinic does not use EHR, the paper encounter form is used by the billing specialist to complete the CMS-1500 (02-12) form. Each insurance carrier has its own thoughts on how the form is to be completed and no two companies agree entirely on the information required, the boxes checked, and the rationale about what information goes in which boxes.

With the transition to an increase in electronic claims submission and the HIPAA regulations, the National Uniform Claim Committee (NUCC) established a standardized data set for use in an electronic environment as well as with paper claim form standards. The NUCC continues to monitor how insurance carriers use the various claim form fields. Additional changes to the CMS-1500 (02-12) form may be required in the future as the NUCC works to create standardized national instructions for completing the form.

To illustrate the completion of a claim form, a fictitious insurance carrier will be used. Insurance carriers often change their rules and regulations for submitting claims. To avoid out-of-date material, we sent this claim for payment to How Much Insurance Company. Using the example given of Leo McKay in the coding section, the CMS-1500 (02-12) in Figure 17-3 shows the properly completed claim form.

Remember, many insurance carriers require some of the boxes to be filled in and others left blank. The billing person for the medical clinic needs to comply with the current requirements of the insurance carrier that is being billed. There is no right or wrong answer for every insurance carrier. If there is a question about billing, check with that carrier about its requirements. There are certain formatting guidelines for completing the claim form that will remain consistent, no matter which insurance company you are dealing with:

PROCEDURE 17–3

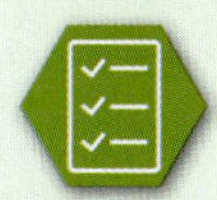

Procedure

Applying Third-Party Guidelines

PURPOSE:

To obtain written authorization to release necessary medical information to third-party payers.

EQUIPMENT/SUPPLIES:

- Patient chart
- CMS-1500 (02-12) claim form

PROCEDURE STEPS:

1. When the patient signs in at the reception desk, check his or her chart to ascertain whether an authorization to release medical information form has been signed and is currently valid. RATIONALE: PHI cannot be released without written authorization from the patient.
2. If there is no record of signature on file, have the patient sign block 12 of the CMS-1500 (02-12) claim form or the offices' customized authorization to release medical information form. RATIONALE: PHI cannot be released without written authorization from the patient.

1. MEDICARE (Medicare#) MEDICAID (Medicaid#) TRICARE (ID#/DoD#) CHAMPVA (Member ID#) GROUP HEALTH PLAN (ID#) FECA BLK LUNG (ID#) OTHER (ID#)

2. PATIENT'S NAME (Last Name, First Name, Middle Initial)		3. PATIENT'S BIRTH DATE MM DD YY SEX M F
5. PATIENT'S ADDRESS (No., Street)		6. PATIENT RELATIONSHIP TO INSURED Self Spouse Child Other
CITY	STATE	8. RESERVED FOR NUCC USE
ZIP CODE	TELEPHONE (Include Area Code) ( )	
9. OTHER INSURED'S NAME (Last Name, First Name, Middle Initial)		10. IS PATIENT'S CONDITION RELATED TO:
a. OTHER INSURED'S POLICY OR GROUP NUMBER		a. EMPLOYMENT? (Current or Previous) YES NO
b. RESERVED FOR NUCC USE		b. AUTO ACCIDENT? YES NO PLACE (State)
c. RESERVED FOR NUCC USE		c. OTHER ACCIDENT? YES NO
d. INSURANCE PLAN NAME OR PROGRAM NAME		10d. CLAIM CODES (Designated by NUCC)

READ BACK OF FORM BEFORE COMPLETING & SIGNING THIS FORM.

12. PATIENT'S OR AUTHORIZED PERSON'S SIGNATURE I authorize the release of any medical or other information necessary to process this claim. I also request payment of government benefits either to myself or to the party who accepts assignment below.

SIGNED ______________________ DATE ______________

Courtesy of the Centers for Medicare & Medicaid Services, www.cms.gov

- The form must *always* be completed in black ink.
- The form must *always* be completed using all capital letters.
- The form must *never* contain any punctuation or symbols of any kind; only letters and numbers may be used.
- Any date entered on the form (DOS, DOB, etc.), must be in eight-digit format. For example, the DOB for our previously mentioned patient, Leo McKay, is April 1, 1963. Therefore, his DOB on the form should appear as 04011963. (Notice there are no hyphens or slashes.)

HEALTH INSURANCE CLAIM FORM

APPROVED BY NATIONAL UNIFORM CLAIM COMMITTEE (NUCC) 02/12

PICA PICA

CARRIER

1. MEDICARE (Medicare#) MEDICAID (Medicaid#) TRICARE (ID#/DoD#) CHAMPVA (Member ID#) GROUP HEALTH PLAN (ID#) FECA BLK LUNG (ID#) OTHER [X] (ID#)

1a. INSURED'S I.D. NUMBER (For Program in Item 1): 555-55-555

2. PATIENT'S NAME (Last Name, First Name, Middle Initial): MCKAY LEO M

3. PATIENT'S BIRTH DATE MM DD YY: 04 01 1963 SEX M [X] F [ ]

4. INSURED'S NAME (Last Name, First Name, Middle Initial): MCKAY, LEO M

5. PATIENT'S ADDRESS (No., Street): 123 W FIRST STREET

CITY: ANYWHERE STATE: XY

ZIP CODE: 01234 TELEPHONE (Include Area Code): (123) 556-6189

6. PATIENT RELATIONSHIP TO INSURED: Self [X] Spouse [ ] Child [ ] Other [ ]

7. INSURED'S ADDRESS (No., Street): 123 W FIRST STREET

CITY: ANYWHERE STATE: XY

ZIP CODE: 01234 TELEPHONE (Include Area Code): (123) 556-6189

8. RESERVED FOR NUCC USE

9. OTHER INSURED'S NAME (Last Name, First Name, Middle Initial)

a. OTHER INSURED'S POLICY OR GROUP NUMBER

b. RESERVED FOR NUCC USE

c. RESERVED FOR NUCC USE

d. INSURANCE PLAN NAME OR PROGRAM NAME

10. IS PATIENT'S CONDITION RELATED TO:

a. EMPLOYMENT? (Current or Previous) [ ] YES [X] NO

b. AUTO ACCIDENT? [ ] YES [X] NO PLACE (State)

c. OTHER ACCIDENT? [ ] YES [X] NO

10d. CLAIM CODES (Designated by NUCC)

11. INSURED'S POLICY GROUP OR FECA NUMBER: 1122334

a. INSURED'S DATE OF BIRTH MM DD YY: 04 01 1963 SEX M [X] F [ ]

b. OTHER CLAIM ID (Designated by NUCC)

c. INSURANCE PLAN NAME OR PROGRAM NAME

d. IS THERE ANOTHER HEALTH BENEFIT PLAN? [ ] YES [X] NO *If yes*, complete items 9, 9a, and 9d.

READ BACK OF FORM BEFORE COMPLETING & SIGNING THIS FORM.

12. PATIENT'S OR AUTHORIZED PERSON'S SIGNATURE I authorize the release of any medical or other information necessary to process this claim. I also request payment of government benefits either to myself or to the party who accepts assignment below.

SIGNED SIGNATURE ON FILE DATE 01 14 20XX

13. INSURED'S OR AUTHORIZED PERSON'S SIGNATURE I authorize payment of medical benefits to the undersigned physician or supplier for services described below.

SIGNED SIGNATURE ON FILE

PATIENT AND INSURED INFORMATION

14. DATE OF CURRENT ILLNESS, INJURY, or PREGNANCY (LMP) MM DD YY: 01 10 20XX QUAL.

15. OTHER DATE QUAL. MM DD YY

16. DATES PATIENT UNABLE TO WORK IN CURRENT OCCUPATION FROM TO

17. NAME OF REFERRING PROVIDER OR OTHER SOURCE 17a. 17b. NPI

18. HOSPITALIZATION DATES RELATED TO CURRENT SERVICES FROM TO

19. ADDITIONAL CLAIM INFORMATION (Designated by NUCC)

20. OUTSIDE LAB? [ ] YES [ ] NO $ CHARGES

21. DIAGNOSIS OR NATURE OF ILLNESS OR INJURY Relate A-L to service line below (24E) ICD Ind. 10

A. R10.9 B. K52.89 C. R63.0 D.
E. F. G. H.
I. J. K. L.

22. RESUBMISSION CODE ORIGINAL REF. NO.

23. PRIOR AUTHORIZATION NUMBER

	24. A. DATE(S) OF SERVICE From MM DD YY	To MM DD YY	B. PLACE OF SERVICE	C. EMG	D. PROCEDURES, SERVICES, OR SUPPLIES (Explain Unusual Circumstances) CPT/HCPCS	MODIFIER	E. DIAGNOSIS POINTER	F. $ CHARGES	G. DAYS OR UNITS	H. EPSDT Family Plan	I. ID. QUAL.	J. RENDERING PROVIDER ID. #
1	01 10 XX		3		99214		123	85 00	1		NPI	1543298760
2	01 10 XX		3		82270		12	13 00	1		NPI	1543298760
3											NPI	
4											NPI	
5											NPI	
6											NPI	

25. FEDERAL TAX I.D. NUMBER: 91-1234432 SSN [ ] EIN [X]

26. PATIENT'S ACCOUNT NO.: MCK111

27. ACCEPT ASSIGNMENT? (For govt. claims, see back) [ ] YES [X] NO

28. TOTAL CHARGE: $ 98 00

29. AMOUNT PAID: $

30. Rsvd for NUCC Use

31. SIGNATURE OF PHYSICIAN OR SUPPLIER INCLUDING DEGREES OR CREDENTIALS (I certify that the statements on the reverse apply to this bill and are made a part thereof.)

SIGNED MARK KING MD DATE 01 14 20XX

32. SERVICE FACILITY LOCATION INFORMATION

a. NPI b.

33. BILLING PROVIDER INFO & PH # (123) 456-7890

INNER CITY HEALTH CARE
8600 MAIN STREET, SUITE 200
RIVER CITY, XY 01234

a. 36640210XX b.

PHYSICIAN OR SUPPLIER INFORMATION

NUCC Instruction Manual available at: www.nucc.org PLEASE PRINT OR TYPE APPROVED OMB-0938-1197 FORM 1500 (02-12)

FIGURE 17-3 Completed CMS-1500 claim form.

The CMS-1500 (02-12) claim form contains all of the identification information that the carrier needs to process or analyze the claim for payment. The new form is distinguishable from the old form in that the 1500 symbol and the date it was approved by the NUCC appear in the top left margin. When completing the PATIENT AND INSURED INFORMATION section, do not use commas to separate the last name, first name, and middle initial. Do not use periods within the name. Do not use commas, periods, or other punctuation in the address. When entering the nine-digit ZIP code, you may include the hyphen. This is the only exception to the punctuation rule. Do not use a hyphen or space as a separator within the telephone number. The top right-hand space, identified as CARRIER, provides space for the carrier's name and address be keyed in. Procedure 17-4 gives instructions for completing a Medicare claim form. Before completing claims for carriers other than Medicare, the medical assistant should verify with a carrier's representative exactly which blocks are required to be filled in for that particular carrier.

PROCEDURE 17–4

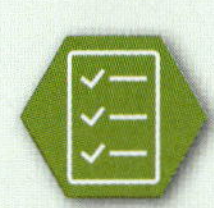

Completing a Medicare CMS-1500 (02-12) Claim Form

PURPOSE:

To complete the CMS-1500 (02-12) insurance claim form for Medicare reimbursement.

EQUIPMENT/SUPPLIES:

- Patient information
- Patient account or ledger card
- Copy of patient's insurance card
- Insurance claim form
- Computer and printer

PROCEDURE STEPS:

1. The CARRIER section of the CMS-1500 (02-12) is in the upper portion of the form. Use the blank space at the top right of the section marked CARRIER to enter the name and address of the payer to whom this claim is being sent. The payer is the carrier, health plan, third-party administrator, or other payer who will handle the claim. The format for this information should be as follows:

   Key on line 4: first line—Name

   Key on line 5: second line—First line of address

   Key on line 6: third line—Second line of address

   Key on line 7: fourth line—City, state (2 letters) and zip code

   Do not use commas, periods, or other punctuation in the address. When entering a nine-digit ZIP code, you may include the hyphen. When printing page numbers on multiple-page claims (generally done by clearinghouses when converting the electronic claim form to the CMS 1500 claim form), print the page numbers in the CARRIER block on line 8 beginning at column 32. Page numbers are to be printed as Page XX of YY. RATIONALE: The claims processor must know who the claim is from.
2. The PATIENT AND INSURED INFORMATION section asks for specific information related to the patient and his or her health insurance plan. The following information is required for this section. Complete each block as directed. RATIONALE: These blocks must be accurately completed or the claim may be denied.

(continues)

HEALTH INSURANCE CLAIM FORM

APPROVED BY NATIONAL UNIFORM CLAIM COMMITTEE (NUCC) 02/12

PICA PICA

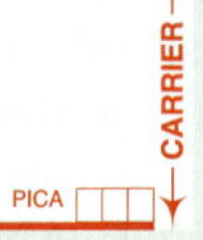

Courtesy of the Centers for Medicare & Medicaid Services, www.cms.gov

Block 1	Indicate the type of health insurance coverage applicable to this claim by placing an *X* in the Medicare box. Only one box can be marked.
Block 1a	Enter insured's ID number as shown on insured's ID card for the payer to whom the claim is being submitted. RATIONALE: The insured's ID number is the identification number of the person who holds the policy. This information identifies the patient to the payer. (For Medicare beneficiaries, this appears as a nine-digit number followed by a letter.)
Block 2	Enter the patient's full last name, first name, and middle initial in this block.
Block 3	Enter the patient's eight-digit birth date (MMDDYYYY). Enter an *X* in the correct box to indicate sex of the patient. Only one box can be marked. If gender is unknown, leave blank.
Block 4	Enter the insured's full last name, first name, and middle initial.
Block 5	Enter the patient's mailing address and telephone number.
Block 6	Enter an *X* in the correct box to indicate the patient's relationship to insured when block 4 has been completed. Only one box can be marked.
Block 7	Enter the insured's address and telephone number. If block 4 has been completed, then this field should also be completed.
Block 8	This is reserved for NUCC use. Leave blank.
Block 9	If block 11d is marked yes (to indicate that the patient carries a secondary insurance plan), complete fields 9 and 9a through 9d with the patient's secondary insurance information; otherwise, leave blank. When additional group health coverage exists, enter other insured's full last name, first name, and middle initial of the enrollee in another health plan if it is different from that shown in block 2.
Block 9a	Enter the policy or group number of the other insured. Do not use a hyphen or space as a separator within the policy or group number.
Block 9b	This is reserved for NUCC use. Leave blank.
Block 9c	This is reserved for NUCC use. Leave blank.
Block 9d	Enter the other insured's insurance plan or program name.
Blocks 10a to 10c	When appropriate, enter an *X* in the correct box to indicate whether one or more of the services described in block 24 are for a condition or injury that occurred on the job or as a result of an automobile or other accident. Only one box on each line can be marked. The two-letter state abbreviation must be shown if YES is marked in 10b. RATIONALE: Any item marked YES indicates there may be other applicable insurance coverage that would be primary.
Block 10d	Refer to the most current instructions from the applicable public or private payer regarding the use of this field.
Block 11	Enter the insured's policy or group number as it appears on the insured's health care ID card. If block 4 has been completed, then this field should also be completed.

(continues)

Block 11a	Enter the eight-digit date of birth (MMDDYYYY) of the insured and an *X* to indicate the sex of the insured. Only one box can be marked. If gender is unknown, leave blank.
Block 11b	This is the other claim ID designated by NUCC. Leave blank.
Block 11c	Enter the insurance plan or program name of the insured. (Some payers require an ID number of the primary insurer rather than the name in this field.)
Block 11d	When appropriate, enter an *X* in the correct box. If marked YES, complete blocks 9, 9a, and d. Only one box can be marked.
Block 12	Enter *Signature on File, SOF,* or legal signature. With a legal signature, enter the date signed in the proper eight-digit format. If there is no signature on file, leave blank or enter *No Signature on File.* RATIONALE: The patient's or authorized person's signature indicates there is an authorization on file for the release of any medical or other information necessary to process or adjudicate the claim.
Block 13	Enter *Signature on File, SOF,* or legal signature. If there is no signature on file, leave blank or enter *No Signature on File.* RATIONALE: The insured's or authorized person's signature indicates that there is a signature on file authorizing payment of medical benefits.

1. MEDICARE (Medicare#) MEDICAID (Medicaid#) TRICARE (ID#/DoD#) CHAMPVA (Member ID#) GROUP HEALTH PLAN (ID#) FECA BLK LUNG (ID#) OTHER (ID#)
1a. INSURED'S I.D. NUMBER (For Program in Item 1)
2. PATIENT'S NAME (Last Name, First Name, Middle Initial)
3. PATIENT'S BIRTH DATE MM DD YY SEX M F
4. INSURED'S NAME (Last Name, First Name, Middle Initial)
5. PATIENT'S ADDRESS (No., Street)
6. PATIENT RELATIONSHIP TO INSURED Self Spouse Child Other
7. INSURED'S ADDRESS (No., Street)
CITY STATE
8. RESERVED FOR NUCC USE
CITY STATE
ZIP CODE TELEPHONE (Include Area Code) ( )
ZIP CODE TELEPHONE (Include Area Code) ( )
9. OTHER INSURED'S NAME (Last Name, First Name, Middle Initial)
10. IS PATIENT'S CONDITION RELATED TO:
11. INSURED'S POLICY GROUP OR FECA NUMBER
a. OTHER INSURED'S POLICY OR GROUP NUMBER
a. EMPLOYMENT? (Current or Previous) YES NO
a. INSURED'S DATE OF BIRTH MM DD YY SEX M F
b. RESERVED FOR NUCC USE
b. AUTO ACCIDENT? YES NO PLACE (State)
b. OTHER CLAIM ID (Designated by NUCC)
c. RESERVED FOR NUCC USE
c. OTHER ACCIDENT? YES NO
c. INSURANCE PLAN NAME OR PROGRAM NAME
d. INSURANCE PLAN NAME OR PROGRAM NAME
10d. CLAIM CODES (Designated by NUCC)
d. IS THERE ANOTHER HEALTH BENEFIT PLAN? YES NO *If yes,* complete items 9, 9a, and 9d.
READ BACK OF FORM BEFORE COMPLETING & SIGNING THIS FORM.
12. PATIENT'S OR AUTHORIZED PERSON'S SIGNATURE I authorize the release of any medical or other information necessary to process this claim. I also request payment of government benefits either to myself or to the party who accepts assignment below.
SIGNED ____ DATE ____
13. INSURED'S OR AUTHORIZED PERSON'S SIGNATURE I authorize payment of medical benefits to the undersigned physician or supplier for services described below.
SIGNED ____
PATIENT AND INSURED INFORMATION

Courtesy of the Centers for Medicare & Medicaid Services, www.cms.gov

3. The PHYSICIAN OR SUPPLIER INFORMATION section must be accurately completed or the claim may be denied. This is the bottom section of the form under the bolded red line.

Block 14	Enter the eight-digit date of the first date of the present illness, injury, or pregnancy. For pregnancy, use the date of the last menstrual period (LMP) as the first date. Leave blank if unknown.
Block 15	Enter the first date the patient had the same or a similar illness. Enter the date in the eight-digit format. Previous pregnancies are not a similar illness. Leave blank if unknown.

(continues)

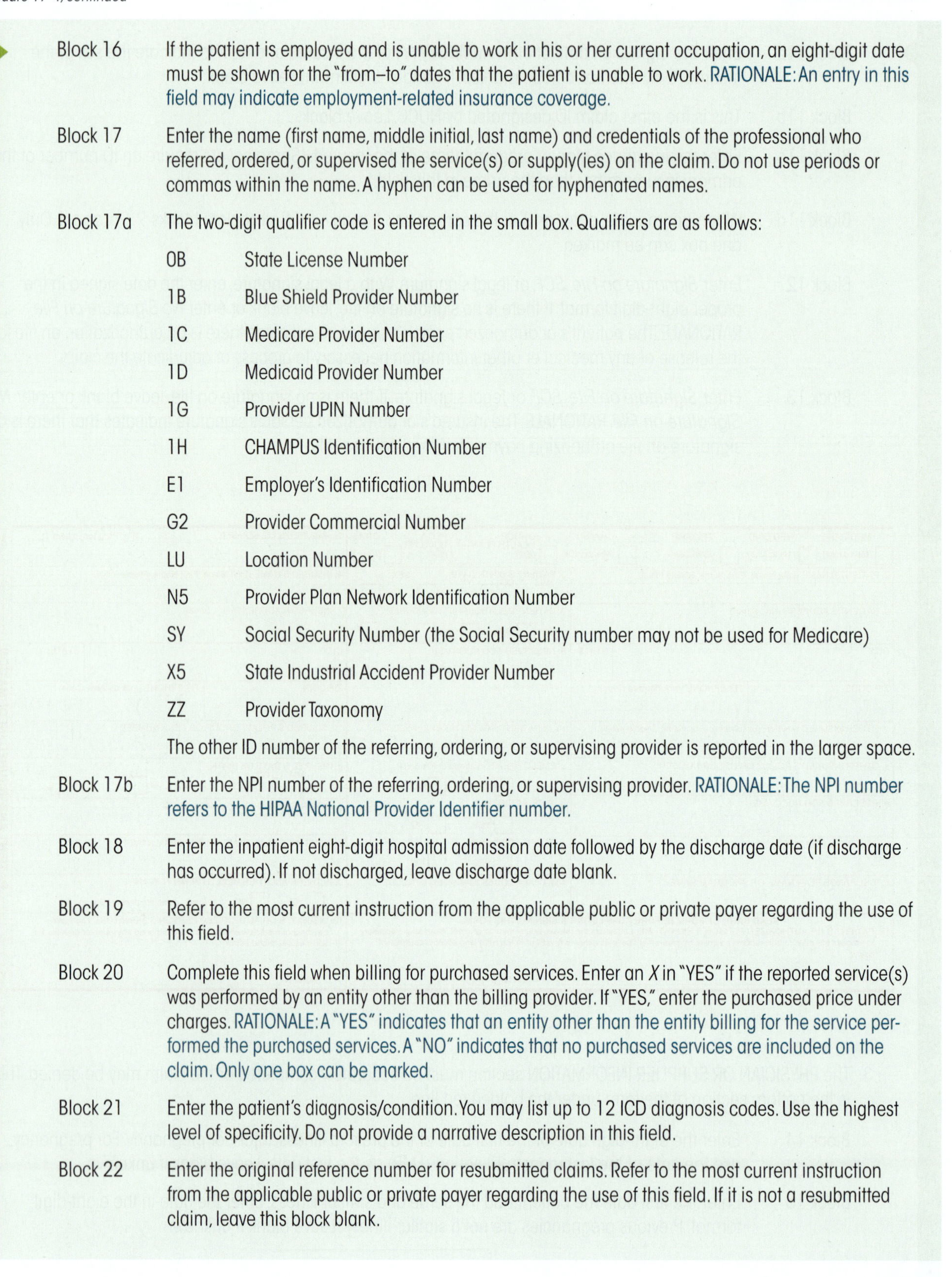

Block 16 If the patient is employed and is unable to work in his or her current occupation, an eight-digit date must be shown for the "from–to" dates that the patient is unable to work. RATIONALE: An entry in this field may indicate employment-related insurance coverage.

Block 17 Enter the name (first name, middle initial, last name) and credentials of the professional who referred, ordered, or supervised the service(s) or supply(ies) on the claim. Do not use periods or commas within the name. A hyphen can be used for hyphenated names.

Block 17a The two-digit qualifier code is entered in the small box. Qualifiers are as follows:

0B	State License Number
1B	Blue Shield Provider Number
1C	Medicare Provider Number
1D	Medicaid Provider Number
1G	Provider UPIN Number
1H	CHAMPUS Identification Number
E1	Employer's Identification Number
G2	Provider Commercial Number
LU	Location Number
N5	Provider Plan Network Identification Number
SY	Social Security Number (the Social Security number may not be used for Medicare)
X5	State Industrial Accident Provider Number
ZZ	Provider Taxonomy

The other ID number of the referring, ordering, or supervising provider is reported in the larger space.

Block 17b Enter the NPI number of the referring, ordering, or supervising provider. RATIONALE: The NPI number refers to the HIPAA National Provider Identifier number.

Block 18 Enter the inpatient eight-digit hospital admission date followed by the discharge date (if discharge has occurred). If not discharged, leave discharge date blank.

Block 19 Refer to the most current instruction from the applicable public or private payer regarding the use of this field.

Block 20 Complete this field when billing for purchased services. Enter an *X* in "YES" if the reported service(s) was performed by an entity other than the billing provider. If "YES," enter the purchased price under charges. RATIONALE: A "YES" indicates that an entity other than the entity billing for the service performed the purchased services. A "NO" indicates that no purchased services are included on the claim. Only one box can be marked.

Block 21 Enter the patient's diagnosis/condition. You may list up to 12 ICD diagnosis codes. Use the highest level of specificity. Do not provide a narrative description in this field.

Block 22 Enter the original reference number for resubmitted claims. Refer to the most current instruction from the applicable public or private payer regarding the use of this field. If it is not a resubmitted claim, leave this block blank.

(continues)

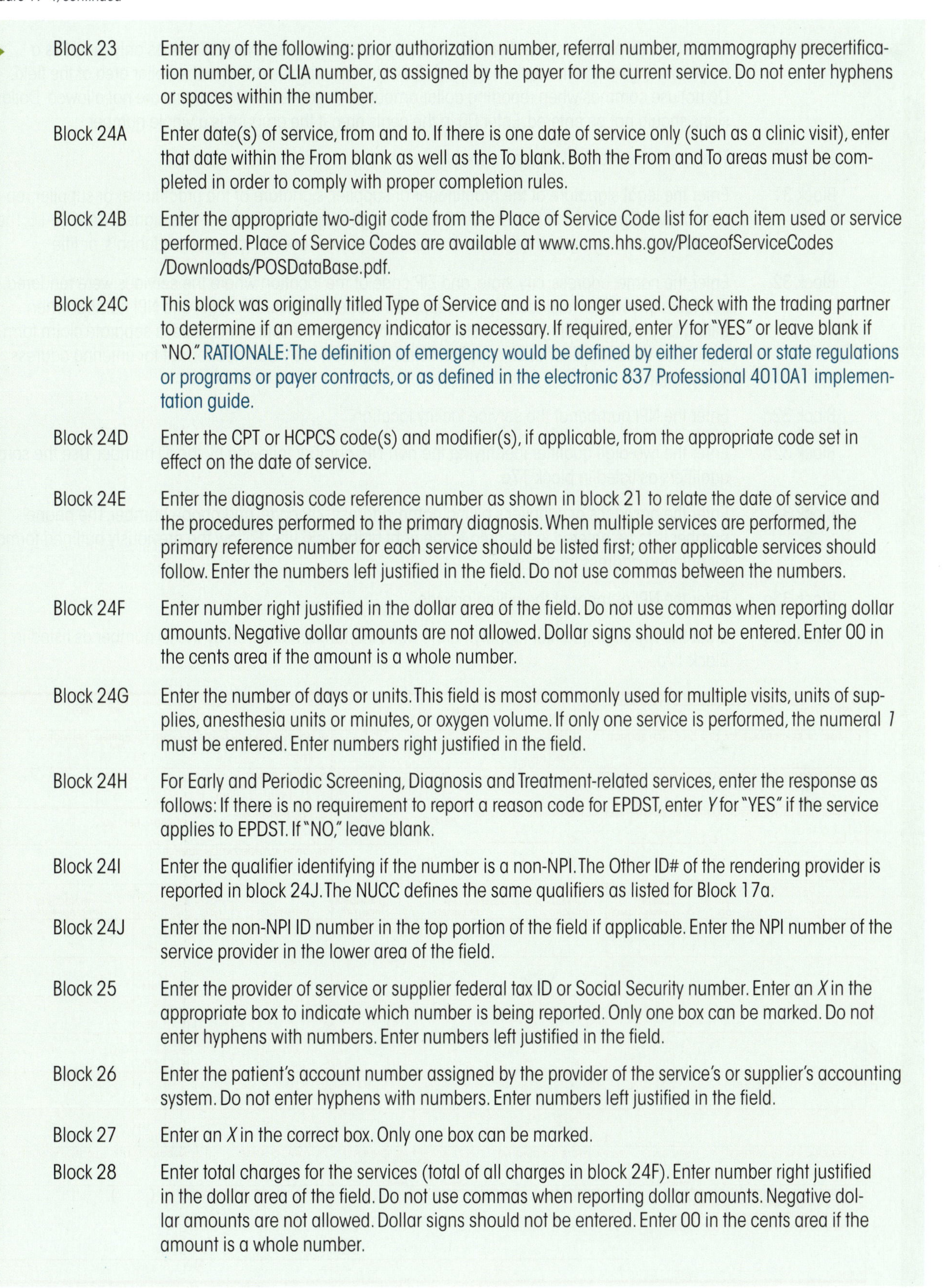

Block 23	Enter any of the following: prior authorization number, referral number, mammography precertification number, or CLIA number, as assigned by the payer for the current service. Do not enter hyphens or spaces within the number.
Block 24A	Enter date(s) of service, from and to. If there is one date of service only (such as a clinic visit), enter that date within the From blank as well as the To blank. Both the From and To areas must be completed in order to comply with proper completion rules.
Block 24B	Enter the appropriate two-digit code from the Place of Service Code list for each item used or service performed. Place of Service Codes are available at www.cms.hhs.gov/PlaceofServiceCodes/Downloads/POSDataBase.pdf.
Block 24C	This block was originally titled Type of Service and is no longer used. Check with the trading partner to determine if an emergency indicator is necessary. If required, enter *Y* for "YES" or leave blank if "NO." RATIONALE: The definition of emergency would be defined by either federal or state regulations or programs or payer contracts, or as defined in the electronic 837 Professional 4010A1 implementation guide.
Block 24D	Enter the CPT or HCPCS code(s) and modifier(s), if applicable, from the appropriate code set in effect on the date of service.
Block 24E	Enter the diagnosis code reference number as shown in block 21 to relate the date of service and the procedures performed to the primary diagnosis. When multiple services are performed, the primary reference number for each service should be listed first; other applicable services should follow. Enter the numbers left justified in the field. Do not use commas between the numbers.
Block 24F	Enter number right justified in the dollar area of the field. Do not use commas when reporting dollar amounts. Negative dollar amounts are not allowed. Dollar signs should not be entered. Enter 00 in the cents area if the amount is a whole number.
Block 24G	Enter the number of days or units. This field is most commonly used for multiple visits, units of supplies, anesthesia units or minutes, or oxygen volume. If only one service is performed, the numeral *1* must be entered. Enter numbers right justified in the field.
Block 24H	For Early and Periodic Screening, Diagnosis and Treatment-related services, enter the response as follows: If there is no requirement to report a reason code for EPDST, enter *Y* for "YES" if the service applies to EPDST. If "NO," leave blank.
Block 24I	Enter the qualifier identifying if the number is a non-NPI. The Other ID# of the rendering provider is reported in block 24J. The NUCC defines the same qualifiers as listed for Block 17a.
Block 24J	Enter the non-NPI ID number in the top portion of the field if applicable. Enter the NPI number of the service provider in the lower area of the field.
Block 25	Enter the provider of service or supplier federal tax ID or Social Security number. Enter an *X* in the appropriate box to indicate which number is being reported. Only one box can be marked. Do not enter hyphens with numbers. Enter numbers left justified in the field.
Block 26	Enter the patient's account number assigned by the provider of the service's or supplier's accounting system. Do not enter hyphens with numbers. Enter numbers left justified in the field.
Block 27	Enter an *X* in the correct box. Only one box can be marked.
Block 28	Enter total charges for the services (total of all charges in block 24F). Enter number right justified in the dollar area of the field. Do not use commas when reporting dollar amounts. Negative dollar amounts are not allowed. Dollar signs should not be entered. Enter 00 in the cents area if the amount is a whole number.

(continues)

Block 29	Enter the total amount the patient or other payers paid on the covered services only (such as a co-payment given on the date of service). Enter number right justified in the dollar area of the field. Do not use commas when reporting dollar amounts. Negative dollar amounts are not allowed. Dollar signs should not be entered. Enter 00 in the cents area if the amount is a whole number.
Block 30	This is reserved for NUCC use. Leave blank.
Block 31	Enter the legal signature of the practitioner or supplier, signature of the practitioner or supplier representative, *Signature on File*, or *SOF*. Enter the eight-digit date the form was signed. RATIONALE: The signature refers to the authorized or accountable person and the degree, credentials, or title.
Block 32	Enter the name, address, city, state, and ZIP code of the location where the services were rendered. Providers of service must identify the supplier's name, address, ZIP code, and NPI number when billing for purchased diagnostic tests. When more than one supplier is used, a separate claim form should be used to bill for each supplier. Follow the previously outlined format for entering address information.
Block 32a	Enter the NPI number of the service facility location.
Block 32b	Enter the two-digit qualifier identifying the non-NPI number followed by the ID number. Use the same qualifiers as listed in block 17a.
Block 33	Enter the provider's or supplier's billing name, address, ZIP code, and phone number. The phone number is to be entered in the area to the right of the field title. Follow the previously outlined format for entering address information.
Block 33a	Enter the NPI number of the billing provider.
Block 33b	Enter the two-digit qualifier identifying the non-NPI number followed by the ID number as listed in Block 17a.

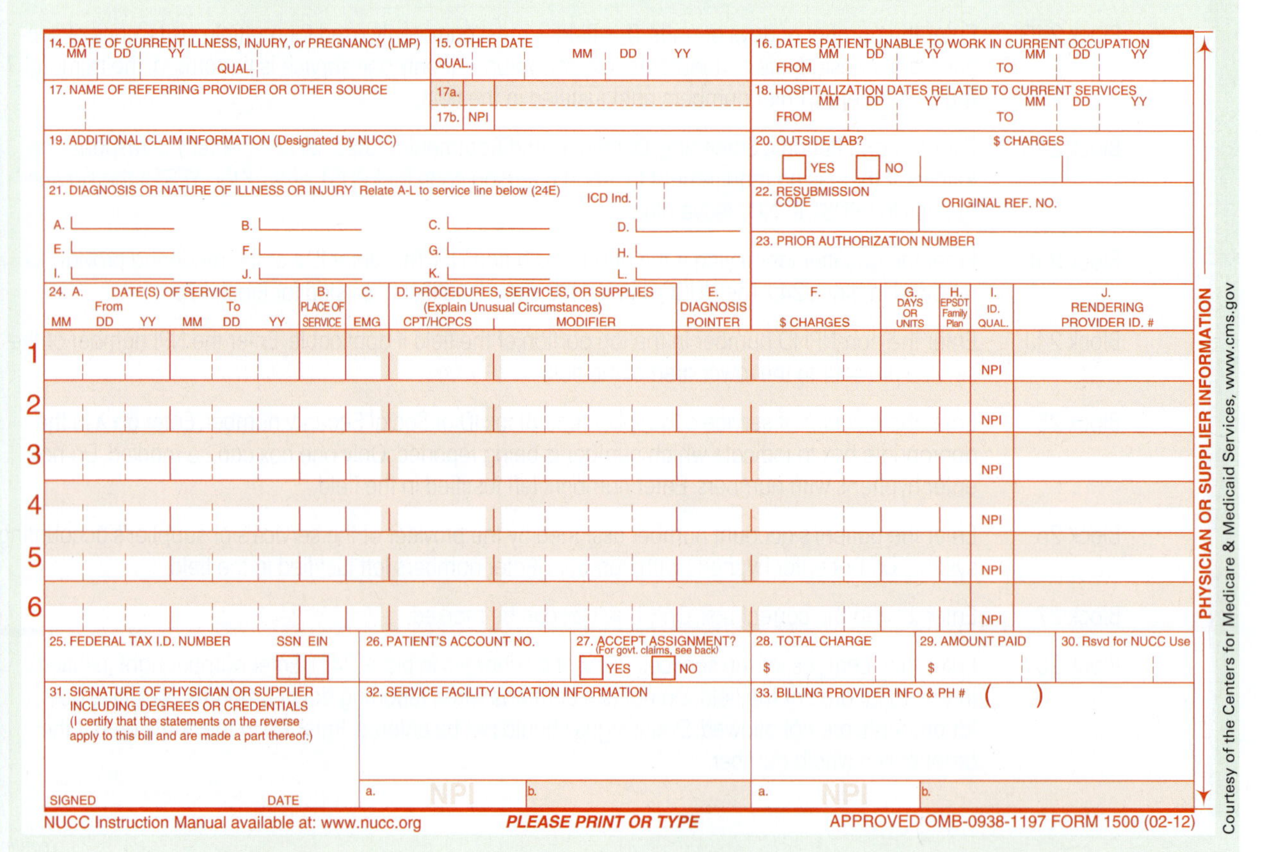

14. DATE OF CURRENT ILLNESS, INJURY, or PREGNANCY (LMP) MM DD YY QUAL.
15. OTHER DATE QUAL. MM DD YY
16. DATES PATIENT UNABLE TO WORK IN CURRENT OCCUPATION FROM MM DD YY TO MM DD YY
17. NAME OF REFERRING PROVIDER OR OTHER SOURCE 17a. 17b. NPI
18. HOSPITALIZATION DATES RELATED TO CURRENT SERVICES FROM MM DD YY TO MM DD YY
19. ADDITIONAL CLAIM INFORMATION (Designated by NUCC)
20. OUTSIDE LAB? YES NO $ CHARGES
21. DIAGNOSIS OR NATURE OF ILLNESS OR INJURY Relate A-L to service line below (24E) ICD Ind.
A. B. C. D.
E. F. G. H.
I. J. K. L.
22. RESUBMISSION CODE ORIGINAL REF. NO.
23. PRIOR AUTHORIZATION NUMBER

24. A. DATE(S) OF SERVICE From MM DD YY To MM DD YY	B. PLACE OF SERVICE	C. EMG	D. PROCEDURES, SERVICES, OR SUPPLIES (Explain Unusual Circumstances) CPT/HCPCS MODIFIER	E. DIAGNOSIS POINTER	F. $ CHARGES	G. DAYS OR UNITS	H. EPSDT Family Plan	I. ID. QUAL.	J. RENDERING PROVIDER ID. #
1								NPI	
2								NPI	
3								NPI	
4								NPI	
5								NPI	
6								NPI	

25. FEDERAL TAX I.D. NUMBER SSN EIN
26. PATIENT'S ACCOUNT NO.
27. ACCEPT ASSIGNMENT? (For govt. claims, see back) YES NO
28. TOTAL CHARGE $
29. AMOUNT PAID $
30. Rsvd for NUCC Use
31. SIGNATURE OF PHYSICIAN OR SUPPLIER INCLUDING DEGREES OR CREDENTIALS (I certify that the statements on the reverse apply to this bill and are made a part thereof.) SIGNED DATE
32. SERVICE FACILITY LOCATION INFORMATION a. NPI b.
33. BILLING PROVIDER INFO & PH # ( ) a. NPI b.

PHYSICIAN OR SUPPLIER INFORMATION

NUCC Instruction Manual available at: www.nucc.org PLEASE PRINT OR TYPE APPROVED OMB-0938-1197 FORM 1500 (02-12)

Courtesy of the Centers for Medicare & Medicaid Services, www.cms.gov

Uniform Bill 04 Form

The NUCC has also updated the CMS-1450 claim form, also known as **Uniform Bill 04 (UB-04)**, to accommodate reporting the National Provider Identifier (NPI) number. The NPI, a requirement of HIPAA legislation, must be used by all HIPAA-covered entities. Figure 17-4 shows a sample of the UB-04 form.

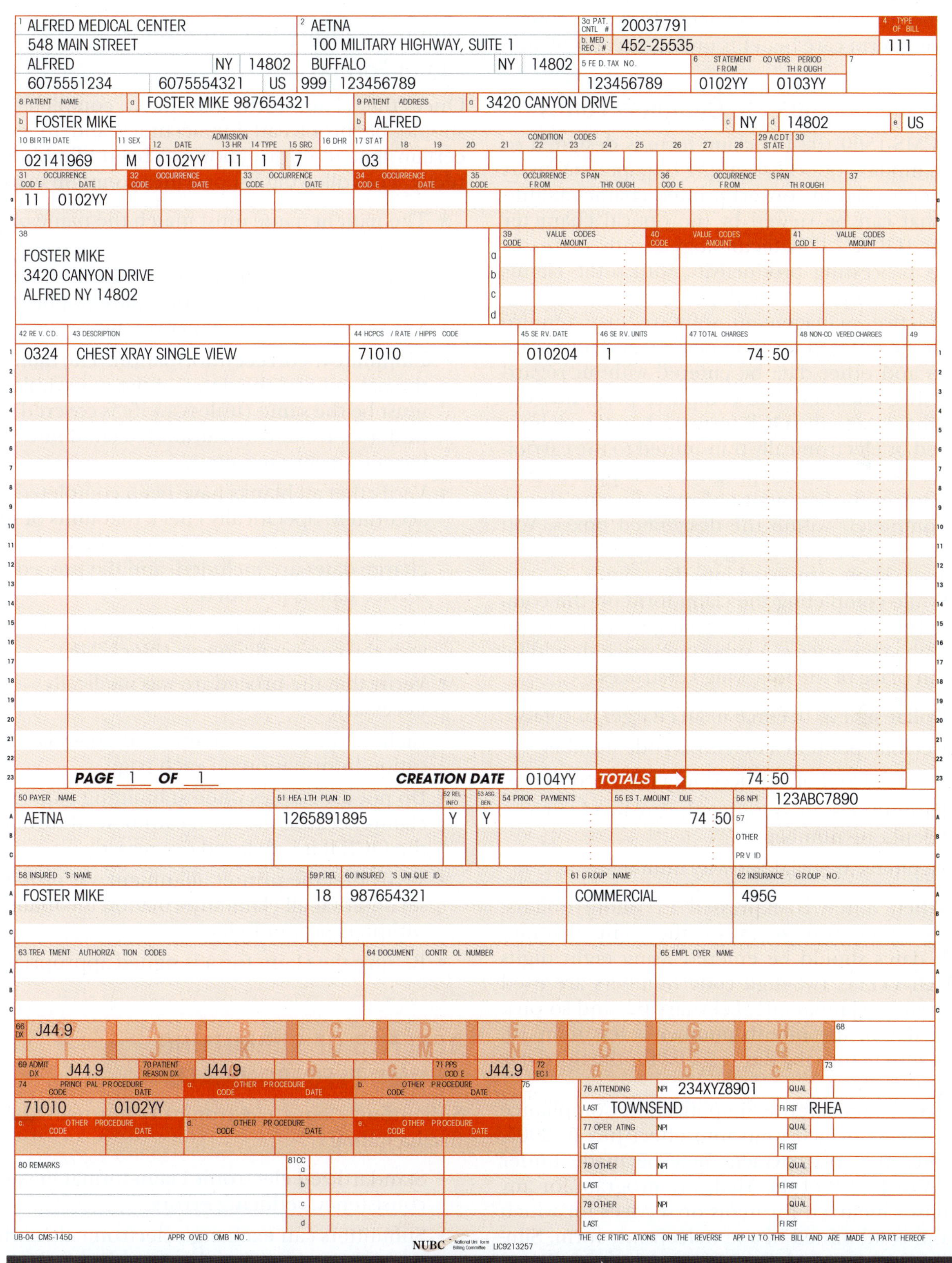

1 ALFRED MEDICAL CENTER
548 MAIN STREET
ALFRED NY 14802
6075551234 6075554321 US

2 AETNA
100 MILITARY HIGHWAY, SUITE 1
BUFFALO NY 14802
999 123456789

3a PAT. CNTL # 20037791
b. MED. REC. # 452-25535
4 TYPE OF BILL 111
5 FED. TAX NO. 123456789
6 STATEMENT COVERS PERIOD FROM 0102YY THROUGH 0103YY
7

8 PATIENT NAME a FOSTER MIKE 987654321
b FOSTER MIKE
9 PATIENT ADDRESS a 3420 CANYON DRIVE
b ALFRED c NY d 14802 e US

10 BIRTH DATE 02141969
11 SEX M
ADMISSION 12 DATE 0102YY 13 HR 11 14 TYPE 1 15 SRC 7
16 DHR
17 STAT 03
CONDITION CODES 18 19 20 21 22 23 24 25 26 27 28
29 ACDT STATE
30

31 OCCURRENCE CODE 11 DATE 0102YY
32 OCCURRENCE CODE DATE
33 OCCURRENCE CODE DATE
34 OCCURRENCE CODE DATE
35 OCCURRENCE SPAN CODE FROM THROUGH
36 OCCURRENCE SPAN CODE FROM THROUGH
37

38
FOSTER MIKE
3420 CANYON DRIVE
ALFRED NY 14802

39 VALUE CODES CODE AMOUNT
40 VALUE CODES CODE AMOUNT
41 VALUE CODES CODE AMOUNT

42 REV. CD.	43 DESCRIPTION	44 HCPCS / RATE / HIPPS CODE	45 SERV. DATE	46 SERV. UNITS	47 TOTAL CHARGES	48 NON-COVERED CHARGES	49
0324	CHEST XRAY SINGLE VIEW	71010	010204	1	74 50		
	PAGE 1 OF 1	CREATION DATE	0104YY	TOTALS	74 50		

50 PAYER NAME	51 HEALTH PLAN ID	52 REL. INFO	53 ASG. BEN.	54 PRIOR PAYMENTS	55 EST. AMOUNT DUE
AETNA	1265891895	Y	Y		74 50

56 NPI 123ABC7890
57 OTHER PRV ID

58 INSURED'S NAME	59 P. REL	60 INSURED'S UNIQUE ID	61 GROUP NAME	62 INSURANCE GROUP NO.
FOSTER MIKE	18	987654321	COMMERCIAL	495G

63 TREATMENT AUTHORIZATION CODES
64 DOCUMENT CONTROL NUMBER
65 EMPLOYER NAME

66 DX J44.9
67 A B C D E F G H I J K L M N O P Q
68

69 ADMIT DX J44.9
70 PATIENT REASON DX J44.9
71 PPS CODE J44.9
72 ECI
73

74 PRINCIPAL PROCEDURE CODE 71010 DATE 0102YY
a. OTHER PROCEDURE CODE DATE
b. OTHER PROCEDURE CODE DATE
c. OTHER PROCEDURE CODE DATE
d. OTHER PROCEDURE CODE DATE
e. OTHER PROCEDURE CODE DATE
75

76 ATTENDING NPI 234XYZ8901 QUAL
LAST TOWNSEND FIRST RHEA
77 OPERATING NPI QUAL
LAST FIRST
78 OTHER NPI QUAL
LAST FIRST
79 OTHER NPI QUAL
LAST FIRST

80 REMARKS
81CC a b c d

UB-04 CMS-1450 APPROVED OMB NO.
NUBC National Uniform Billing Committee LIC9213257
THE CERTIFICATIONS ON THE REVERSE APPLY TO THIS BILL AND ARE MADE A PART HEREOF.

FIGURE 17-4 UB-04 claim containing sample patient data (with highlighted form locators that contain ICD and CPT codes).

The UB-04 form is the standard form used for inpatient admissions, outpatient and emergency department services and procedures, psychiatric facilities, drug and alcohol facilities, clinical and laboratory services, walk-in centers, nursing facilities, home health care agencies, hospice centers, and long-term care benefits under a health plan.

Using the Computer to Complete Forms

The CMS-1500 (02-12) claim form is designed to accommodate optical scanning of paper claims. A scanner is used to convert printed characters into text that can be viewed by the optical character reader (OCR). This technology greatly increases claims processing productivity, with some claims being paid within 7 to 10 days.

Practice management software may require data to be entered using uppercase and lowercase letters and other data be entered without regard to OCR guidelines. The computer program converts the data to the OCR format when the claim is printed or electronically transmitted to the carrier. Always use the software program's test pattern program to verify alignment of forms. Be sure the *X*s are completely within the designated boxes. You may need to check this alignment each time a new batch of claims is inserted into the printer.

While completing the claim form on the computer, remember not to interchange a zero (*0*) with the alpha character *o*. A substitute space should be used in place of the following keystrokes:

- Dollar sign or decimal in all charges or totals
- Decimal point in a diagnosis code number
- Dash in front of a procedure code modifier
- Parentheses surrounding the area code in a telephone number
- Hyphens in Social Security numbers

When a fee is expressed in whole dollars, always enter two zeros in the cent column. Birth dates should be entered using eight digits (MMDDYYYY). Two-digit code numbers are used for months (January 01, February 02, and so on). If the day of the month number is less than 10, add a zero before the day (e.g., 03 for the third day of the month).

The Administrative Simplification Compliance Act (ASCA), which went into effect July 5, 2005, specifies that no payment may be made under Part A or Part B of the Medicare program for any expenses incurred for items or services for which a claim is submitted in a nonelectronic form. Simply stated, paper claims submitted to Medicare will not be paid. Some exceptions to this rule can be found in the *Medlearn Matters* article MM3440 available at the CMS website (http://www.cms.gov by searching for "Medlearn Matters").

Common Errors in Completing Claim Forms

Once the claim form has been completed, it should be proofread for accuracy and to make certain that all information has been filled in correctly. The following list provides common errors:

- The patient name must match the name on the insurance card.
- Eliminate typographic errors. Check all numbers carefully to be sure they have not been transposed or entered incorrectly.
- Eliminate incorrect information. The name of the patient and the name of the policyholder must be the same (unless a wife is covered under a husband's insurance, a child under a parent's insurance, etc.).
- Verify that all blanks have been completed accurately. Specifically check that units of service are entered, hospital admission and discharge dates are included, and the procedure service date is provided.
- Verify that each procedure links correctly with the correct diagnosis (block 24E).
- Verify that the procedure was medically necessary.
- Include the patient's name and policy identification information on each page.
- Do not use staples when submitting paper claims because the form cannot feed through the OCR if it is defaced or creased.
- Verify that the printer alignment was properly set and that all claim information is contained within its proper field.
- Be sure the claim form is signed appropriately.

BENEFITS OF SUBMITTING CLAIMS ELECTRONICALLY

Submitting claims electronically has many benefits, including:

- Standardized electronic claim format ensures consistency, reducing errors.
- Submitters can exchange electronic data with multiple payers using the same data format.

- Supplies required (e.g., paper, postage) and administrative costs are reduced.
- Cash flow can be significantly improved because Medicare pays 14 days after receipt of complete and accurate electronically submitted claims (paper claims may take a minimum of 29 days to process).

MANAGING THE CLAIMS PROCESS

Once the claim form has been completed, a series of events take place. The medical assistant or administrative staff, who may have used a referral number generated by a point-of-service device, enters the claim into the office register (or practice management software) of submitted claims; the insurance carrier processes the claim; an explanation of benefits letter is sent to the insured person and the medical provider; and, if necessary, follow-up procedures are instituted if payment is not received from the carrier within a specified time period. Each of these events is discussed in detail in the following sections.

Documentation of Referrals

Many insurance plans require that a referral be preapproved by the plan before scheduling an appointment with someone other than the primary care provider. This is particularly true for managed care plans, especially HMOs. The medical assistant working in both the primary care facility and specialist facility must make sure that when an approval is required, the necessary authorization has been obtained and the referral number is recorded in the patient's file. The referral number must be submitted as part of the claim submitted to the carrier by the specialist. This piece of information would be entered in block 23 of the CMS-1500 (02-12).

Point-of-Service Device

An electronic device available to some health care providers is a **point-of-service (POS) device**. This device provides immediate and direct access to patient eligibility information and managed care functions through an electronic network connecting the medical clinic and the health plan's computer.

The POS device is a small card-swipe box similar in design and function to a credit card terminal (Figure 17-5). It allows medical clinic personnel to:

- Record a patient visit
- Check eligibility for patients in the health plan

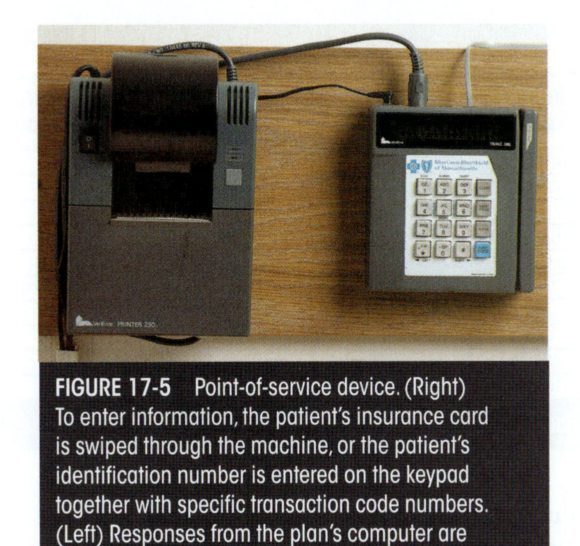

FIGURE 17-5 Point-of-service device. (Right) To enter information, the patient's insurance card is swiped through the machine, or the patient's identification number is entered on the keypad together with specific transaction code numbers. (Left) Responses from the plan's computer are printed directly in the medical office.

- Enter referrals for patients in managed care plans
- Verify referral information
- Check authorization status
- Enter inpatient authorization requests
- Enter outpatient authorization requests

After the necessary information is entered by the medical assistant, the POS device communicates with the health plan's computer system. The computer then returns an acknowledgment to the medical clinic confirming the transaction or giving an error message code. For example, when visits are recorded accurately, a reference number is generated that is used as the medical clinic's confirmation that the transaction is complete. On successful entry of a referral, a referral number is generated. Specialists may use this number on claims they submit for services they render under the referral.

Maintaining a Claims Registry or Claims Tracking System

When claim forms are sent to the appropriate insurance carrier, it is wise and necessary for the medical clinic personnel to keep a diary or register of submitted claims (Figure 17-6). This **claim register**, created with a spreadsheet or software, should include the patient's name, the insured's name if it is different from the patient's name, the dates of service for which the claim is being made, the amount of the claim, and the date the claim is submitted. When payment is received, the date of payment should be entered. When aging and

INSURANCE CLAIMS STATUS

ACTION DATE	LAST NAME	FIRST NAME	INSURANCE COMPANY	ORIGINAL BILLING DATE	TOTAL CHARGES $	AMOUNT RECEIVED	STATUS / ACTION TAKEN
1/30/2008	McKay	Leo	Nationwide	1/30/2008	$ 88.00	$ -	Submitted
2/14/2008	Lovelace	Terry	World Health	9/24/2007	$ 128.00	$ -	Add'l data submitted
4/15/2008	Taxman	William	US Health	12/15/2007	$ 640.00	$ 640.00	Paid in full
5/1/2008	Fooler	April	Surprise Health	4/1/2007	$ 375.98	$ -	Collection
5/16/2008	Zonker	James	Gotcha Covered	4/3/2008	$ 236.00	$ 136.00	Patient billed $100.00
7/5/2008	Stripes	Stanley	Bangor Insurance				

FIGURE 17-6 Sample claim register.

reconciling accounts, the bookkeeper then can check the diary to note where the claim is in the process.

Following Up on Claims

Occasionally, claims are denied because the claim form was incomplete. However, if there is no payment from the carrier and no other notification after a period of 1 to 6 weeks, it is necessary to follow up on the claim. The claim register will enable the clinic to keep track of the progress of claims (Figure 17-6).

To follow up, a toll-free number is provided by most carriers. The necessary information to have on hand before making the call includes a copy of the claim form and the patient's name and insurance identification number. The carrier should be able to give the status of the claim. If payment is delayed, the carrier should be able to give the date when it can be expected. It is possible that payment was sent to the insured person, in which case a statement should be sent to the patient. If there is a problem with the claim, the medical assistant may need to investigate the cause of the error and submit a revised claim.

See Chapter 19 for information on billing and collection procedures.

THE INSURANCE CARRIER'S ROLE

The claims processor at the insurance carrier checks the codes to confirm that the procedures and accompanying diagnoses link properly with one another. The processor then analyzes the information to confirm that:

1. The coverage was in force at the time of treatment.
2. The provider has contracted with the insurance carrier.
3. There are no exclusions or restrictions on the policy for payment of the diagnosis, service, or procedure.
4. There are no preexisting condition restrictions.
5. The diagnosis and procedures done are reasonable and meet medical necessity.

The processor also checks to make sure that the billed amount falls within the usual, customary, and reasonable fee that the insurance carrier has developed for that specific procedure CPT code.

Explanation of Benefits Letter

On completion of the processing of the claim, the insurance company sends an **explanation of benefits (EOB)** letter to the insured person. Figure 16-1 shows a sample EOB. This form includes the dates; charges; amounts applied toward the deductible; amounts not covered either because of an exclusion or excess over the usual, customary, and reasonable charge; and the amount the company is paying for this claim. Some EOB letters even serve as a "bill" or "notice" in that they indicate the amount the insured must forward to the provider for payment of the account in full.

LEGAL AND ETHICAL ISSUES

Legal

Issues of insurance fraud and abuse must be understood before accurate codes can be assigned to medical procedures, services, and diagnosis of disease. See Chapter 16 for a complete discussion regarding insurance fraud and abuse.

The Omnibus Budget Reconciliation Acts of 1986 and 1987 state that providers can be assessed civil penalties if they "know of or should know that claims filed with Medicare or Medicaid on their behalf are not true and accurate representations of the items or services actually provided." This means that providers can be held responsible not only for negligent mistakes they make but also for mistakes made on their behalf by their medical assistants or administrative staff who complete insurance claim forms. The penalties assessed are usually in the form of a monetary fine and may also involve exclusion from Medicare and Medicaid programs for a specified period of time.

Compliance Programs

Compliance programs based on guidelines issued by the Office of the U.S. Inspector General are not mandatory; however, they help prevent violations that can be financially costly and that may carry criminal penalties for the provider and clinic personnel. Participation in a compliance program demonstrates that the practice is making a good-faith effort to submit claims appropriately and is considered equivalent to practicing preventative medicine. The following are basic elements of a compliance program:

1. Have a designated compliance officer.
2. Develop and use written standards and procedures for coding.
3. Develop a plan for communicating coding standards and procedures.
4. Train personnel in standards and procedures.
5. Conduct periodic audits.
6. Respond to detected violations and notify appropriate government agencies.
7. Make personnel aware that they have an ethical duty to report suspected or observed fraudulent or erroneous coding practices so that they can be corrected. Publicize and enforce disciplinary standards on coding violations.

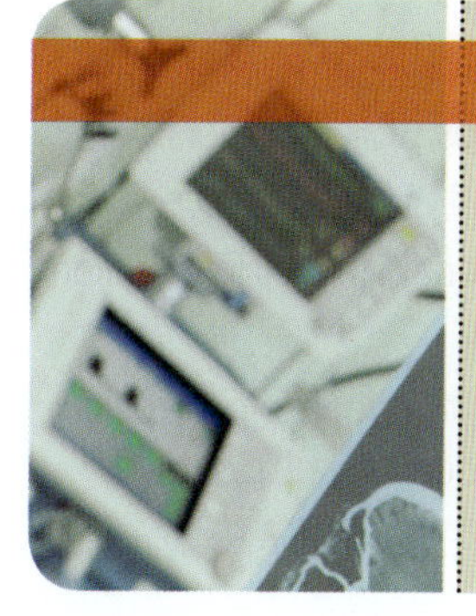

CASE STUDY 17-1

Refer to the scenario at the beginning of the chapter.

CASE STUDY REVIEW

1. Explain why coding accurately is important to health care providers and insurance companies that act as third-party payers for health care services rendered to patients.
2. List ways to ensure accurate coding.
3. Recall common errors in completing insurance claim forms.

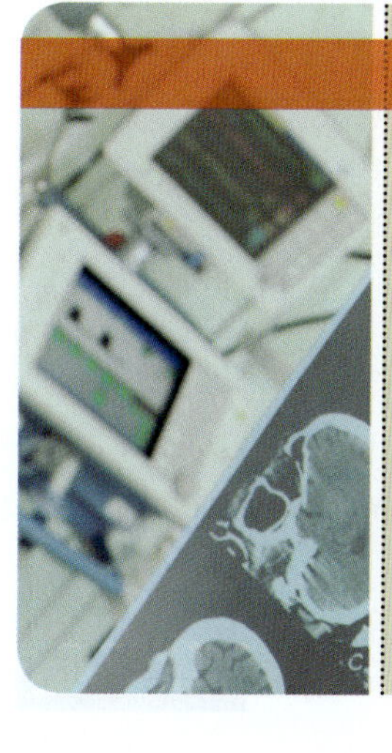

CASE STUDY 17-2

Leo McKay, an established patient at Inner City Health Care, schedules a visit, reporting nausea and severe abdominal pain. Dr. Winston Lewis spends 30 minutes taking a history and doing an examination. He suspects an ulcer and orders laboratory tests (complete blood count [CBC], guaiac, lipid panel, and urinalysis [UA]) to be done in the clinic and sends Mr. McKay for an upper GI series. Mr. McKay returns in 10 days to learn that the test results show a duodenal ulcer.

CASE STUDY REVIEW

1. What are the proper diagnosis codes for Mr. McKay?
2. What are the proper procedure codes for Mr. McKay?
3. In coding the claim form for Mr. McKay's visit, what ethical principle and legal principle should guide the medical assistant?

Summary

- Coding is the application of alphanumeric characters selected from standard terms used to describe a condition, disease, or service in health care.
- Coding is done in order to process demographic, insurance, and coded medical diagnoses and procedures in order to request reimbursement for services and supplies used in health care.
- The coding systems used within the United States include Current Procedural Terminology (CPT); Healthcare Common Procedure Coding System (HCPCS); International Classification of Diseases, 10th Revision, Clinical Modification (ICD-10-CM); and ICD-10-PCS.
- When performing billing procedures, medical assistants and medical administrative staff are expected to adhere to ethical standards and legal practices.
- Imprecise coding affects how quickly the provider is reimbursed and the correct amount of the reimbursement. Common types of coding errors and abuse include down-coding, up-coding, assumptive coding, and unbundling.
- The National Correct Coding Initiative (NCCI) promotes national correct coding methodologies.
- The claim form is completed by the medical assistant, administrative office staff, or billing clerk in the ambulatory care setting.
- Coding the claim form is a precise way to communicate with the insurance carrier. Coding indicates the complexity of the visit, the diagnosis for the visit, and the specific procedures performed.
- The CMS-1500 (02-12) is the claim form accepted by all insurance carriers.
- Security and confidentiality measures must be in place in medical clinics to protect patient information.
- Authorization to release necessary medical information to payers, such as insurance carriers, must be obtained from the patient, the parent, or the guardian before any information is released.
- The UB-04 form is the standard form used for inpatient admissions, outpatient and emergency department services and procedures, psychiatric facilities, drug and alcohol facilities, clinical and laboratory services, walk-in centers, nursing facilities, home health care agencies, hospice centers, and long-term care benefits under a health plan.
- Once the claim form has been completed, it should be proofread for accuracy and to make certain that all information has been filled in correctly.
- Once the claim form has been completed, the medical assistant or administrative staff enters the claim into the office register (or practice management software) of submitted claims and the insurance carrier processes the claim.
- The claims processor at the insurance carrier checks the codes to confirm that the procedures and accompanying diagnoses link properly with one another.
- Providers can be held responsible not only for negligent mistakes they make but also for mistakes made on their behalf by their medical assistants or administrative staff who complete insurance claim forms.

Study for Success

To reinforce your knowledge and skills of information presented in this chapter:

- Review the *Key Terms* and *Learning Outcomes*
- Consider the *Critical Thinking* features and *Case Studies* and discuss your conclusions
- Answer the questions in the *Certification Review*

Procedure

- Perform the *Procedures* using the *Competency Assessment Checklists* on the *Student Companion Website*

CERTIFICATION REVIEW

1. What is a description of CPT Codes?
   a. They are for diagnosis coding.
   b. They have five digits and may have two-digit modifiers.
   c. They have three-digit codes with a decimal point and one to two additional digits.
   d. They are updated semiannually.
2. What is the first reference that should be used when coding a diagnosis?
   a. CPT
   b. ICD-10-CM alphabetical index
   c. Z codes in ICD-10-CM
   d. V codes in ICD-10-CM
   e. HCPCS
3. What is an accurate description of Level II of HCPCS?
   a. It provides codes to enable the provider to report nonprovider services.
   b. It is the same as the regular CPT system.
   c. It is assigned by the fiscal intermediary.
   d. It uses the letter codes *W*, *X*, *Y* and *Z*.
4. What statement is true about ICD-10-CM codes?
   a. They were developed by the AMA as uniform descriptions of medical, surgical, and diagnostic services.
   b. They are divided into seven sections.
   c. They use modifiers.
   d. They code every disease, illness, condition, injury, and cause of injury known.
   e. They include codes for new and established patients.
5. Most insurance carriers accept which claim form?
   a. UB-04
   b. CMS-1500 (02-12)
   c. CPT
   d. HCFA-1450
6. What is the purpose of maintaining a claim tracking system?
   a. To anticipate claims to be sent to insurance companies for processing
   b. To check how many claims are sent to Medicare
   c. To monitor claims that have been sent to insurance companies for processing
   d. To help in aging accounts
   e. To record the amount of co-payments
7. What information is *NOT* included in the CARRIER section of the CMS-1500 (02-12) insurance claim form?
   a. The payer's name
   b. The patient's name
   c. The payer's address
   d. The payer's city, state, and ZIP code
8. What information is included in the PATIENT AND INSURED section of the CMS-1500 (02-12) insurance claim form?
   a. Health insurance plan
   b. Patient's name and address
   c. Insured's name and address
   d. NPI number of the billing provider
   e. Address and telephone number of the billing provider
9. Which of the following codes is an example of a CPT code?
   a. Irregular menstrual cycle, A99901
   b. Biopsy, soft tissue of neck, A98.5
   c. Dissection of the renal artery, A00.00
   d. Adenitis, lymph gland, except mesenteric, 99205
10. What unique billing form is used extensively by acute care facilities for processing inpatient and outpatient claims?
    a. UB-04
    b. CMS-1500 (02-12)
    c. CPT
    d. HCFA-1450
    e. Superbill

CHAPTER 18

Daily Financial Practices

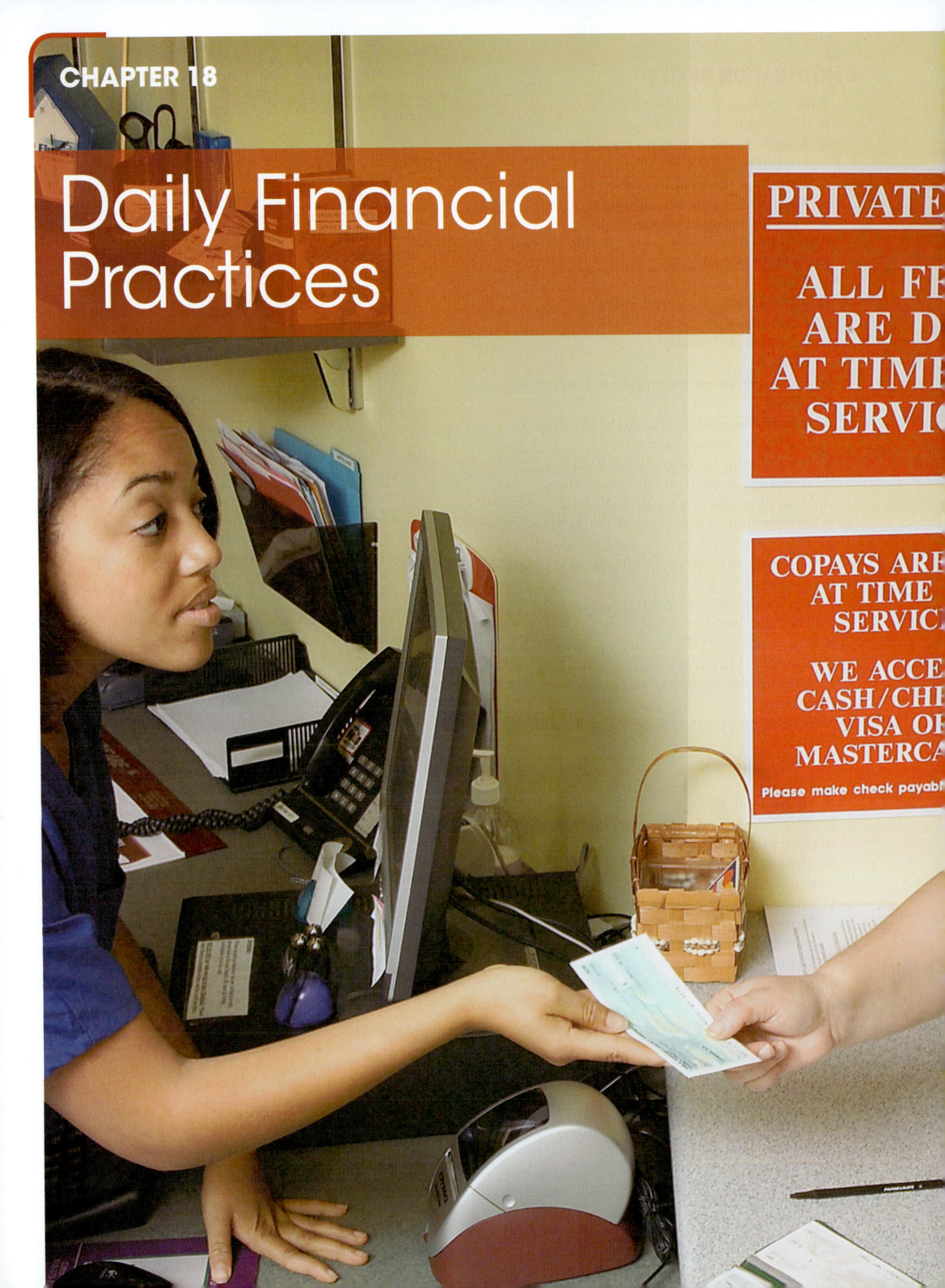

LEARNING OUTCOMES

1. Define and spell the key terms as presented in the glossary.
2. Practice effective communication in regard to establishing patient fees.
3. Identify circumstances that require adjustment of fees and post accordingly.
4. Develop knowledge of various credit arrangements for patient fees.
5. Differentiate between bookkeeping and accounting.
6. Compare manual and computerized bookkeeping systems in ambulatory health care.
7. Describe the pegboard system.
8. State the advantages of computerized systems for financial practices.
9. List six good working habits for financial records.
10. Describe the encounter form.
11. Identify the parts of the patient account or ledger.
12. Discuss preparation of patient receipts.
13. Describe month-end activities.
14. Describe banking procedures, including types of accounts and services.
15. Show proficiency in preparing deposits and checks and reconciling accounts.
16. Explain the process of purchasing equipment and supplies for the ambulatory care setting.
17. Demonstrate proficiency in establishing and maintaining a petty cash system.

KEY TERMS

accounts payable	encounter form
accounts receivable	guarantor
adjustments	ledger
balance	money market savings account
cashier's check	notary
certified check	payee
credit	pegboard system
day sheet	petty cash
debit	posting
electronic check	remote deposit capture
electronic check conversion	voucher check

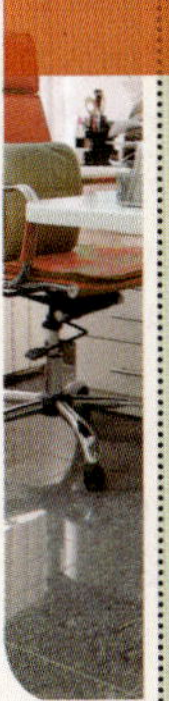

SCENARIO

At Inner City Health Care, many different types of patients are seen. Most have some kind of insurance, either a private or employer plan or an HMO plan; some are on Medicare; a few are on Medicaid; and occasionally a patient does not have any insurance or any financial resources to pay for treatment. Whoever schedules the first patient appointment also opens a courteous discussion with the patient about provider fees and the patient's anticipated method of payment. Initiating this discussion of fees at the beginning of the provider–patient relationship keeps patients informed of their responsibility for payment and helps the medical assistants at Inner City Health Care make any necessary credit arrangements with the patient before treatment begins.

Chapter Portal

Clinic settings are primarily designed to serve the patient. However, without sound financial practices, patient care will suffer and the practice will not thrive and grow. The health care industry is complex and complicated. The impact of managed care and the many detailed insurance plans affect not only the way patients receive treatment, but the manner in which the ambulatory care center is administered from a financial point of view.

The discussion of fees is only a small part of the clinic setting's daily financial practices. Selecting an appropriate system for tracking patient accounts, overseeing banking procedures, managing the purchase of supplies, controlling patient accounts, and establishing a petty cash system all are important to the smooth functioning of the modern clinic.

PATIENT FEES

All providers receive education, training, and experience in diagnosing and treating the health issues of their patients. That is their major concern; therefore, the management of the business details usually becomes the responsibility of the medical assisting staff. This includes but is not limited to informing the patients about charges, collecting payments, making credit arrangements if necessary, and making certain that patients and their providers receive the full benefit of medical insurance. An attitude that anticipates that the majority of patients pay their medical bills in a timely and responsible manner is helpful in completing these tasks.

Helping Patients Who Cannot Pay

Communication

Integrity

There are times when patients may have difficulty paying their bills. The economy is constantly changing, and with its fluctuations, individuals lose their jobs and often their medical insurance. The majority of today's employment force does not recall a time without medical insurance when patients expected to pay the total fee for medical services. These same patients may not fully comprehend what medical services cost. They likely do not understand the explanation of benefits (EOB) from their insurance reports. There is also a growing number of "working poor" in society, who may work two or more part-time jobs but never qualify for company insurance benefits and struggle daily to pay necessary bills. Some patients must decide whether to put food on the table or pay the provider. Emergencies can deplete an individual's financial resources as well. These are the times when the administrative medical assistant might make financial arrangements with patients allowing full payment for the services provided. Patients will appreciate the assistance, and the administrative medical assistant can expect the patient to abide by the agreed plan. Such an agreement fosters a climate where patients are less likely to withdraw from any necessary medical treatment when their finances are low.

Determining Patient Fees

Providers place a value on their services. In today's managed care environment, the clinic has many different arrangements with patients, insurance carriers, and health maintenance organization (HMO) insurance contracts. Managed care contracts pay predetermined fees for specific procedures and services. Providers who practice in a concierge-type medical group collect an additional fee. This usually is a flat fee at the beginning of each year for the specialized service; many do not accept the insurance carrier's required co-payment. Patients who choose concierge medical services are willing to pay the additional fee and generally have the resources to do so. Provider fees for procedures, however, are billed and reimbursed according to standard insurance guidelines.

Discussion of Fees

The manner in which billing is done and fees are established varies depending on the type of medical facility, the needs of the practice, and the professional services rendered. Today, the fee for the visit is simply stated, and if a person does not have cash or a check, the option of credit or debit card payment is often provided. If a patient is a member of an HMO, the patient is expected to pay any established co-payment amount at the time of service.

Inherent to the total billing process is the necessity of informing patients of charges and exactly what portion of the bill they are expected to pay. Ideally, the patient should be told the approximate cost of the procedures at the start of treatment. For Medicare and Medicaid patients, a form officially known by Medicare as an Advanced Beneficiary Notification (ABN) or by Medicaid as a waiver is the only legal means a clinic has to collect payment on charges not allowed by Medicare or Medicaid (Figure 18-1). These forms are to be in writing, and should indicate the type of procedure(s), the total responsibility of the patient, and the reason why this payment is the patient's responsibility.

Charges for some routine visits may be submitted to an insurance carrier, and the clinic may not always know what portions are covered until information is received from the carrier. The facility may contract with numerous insurance plans, including private carriers, and participation in these plans determines the amount the patient owes. Many misunderstandings can be prevented and subsequent collection of delinquent accounts expedited when the clinic staff is well informed about insurance reimbursement and carefully explains fees to the patients.

Adjustment of Fees

Providers who accept assignment with Medicare and Medicaid are mandated to charge every patient the same amount for similar services rendered. If a professional courtesy is extended, then it is considered insurance fraud, because the clinic would be billing insurance an increased rate over what others are charged. Deductibles are to be collected from patients as part of their premium expectation. Unless you follow government guidelines for establishing when patients are financially unable to pay their portion of the bill, you cannot give discounts to patients for cash payments.

Adjustments may be made for patients with limited income. For example, for patients who recently lost a job or ran into unfortunate financial circumstances, the provider may write off a portion of the bill. This sum will be written off against the provider's income, and the patients do not pay that portion.

Adjustments also may occur with Medicare, Medicaid, Blue Cross/Blue Shield, and private health insurance patients. Providers who accept assignment in these programs agree to accept as payment in full what the insurer allows. For instance, a fee of $150 may be charged, but $95 is accepted as payment in full by the provider after deductibles and co-payments are satisfied. The remainder of the bill, $55, is written off so that the patient is not responsible for the nonallowed amount.

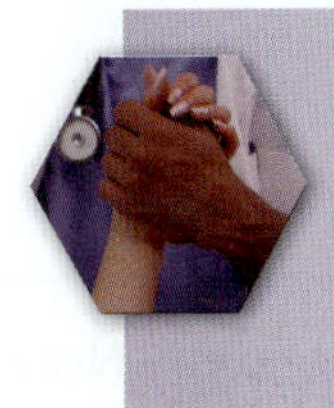

Patient Education

One way to easily provide information to patients regarding fees is to include in the clinic brochure policies regarding fees, insurance, co-payments, and how third-party payments are handled. If credit and debit cards are allowed, include that information as well.

Medical assistants must be aware, however, of the pitfalls of adjusting or reducing fees. It is difficult to accept all hardship cases and still remain a viable practice. It is always a helpful resource to patients who cannot pay to be given the names and telephone numbers of local health care clinics that may be able to accept them as patients on a sliding scale or no-fee basis.

Refunds. On rare occasion, a refund will be necessary. It usually occurs when the insurance carrier pays more than anticipated, double pays for the same charges, or the patient paid and the insurance covered the charges. Notably, there are a few members of the older adult population who may still be a little uncomfortable with Medicare and are accustomed to paying for all their medical expenses out of pocket; therefore, they will pay their entire bill when the statement is received. When Medicare payments arrive, an overpayment is created. The financial transaction required is to prepare a check for the amount due to the patient and enter the transaction on the **day sheet** and patient account or ledger.

CREDIT ARRANGEMENTS

If the patient will need to pay a substantial out-of-pocket amount, it is beneficial to make the patient aware of this and discuss different credit arrangements that can be made. Many clinics will accept prearranged installment payments, usually without finance charges, to spread the cost of services over a preagreed period. This eases the financial burden on the patient and also makes it more likely that the balance due will be collected.

A. Notifier:

B. Patient Name: **C. Identification Number:**

Advance Beneficiary Notice of Noncoverage (ABN)

NOTE: If Medicare doesn't pay for **D.** ___________ below, you may have to pay.
Medicare does not pay for everything, even some care that you or your health care provider have good reason to think you need. We expect Medicare may not pay for the **D.** ___________ below.

D.	E. Reason Medicare May Not Pay:	F. Estimated Cost

WHAT YOU NEED TO DO NOW:

- Read this notice, so you can make an informed decision about your care.
- Ask us any questions that you may have after you finish reading.
- Choose an option below about whether to receive the **D.** ___________ listed above.

Note: If you choose Option 1 or 2, we may help you to use any other insurance that you might have, but Medicare cannot require us to do this.

G. OPTIONS: Check only one box. We cannot choose a box for you.

☐ **OPTION 1.** I want the **D.** ___________ listed above. You may ask to be paid now, but I also want Medicare billed for an official decision on payment, which is sent to me on a Medicare Summary Notice (MSN). I understand that if Medicare doesn't pay, I am responsible for payment, but **I can appeal to Medicare** by following the directions on the MSN. If Medicare does pay, you will refund any payments I made to you, less co-pays or deductibles.

☐ **OPTION 2.** I want the **D.** ___________ listed above, but do not bill Medicare. You may ask to be paid now as I am responsible for payment. **I cannot appeal if Medicare is not billed**.

☐ **OPTION 3.** I don't want the **D.** ___________ listed above. I understand with this choice I am **not** responsible for payment, and **I cannot appeal to see if Medicare would pay**.

H. Additional Information:

This notice gives our opinion, not an official Medicare decision. If you have other questions on this notice or Medicare billing, call **1-800-MEDICARE** (1-800-633-4227/**TTY:** 1-877-486-2048). Signing below means that you have received and understand this notice. You also receive a copy.

I. Signature:	J. Date:

According to the Paperwork Reduction Act of 1995, no persons are required to respond to a collection of information unless it displays a valid OMB control number. The valid OMB control number for this information collection is 0938-0566. The time required to complete this information collection is estimated to average 7 minutes per response, including the time to review instructions, search existing data resources, gather the data needed, and complete and review the information collection. If you have comments concerning the accuracy of the time estimate or suggestions for improving this form, please write to: CMS, 7500 Security Boulevard, Attn: PRA Reports Clearance Officer, Baltimore, Maryland 21244-1850.

Form CMS-R-131 (03/11) Form Approved OMB No. 0938-0566

FIGURE 18-1 Advance Beneficiary Notice.

Payment Planning

Medical assistants can help patients plan for anticipated medical expenses (e.g., having a baby, surgery, extensive therapy). When patient and provider know in advance that there will be costly medical expenses, the medical assistant should review the patient's insurance coverage. It is helpful to prepare an estimate sheet, which will give the patient an idea of the cost of the medical services for the planned treatment. The estimate may also include the anticipated cost of anesthetist, consultants, and hospital charges.

Many clinics accept credit and debit cards as a means of payment. Remember, this service is strictly for the convenience of the patient, and providers cannot increase their charges for patients who wish to use these cards even though the provider is charged a fee for this service. Credit and debit cards are convenient and ensure payment; therefore, the practice may wish to encourage their use.

The one advantage to accepting credit/debit cards is that monies for fees charged usually are available within 24 hours. Also, the provider is relieved of the responsibility of collection. However, credit card companies do assess a fee for every charge made, which the clinic must pay.

Integrity

When a patient decides to use a credit or debit card, it is extremely important that confidentiality be maintained to the fullest extent possible. When writing a description of the services on the credit card receipt, the medical assistant should be as vague as possible to preserve patient confidentiality. For example, "medical services" is often used.

THE BOOKKEEPING FUNCTION

Daily financial management in the clinic is important to the functioning of the clinic, because it directly affects overall accounting and bookkeeping procedures. *Accounting* generates financial information for the ambulatory care setting and is defined as a system of monitoring the financial status of a facility and the specific results of its activities. Accounting provides financial information for decision making (see Chapter 20). *Bookkeeping*, the actual daily recording of the accounts or transactions of the business, is a major part of this accounting process. This chapter deals with daily bookkeeping (or recording) functions necessary to manage the income and expenses of an ambulatory care setting.

Managing Patient Accounts

Legal

All businesses must keep careful records of income and expenses for tax and legal purposes. One aspect of this recordkeeping in a medical practice is maintaining patient accounts. Because few patients are able to pay in full each time they are seen by the provider, it is necessary to maintain account records for each individual or family as opposed to simply keeping a record of cash received, as is done in many other types of business. The total amount of money owed to the medical facility by patients is known as **accounts receivable**; this must be carefully monitored to ensure that the provider is paid for services provided in a timely manner and that patients are properly credited for payments made.

There are various ways to track patients' balances. This chapter discusses the two most common methods:

- Computerized financial systems
- The **pegboard system** (also known as the write-it-once method)

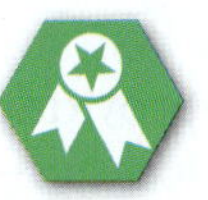
Competency

Although the financial records of most practices are fully automated, many practices probably started with some sort of manual system (generally pegboard). Converting from manual to computerized recordkeeping seems cumbersome at the beginning, but it offers great versatility and reduces the need to record and re-record entries. A knowledgeable medical assistant will understand both the manual and computerized systems. In an emergency, when the computer system is down, or if the front desk staff needs to record payments quickly and batch them for input into the software later, modified use of a write-it-once daysheet accommodates this.

Pegboard System. A complete pegboard or write-it-once system consists of day sheets, ledger cards, **encounter forms** or charge slips, and receipt forms. The forms are designed to work together to simplify the task and to avoid mistakes in patient accounts. All forms have matching columns that align and are held in place on the pegboard when the system is in use (Figure 18-2). The forms are on NCR (no carbon required) paper, which permits entering of charges, credits, or adjustments, called **posting**, onto the day sheet, encounter form, or receipt and the patient's ledger simultaneously. The day sheet provides complete and up-to-date information about accounts receivable status at a glance. Also, a pegboard system is relatively inexpensive.

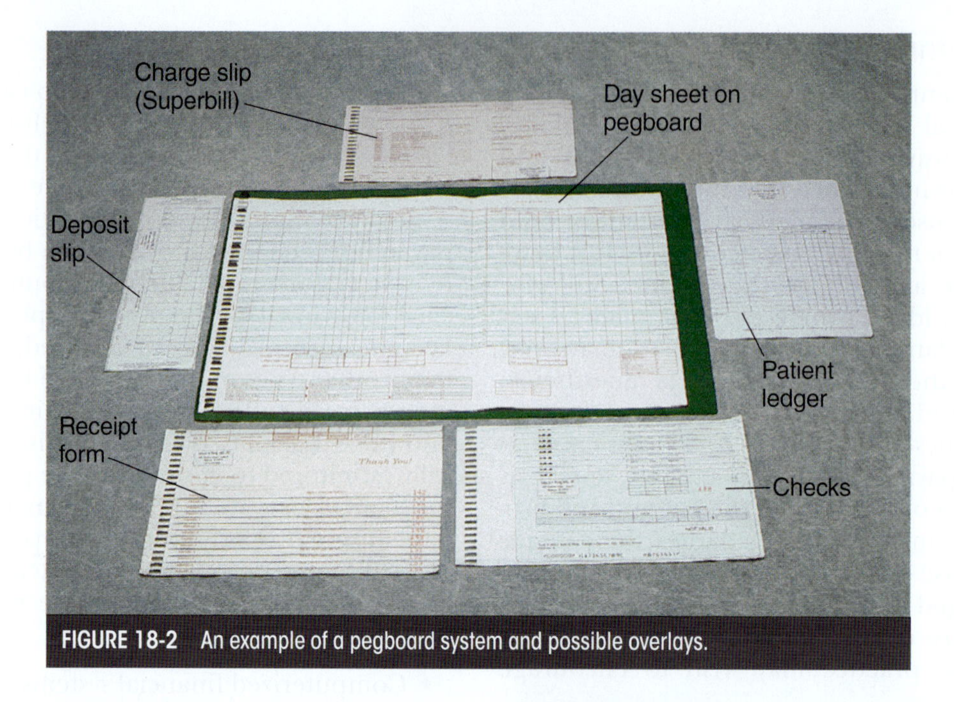

FIGURE 18-2 An example of a pegboard system and possible overlays.

Computerized Financial Systems. The majority of medical facilities use computers for bookkeeping. A number of medical practice software packages are available on the market. These ready-made systems are available for both single or multiple-provider partnerships and large group practices. Occasionally, a consultant is hired to design a customized program, although this can be more expensive than purchasing mass-produced software.

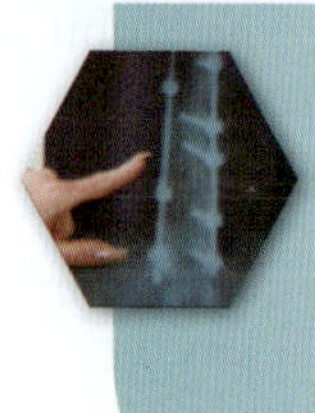

Critical Thinking

Discuss with another student the advantages and disadvantages of adopting a computer system that allows the practice to start with one component and add more components at a later time.

The Importance of Good Working Habits in Financial Transactions. In managing the day-today finances of the clinic, always observe the following guidelines:

1. Competency Always work with care and accuracy; it is extremely easy to transpose numbers (e.g., entering 23 instead of 32) or make other posting errors. A moment of carelessness can result in hours spent trying to find the mistake.
2. The work must be kept current or it may become an overwhelming chore.
3. Double-check all entries made for accuracy.

In a manual bookkeeping system, follow these additional rules:

- Use a consistent ink color; black or blue is preferred.
- Form your numbers and letters carefully, using neat and clear writing.
- Align your columns carefully, preferably using paper with grid lines.
- Write small enough to stay within the columns.
- Be careful when placing or carrying decimal points.
- Double-check all math.
- If a mistake is found, draw one line through the error and write "Corr." or "Correction" above it. Red ink may be used in correcting errors on a paper copy.

RECORDING PATIENT TRANSACTIONS

The administrative medical assistant is largely responsible for recording patient transactions for the practice. Bookkeeping activities must be exact. Either they are right or they are wrong, and in any form of business, they have to be right to be correct and to be "in balance." In the pegboard or manual system, if an error is made during entry, it will carry through to all the other documents, thus compounding the error. In a computerized system, there is the old but true statement, "garbage in, garbage out." All entries must be correct; there is no room for just a "slight" mistake.

In one way or another, the forms and procedures discussed in the following sections are common elements to any system of bookkeeping for a medical practice.

Encounter Form

The encounter form (see Figure 17-1), also known as the charge slip, superbill, or multipurpose billing form, is used in both manual and computerized bookkeeping systems. It often is a two-part form that has the following functions:

1. Provides patients one copy with a record of account activity for the day (usually a pink form)
2. Provides a second copy that serves as the clinic's permanent copy of account activity (usually the original, white form)

The encounter forms can be custom designed to fit the particular practice, computer system, or pegboard. Often, the encounter form is attached to the patient's chart so that the provider is able to indicate the day's activities and charges; the provider can also use this form to indicate a requested return visit. The encounter form will typically include procedure and diagnosis codes. The most applicable procedure codes can be preselected and printed on the encounter form to fit the practice, with blank lines added for infrequently used procedures. Often, providers use the form to check the appropriate procedures and diagnoses while they are still with the patient in the examination room.

Encounter forms are designed to fit over the pegs of a pegboard system when a manual system is used. In a computerized system, an encounter form carrying the same information is prepared for the patient, printed, and attached to the patient chart. Some computer systems automatically match the correct charge to the procedure code identified. When a facility is totally automated (including medical records), the provider identifies patient procedures in the medical record on the computer. The computer software assigns appropriate codes and charges to create the encounter form, which can be printed for the patient at the completion of the service.

Patient Account or Ledger

The financial record of the patient is known as that patient's account. All the patient accounts with outstanding balances make up the accounts receivable. Patient accounts are recorded in an accounts receivable **ledger**. (Figure 18-3 illustrates a typewritten ledger.) The ledger, or record of services, lists payments and balances due. In family practice, each adult has his or her own ledger or account that carries insurance information, name of subscriber, and patient's relationship to the subscriber. A responsible party is identified for each minor or patient who does not have insurance, and that name also appears on the ledger. Charges for any members of the family seen in the clinic are entered on their own ledger. It is important that charges and credits be applied to the correct family member for insurance purposes and accurate bookkeeping practices.

In cases of divorced parents and blended families, the parent with physical custody of the child is considered to be the **guarantor** and the one responsible for payment if the child is not insured with a contracted insurance carrier or if there is any amount left over once the insurance has paid. This prevents the staff from having to interpret divorce decrees and parenting plan documents. This information should be clearly identified and discussed with the parent when appointments are made.

In the manual system of bookkeeping, ledger cards are used. They have a minimum of three columns for entering figures:

1. **Debit** column is on the left and is used for entering charges and a brief description of services, including a procedure code.
2. **Credit** column is to the right of the debit column and is used for entering payments.
3. **Balance** column is at the far right and is used to record the difference between the debit and credit columns and shows any amount due.

Most ledger cards have space for another column called **adjustments**, which are used to indicate any insurance payments, personal discounts or write-offs, or any other subtractions for the account that need to be recorded.

The adjustment column is a credit column; therefore, entries here normally reduce the balance due. When making an adjustment intended to increase the balance, a negative entry (in parentheses) is made to show that you reverse the function when you balance. (Add instead of subtract the amount.) For example, Edith Leonard had surgery, and because of a hardship, the provider agreed to reduce the fee by half of the balance remaining after insurance has paid. At the time of surgery, a charge of $2,500 is entered on her ledger and the day sheet. Today, payment is received from her

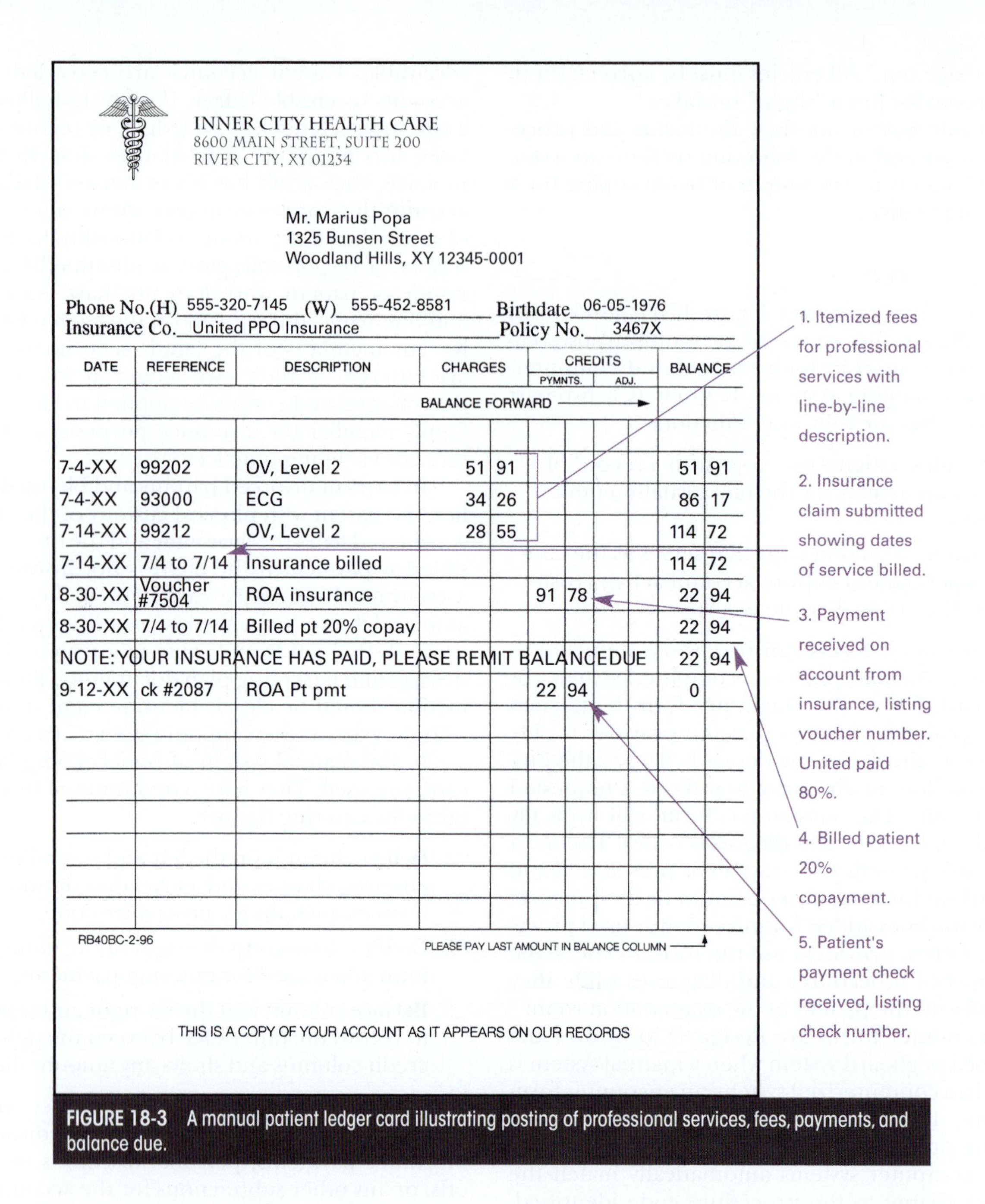

INNER CITY HEALTH CARE
8600 MAIN STREET, SUITE 200
RIVER CITY, XY 01234

Mr. Marius Popa
1325 Bunsen Street
Woodland Hills, XY 12345-0001

Phone No.(H) 555-320-7145 (W) 555-452-8581 Birthdate 06-05-1976
Insurance Co. United PPO Insurance Policy No. 3467X

DATE	REFERENCE	DESCRIPTION	CHARGES	CREDITS PYMNTS.	CREDITS ADJ.	BALANCE
		BALANCE FORWARD →				
7-4-XX	99202	OV, Level 2	51 91			51 91
7-4-XX	93000	ECG	34 26			86 17
7-14-XX	99212	OV, Level 2	28 55			114 72
7-14-XX	7/4 to 7/14	Insurance billed				114 72
8-30-XX	Voucher #7504	ROA insurance		91 78		22 94
8-30-XX	7/4 to 7/14	Billed pt 20% copay				22 94
NOTE: YOUR INSURANCE HAS PAID, PLEASE REMIT BALANCE DUE						22 94
9-12-XX	ck #2087	ROA Pt pmt		22 94		0

RB40BC-2-96

PLEASE PAY LAST AMOUNT IN BALANCE COLUMN

THIS IS A COPY OF YOUR ACCOUNT AS IT APPEARS ON OUR RECORDS

FIGURE 18-3 A manual patient ledger card illustrating posting of professional services, fees, payments, and balance due.

insurance company in the amount of $2,000, which would normally leave a balance of $500. However, because the provider agreed to write off half of that amount ($250), you enter $250 in the adjustment column when posting the insurance payment. That amount is subtracted from the previous balance to get the new total of $250.

Procedure

The ledger is placed under the charge slip or encounter form in a pegboard system and aligned before posting. Never post any patient entry in this manual system without the patient's ledger in place. This prevents recording information on the day sheet while inadvertently omitting it from the JB patient's ledger. Procedure 18-1 identifies steps in recording/posting patient charges and adjustments.

In the computerized system, a patient's account or ledger can be printed with the same information by just entering the patient's name and usually an identification number. The computerized patient account ledger provides more room for helpful detail and is much faster to create than the manual paper ledger (Figure 18-4).

PROCEDURE 18-1

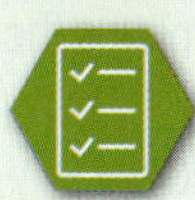
Procedure

Recording/Posting Patient Charges, Payments, and Adjustments

PURPOSE:

To record information including services rendered, fees charged, any adjustments made, and balances pertaining to a patient's clinic visit and patient's account.

EQUIPMENT/SUPPLIES:

- Calculator
- Patient's account or ledger
- Computerized PM System

PROCEDURE STEPS:

1. Check the patient's account before the patient's appointment to make certain it is current. The account will indicate any recent insurance payments, any amount received on the account, and any balance due. RATIONALE: Allows the medical assistant to focus entirely on the patient at arrival time and gives a current picture of the patient's account.
2. When the patient arrives, check for name, address, telephone numbers, and any changes regarding medical insurance. Make any changes in the PM system account for the patient, or on the ledger. RATIONALE: Ensures that information is current and up to date.
3. On the encounter form or superbill, complete any necessary items such as the date of service and the responsible party's name. RATIONALE: The encounter form allows the provider to indicate appropriate procedure and diagnosis codes.
4. When the provider completes the treatment or examination, he or she will check the procedures and diagnosis on the encounter form. RATIONALE: Provider marks the appropriate codes and signs the encounter form, indicating it is correct. The provider or licensed caregiver is the only one authorized to select the appropriate procedure codes.
5. When the patient returns to the front desk, refer to the provider's fee schedule, enter the charge next to each procedure, and calculate the total. If the procedure description is not indicated, one is to be provided. A description is necessary for each service. Check to see if the codes match the services provided. If they do not match, refer it back to the provider or licensed caregiver for correction. RATIONALE: Medical clinic staff and the patient can identify the charge to the particular service given and know that the coding and charges will match.
6. If using the manual pegboard system, post charges for today's services or procedures, any payments received, and adjustments applied, in the Charges, Payments, and Adjustment columns respectively. If using a PM system, open the module to post charges and open the patient's account. Post each service or procedure and any payments received and adjustments applied. Save the data to update the record. RATIONALE: Clearly indicates charges made and payments received, creating an updated account.
7. If any adjustment applies to the account, enter the amount in the adjustment column. If there is no adjustment column and the adjustment will *reduce* the bill, enter the amount in the payment column enclosed by parentheses. If the adjustment will *increase* the bill, place the amount in the charge column (no parentheses) with an explanation in the description column. In the *manual system,* the adjustment amount will be either added to or subtracted from the totaled figures. RATIONALE: Adjustment is shown as separate from basic charge so that the provider's fee profile is unaffected.
8. Using a manual system, determine current balance by adding credits and subtracting debits to the running balance and determine the amount in the current balance. Always use a calculator (one with a tape is recommended) to calculate and verify your mathematics. When using a PM system, the software will automatically calculate the

(continues)

balance. Verifying accuracy of the posting is integral for a properly updated balance. RATIONALE: Completes the recording of patient charges, payments, and adjustments.

9. If the posting includes a payment from the patient, place a restrictive endorsement on the check. RATIONALE: Ensures that the check can only be cashed by the authorized party.
10. In a manual pegboard system, enter the amount in the payment column. In the description column, identify as cash, check, or insurance payment. If payment is a check, enter the number of the check. When using a PM system, follow the guidelines for the payment posting module to indicate type of payment. RATIONALE: This information is necessary in making the bank deposit slip.
11. Place the cash or processed check in the appointed secure place awaiting deposit. RATIONALE: Keeps receivables together and ready for deposit.

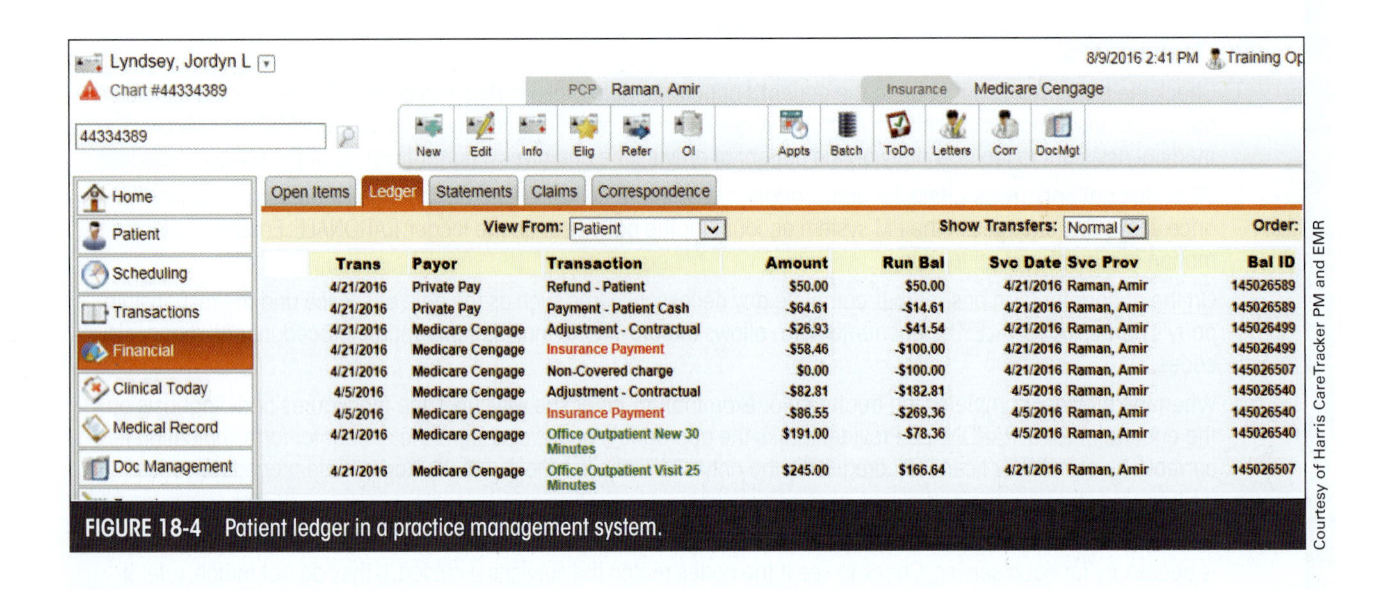

FIGURE 18-4 Patient ledger in a practice management system.

Courtesy of Harris CareTracker PM and EMR

See Table 18-1 for more information on the necessary components of a bookkeeping system including the day sheet and receipt forms. Procedure 18-2 describes the process for balancing a day sheet.

Month-End Activities

In the pegboard system, when the last day sheet for the month has been balanced, it is then necessary to verify that the month-end figures on the day sheet agree with patient accounts. Although this may be a time-consuming process in the manual system, it will find mistakes before they grow into major accounting or collection problems.

Reconciling the month-end sheet to the patient ledgers is accomplished by adding all the open balances on the ledgers and verifying that the total agrees with the end-of-month accounts receivable balance on the last day sheet of the month. When these figures agree, the accounts receivable balance is correct.

By following these procedures of "checks and balances," it is likely that all payments have been properly credited to patient accounts and deposited, and that all charges shown as outstanding on the day sheet agree with the outstanding balances of the individual patient accounts. If a payment is somehow misplaced, the deposits will not agree with the credits or with the patient ledgers, and an error will be revealed immediately. Not only does this catch errors, it also eliminates the possibility of loss of a check or undetected theft of funds, because when a mistake is caught immediately, the payer can stop payment on the missing check or credit or debit card slip and a new payment can be made.

TABLE 18-1

COMPONENTS OF THE BOOKKEEPING SYSTEM

COMPONENT	DESCRIPTION
Pegboard	A hard writing surface with a margin of "pegs" that hold documents in place while using the components of the system (superbill, ledger, receipts, etc.).
Encounter form	The encounter form, also known as the charge slip, superbill, or multipurpose billing form, is used in both manual and computerized systems. It provides the codes for the procedures performed and for which diagnoses during an encounter with the provider. The form serves as an itemized statement for insurance billing and a receipt for payments.
Ledger	The ledger, or record of services, lists payments and balances due from an individual patient, or the individuals of a family represented on a single ledger.
Day sheet	The pegboard write-it-once section is where individual transactions are posted for the day, using the ledger card and encounter form on top of the day sheet. The information in this section includes the date, patient name, description of transaction or service, charges, credits, and previous and current balances. At the bottom of the day sheet, transactions are totaled and balanced to be carried forward to the next day, or closed at the end of each month.
Receipt forms	Receipt forms used for payments on accounts usually are not customized with other than the name, address, and telephone number of the practice preprinted. The receipt form is used only when someone makes a payment on an account on a day when no services were rendered. It is not necessary to use a receipt form for payment received in the mail.

PROCEDURE 18-2

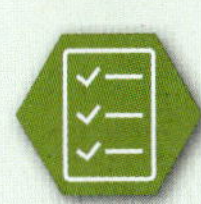

Procedure

Balancing Day Sheets in a Manual System

PURPOSE:

To verify that all entries to the day sheet are correct and that the totals balance.

EQUIPMENT/SUPPLIES:

- Day sheet
- Calculator

PROCEDURE STEPS:

1. *Column totals.* The first step in balancing a day sheet is to total columns A, B_1, B_2, C, and D, and enter the total for each column in the boxes marked Totals This Page. The column totals are then added to the figures entered in the Previous Page column boxes to arrive at the Month to Date totals, which provide the total charges, credits, and so forth entered from the first working day of the month to the present. RATIONALE: Establishes column totals.
2. *Proof of posting.* This box is used to verify that entries have been made correctly and that the column totals are accurate. *All figures entered here are taken from the "Totals This Page" column boxes.*
   a. Enter today's column D total, which shows the sum of all the previous balances entered when the transactions were posted.
   b. Added to this is the column A total of all charges for that day, to arrive at a subtotal. Enter the amount where indicated in the box.

(continues)

c. Because columns B_1 and B_2 are both credit columns that reduce balances, they are added together and entered in the box labeled Less Cols B_1 and B_2; the total of credits is subtracted from the subtotal. If all entries and addition are correct in the posting area, the result should equal the amount in column C and the transactions for that day are balanced. RATIONALE: Verifies entries have been made correctly and that the totals are accurate.

Overview: When an individual transaction is entered, the patient's previous balance (D) is added to the charges for the day (A). If there are any payments or adjustments made at that time, they are entered in the B columns and subtracted from the A + D amount to achieve the new balance (C). Because each transaction is actually D + A – B = C, the column totals of D + A – B will always equal the C total.

	D		A		B		C
	10	+	5	–	2	=	13
	2	+	7	–	1	=	8
Column Totals	12	+	12	–	3	=	21

3. *Accounts Receivable (A/R) Control.* This box simply adds the previous day's A/R balance to the current day's totals to include the current day's business and arrive at the new A/R total.
   a. The column A and column B totals are carried straight across from the Proof of Posting box to the corresponding blanks in the A/R Control box.
   b. Add the amount already entered in the Previous Day's Total space to the Column A amount to arrive at a subtotal.
   c. Subtract the amount carried over from the Less Columns B_1 and B_2 box to find the new A/R amount. RATIONALE: Determines new accounts receivable balance.
4. *A/R Proof* verifies, or proves, the A/R balance in the A/R Control box. *The figure entered on the first line of this box will not change during a calendar month* because it shows how much the A/R balance was on the first working day of the month. *All other figures entered will be taken from the Month-To-Date column boxes.*
   a. Enter the amount from column A (month-to-date) where shown.
   b. Add the column A amount to the A/R 1st of Month figure and enter the sum in the subtotal space.
   c. Enter the B_1 and B_2 month-to-date amounts and subtract from the subtotal. This amount goes in the Total A/R space.

   If all posting and addition are correct, the Total A/R amounts in the A/R Control and A/R Proof boxes will match and the day is balanced. RATIONALE: Verifies the accounts receivable balance in the accounts receivable control box.
5. *Deposit verification* involves totaling the columns in Section 2 and entering the sum of the columns in the space marked Total Deposit.

   NOTE: The Total Deposit and the Total of Payments Received in column B_1 should match. RATIONALE: Verifies deposit total.
6. *Business Analysis Summary.* If this section is used, total each column in the summary section.

   NOTE: If the Business Analysis Summary is used to break out charges by type or by provider, the sum of the columns should equal today's column A total. If it is used to credit payments to different providers, the sum of the columns will equal today's payment column.

   RATIONALE: The total deposit and the total of payments received in column B_1 should match to prove totals.
7. *After the day sheet is balanced,* there is one step remaining: the transfer of balances.
   a. Take out a new day sheet for the next day.
   b. Transfer the Month-To-Date column totals to the Previous Page columns boxes on the new sheet.
   c. Enter the Total A/R amount from the last day sheet in the Previous Day's Total space of the A/R Control box on the new day sheet.
   d. Enter the A/R 1st of Month Amount in the A/R Proof box on the new sheet. RATIONALE: Transfers balances to prepare a new day sheet for the next day's activities.

   The new day sheet is now ready for posting.

Computerized Patient Accounts

A practice management system offers many advantages in managing patient accounts. The program automatically creates an encounter form the day before the patient is seen or when the administrative medical assistant prints out the schedule. After the patient's examination, the program calculates the charges for the monthly billing statement (Figure 18-5). The management program also creates and updates the patient account, adds new names to the list of patients and to the daily log, and transfers data to produce insurance forms, statements, a list of checks received each day, and deposit slips. In addition, the program automatically ages accounts at each billing cycle and creates billing statements. As a result, when patient accounts are computerized, practice collections usually increase.

The computerized patient account contains personal information about each patient, including name, address, and telephone number; email address; the person responsible for payment; and all insurance carriers. The account also lists all previous clinic visits and the procedures, procedure codes, charges, payments, and adjustments for each visit. Most account management software can be customized to meet the special needs of the individual clinic.

As billing information is entered from the encounter forms, the computer automatically updates the account by adding a description of each procedure and procedure code and each diagnosis and diagnosis code. The computer software automatically posts the charges and calculates the balance after credits and adjustments are entered.

Procedure

Once charges and payments have been entered and the day has been closed, they are not easily removed or changed. This is an important software design because it ensures that monies are not removed from receivables credited to a previous month. This procedure would cause the practice year-end balance to be unresolved. Procedure 18-3 describes the steps for electronically processing patient credit balances and refunds.

As useful and efficient as a computerized bookkeeping system can be, it is important to recognize that an inadequate manual system will not get better once computerized. Also, it takes time to move to a computerized system, train personnel, and enter existing patient data. Manual and computer systems may need to run concurrently for a month or two.

BANKING PROCEDURES

Understanding bank accounts and services, making deposits, preparing checks, and reconciling accounts are all a part of daily financial practices. Although many banking services are similar from one bank to another, it is a good idea for the medical assistant in charge of maintaining daily accounts to investigate the banking resources of the local community. In an effort to secure new business, many banks compete for customers by offering special services that can be of use to the medical practice.

Online Banking

Use of the Internet has changed banking and the services it provides. Online banking allows individuals to check account balances, transfer funds between accounts, pay bills electronically, check credit card balances, view images of checks and deposits, and download account information 24 hours a day, 7 days a week. Considerable time and expense can be saved with online banking, but remember that any online banking should be completed only through the use of secure and unique passwords granted to only those individuals deemed necessary.

Types of Accounts

Checking and savings accounts are the two primary types of accounts used in the medical practice.

Checking Accounts. The checking account is the primary account type the medical assistant will use in the clinic. Today, there are many variations on checking accounts. In the event that the medical assistant is responsible for establishing a new account, it is worthwhile to investigate features of different checking accounts both within the same bank and at competing banks.

Some features that may differ include:

- Interest paid
- Monthly fees
- Check charges
- Automated teller machine (ATM) access and fees
- After-hours deposit capabilities
- Initial deposit and balance requirements
- Overdraft protection
- Fees for checks

Napa Valley Family Associates

ACCOUNT #	38803-42539489	STATEMENT DATE	3/15/2014
LAST PAYMENT	$14.61	STATEMENT TOTAL	$266.64

Statement - Page 1

DATE OF SERVICE	PATIENT	DESCRIPTION OF SERVICES	PROCEDURE CODE	SERVICING PROVIDER	AMOUNT	PATIENT AMT DUE
3/10/2014	Lyndsey, Jordyn L (42539489)	Office Outpatient New 30 Minutes	99203	Raman, Amir	-$86.55	**$21.64**
		Per Your Insurance Company, Your Copay Has Not Been Paid In Full. The Balance Is Your Responsibility. Thank You.				
		Transaction 03/10/2014, Adjustment - Contractual			-$82.81	
		Transaction 03/10/2014, Charges			$191.00	
3/13/2014	Lyndsey, Jordyn L (42539489)	Office Outpatient Visit 25 Minutes	99214	Raman, Amir	$245.00	**$245.00**
		See Billing Note				
		Transaction 03/13/2014, Non-Covered charge			$0.00	

MAKE CHECKS PAYABLE TO: Napa Valley Family Associates

PLEASE PAY THIS AMOUNT | **$266.64**

TO ENSURE PROPER CREDIT, PLEASE DETACH AND RETURN BOTTOM PORTION WITH YOUR PAYMENT

Napa Valley Family Associates
101 Vine Street
Napa, CA 94558

707- 555-1212 Ext:

ACCOUNT #	38803-42539489	STATEMENT DATE	3/15/2014
AMOUNT ENCLOSED $		STATEMENT TOTAL	$266.64

☐ CHECK BOX AND ENTER ADDRESS OR INSURANCE CORRECTIONS ON THE REVERSE SIDE

☐ IF PAYING BY CREDIT CARD, FILL OUT THE INFORMATION ON THE REVERSE SIDE

ADDRESSEE:
JORDYN L LYNDSEY
PO BOX 84557
FAIRFIELD, CA 94533

REMIT TO:
NAPA VALLEY FAMILY ASSOCIATES
101 VINE STREET
NAPA, CA 94558

IF ANY OF THE INFORMATION HAS BEEN CHANGED SINCE YOUR LAST STATEMENT, PLEASE INDICATE...

ABOUT YOU:

YOUR NAME (Last, First, Middle Initial)

ADDRESS

CITY | STATE | ZIP

TELEPHONE ( ) | MARITAL STATUS ☐ Single ☐ Divorced ☐ Married ☐ Widowed

EMPLOYER'S NAME | TELEPHONE ( )

EMPLOYER'S ADDRESS | CITY | STATE | ZIP

IF PAYING BY CREDIT CARD, FILL OUT BELOW

☐ AMERICAN EXPRESS ☐ MASTERCARD ☐ VISA

CARD NUMBER

CHARGE THIS AMOUNT | EXPIRATION DATE

SIGNATURE | CARDHOLDER NAME

ABOUT YOUR INSURANCE:

YOUR PRIMARY INSURANCE COMPANY'S NAME | EFFECTIVE DATE

PRIMARY INSURANCE COMPANY'S ADDRESS | PHONE

CITY | STATE | ZIP

POLICYHOLDER'S ID NUMBER | GROUP PLAN NUMBER

YOUR SECONDARY INSURANCE COMPANY'S NAME | EFFECTIVE DATE

SECONDARY INSURANCE COMPANY'S ADDRESS | PHONE

CITY | STATE | ZIP

POLICYHOLDER'S ID NUMBER | GROUP PLAN NUMBER

FIGURE 18-5 Computerized patient statement.

Courtesy of Harris CareTracker PM and EMR

PROCEDURE 18-3

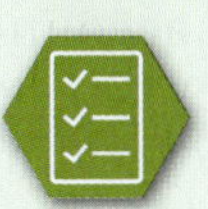

Processing Credit Balances and Refunds Using a Computerized PM System

PURPOSE:

To post overpayment refunds to patient accounts with a credit balance.

EQUIPMENT/SUPPLIES:

Computer and PM system

PROCEDURE STEPS:

To post overpayment refunds to patient accounts with a credit balance.

1. Using your chosen PM system, navigate to the payment posting module and open the patient account.
2. Click on the line item for the date and procedure for which a refund shall be posted. *Hint:* If more than one service needs to be refunded, apply it to each separately. Check balances as you post to verify these are correct.
3. In the *Description* field, enter "Refund overpayment."
4. Enter the amount to be refunded. Save to apply the refund to the balance.
5. If applicable, apply a refund to the next service in the same manner.

- Special services extended free of charge such as **notary**, cashier's checks, traveler's checks, and online banking

When selecting an account, rather than choosing the account with the lowest fees, consider convenience, the relationship possible with a given bank, bank hours, number of bank locations, and other factors.

Savings Accounts. Savings accounts initially were distinguished from checking accounts because they paid interest on the money deposited. However, many checking accounts now pay interest as well. In either case, the interest is minimal on accounts that give immediate access to the deposit. **Money market savings accounts** often pay a higher rate of interest, although they may require a higher initial deposit and maintenance of a higher balance. Access to the account may require 24-hour turnaround time. Such accounts are useful when access to money is not needed frequently or when accumulating an amount necessary to invest for long-term goals.

Types of Checks

For the most part, the clinic setting uses a standard business check. However, for special purposes, it is useful to understand the other check types available:

- A **cashier's check** is occasionally used when a check must be guaranteed for the amount in which it is written. Because a cashier's check is the bank's own check drawn against the bank's accounts, the recipient has the assurance that the check will clear. Cashier's checks are obtained at the bank by paying the bank representative cash or sometimes a personal check for the amount of the cashier's check. It is important to understand, however, that not all facilities will accept a cashier's check. Be sure to check with the office manager about accepted policy.
- A **certified check** is the depositor's own check that the bank has "certified" with a date and signature to indicate that the check is good for the amount in which it is written.
- Money orders are available from a number of places, even online. The U.S. Postal Service and Western Union are common sites for the purchase of money orders. They are purchased with cash and are similar to cashier's checks. A few patients may use money orders to pay their bills.

- A **voucher check** is a type of check with a stub attached that can be used to indicate invoice dates, services provided, and so on. Some payroll checks are written on voucher checks.
- **Electronic checks** have become widely used in clinic settings. Although performing the same purpose as a paper check, electronic checks give the added convenience of faster processing, security, and guaranteed value.

Depositing Checks

Deposits are usually made daily because they serve as another proof of posting and because leaving large sums of money in the facility overnight is unwise. A rubber endorsement stamp from the bank should be used to immediately imprint the back of all checks received directly from patients and in the mail. Be sure all checks are stamped before depositing them. Scanning or photocopying all checks before deposit is one way to ensure accuracy, although with online banking images of deposited checks are available with the account statements.

Because the endorsement transfers rights to whoever holds the check, it is important to take certain precautions. A blank endorsement consists of a signature only (whether in pen or with a stamp) and presents a danger in that, if the check is lost or stolen, someone else could endorse the check below the signature and cash it. A restrictive endorsement should be used on all checks received in the clinic. Restrictive endorsements include the signature and the words *for deposit only* or *pay to the order of*. . . (include the name of bank and account number; in addition, all possible payees' names should be listed under the company name, with the clinic address). This restricts the use of the check should it be lost or stolen.

Deposits and Technology. Online banking affords many conveniences, and there are multiple ways to make deposits using technology. By using these methods, deposit preparation can be streamlined, speeding up receivables to account, and eliminating trips to the bank. Money is becoming more digital, and with the advent of online-only banks and money transfer apps, there are new ways to handle paper checks. Instead of using bank tellers or ATMs, making a deposit can be as easy as taking a picture of the front and back of endorsed checks and uploading images to the bank account. Two common deposit methods are remote deposit capture and electronic check conversion.

- **Remote deposit capture** is a process by which consumer and business check payments are deposited using a check scanner and PC at the clinic, or capturing images of endorsed checks via a smart phone and apps.
- **Electronic check conversion** is a process by which a paper check is used as a source of information. The check number, account number, and the number that identifies the financial institution are used to make a one-time electronic payment from the account. In effect, this is an electronic fund transfer, even though the check itself is not the method of payment. As such, the check is given back to the payer (even a blank check will suffice), but the check should not be used again for a different transaction. Businesses using this method are required to disclose to the payer that the check will be used for electronic transfer of funds.

Other methods of depositing or transferring money digitally would include direct deposit, pay-by-phone, bank pay, and person-to-person payments (various financial institutions have adopted proprietary names for person-to-person electronic fund transfer).

Critical Thinking

How does a practice management system save time, human resources, and increase efficiency in a clinical setting? Give three examples.

Cash on Hand

Most medical practices need to have cash available on a daily basis. If it is the practice to collect co-payments and any coinsurance at the time of service, some patients will pay in cash and need change. Cash usually is kept in a locked change drawer that contains up to $200 in small bills at the beginning of each day. Any time a patient pays cash for the service, a receipt is prepared. Receipts are prenumbered, thus monitoring loss or theft. Cash amounts paid by patients must also be noted in their account or ledger. The term *received on account (ROA) cash* is usually indicated in the description column. If payment is made by check, follow the same procedure except the word *check* is used instead of *cash*.

At the end of each day, the cash drawer is balanced. The amount of cash received will be noted on the deposit slip as "currency." The remaining amount in the cash drawer will be the same as the beginning amount. Also, the day's cash received must match the cash control on the daily sheet. It is a good idea for only one person to handle the cash in the cash drawer; thus, it is not necessary for more than one person to balance the cash drawer at the end of the day. The cash drawer is not to be confused with petty cash, which is discussed later in this chapter. Petty cash is used to purchase small items such as postage, clinic refreshments, and so on. Checks are always written for major purchases, with the cash drawer used only to accommodate patient needs when payment is made in cash.

Most business accounts use deposit slips similar to the one shown in Figure 18-6. They are always completed in duplicate or a copy is made—one copy to accompany the deposit and one to be retained for clinic records. As shown, these deposit slips are longer than those generally used for personal accounts and have room for more entries and more information. If your manual day sheet has a built-in duplicate deposit slip, it will have been completed during posting.

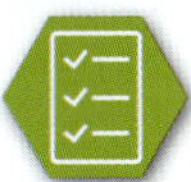

A computerized system of financial records can provide deposit slips that may be used. The same procedure is followed as previously discussed. Procedure 18-4 outlines the steps in preparing a deposit.

Accepting Checks

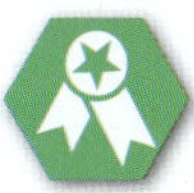

When accepting checks from patients and other individuals, take time to inspect the check. This may eliminate checks returned from the bank for various reasons:

- Inspect the check for correct date, amount, and signature.
- Do not accept a third-party check (a check written to the patient from another person or company) unless it is from the insurance carrier.

- If a deposited check is returned marked *non-sufficient funds* (*NSF*), call the bank that returned it and verify availability of funds. If funds are available, immediately redeposit the check for processing. If the check is returned a second time marked

Inner City Health Care
8600 Main Street, Suite 201
River City, NY 01234
(123) 555-0326

DEPOSIT SLIP

_______________ 20 ____

First Bank
5411 Brown Rd.
River City, NY 01234

⑆1220149321⑆

CURRENCY		
COIN		
CHECKS		
TOTAL FROM OTHER SIDE		
TOTAL		

Front

List all items separately		
Total Enter on front side		

Back

FIGURE 18-6 Sample deposit slip.

PROCEDURE 18-4

Preparing a Deposit

PURPOSE:

To create a deposit slip for the day's receipts.

EQUIPMENT/SUPPLIES:

- New deposit slip
- Check endorsement stamp
- Calculator
- Cash and checks received for the day

PROCEDURE STEPS:

1. Separate all checks from currency (paper money). RATIONALE: Each must be entered as a separate total.
2. Count all currency to be deposited and enter the amount in the space provided. Gather bills facing the same direction in order (i.e., 50s, 20s, 10s, and so on). RATIONALE: Follows bank procedure.
3. Count all coins to be deposited and enter the amount in the space provided. Coins may need to be wrapped. RATIONALE: Follows bank procedure.
4. On the back of the deposit slip list each check separately. Include the patient name in the left-hand column and enter the amount of the check in the right-hand column. RATIONALE: Follows bank procedure.
5. Total the checks listed and copy the total on the front where it is indicated to place the total from the other side. RATIONALE: Follows bank procedure.
6. The sum of currency, coins, and checks should always equal the total in the Payments column on that day's day sheet. RATIONALE: Proof of accuracy.
7. Attach the top copy of the deposit slip to the deposit, leaving the carbon on the pad. RATIONALE: Provides the clinic and bank with a record of deposit.
8. Enter the date and amount of the deposit in the space provided on the checkbook stubs. RATIONALE: Keeps checkbook register current with money in account.
9. Add the amount of the deposit to the checkbook balance. RATIONALE: Keeps checkbook register current with money in account.
10. Deposit at the bank, either in person or at the night deposit. In either case, be sure a record of deposit is received (it will be mailed if the night deposit is used). It is not recommended that deposits be made through ATMs; currency should never be deposited in an ATM. RATIONALE: Proves bank processed the deposit as indicated.

NSF, it is necessary to perform two bookkeeping functions. First, deduct the amount from the checking account balance of the practice. Second, add the amount back into the amount due by the patient in his or her account balance by entering the amount in the paid column in parentheses and increase the balance by the same amount. Place a brief explanation in the description column. Follow the clinic procedure for notifying the patient that the check was returned. See Procedure 18-5.

Lost or Stolen Checks

In the event that a check is missing and is thought to be lost or stolen, report this to your bank immediately. In some cases, you may be advised to stop payment to prevent unauthorized cashing of the check. In other situations, the bank may place a warning on the account, advising bank representatives to be especially careful about checking signatures to detect any attempt at a forged signature.

PROCEDURE 18-5

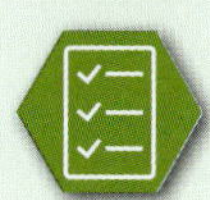
Procedure

Recording a Nonsufficient Funds Check

PURPOSE:

To perform bookkeeping functions that keep accounts in proper balance.

EQUIPMENT/SUPPLIES:

- The practice's account balance
- Manual day sheet
- Manual ledger
- Nonsufficient funds (NSF) check

PROCEDURE STEPS:

1. Follow the clinic policy for notifying the patient of the returned check. RATIONALE: Policy may vary from clinic to clinic.
2. When the NSF check has been returned the second time, deduct the check amount from the account balance of the clinic. RATIONALE: The funds can no longer be counted as earnings received.
3. Add the amount of the NSF check back into the patient's ledger. Place the amount in parentheses in the paid column and increase the total by the same amount. In a manual system, the entry and math are performed by the medical assistant. RATIONALE: The amount is still owed by the patient, is not considered paid, and must be reflected in the amount due.
4. Place a brief explanation in the description of the column such as "NSF 12/09/20XX."

Writing and Recording Checks

Part of daily financial practices includes writing checks to pay bills (**accounts payable**), refunding overpayment, and replenishing petty cash. Writing the checks and paying the bills is usually done systematically. Chapter 20 discusses accounts payable and disbursement records in greater detail. It is important that checks be prepared either electronically or written legibly to avoid bank errors. Checks should be dated and must include the name of the **payee**. The amount of payment entered both in figures and in words should match exactly. If there is a discrepancy, the bank will not accept the check or may pay the incorrect amount. It is also advisable that the "memo" line indicates what the check is for and includes any account or invoice number for reference. Figure 18-7 shows a sample of a properly completed check.

Procedure

Rules for Preparing Checks. Follow these rules to ensure that checks are properly prepared and recorded (see Procedure 18-6).

- Confirm that the numeric and written amounts agree.
- Confirm that everything is spelled correctly.
- Follow clinic procedure for having the provider or office manager approve all expenditures and sign all outgoing checks.
- Determine that the check has been signed by an individual with signature privileges.
- Confirm that the check is payable to the correct payee and that the current date is used.

Chapter 20 provides information on electronic check writing.

Reconciling a Bank Statement

Each month the bank will send a statement for the checking account (Figure 18-8). With online banking, a bank statement can be accessed electronically at any time. It also can be printed and used similar to a standard printed bank statement. The statement will show the account

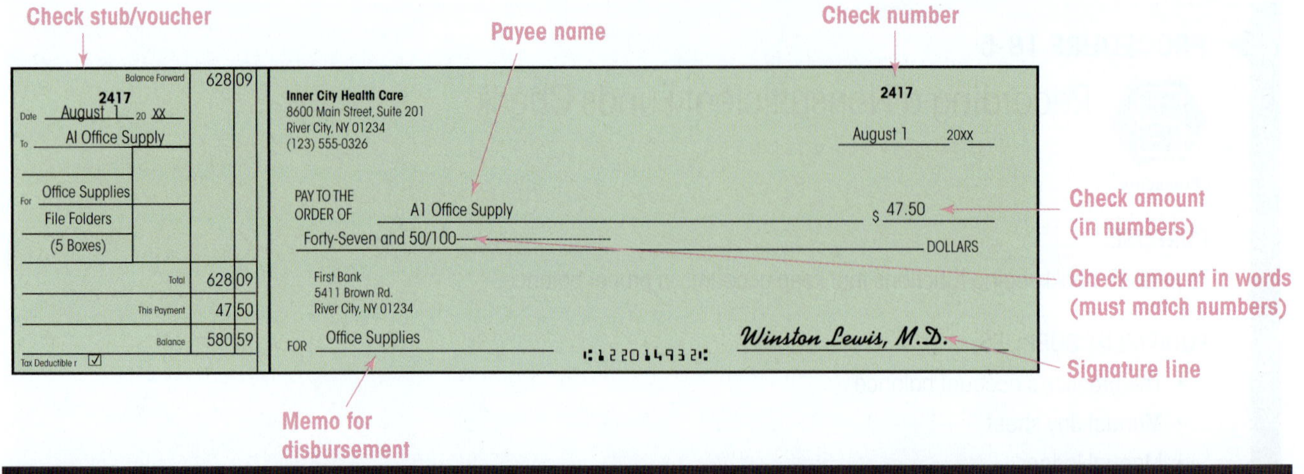

FIGURE 18-7 Sample of properly completed check and check stub voucher.

PROCEDURE 18-6

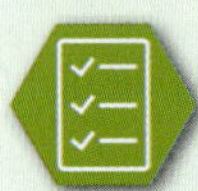

Writing a Manual Check

PURPOSE:

To write a check to pay for expenses incurred and provide proof of payment. (Never written a check before? Go to http://www.checkright.org for practice.)

EQUIPMENT/SUPPLIES:

- Checkbook and check register with balance of $7,298.35
- Pen with black ink
- Calculator

CHECKING WRITING EXERCISES:

Write checks for the following invoices using the current date:

1. $54.99 for case of printer paper to Landau Products
2. $450.00 for last month's janitorial services to MJB Services
3. $1,335.38 for clinical supplies to Redding Medical Supply House
4. $687.19 to Atlantic Electric for last month's heat and electricity
5. $350 to American Association of Medical Assistants for AAMA membership for the four medical assistants in the clinic

PROCEDURE STEPS:

1. Gather all invoices to be paid.
2. For the check register, use black ink:
   a. Enter check number 101 in the register if not preprinted.
   b. Enter the current date and year (usually in numbers, i.e., 02/14/20XX).
   c. Enter the individual or company the check is to be paid to: Landau Products.
   d. Enter the amount to be paid on the check: $54.99.

(continues)

e. Subtract check amount from the present balance. Total $7,243.36 appears as the available balance. RATIONALE: These steps ensure that the check register is not overlooked when writing a check and establishes a well-recognized routine.

3. To write the check, use black ink:
   a. Enter check number 101 if not preprinted.
   b. Enter the current date and year (usually written out, e.g., February 14, 20XX).
   c. Enter the individual or company the check is to be paid to: Landau Products.
   d. Enter the amount to be paid on the check: $54.99. Do not leave spaces between numbers or between the dollar sign and the first number. RATIONALE: This helps to prevent any tampering of the check by adding numbers.
   e. Write out the amount to be paid by check (Fifty-four dollars and 99/100). Fill in any space left between the last number or word and draw a wiggly line over to the amount entered in numbers. RATIONALE: When the written amount and the number amount match, errors are prevented. The wiggly line makes it more difficult for anyone to tamper with the check.
   f. Describe what the check is written for in the bottom left corner (Printer paper, case). RATIONALE: Explains the purpose of the check.
   g. If you have check-writing authority in the clinic, sign the check with your name the same as indicated on the bank's records. If you do not have check-writing authority, hold this check and the others to give to the individual with that authority. RATIONALE: The person responsible can review the checks with the invoices to verify valid expenses.
4. Continue writing checks for items 2 through 5 in the Check Writing Exercises, being certain to number checks consecutively and to subtract each check. Submit checks and check register with final balance to your instructor for evaluation.

Summary of Account Balance — Closing Date 1/15/XX

Account # 1257-164013 — Ending Balance $8,347.62

Beginning Balance	$7,152.18
Total Deposits and Additions	$8,643.86
Total Withdrawals	$7,433.21
Service Charge	$ 15.24

Number	Date	Amount	Number	Date	Amount
201	12/18/XX	173.82	234	1/4/XX	96.31
223*	12/18/XX	44.12	235	1/4/XX	73.48
224	12/20/XX	586.00	236	1/6/XX	325.40
225	12/21/XX	24.15	237	1/7/XX	40.00
226	12/22/XX	33.90	238	1/8/XX	66.77
228*	12/23/XX	1250.00	241*	1/9/XX	15.55
229	12/24/XX	11.75	242	1/10/XX	12.45
230	12/24/XX	19.02	243	1/10/XX	4441.25
231	1/2/XX	43.80	244	1/10/XX	64.55
232	1/3/XX	39.00			
233	1/4/XX	71.50			

*Denotes gap in check sequence

Date	Deposit Amount	Date	Deposit Amount
18-Dec	361.75	4-Jan	825.00
19-Dec	586.00	5-Jan	1286.71
20-Dec	918.21	7-Jan	608.00
21-Dec	201.00	8-Jan	811.15
2-Jan	475.00	9-Jan	1092.68
3-Jan	1478.36		

Front

1. Enter Ending Balance from the front of this statement
$ 8,347.62

2. Enter deposits not shown on this statement
$ 3,162.50

3. Subtotal (add 1 & 2)
$ 11,510.12

4. List outstanding checks or other withdrawals here

Check #	Amount
222	37.89
227	161.15
239	11.50
240	92.12
245	835.17
246	21.75
247	586.00

5. Total outstanding checks
$ 1,745.58

Balance (subtract #5 from #3)
$ 9,764.54
This should equal your checkbook balance

Back

FIGURE 18-8 Sample bank statement with check reconciliation.

balance according to the bank's records, a listing of all checks that have cleared the bank, deposits received by the bank, and any service charges deducted from the account. It is necessary to reconcile the entries in the checkbook against this statement to be sure there are no errors either in the checkbook or in the bank's records. Your bank statement is another means of ensuring that the accounts receivable is accurate for the previous month. If you use an accounting software package, this will also have a computerized option for reconciling.

Procedure

Procedure 18-7 details the steps involved in reconciling the statement.

PURCHASING SUPPLIES AND EQUIPMENT

It is important to ensure proper control over purchasing of supplies and equipment for several reasons:

1. To avoid purchase of unnecessary items
2. To avoid duplication of items purchased
3. To provide a system for payment of only those items properly ordered and received

To accomplish these things, you should follow the first rule of purchasing: nothing is ordered or paid for without a purchase order or purchase order number. A copy of the purchase order is sent to the supplier and a copy is retained by the

PROCEDURE 18-7

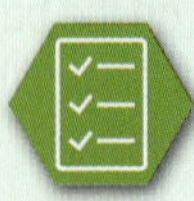
Procedure

Reconciling a Bank Statement

PURPOSE:

To verify that the balance listed in the checkbook agrees with the balance shown by the bank.

EQUIPMENT/SUPPLIES:

- Checkbook
- Bank statement
- Calculator

PROCEDURE STEPS:

1. Make sure the balance in the checkbook is current (all deposits and checks entered have been added or subtracted). RATIONALE: Ensures totals are accurate.
2. If a service charge is listed on the statement, subtract that amount from the last balance listed in the checkbook. RATIONALE: Reconciles current balance.
3. In the checkbook, check off each check listed on the statement and verify the amount against the check stub. RATIONALE: Verifies accuracy.
4. In the checkbook, check off each deposit listed on the statement. RATIONALE: Verifies accuracy.
5. The back of the statement contains a worksheet to be used for balancing.
6. Copy the ending balance from the front of the statement to the area indicated on the back.
7. Go through the check stubs and list on the back of the statement in the area provided any checks that have not cleared and any deposits that were not shown as received on the statement.
8. Total the checks not cleared on the statement worksheet.
9. Total the deposits not credited on the worksheet.
10. Add together the statement balance and the total of deposits not credited.
11. Subtract the total of checks not cleared. This amount should agree with the balance in the checkbook. If so, the checkbook is balanced and the statement should be filed in the appropriate place. RATIONALE: Following procedure steps 5 through 11 completes verification of accuracy.

clinic for verification of shipment and payment of invoice.

Preparing a Purchase Order

Purchase order forms are available from office supply companies or can be ordered from a printer and customized to the needs of the clinic setting. As an alternative to ordering preprinted purchase order forms, the clinic staff may choose to create their own forms using Microsoft Excel software. This enables the clinic to have electronic access to the form with embedded formulas. Figure 18-9 shows a typical purchase order form properly completed, which is reviewed here section by section.

The purchase order form can vary greatly; some have more or less information. The form shown in Figure 18-9 contains the usual information required. The important thing is that the purchase order is used consistently.

- *Date.* The day the purchase order is created.
- *Purchase order number.* A preprinted number that is used on invoices and statements from the supplier and on the check used to pay the invoice. It is also important for tracking the status of the order. In smaller practices, the purchase order number may simply be the name of the person ordering with the date the order was placed immediately following.
- *Bill to address.* This is generally used when items are to be shipped to an address different from the address where the supplier will send the bill for goods or services.
- *Ship to address.* When items are to be sent by supplier, this must always be completed.
- *Vendor information.* The name and address of the supplier where the purchase order is to be sent.
- *Req. by* ("Requested by"). States which individual or department has requested the item(s).

PURCHASE ORDER

NO. 1742

Date:

Bill To:	Ship To:	Vendor:
Inner City Health Care 8600 Main Street, Suite 201 River City, NY 01234 (123) 555-0326	**Inner City Health Care** 8600 Main Street, Suite 201 River City, NY 01234 (123) 555-0326	**AZ Medical Supply** 4721 E. Camelback Rd. Phoenix, AZ 85252 (602) 555-3246

REQ BY	BUYER	TERMS
Ellen Armstrong	Marilyn Johnson	Net 30

QTY	ITEM	UNITS	DESCRIPTION	UNIT PR	TOTAL
10	427A	Box	Surgical gloves - Sz 7	9.20	92.00
1	327DC	Case	2" gauze pads	60.30	60.30
5	1943C	Box	Tongue depressors	5.80	29.00
15	7433	Ea	Examination table paper (roll)	10.50	159.50
				SUBTOTAL	338.80
				TAX	28.80
				FREIGHT	Prepaid
				BAL DUE	376.60

FIGURE 18-9 Purchase order form.

- *Buyer.* States the individual in the clinic who is authorized to issue a purchase order.
- *Terms.* Agreement between buyer and seller as to when payment is due.
- *Qty.* Quantity of item being ordered (number of units).
- *Item.* Vendor's catalogue part or item number.
- *Units.* How the item is sold—individually (ea.), by the box, case, or dozen. Many suppliers will not split units (i.e., will not sell less than a full case).
- *Description.* Brief description of item (helps as a cross-check for the vendor in the event that an item number is entered incorrectly).
- *Unit price.* How much *one* unit (ea., box, case, dozen) costs.
- *Total.* Cost of one unit multiplied by the number of units being ordered.
- *Discount.* If any discount is allowed for quick and early payment, it is noted here. For instance, there might be a 10% discount for paying within 10 days. The discount amount is entered before the Total column is summed.
- *Subtotal.* Sum of the Total column.
- *Tax.* Sales tax required by the state.
- *Freight.* How much the customer must pay to have the order delivered (not always applicable).
- *Bal. Due.* The sum of the subtotal, tax, and freight charges; this is how much the clinic will be billed.

Verifying Goods Received

Proper purchasing procedure does not stop with the completion and mailing of the purchase order. When goods are received, it is necessary to verify that the correct items and quantities were shipped by the vendor. Chapter 20 discusses accounts payable.

PETTY CASH

Petty cash is money kept in the clinic for minor, routine, or unexpected expenses such as postage-due mail or coffee supplies. Keep petty cash totally separate from the cash drawer that is used to make change for patients paying their co-payment. Keeping this cash on hand eliminates the necessity of the provider or office manager having to sign checks for such items. Petty cash is not used to pay bills or make large routine purchases.

The amount of cash on hand for this purpose is small, usually $75 to $100, and is usually kept in small denominations. However, records must be as carefully maintained as for any other financial transactions and balanced each day before closing.

Establishing a Petty Cash Fund

If your clinic does not already have a petty cash fund or if you are in a new practice that has not yet established a fund, determine how much the fund should be and write a check to "Cash" for that amount. The amount should be enough to cover several days of incidental expenses.

Tracking, Balancing, and Replenishing Petty Cash

Tracking. Keep a supply of petty cash vouchers on hand to track how petty cash is used. When money is taken from petty cash, a voucher must always be completed and the receipt from the purchase attached. Vouchers and receipts are kept in the petty cash box with the money until the fund is replenished. Figure 18-10 shows an example of a petty cash form used to track funds.

Balancing and Replenishing. When the fund gets low, write another check to "Cash" to bring it back up to the original amount. To determine the amount of the check, it is necessary to first balance the account. After the account is balanced, list how funds were spent in such a way that the bookkeeper can disburse the check properly.

Procedure 18-8 outlines the steps involved in establishing and maintaining a petty cash account.

DOCUMENTATION

Financial records of patients are to be kept separate from the patients medical charts. Except for the attachment of the encounter form or superbill at the time of the visit, they rarely are seen together. Often, only the patient's medical record is necessary for documentation; other times, only the financial information is necessary. This policy also serves as a reminder that the care given to patients has nothing to do with their ability to pay.

Petty Cash Voucher Forms

Petty Cash Voucher

Ref:				Date ________
Details				Received (dollar amount) $ ________
Acct No.	Account Name	Total		For: ________
				________
				________
	Total			Approved By / Received By

FIGURE 18-10 Petty cash voucher.

PROCEDURE 18-8

Establishing and Maintaining a Petty Cash Fund

PURPOSE:

To establish and maintain a petty cash fund for incidental expenses, making certain that receipts match the difference between the beginning and ending balance of the fund.

EQUIPMENT/SUPPLIES:

- Petty cash box with cash balance
- Vouchers
- Calculator

PETTY CASH EXERCISES:

1. Write a check to "Cash" for $100 to be taken to the bank.
2. Vouchers are made for the following incidentals:
   a. $20 to staff employee to purchase coffee supplies. Actual amount for supplies is $13.87; employee returns $6.13 cash
   b. $2.24 for postage due to postal employee
   c. $3.18 to postal employee for guaranteed forwarding address
   d. $35.00 to Shannon's Pizza delivery for staff meeting lunch

PROCEDURE STEPS:

Establish the Fund:

1. Cash the check for $100 and receive the money in denominations of 1s, 5s, 10s, and 20s. Place the cash in the cash box at the clinic. RATIONALE: The amount establishes petty cash and provides bills for the incidental purchases.

(continues)

2. When cash is needed for an incidental expense, such as postage due, prepare a voucher for the amount needed. No cash is taken from the fund without a voucher. RATIONALE: The written voucher indicates what the money is used for.
3. After the purchase, attach the receipt for the purchase to the voucher. RATIONALE: This step provides proof of the purchase.

Balance Petty Cash Fund:

1. After the activity identified in the Petty Cash Exercises, count the money remaining in the box. RATIONALE: Verifies the amount of cash remaining in petty cash.
2. Total the amounts of all vouchers in the petty cash box. RATIONALE: Determines amount of expenditures.
3. Subtract the amount of receipts from the original amount in petty cash. This should equal the amount of cash remaining in the box. RATIONALE: Proves that the amount of expenditures deducted from the beginning amount equals the amount left in the box.
4. When the cash has been balanced against the receipts, write a check *only for the amount that was used.* RATIONALE: Brings dollar amount back to original petty cash amount.

Petty Cash Check Disbursement:

1. Sort all vouchers by account.
2. On a sheet of paper list the accounts involved.
3. Total vouchers for each account and record individual totals on the list.
4. Copy this list with its totals on the memo portion of the stub for the check written to replenish petty cash.
5. File the list with the vouchers and receipts attached, after noting the check number on the list.

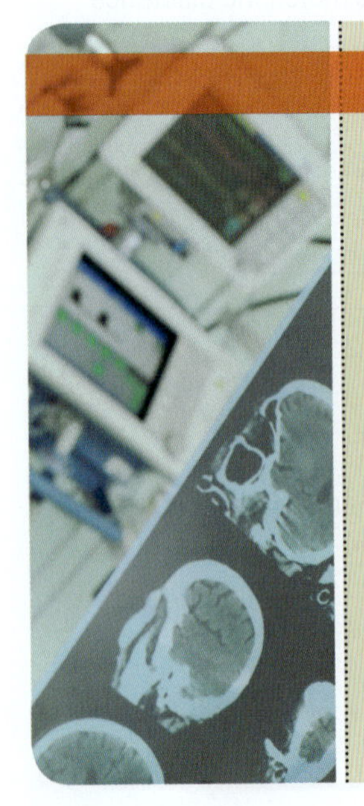

CASE STUDY 18-1

Refer to the scenario at the beginning of the chapter. As you consider the discussion of patient fees, determine what steps to take in the following situations.

CASE STUDY REVIEW

1. The clinic's patient has been diagnosed with non-Hodgkin's lymphoma (diffuse large B-cell lymphoma) in stage 3. Surgery and aggressive chemotherapy are in process. The patient has Medicare and a small Medigap policy. You know there are expenses coming soon that neither insurance will cover. What can you suggest?
2. This patient has been with the clinic for 11 years and was covered most of the time by excellent private insurance. The circumstances have changed, however. Today the patient works part time, has only Medicaid insurance, and has very few private funds. The provider's diagnosis is severe depression, and the provider instructs the patient to make two appointments weekly until the medication prescribed begins to make a significant difference in this patient's life. You know there are severe limitations to reimbursement from the state regarding this diagnosis. What steps will you take?

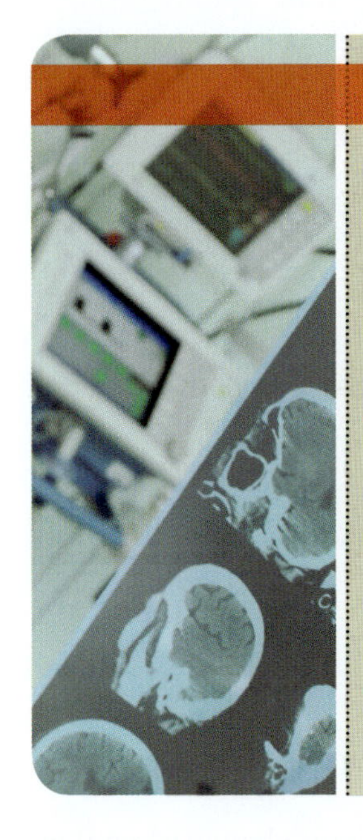

CASE STUDY 18-2

Joann Crier has completed her 3-month probation period with Inner City Health Care. She is doing quite well and has demonstrated skill in accurate financial documentation. She has been asked to take over reconciling the monthly bank statements and managing all the accounts payable, including getting the checks ready for the provider's signature. She has difficulty, however, completing these tasks until after hours when the clinic is closed and quiet. Clinic manager Marilyn Johnson, CMA (AAMA), has told her that it must be done within normal working hours unless special permission is granted.

CASE STUDY REVIEW

1. What suggestions can you make to Joann to allow her to complete these tasks during normal working hours?
2. What impact does the time of day, day(s) of the month, or place where the tasks are completed have on your suggestions?
3. Are there any circumstances you can identify when overtime might be warranted to allow Joann to complete the tasks after hours?

Summary

- The daily financial responsibilities of a medical clinic include patient bookkeeping, purchasing supplies and equipment, and petty cash.
- Proficiency in these functions is integral for a solvent practice that has the proper income, resources, and supplies available to provide appropriate patient care, and a healthy business in which to provide services, including a well-stocked and equipped clinic.
- The medical assistant must be familiar with using a system to post and track income data, as well as other types of financial transactions required by the practice.
- Clinics may use a pegboard system as a comprehensive manual system for tracking these data. Computerized bookkeeping offers many advantages related to speed, high accuracy, and elimination of some routine tasks while providing the same important financial data.
- Accurate and scrupulous maintenance of the accounts payable system ensures that bills are paid on time and those payments are properly documented for tax purposes.
- Practicing maximum accuracy in all bookkeeping functions is vital for the medical clinic.
- All charges and receipts must be recorded immediately.
- It is best practice for medical clinic personnel to make deposits of checks and currency the same day they are received.
- The medical assistant must always verify and recheck totals of all deposits and expenditures.
- Medical clinic personnel must stay current with all checking account duties such as account reconciliation.
- Medical clinic personnel must be prompt with all accounts payable.
- The medical assistant will likely be expected to maintain a petty cash fund and the clinic cash drawer for small daily cash transactions.

Study for Success

To reinforce your knowledge and skills of information presented in this chapter:

- Review the *Key Terms* and *Learning Outcomes*
- Consider the *Critical Thinking* features and *Case Studies* and discuss your conclusions
- Answer the questions in the *Certification Review*

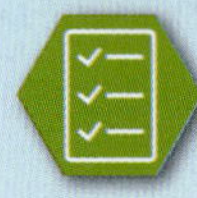
Procedure

- Perform the *Procedures* using the *Competency Assessment Checklists* on the *Student Companion Website*

CERTIFICATION REVIEW

1. Which of the following is an accurate description of the debit column of a ledger ?
   a. It is the column to the right of the balance column.
   b. It is the column on the left; used to enter charges, procedure codes, and description of services.
   c. It is the column at the far right that records the difference between the debit and credit columns.
   d. It is the column that indicates the patient's debt to the practice.
2. Which of the following statements regarding the use of debit/credit cards by patients to pay for services in ambulatory care settings is accurate?
   a. It is never done.
   b. It is unethical.
   c. It is sure to compromise the integrity of the clinic.
   d. It is a financial arrangement increasingly being used.
   e. It is done because most people carry no cash.
3. What is the purpose of the first section of the manual day sheet?
   a. To record deposits
   b. For business analysis
   c. To post individual transactions
   d. To total transactions
4. Which method is identified as a good working habit for financial transactions?
   a. Double-checking all entries for accuracy
   b. Keeping the bookkeeping tasks current and up to date
   c. Allowing the computer to create all the entries
   d. Managing the accounts on a weekly basis
   e. Both a and b
5. Which of the following statements is an accurate description of petty cash?
   a. It is necessary to give patients change when they pay in cash.
   b. It is used by the provider when taking a colleague to lunch.
   c. It pays for routine and unexpected minor expenses of the clinic.
   d. It comes from the provider's personal account.
6. Which of the following is true regarding encounter forms?
   a. They can be ordered to fit the practice.
   b. They provide a separate ledger for each patient household.
   c. They list common services provided, procedural code, and diagnosis code.
   d. They should be destroyed after processing.
   e. Both a and c
7. Which of the following is an accurate description of receipts?
   a. They are used for payments on accounts.
   b. They are not given unless services are rendered the same day.
   c. They are mailed to patients when payment is made by mail.
   d. They are unnecessary, especially in the computerized system.
8. What is a necessary step when accepting checks from patients?
   a. Inspect for correct date, amount, and signature
   b. Immediately stamp with a restrictive endorsement
   c. Automatically accept third-party checks
   d. Both a and b
   e. None of these

9. What is the name for a check with an attached stub for recording information?
   a. Certified check
   b. Cashier's check
   c. Voucher check
   d. Money order

10. Why is it important to ensure proper control over purchasing of supplies and equipment?
    a. To avoid purchase of unnecessary items
    b. To avoid duplication of items purchased
    c. To provide a system for payment of only those items properly ordered and received
    d. All of these
    e. None of these

CHAPTER 19

Billing and Collections

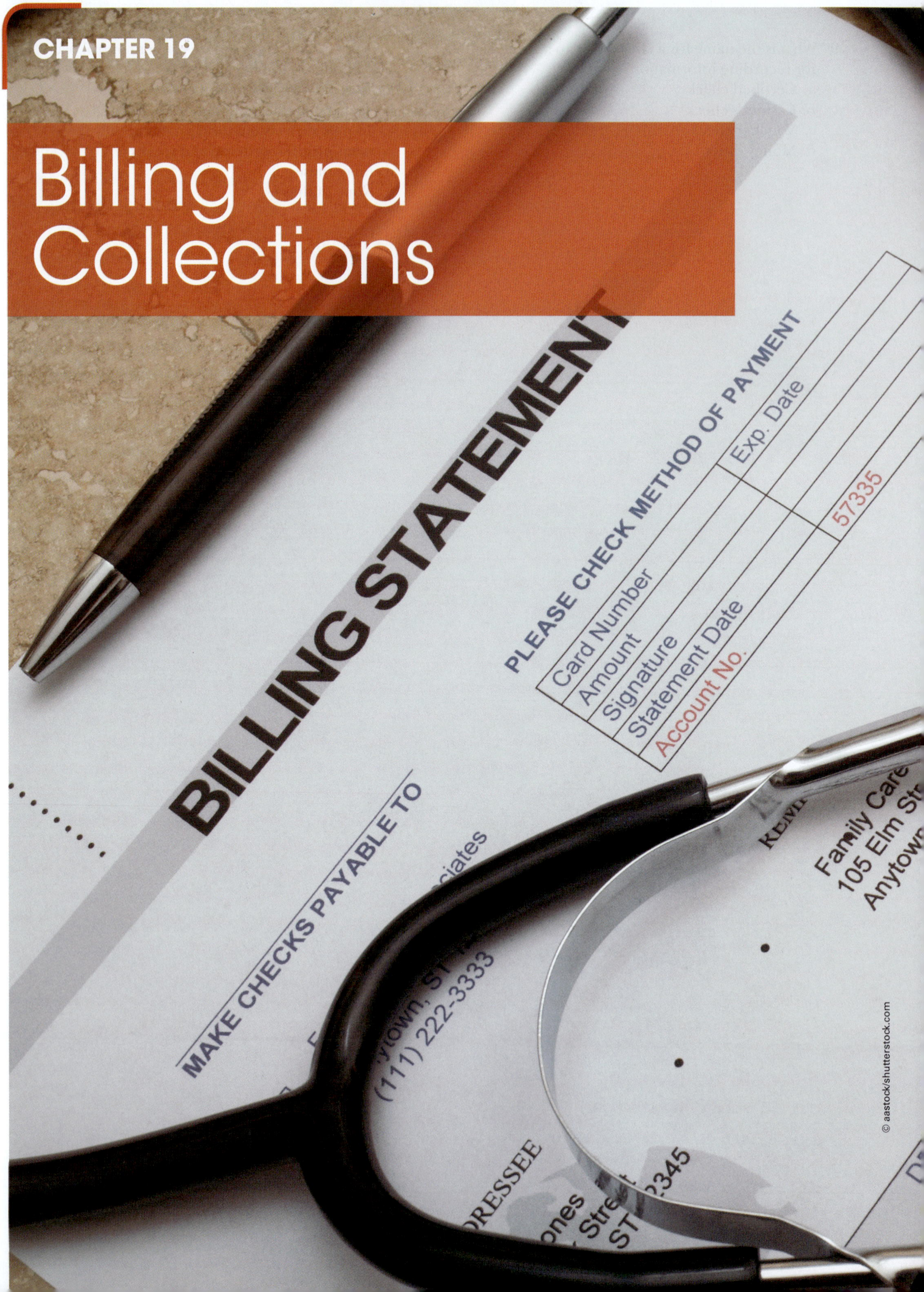

LEARNING OUTCOMES

1. Define and spell the key terms as presented in the glossary.
2. Analyze the importance of billing and collections to the clinic.
3. Describe the advantages of billing at least the co-payment and co-insurance at time of service.
4. Describe the impact of the Truth-In-Lending Act as it applies to collections.
5. Compare computerized billing and manual billing.
6. Recall the components of a complete statement.
7. Differentiate between monthly and cycle billing.
8. Explain the process of aging accounts.
9. Describe the importance of a courteous manner in telephone collections.
10. State legal and ethical guidelines for telephone collections.
11. Describe the impact of the Fair Debt Collection Practice Act as it applies to collections.
12. Describe the process of sending a series of collection letters.
13. List points to consider when using a collection agency.
14. Recall three special collections problems encountered in the clinic.
15. Explain how the statute of limitations impacts the medical assistant's practice.
16. Discuss the merits of a professional attitude in collections.

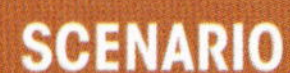

KEY TERMS

accounts receivable ratio
collection ratio
Fair Debt Collection Practice Act (FDCPA)
probate court
statute of limitations
Truth-in-Lending Act

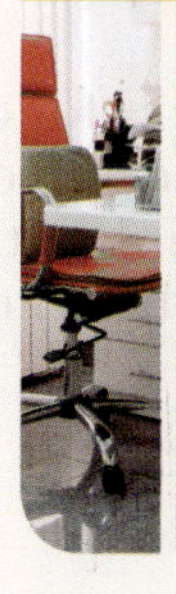

SCENARIO

At Inner City Health Care, patient billing is typically done at time of service, and a charge slip noting date, description of charges, and fees is given to the patient on leaving the clinic. Clinic policy states that, if possible, patients should pay their part of the fee, or their co-pay, at time of service. Marilyn Johnson, CMA (AAMA), the clinic manager, has found that this is the most efficient way to ensure timely payment and eliminates the need to mail a separate statement. However, the clinic is flexible, and if the patient cannot pay all or part of the charge at the visit, Marilyn works out a payment schedule that is acceptable to both the clinic and the patient.

Chapter Portal

In the clinic, patient billing is a critical administrative function that helps to maintain a healthy, viable practice. Timeliness is essential in billing, because the clinic depends on its accounts receivable to pay its bills in a responsible manner. Billing need not be a complex activity, but it must be completely accurate. In the few clinics still using pegboard accounting, billing and collection procedures are done manually, often using the patient's ledger as the basis for the statement. When the facility is computerized, patient bills and collection notices are computer generated.

The best method of patient billing and collections is a method that is customized to the practice and that regards the patient as a consumer who should be respected. Patients appreciate knowing in advance what charges and fees they are expected to pay.

BILLING PROCEDURES

The clinic's cash flow and collection process are dependent on up-to-date and accurate billing techniques. The financial status of the practice is reflected in monthly financial statements indicating unpaid patient balances, which, if they persist, are reviewed for appropriate action, including possible referral to a collection agency. Copies of all billing forms will be retained in the patient account record.

Timeliness and accuracy have a significant influence on prompt payment and how soon collection of the patient account will be finalized. In other words, billing performance can be measured by the time it takes to generate and submit a complete statement, that is, a statement with full documentation. If a facility is experiencing problems generating patient bills, a billing timeliness analysis worksheet can be constructed to identify internal delays that affect how quickly an account is billed, and thus paid. By focusing on inefficiencies in the revenue cycle, processes may be identified that need to be streamlined. For example, the date of service and insurance verification, the date the bill was generated, and the date the bill was submitted to the patient or third party can determine the efficiency of the billing process.

A billing efficiency report is another instrument that may be used to monitor the efficiency of the billing process. This report lists the previous month's billing backlog, which is added to the number of new accounts. The number of processed accounts is then subtracted. The weekly number of accounts that were rebilled also is noted, and the amount of time billing personnel spent on billing accounts is recorded. Production efficiency is calculated from these data. Inherent to this system is the careful monitoring of follow-up bills, including whether they were paid, whether the insurance paid, and an assessment of the patient's responsibility for payment.

CREDIT AND COLLECTION POLICIES

It is important that patients understand the billing policy and are educated about their accounts, how they are paid, and what their responsibility is toward payment. This is most easily accomplished in a patient information brochure (see Chapter 21) identifying all aspects of the medical practice, including how bills are paid. The clinic staff also must have a well-defined policy related to patient billing and collecting.

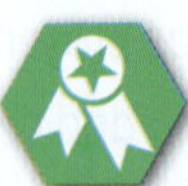

Even uncomplicated patient billing should be done according to credit and collection policies established by the provider-employers of the clinic. Having a formalized policy makes decision making easier and gives the medical assistant or office manager responsible for billing and collections authority to act. For example, some questions the providers and office manager may want to address include:

- When will payment be due from the patient?
- What kind of payment arrangements can be made if the patient does not pay at time of service?
- Will the patient be responsible for obtaining referrals, and if so, how will patients who did not obtain one prior to the visit be handled?
- At what point should a patient be reminded of an overdue bill?
- How is the reminder initially managed: by telephone, a note on the statement, or a letter?
- At what point will a patient bill be considered delinquent?
- Will a collection agency be used? Who decides?
- If exceptions to the policy are to be made, who makes these exceptions and what steps are taken?

By answering these and other questions, a straightforward credit and collection policy can be devised that is a guide to both patients and the medical assistant in charge of billing.

PAYMENT AT TIME OF SERVICE

The best opportunity for collection is at the time of service. This process begins with the medical assistant who schedules

Patient Education

Patients appreciate knowing their responsibility in terms of payment. Whoever schedules the first appointment with a new patient should diplomatically inform the patient of clinic policy on payment of fees. If the patient anticipates a problem in paying promptly, a schedule can be established that is agreeable to both parties.

appointments. Make certain all patients have the information they need. After determining the urgency and reason for the appointment, collecting information regarding a chief complaint, and assigning a time for the appointment, it is appropriate to discuss the financial concerns of patients (Procedure 19-1). Patients may be shy in asking certain questions, but they have questions about most of the following issues:

- Whether the providers contract with their insurance carrier
- How payment is made if insurance does not cover certain procedures
- Whether they can be billed for co-payments and coinsurance
- How payment is made for services if they have no insurance
- An approximate cost of a particular service

PROCEDURE 19-1

Procedure

Explaining Fees in the First Telephone Interview

PURPOSE:

To establish rapport with patients, to discuss providers' fees, and to identify the patient's responsibility before the first visit.

EQUIPMENT/SUPPLIES:

- Provider's fee schedule
- Appointment schedule
- Telephone

PROCEDURE STEPS:

1. Place the providers' fee schedule and the appointment schedule close to the telephone. RATIONALE: Prepared clinic staff do not have to search for something vital to the phone conversation.
2. Answer the phone before the third ring. ***Identify the name of the clinic and yourself.*** RATIONALE: The person calling feels attended to and knows the call has been correctly placed.
3. ***Acknowledge the patient*** and offer assistance; for example, a comment such as "How can I help you?" RATIONALE: Sets the tone for the patient to continue with the request.
4. After the patient is identified as a new patient and the nature of the visit is determined appropriate, discuss possible dates for the appointment. A statement such as, "Our next available appointment is Thursday at 11:30 AM. Can you make it then?" is a good way to begin.
5. Tell the patient that you will be discussing clinic policies briefly now and will mail the patient information brochure before the appointment. RATIONALE: The patient brochure details some of the information discussed in the telephone conversation and further verifies the clinic's policies.
6. Ask about medical insurance. If the patient is insured, get the identification number, the name of the subscriber, the employer, and a telephone number of the insurance carrier if possible. RATIONALE: This allows you to check for any preauthorization required and for the currency of the plan.
7. Explain that the clinic policy requires any co-payment and co-insurance to be paid at the time of the visit. RATIONALE: Establishes patient's financial responsibility immediately.
8. Check to see if the patient has transportation and knows how to get to the clinic, and provide directions if necessary. RATIONALE: Ensures that there is no confusion about location and accessibility.
9. Request that the patient arrive about 15 minutes before the appointment to complete some forms. RATIONALE: Ensures that the patient has time to complete information and can ask any questions that might occur.
10. After closing the telephone interview, promptly mail the patient information brochure.

Do not tell a patient, "We do not take your insurance." It is much better to make a statement such as, "Our providers do not contract with that insurance. However, we can work with you on a fee-for-service basis and help make finances workable for you." The atmosphere has now been created to ensure prompt collection and increased cash flow for the practice. To accommodate patients, clinics now increasingly accept debit and credit card payments. Remember, also, that if your facility does use a sign-in method as patients arrive, then the all-important personal contact may be missed. With that missed opportunity also goes the opportunity to discuss finances.

Most insurance contracts require the provider to bill the insurance company *before* billing the patient, except for the co-payment. It is critical to abide by each contract to protect the provider. If the patient is a member of a health maintenance organization (HMO) and the clinic is a participating provider, it is bound to the terms of that agreement. If not restricted by the insurance contract, be certain to explain to the patient at the time of service that any payment owed will be adjusted according to the patient's insurance and the terms of that policy. Also remember that all patients must be treated the same and charged the same for services.

With the knowledge of what portion of the fee can be collected at the time of service, the medical assistant says to the patient prior to leaving the facility, "The fee for your services today is $85. Will you be paying by cash, check, or credit/debit card?" When the policy for collecting fees is shared when the appointment is made, patients are not surprised by this approach. Allow the patient to be the next person to speak in response to the question asked. If for some reason a fee cannot be immediately paid, the patient will respond by asking what kind of arrangements might be made. Even if financial arrangements are necessary, the discussion of the day's fee for the service is in process.

TRUTH-IN-LENDING ACT

In those situations where a payment schedule is arranged, clinic policy will dictate if any interest is charged. Although it is not illegal to charge interest on patient accounts, many providers still prefer not to assign any interest on installment payments or past-due accounts.

Competency

For installment payments (such as prenatal care or surgery), medical assistants need to be aware of the conditions of the **Truth-in-Lending Act**, Regulation Z of the Consumer Protection Act of 1967 (see Chapter 6). If there is bilateral agreement between providers and their patients for payment of medical services in more than four installments, that agreement must be in writing and must provide information on any finance charges. The information must be in writing even if there are no finance charges made (Figure 19-1). The patient is given the original copy of the disclosure statement; a second copy is kept in the clinic.

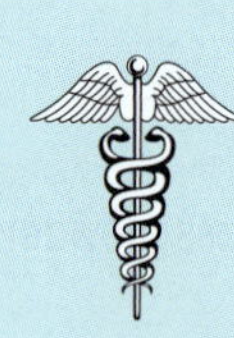

INNER CITY HEALTH CARE
8600 Main Street, Suite 200
River City, XY 01234
(123) 456-7890

FEDERAL TRUTH-IN-LENDING STATEMENT
For Professional Services

Patient: Cari R. Jacobson
Address: 913 Swanson Street
River City, XY 61820
Parent: ______

1. Cost of services rendered	$1,500.00
2. Down Payment	225.00
3. Unpaid Balance	1,275.00
4. Amount Financed	1,275.00
5. Finance Charge	-0-
6. Annual Percentage Rate of Finance Charge	-0-
7. Total of Payments (4 + 5 above)	1,275.00
8. Total Amount After Payments	1,500.00

Total payment due is payable to Dr. Winston Lewis at above address in 5 monthly installments of $ 255. The first installment is payable on August 1, 20XX, and each subsequent payment is due on the same day of each consecutive month until paid in full.

07-24-XX
Date of Agreement

______
Signature of Patient;
Parent if Patient is Minor

FIGURE 19-1 Truth-in-Lending Act document showing installment and interest agreement.

COMPONENTS OF A COMPLETE STATEMENT

Once a patient has been accepted for treatment, it is important to maintain accurate and timely records of his or her account and payment history. That information is just as vital to the healthy management of the practice as the patient's medical record. Invoice patient services promptly according to the clinic policy, send statements regularly, and make certain they are complete and accurate. Statements to patients must be professional looking, neat, inclusive of all services and charges, and easily understood. Procedure and diagnosis codes are necessary for insurance and reimbursement, but they usually mean nothing to patients. Make certain patients can understand the terminology used to explain the procedures they received.

Billing occurs in a number of different ways, with the computer-generated statement the most widely used. As mentioned in Chapter 18, an encounter form may be used as the statement, especially if payment is made at the time of the service (Figure 19-2). Typewritten statements will likely use the continuous-form billing statement that is printed on a roll with perforated edges for separation. Photocopied statements are often used with a pegboard system. The ledger cards are coordinated with the same-size copy paper. These photocopied ledgers are placed in a window envelope so that the address on the ledger card shows through the window.

If the statement is to be mailed, an enclosed self-addressed envelope is appreciated by the patient and may result in a faster turnaround of payment. Stamp the words *Address Service Requested* on the envelope just below the return address. When this statement is stamped on the envelope, a valuable tool in collections is available at minimum cost. If the statement cannot be delivered as addressed (the patient has moved or "skipped" and has left no forwarding address), the post office researches this information and returns the envelope to you with a yellow sticker providing the new address and any other updated information. If the patient has ordered that mail be forwarded, the post office will forward the statement to the patient and send the medical facility a form with the new address. There is a fee for this service.

DATE	PATIENT	SERVICE CODE	FEES CHARGED	CREDITS PAID	CREDITS ADJ.	BALANCE DUE		PREVIOUS BALANCE	NAME	RECEIPT NO.

THIS IS YOUR RECEIPT
AND/OR A STATEMENT OF YOUR ACCOUNT TO DATE

PATIENTS NAME ☐ M ☐ F
ADDRESS
CITY STATE ZIP
RELATIONSHIP BIRTHDATE
SUBSCRIBER OR POLICY HOLDER
☐ MEDICARE ☐ MEDICAID ☐ BLUE SHIELD ☐ 65-SP.
INSURANCE CARRIER
AGREEMENT #
GROUP #

OFFICE VISITS AND PROCEDURES

99211	EST PT - MINIMAL OV	1				HOSPITAL VISIT	14	
99212	EST PT - BRIEF OV	2				EMERGENCY	15	
99213	EST PT - INTERMEDIATE OV	3				CONSULTATION	16	
99214	EST PT - EXTENDED OV	4			93000	EKG	17	
99215	EST PT - COMPREHENSIVE OV	5			93224	ELECTROCARDIOGRAPHIC MONITORING	18	
99201	NEW PT - BRIEF OV	6			93307	ECHOCARDIOGRAPHY	19	
99202	NEW PT - INTERMEDIATE OV	7			85025	CBC	20	
99203	NEW PT - EXTENDED OV	8			81000	URINALYSIS WITH MICROSCOPY	21	
99204	NEW PT - COMPLEX OV	9			36415	ROUTINE VENIPUNCTURE	22	
99205	NEW PT - COMPREHENSIVE OV	10			71020	RADIOLOGY EXAM-CHEST-2 VIEWS	23	
99238	HOSPITAL DISCHARGE	11			30300	REMOVE FOR. BODY-INTRANASAL	24	
99025	NEW PT - SURGERY PROC. PRIMARY	12					25	
	NURSING HOME VISIT	13					26	

D - OTHER SERVICES

AUTHORIZATION TO RELEASE INFORMATION: I HEREBY AUTHORIZE THE UNDERSIGNED PHYSICIAN TO RELEASE ANY INFORMATION ACQUIRED IN THE COURSE OF MY EXAMINATION OR TREATMENT.
SIGNED (PATIENT, OR PARENT IF MINOR) DATE

NEXT APPOINTMENT AT AM PM
RETURN DAYS WEEKS MONTHS

PLACE OF SERVICE ☐ OFFICE ☐ OTHER
DIAGNOSIS OR SYMPTOMS
DOCTOR'S SIGNATURE

INNER CITY HEALTH CARE
8600 MAIN STREET, SUITE 200
RIVER CITY, XY 01234
(123) 456-7890

03626

FIGURE 19-2 The sample encounter form (charge slip) is a multipurpose form used to document information for insurance claims as well as to provide the patient with a receipt and documentation of procedures, diagnoses, and fees. It can be used as the patient's first bill.

A well-prepared patient statement should contain not only information for the patient but information needed to process medical insurance claims as well. The following information should be included (see Procedure 19-2):

- Patient's name and address
- Patient's insurance carrier and identification number
- Date and place of service
- Description of service and fee for each service
- Accurate procedure and diagnosis codes for insurance processing (see Chapters 16 and 17)
- Provider's signature and identification code or National Provider Identifier (NPI)
- Clinic name, address, telephone number, fax number, and Web site when applicable

Computerized Statements

By far the most common statements are computer generated. Typically, the medical assistant keys the computer command to search the patient database for outstanding balances and directs the computer to print statements.

Financial management software will age accounts (see the "Aging Accounts" section) and can generate collection letters that have been specifically designed for the practice, allowing the medical assistant to key in the appropriate specific information.

All provider orders, prescriptions, recommendations, and a copy of the visit and health summary can be waiting for the patient at the time of

PROCEDURE 19-2

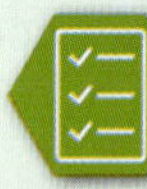

Preparing Itemized Patient Accounts for Billing

PURPOSE:

To notify patients of the fees for services rendered and collect on those accounts.

EQUIPMENT/SUPPLIES:

- Computer
- Calculator
- Electronic patient account or ledger cards
- Billing statement forms

PROCEDURE STEPS:

1. Gather all accounts and ledgers with outstanding balances. RATIONALE: Everything in one place saves time and energy.
2. Separate any accounts that are labeled as overdue. RATIONALE: Individual decisions on these accounts are necessary before taking action.
3. ***Paying attention to detail,*** and for each account, perform the following:
   a. Verify the name and address of the patient and the person responsible for payment.
   b. Place current date on the statement.
   c. Scan the account information for any possible errors.
   d. Itemize the procedures in terms patients understand and indicate charges.
   e. Identify and subtract any payments (co-payment, co-insurance, down payment) that have been made.
   f. Verify the unpaid balance that is carried forward and is due.
4. Discuss with the clinic manager any action to be taken on past-due accounts. Follow through with those instructions. RATIONALE: More than one person is involved in the collection process.
5. Place statements in envelopes and mail. RATIONALE: Ensures timely delivery of statements.

checkout, if desired. With a single key entry, an electronic invoice is generated with appropriate diagnostic and procedural codes already applied. If insurance is to be billed, the claim is automatically placed in the insurance queue to be uploaded electronically to third-party payers.

Any payments made can be posted electronically and statements can then be printed for the patient. The collection portion of the financial management software keeps up with the daily billing tasks.

MONTHLY AND CYCLE BILLING

The billing schedule is often determined by the size of the medical practice. Monthly billing is a system in which all accounts are billed at the same time each month. In a smaller clinic, monthly billing may be the most efficient method. Cycle billing staggers bills during the month and is a flexible system for larger practices.

Monthly Billing

In a monthly billing system, one or two days of each month are devoted to billing and mailing all statements. Typically, statements should leave the clinic no later than the 25th of the month to be received by the first of the following month. The major disadvantage of monthly billing is that a medical assistant may neglect other activities during this time-consuming period. To avoid these problems, billing statements may be prepared intermittently over a one- or two-week period and stored until the mailing date. To avoid confusion caused by delays in mailing, a message to "Disregard if payment has already been made" should be printed on the form. Patients become annoyed and the practice appears disorganized if a statement arrives several days after payment has been made.

Cycle Billing

In a cycle billing system, all accounts usually are divided alphabetically into groups, with each group billed at a different time. In this way, administrative personnel with numerous bills to process each month will be able to handle them in a more efficient manner. Statements are prepared on the same schedule each month. They can be mailed as they are completed, or held and mailed at one time. A typical cycle billing schedule is shown in Figure 19-3. The system can be varied to suit the needs of the individual practice.

Sample of Cycle Billing

1. Divide the alphabet into four sections: A to F, G to L, M to R, S to Z.
2. Prepare statements for patients whose last names begin with A through F on Wednesday and mail them on Thursday of Week 1.
3. Prepare statements for patients whose last names begin with G through L on Wednesday and mail them on Thursday of Week 2.
4. Prepare statements for patients whose last names begin with M through R on Wednesday and mail them on Thursday of Week 3.
5. Prepare statements for patients whose last names begin with S through Z on Wednesday and mail them on Thursday of Week 4.

FIGURE 19-3 Typical schedule for cycle billing system.

PAST-DUE ACCOUNTS

As efficient and effective as the billing process may be, there will still be collections on some accounts. The most common reasons for past-due accounts include:

- *Inability to pay.* People may have financial hardships from time to time (see Chapter 18).
- *Negligence.* People may forget to make a payment because they have been away or dealing with a family emergency.
- *Unwillingness to pay.* When a patient complains about a charge or refuses to pay, it may have nothing to do with finances. Often, they are dissatisfied with the care or treatment they have received. These patients should be referred to the provider or office manager for immediate attention.
- *Third-party payers.* Past-due accounts may result because of inaccurate or insufficient insurance information. Claims can be rejected because of many varied reasons, and time limits must be observed.
- *Minors.* Minors who are not legally emancipated may seek and receive treatment, but they are not responsible for paying the bill (see Chapter 6). If the medical practice treats minors who are not emancipated, a clinic policy should determine how these minors pay for their services. Emancipated minors are responsible for their bills. Many facilities ask for cash at the time of the service.

COLLECTION PROCESS

The process of collecting delinquent accounts begins with first establishing how much has been owed and for how long.

Ideally, collection of accounts receivable should be prompt and conducted in a timely fashion. Management consultants recommend collecting at least a portion of the fees at the time of service and that a **collection ratio** of 90% or better should be maintained. Another important factor is the **accounts receivable ratio**, which measures the speed with which outstanding accounts are paid. The desirable accounts receivable ratio is less than 2 months for collection of accounts receivable.

Collection Ratio

A collection ratio is a method used to gauge the effectiveness of the clinic's billing practices. This ratio shows the status of collections and the possible losses in the medical facility. It is a good idea to obtain the ratio monthly, quarterly, and yearly. Typically, the collection ratio is calculated by dividing the total collections by the net charges (gross or total charges minus any adjustments). This yields a percentage that is referred to as the collection ratio. See the following example:

$$\frac{\text{Total Amount Collected This Month}}{\text{Total Monthly Charges Minus Adjustments}} = \text{Monthly Collection Ratio}$$

$$\frac{\$34{,}650}{\$44{,}928} = .7712 \text{ or } 77\%$$

In this sample, you can determine that more time and energy needs to be spent in collecting accounts. The practice is losing almost 25% of its income potential. Not only is the income potential being lost but also the ability to invest that income is lost, making the potential loss even greater.

Accounts Receivable Ratio

An accounts receivable ratio indicates how quickly outstanding accounts are paid. It can also be a measure of how effective the collections are. To calculate the accounts receivable ratio, divide the current accounts receivable balance by the average monthly gross charges. This yields the typical turnaround for collecting accounts receivable. See the following example:

$$\frac{\text{Current Accounts Receivable}}{\text{Average Monthly Gross Charges}} = \text{Accounts Receivable Ratio}$$

$$\frac{\$145{,}048}{\$44{,}928} = 3.2$$

Because the goal of the accounts receivable ratio is payment in less than 2 months, you can quickly observe that this practice is over 1 month behind in collections. Chapter 20 gives additional information on accounts receivable and collection ratios.

The longer a practice delays attempting to collect delinquent accounts, the less chance there is of receiving payment. Statistics show that the value of the dollar decreases rapidly in the collection process. That is, the more time and energy put into collections, the less value received in return. You may manage to collect the full amount due, but when you consider the time and expense involved, it may not have been worth the effort and expense. Therefore, the value of the debt to be received after successful collection must be considered when determining how aggressive to be in debt collections.

AGING ACCOUNTS

Account aging is a method of identifying how long an account has been overdue. This means that past-due accounts are identified according to the length of time they have been unpaid. When using a pegboard bookkeeping system, color-coded strips are attached to the ledger cards to show the age of an account, or the cards can be stored behind a color-coded divider in a separate file labeled "Unpaid." For example, a red strip might be used for accounts 1 month overdue, a blue strip for accounts 2 months overdue, and other colors for additional months overdue. A written code such as "OD3/2/23" should be written on the ledger card to indicate when the overdue notice was mailed, meaning "Overdue notice No. 3 mailed on February 23."

Depending on the type of patient served, different aging systems are used. In a computerized billing system, the accounts are automatically aged, and the aging schedule or process is shown on the computerized ledger.

Computerized Aging

Aging accounts using a computer software system is simple. Before printing billing statements, the medical assistant keys the appropriate commands to age the accounts. The program can age accounts according to several criteria: for example, by past due balance, zero balance, or credit balance accounts. Accounts can also be aged by government agency category or by insurance carrier. All Medicare or Medicaid accounts might be aged separately from other accounts. Sorting out Medicare and Medicaid accounts may also be done when computing the accounts receivable ratio and the collection ratio.

The computer can also generate and print an accounts receivable report showing each overdue account, the balance overdue, and a breakdown showing how long the account has been overdue. This breakdown is usually divided into accounts 0 to 30 days overdue, 31 to 60 days overdue, 61 to 90 days overdue, and 90 days or more overdue. Additional reports can be generated from the accounts receivable report. For example, the clinic staff may wish to print a report showing accounts that have been delinquent for more than 90 days or accounts that are delinquent by more than a certain dollar amount.

COLLECTION TECHNIQUES

Clinic settings use both telephone and written communications in their collection techniques. Although both have some measure of effectiveness, some practices prefer to call the patient with a past-due account before officially initiating collection proceedings. The patient may have misplaced the statement, forgotten a payment, or been away on an extended vacation; a quick telephone call can often resolve the situation without the time and expense involved in collections. Also, the patient usually appreciates the courtesy and personal approach.

Many patients work part or full time, which sometimes makes telephone calls difficult to complete. It is often beneficial for providers to ask the office manager or the medical assistant in charge of collections to work 2 or more hours one evening a week for the purpose of making collection telephone calls. Calls are more likely to be answered in the time period from 5 PM to 8 PM than during the middle of the day. Figure 19-4 shows a sample collections policy.

SAMPLE COLLECTION POLICY SCHEDULE

- Encounter form (if used) given to patient at time of visit.
- Itemized statement sent no later than the end of that month.
- Itemized statement with overdue notice no later than the end of the second month.
- Telephone call reminding the patient of the bill. "We've sent two statements and we haven't received payment. Do you need more information from us?" Offer help at this point in establishing a payment schedule, and seek to get a commitment from the patient.
- If a financial schedule is to be established, prepare it and mail to the patient within a day of the phone conversation. Follow up on that commitment within 15 days. The follow-up message may be a thank you for sending the first payment. Carefully monitor payments and their timeliness.
- If no payment schedule is made by the patient, send a letter stating the amount due before the account is past due three months. Discuss with office manager and/or physician regarding the merit of continued collection at this time.
- If collections are to continue, notify the patient one more time of his or her responsibility and ask for payment.
- If no payment is received, send a letter stating that "Your account has been turned over to a collection agency" if outside collectors are used. Make no more phone calls.*

*Some physicians send a letter of discharge to patients at this time via certified mail. (See Chapter 6.)

FIGURE 19-4 Sample collection policy.

Billing Insurance Carriers

Many patients have some form of medical insurance (see Chapter 16). Make it a practice to send each computer claim within 2 days or less of the patient account data being entered into the computer. Batches of claims to insurance carriers should be forwarded at the end of each day. In the era of electronic claims processing, much time is saved in not having to prepare hard copies of the forms for mailing. Electronic claims transmission (ECT; also known as electronic medical claims, or EMC, and electronic claims submission, or ECS) dictates that the practice's computer system must be able to communicate with the insurance carrier's computer. This paperless process yields fewer errors than the manual process because ECT software includes some built-in checks to determine any invalid codes, sex or age conflicts, and correct procedure and diagnostic code linkages to the services provided. Insurance claims sent via the paper route will take more time to process, and the turnaround time for payment is also longer. Most claim departments of insurance carriers and government agencies have large numbers of employees with varying levels of experience. Payment can be delayed because of an overburdened claim department, a form that has been lost in transit, a misfiled form, an inexperienced employee, or numerous other reasons.

The medical assistant should maintain an up-to-date claims register or insurance-pending report and take firm control of the practice's collection procedures to ensure that claims are paid promptly.

This claims register or insurance-pending report may be a part of the computerized billing system. If so, the printout will show how much the practice charged insurance carriers and how much was received. This clearly shows which carriers are slower than others and where other problems might arise. For any claim pending more than 45 days, it is a good idea to make a call to the carrier to find out whether the claim has been received, where it is in the process, and whether the clinic staff might have done something to delay the process. Such phone calls can become carefully cultivated personal contacts with insurance representatives to pave the way for cooperation in the future.

In clinics where the medical assistant files claims for patients, a follow-up collection policy is important to maintain strong cash flow. When carriers do not pay in full or question or deny a claim, the medical assistant should determine the nature of the problem and rebill or appeal the decision, whichever action is appropriate.

Telephone Collections

Presentation

The medical assistant is likely to use the telephone for collection procedures. Telephoning is often an effective measure because a patient may respond to a call more than to a bill received in the mail.

A successful telephone collection call is enhanced by keeping to the facts and being tactful, pleasant, and diplomatic. When making calls to patients regarding past-due accounts, there are some things to keep in mind to maintain the desired relationship with patients. Always remain courteous and respectful. Do not treat patients with suspicion or threats. Remember, the health profession is dedicated to helping people; avoid antagonizing patients.

Most people do not let their bills become past due on purpose or out of spite. Keep this in mind when making calls. Work with patients to encourage and enable them to pay any fees they owe.

Legal

Integrity

Certain legal rules and ethical guidelines govern telephone collections:

- When making collection calls, callers must identify themselves and ascertain that they are talking to the person who is responsible for the account.
- A collection call could be embarrassing to the patient; therefore, it should not be made to the patient's place of employment.
- In most states, a debtor may be contacted only between 8 AM and 9 PM.
- Do not make telephone calls at odd hours or make repeated calls to the debtor's friends, employers, or relatives.
- If a contact must be made to the debtor's place of business, do not reveal to any third party the nature of the call. Patients have a right to confidentiality and privacy.
- Do not threaten to turn the person's account over to collection agencies.

When collecting by telephone, it is helpful to keep complete, accurate records of the process indicating who said what and how much was promised as payment. If after 2 weeks nothing has been resolved as a result of the calls, then another course of action may be the solution, especially for large sums of money owed. Collection letters may be necessary.

Fair Debt Collection Practices Act. Violating rules regarding harassment makes the caller vulnerable to charges under the **Fair Debt Collection Practices Act (FDCPA)**. According to the guidelines set by the FDCPA, which is overseen by the Federal Trade Commission (FTC), debt collectors are not allowed to use their positions to collect a debt using any manner of work performance that is found to be abusive, deceptive, or unethical. The collectors must abide by certain guidelines, such as not calling a debtor at work without written consent and keeping calls to debtors between the hours of 8 AM and 9 PM. Under the FDCPA, debts that are created by medical expenses are a type of debt that can be sent to collection agencies and subsequently collected upon. The collectors are strictly prohibited from using profane language or any language that indicates a threat (such as wage or tax refund garnishment). It is very important that the administrative medical assistant abide by such guidelines as given within the FDCPA.

Collection Letters

Collection letters are sent to encourage patients to pay overdue balances. After two statements are mailed to patients and the charge slip or encounter form has brought no response, the clinic begins sending collection letters.

Lack of payment from a patient may not be considered serious until after 60 days. When the patient fails to respond to the encounter form, to the statement, or to a 60-day statement with an "Overdue" remark, a series of collection letters begins. One typical collection letter series is shown in Figures 19-5A through Figure 19-5C. Collection letters and notes are kept separate from a patient's chart.

USE OF AN OUTSIDE COLLECTION AGENCY

Occasionally, the clinic turns over highly delinquent accounts to an outside collection agency. Discretion is always advised here, however, because the fees to be collected may not justify the expense of collection. For unpaid accounts with large balances, however, this is often a viable solution.

One service provided by a collection agency is an intercept letter. For a nominal fee, this letter may be sent from the agency as the last resort before the account is turned over to collection. This communication alerts patients to the fact that if a response is not received, their account will go to collection. This often is the only action needed for the patient to pay the outstanding bill. Another service of a credit bureau or collection agency is to provide credit ratings of patients at the provider's request. Providers who pay for this service are able to monitor patients' ability to pay their bills, as well as to trace a "skip," someone who leaves with an outstanding bill and no forwarding address.

When selecting a collection agency, be certain to hire one that is compatible with the medical practice's philosophy. Questions that might be asked of potential collection agencies include the following:

- Does the agency handle only medical and dental accounts?
- What methods are used to make collections?
- Is the agency fee a flat charge per account or a percentage of the account recovered?
- How promptly does the agency settle accounts?
- Will the agency supply a list of satisfied customers or references?
- What ability does the medical practice have to end the agency's collection efforts?

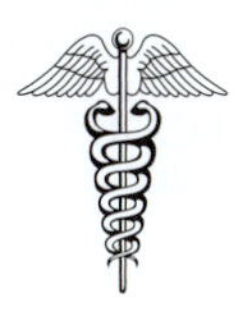

INNER CITY HEALTH CARE
8600 MAIN STREET, SUITE 200
RIVER CITY, XY 01234

June 14, 20XX

Mr. John O'Keefe
12 Gravers Lane
Northborough, XY 12345

Dear Mr. O'Keefe:

Your account with our clinic is three months past due, and you have not responded to our previous requests for payment. Please pay your balance of $852 at this time, or contact us with a plan for payment.

Please call me at (123) 456-7890 if you have a question about your account or a plan for payment. Otherwise, we expect your payment immediately.

Sincerely,

Marilyn Johnson
Clinic Manager

A

FIGURE 19-5 Sample collection letters. (A) First letter. *(continues)*

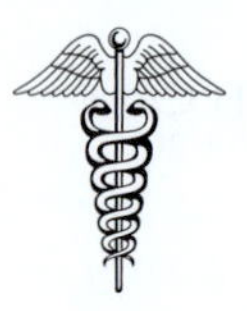

INNER CITY HEALTH CARE
8600 MAIN STREET, SUITE 200
RIVER CITY, XY 01234

July 15, 20XX

Mr. John O'Keefe
12 Gravers Lane
Northborough, XY 12345

Dear Mr. O'Keefe:

Your son, Chris, was seriously ill in March when he was seen by Dr. King. Dr. King used her experience and education to treat Chris, believing you would pay your account within a reasonable amount of time.

Four months have passed and you have still not remitted the $852 outstanding balance on your account. We cannot continue to keep your unpaid account on our books. If you are experiencing financial difficulties, please call the clinic at (123) 456-7890 so we can arrange a payment schedule that is agreeable to both of us.

Sincerely,

Marilyn Johnson
Clinic Manager

B

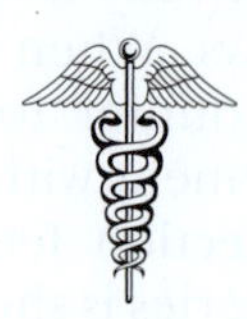

INNER CITY HEALTH CARE
8600 MAIN STREET, SUITE 200
RIVER CITY, XY 01234

August 17, 20XX

CERTIFIED MAIL

Mr. John O'Keefe
12 Gravers Lane
Northborough, XY 12345

Dear Mr. O'Keefe:

This is our final attempt to collect your account of $852, which is five months past due. You have not responded to all our previous letters [or letters and phone calls], so we have no alternative but to turn over your account to a collection company.

Your account is being assigned to Ambler Medical Collection Service, which will pursue whatever legal means is necessary to collect this debt. If you contact me at (123) 456-7890 within seven days, we can prevent the account from this assignment and resolve the balance.

Sincerely,

Marilyn Johnson
Clinic Manager

C

FIGURE 19-5 *(continued)* (B) Second letter. (C) Third letter.

Once a collection agency has been selected, carefully follow their instructions about any contact patients make with the medical clinic regarding their account as well as any other guidelines in their contract with the practice. Keep a record of accounts given to the agency, as well as their rate of return. Hopefully, the agency will be able to motivate patients to pay for the health care services they have received while still maintaining the practice's good reputation and increasing your profit margin. Medical collections let your patients know that the practice is serious about collecting past-due accounts.

There is often a question about how payments from collection agencies are posted. This is one purpose of the adjustment column. Place the amount received in the adjustment column because it is a subtraction from the amount due. If there is no adjustment column, put the amount in the charge column and put red parentheses around it or circle in red so the amount is actually subtracted from the balance. The remaining balance after collections are paid is written off (Procedure 19-3).

USE OF SMALL CLAIMS COURT

In certain circumstances, a clinic's manager may consider bringing a case to small claims court. Typically, small claims courts handle cases that involve only limited amounts of debt (these vary from state to state), they usually do not permit representation by an attorney, and they are generally efficient and streamlined in their proceedings. Nonetheless, preparing for small claims courts and taking time to appear will require a certain investment of staff. It is important to note that if the court finds in the clinic's favor,

PROCEDURE 19-3

Posting/Recording Collection Agency Adjustments

PURPOSE:

To keep track of financial adjustments.

EQUIPMENT/SUPPLIES:

- Manual bookkeeping system or computerized system
- Patient's account
- Black and red ink pens for use in manual bookkeeping system
- Computerized PM system

PROCEDURE STEPS:

1. If using a manual system, use the daily schedule of services/charges in front of you (the manual daily sheet), enter amount received from the collection agency on a patient's account and a note such as "Payment from ABC Collection Agency" in the explanation section. If using a PM system, use the payment posting module and locate the patient record. RATIONALE: Indicates funds received on a collection contract.
2. Record the amount received and the explanation in the patient's account as well.
   a. Using a manual system, post the amount received by subtracting from the account balance. Use the adjustment column to write off the balance amount. This should zero out the account.
   b. In a PM system, post the amount received to the patient account from the collection agency, and adjust the balance to zero out the account. RATIONALE: Clearly indicates what portion of the account the patient has paid and the amount that is not collectible. In a manual system, the difference between the amount collected and amount paid by the collection agency (including the agency's fee) is entered as a negative adjustment. In a PM system, this is tracked within the software. At the end of the year, totals can be obtained for the practice's income tax preparation.

the clinic still must collect the money from the defendant. An account assigned to a collection agency cannot be addressed in small claims court.

SPECIAL COLLECTION SITUATIONS

In patient billing and collections, a number of special situations may arise.

Bankruptcy

If a patient has declared bankruptcy, statements may no longer be sent nor may any attempts be made to collect delinquent accounts. A patient declaring bankruptcy usually does so under Chapter 7 or Chapter 13 bankruptcy law. In a Chapter 7 bankruptcy, a patient declares bankruptcy to all debtors and is allowed to clear all debts and start fresh. The medical clinic should file a proof-of-claim form and provide a copy of the patient's outstanding account to the bankruptcy court. In a Chapter 13 bankruptcy, also known as a "wage-earner's bankruptcy," patients (wage-earners) are protected from bill collectors and are allowed to pay their bills over a specified time. The court determines a monthly amount that the debtor can pay, collects that sum, and parcels it out to the creditors over a period as long as five years. The clinic must file a claim as directed by the debtor's attorney to collect any fees outstanding. Because a provider's fee is an unsecured debt, it is one of the last to be paid. Bankruptcy laws are federal and are subject to the Federal Wage Garnishment Law regarding attaching property to satisfy debt.

Estates

Collection of fees when a patient has died must be directed to the executor of the estate or the one responsible for overseeing the estate. Some general guidelines to follow include:

- Show courtesy by not sending a statement in the first week or so after a death.
- Prepare an itemized statement of the deceased patient's account. (In some cases, a special form is required for this.)
- Mail the account information via certified mail with a return receipt requested to the administrator of the estate. The name can be obtained by calling the probate department of the superior court.
- If there is no known or identified administrator, send a copy of the itemized statement to the "Estate of (name of patient)" at the patient's last known address. Often, a family member has assumed the responsibility for paying the patient's account balances.
- If unsure of how to proceed, contact the clinic's attorney or the clerk of the **probate court** for advice.

Tracing "Skips"

Legal

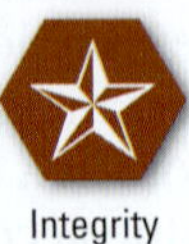
Integrity

A "skip" is a patient with an unpaid bill who has apparently moved with no forwarding address. If a statement is returned to your clinic marked "no forwarding address," first determine if any internal errors were made in addressing the envelope. If the address is determined to be correct, the medical assistant may try to call the patient at the telephone number on the patient ledger; it is possible that the patient has retained the same number, or there may be a new number given. If the medical assistant is unable to secure a telephone number, the facility needs to decide whether to pursue the unpaid debt. This will depend on clinic policy and the amount that is owed. If it is decided to pursue an unpaid account, it can be turned over to a collection agency. If the medical assistant attempts to trace the skip by calling employers or relatives, it is important not to violate any laws in doing so and to maintain the patient's confidentiality.

STATUTE OF LIMITATIONS

Legal

A **statute of limitations** is a statute that defines the period in which legal action may take place. When applying this concept to collections, the time period is usually defined by the class into which the account falls. These include open book accounts, which may have periodic charges against them; written contracts; and single-entry accounts, which have only one charge against them. The time period in which legal action must take place against any of these accounts varies from state to state. If an unpaid account is more than 3 years old, it is wise to investigate the statute of limitations in your state before spending time and effort in collections. (For state-by-state information on the statute of limitations on debts, see www.creditinfocenter.com, under "Debts.")

MAINTAIN A PROFESSIONAL ATTITUDE

Presentation

Collecting past-due accounts is one of the most difficult tasks delegated to medical assistants. Not everyone is able to perform this task. Placing calls can be discouraging, especially if the results seem less than anticipated. Not all accounts can be collected. Identify these accounts early, write them off, and save the medical practice time and money. Keep any bias and your emotions out of the process. Rely only on your information, the aged account, and the realization that the clinic policy is well thought out and provides a win–win solution for both the patient and the provider as much as possible. When dealing with a "true deadbeat" who has no intention of paying the bill, be proud of your provider's attention to that patient's need, but discuss with the provider the possibility of discharging the patient. Staff may need additional training and education from time to time to update skills on patient service and how to maintain goodwill during the collection process.

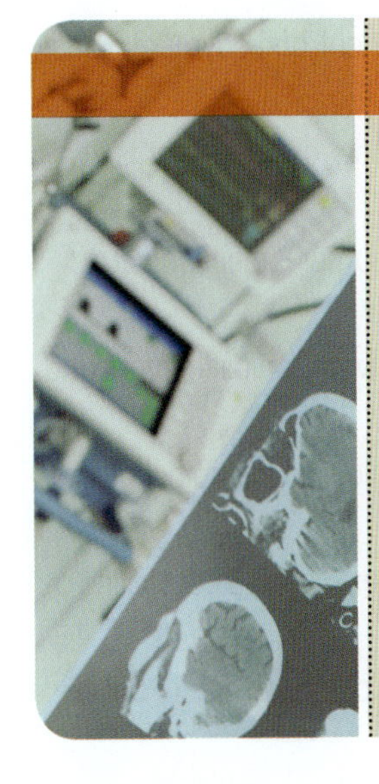

CASE STUDY 19-1

Refer to the scenario at the beginning of the chapter. For patient accounts more than 60 days overdue, Inner City Health Care begins a series of collection proceedings to attempt to collect the monies. Initially, they place a telephone call to the patient to determine whether a billing problem might be present that can be clarified over the telephone. If they cannot reach the patient or the patient does not respond to the call, then collections begin. Marilyn has assigned this function of the billing process to Ellen Armstrong, CMAS (AMT), because Ellen has a warm telephone manner and is good with patients.

CASE STUDY REVIEW

1. Why is Ellen's telephone manner important in the collection process?
2. In addition to telephone collections, what patient letters might Ellen send?
3. Ellen has come across an account that is delinquent and discovers that the patient has declared bankruptcy. What can Ellen do now?

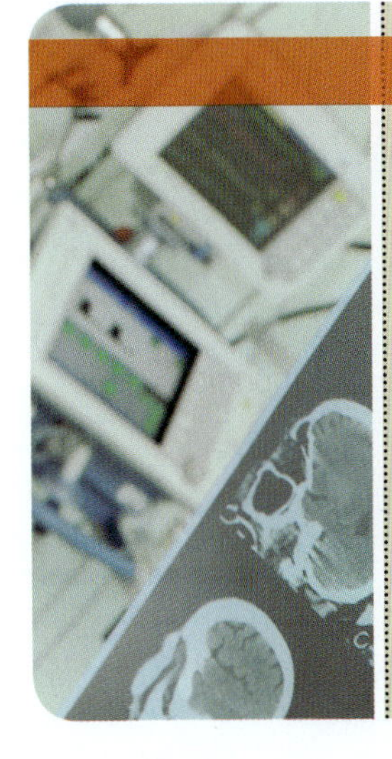

CASE STUDY 19-2

Morgan Bryant is the custodial parent and single mother of her 5-year-old son Custer, who has been a patient of Inner City Pediatric Clinic since his birth. Custer's father's insurance covered his medical expenses. During a separation and the resulting divorce, the medical bills continued to go to Custer's father. Morgan comes to the reception desk to discuss the collection letter she received. Her parenting plan requires her former husband to provide medical coverage for their son. However, it appears he canceled his policy coverage on his son 4 months ago and Morgan did not know this until she received the letter. Morgan is in tears.

CASE STUDY REVIEW

1. What is the first step the administrative medical assistant should take?
2. Is there anything the clinic staff might have done differently in collecting this account?
3. What might be done for Morgan now? Are any resources available to Morgan?

Summary

- The cash flow and collection process are dependent on up-to-date and accurate billing techniques.
- The financial status of the practice is reflected in monthly statements indicating unpaid patient balances, which will need to be reviewed regularly for appropriate action, including possible referral to a collection agency.
- Timeliness and accuracy have a significant influence on prompt payment and how soon collection of the patient account will be finalized.
- Understanding the formal credit and collections protocols of the clinic in order to educate patients of their financial responsibilities, thereby promoting cooperation and compliance from patients when collecting payments, is the responsibility of the medical assistant.
- Co-payments and other payments should be collected at the time of service.
- Medical assistants must have knowledge of the insurance plans accepted by the clinic, and alert patients when benefits are being used out of network, or are noncovered benefits.
- The medical assistant should discuss services not covered by the insurance plan with the patient, and payment plans that may be available to the patient if needed.
- The medical assistant should have knowledge of solutions and resources for uninsured or underinsured patients, including payment plans, when available.
- The medical assistant must be familiar with the Truth-in-Lending Act, Regulation Z of the Consumer Protection Act of 1967, as it applies to credit and collections in the clinic.
- The medical assistant is responsible for gathering data on collection ratios and account receivable ratios to target and achieve goals that keep outstanding balances to a minimum, and cash flow at a maximum.
- Medical personnel must use proper collection techniques, both by telephone and by letter, following the guidelines of the Fair Debt Collections Practices Act.
- Special collection resources can be used when needed, including small claims court, billing estates and contacting a probate court, and tracing skips properly, within the law.
- You must be aware of state laws regarding the statue of limitations for collection outstanding balances, and of bankruptcy laws for Chapter 7 and Chapter 13, the two most common types.

Study for Success

To reinforce your knowledge and skills of information presented in this chapter:

- Review the *Key Terms* and *Learning Outcomes*
- Consider the *Case Studies* and discuss your conclusions
- Answer the questions in the *Certification Review*

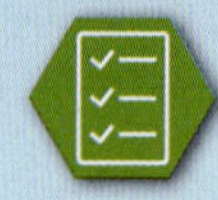

Procedure

- Perform the *Procedures* using the *Competency Assessment Checklists* on the *Student Companion Website*

CERTIFICATION REVIEW

1. Which of the following is true of the Truth-In-Lending Act?
   a. It is designed to place limits on the amount of debt for which consumers are liable.
   b. It is also known as the statute of limitations.
   c. It is also known as Regulation Z.
   d. It does not apply to medical facilities.
2. Which of the following is an accurate description of cycle billing?
   a. It is completed every fourth month.
   b. It is done only by computer.
   c. It is completed by the 25th of the month.
   d. It is a system in which accounts are divided into sections for billing purposes.
   e. It is done on a daily basis.
3. What is one of the most common reasons why patient bills go unpaid?
   a. Inability to pay because of financial hardship
   b. Patients consider the cost of medical care too high
   c. Patients think their insurance should cover all medical bills
   d. Patients think providers make too much money
4. What is the definition of aging accounts?
   a. It is a process of identifying overdue patient accounts.
   b. It describes patients who have a long-term relationship with the ambulatory care center.
   c. It describes older adult patients with Medicare.
   d. It applies to accounts considered inactive.
   e. It is the date the account is paid in full.
5. What happens when an unpaid account goes to small claims court?
   a. The medical clinic must engage an attorney representative.
   b. The medical clinic is still responsible for collecting even if the court finds in its favor.
   c. There is no need to show up at court.
   d. A large sum of money must be at issue.
6. Which of the following is true of a collection ratio?
   a. It shows status of collections and possible losses.
   b. It divides the current accounts receivable by the average monthly gross charges.
   c. It should be 90% or better.
   d. It is the amount of cash collected each day.
   e. Both a and c
7. What is a claims register?
   a. It identifies how many past-due claims have been collected.
   b. It may also be called the insurance-pending report.
   c. It is maintained by each insurance carrier for the provider.
   d. It is a tickler file that maintains all patients' insurance information.
8. Which statement below is true about using the telephone to help collect money from patients?
   a. Calls are best made after 8 PM when patients are home.
   b. Collections must abide by the Fair Debt Collection Practice Act.
   c. Collections are usually successful after numerous calls at the patient's place of employment.
   d. The collections process will require overtime pay for the medical clinic staff.
   e. Telephone collections are not an effective tool.
9. What is the definition of a "skip"?
   a. The time period when legal action cannot be taken
   b. An estate involved in probate
   c. One who moves without a forwarding address and leaves an unpaid bill
   d. One who has paid a portion of a debt
10. Which of the following is true regarding using a collection agency for patient accounts?
    a. It is better if the agency handles only medical and dental accounts.
    b. It creates a bad feeling between patients and providers.
    c. It cannot possibly do as good a job as the medical clinic staff.
    d. The agency seldom describes its methods for collections.
    e. The agency is used to collect highly delinquent accounts.

CHAPTER 20

Accounting Practices

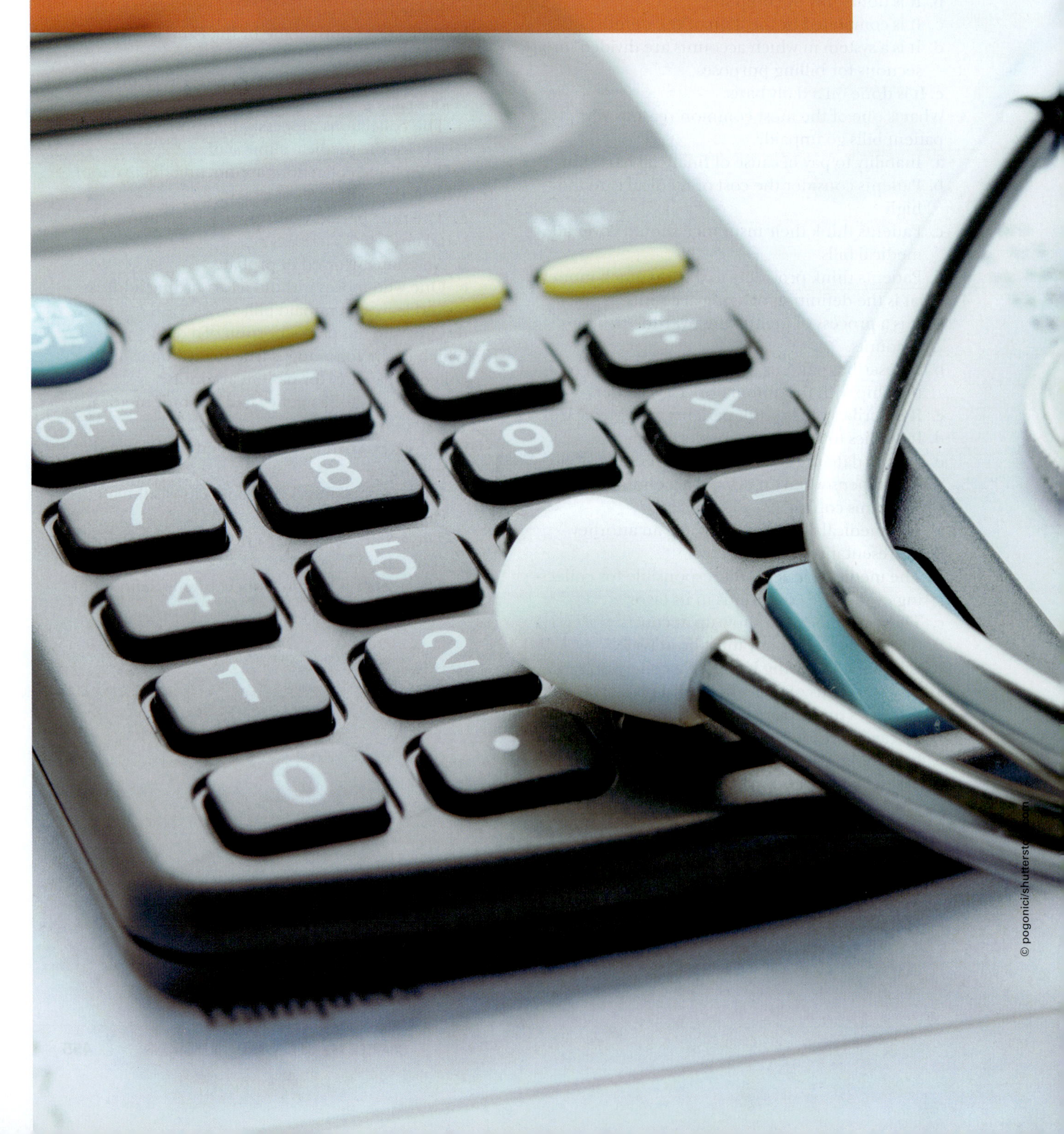

LEARNING OUTCOMES

1. Define and spell the key terms as presented in the glossary.
2. Explain basic bookkeeping computations.
3. Explain the purpose and range of the accounting function in the clinic.
4. Describe the four different types of bookkeeping and accounting systems.
5. Recall the importance of the day-end summary and the accounts receivable trial balance.
6. Compare and contrast financial, managerial, and cost accounting.
7. Explain the use and validity of the income statement and the balance sheet.
8. Recall three useful financial ratios and explain them in detail.
9. Identify the proper steps in accounts payable management.
10. Discuss the impact of utilization review on reimbursement.
11. Discuss legal and ethical guidelines in accounting practices.

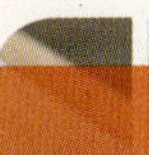

KEY TERMS

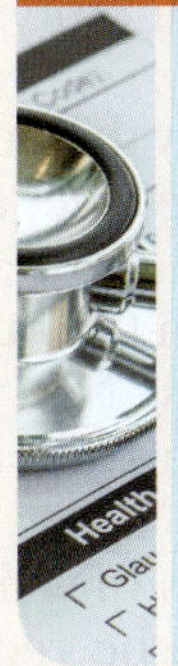

- accounting
- accounts payable
- accounts receivable (A/R) ratio
- accrual basis
- assets
- balance sheet
- cash basis
- check register
- collection ratio
- cost accounting
- cost analysis
- cost ratio
- financial accounting
- fixed cost
- income statement
- liability
- managerial accounting
- owner's equity
- trial balance
- utilization review (UR)
- variable cost

SCENARIO

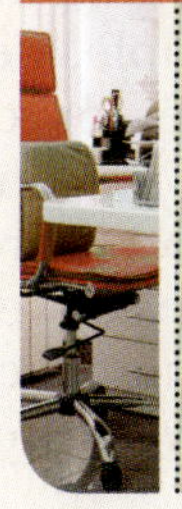

When Mark King, one of the owners at Inner City Health Care, and clinic manager Marilyn Johnson, CMA (AAMA), decided to add a new medical assistant to the staff, they first reviewed the financial records for the previous year. Although the volume of work in the center generated the need for an additional employee, King and Johnson had to be sure it was financially feasible. In addition to past records, they also had to make some projections for the upcoming year; with certain new managed care fees, they had to be sure that anticipated revenues would be sufficient to sustain the salary of a new employee.

Chapter Portal

Medical financial management in the private practice setting is vitally important in the daily functioning of the medical clinic business. It directly affects overall bookkeeping and accounting procedures. Accounting generates financial information for the clinic and is defined as a system of monitoring the financial status of a facility and the specific results of its activities. It provides financial information for decision making.

Previous chapters have included the topics of proper daily bookkeeping financial practices (see Chapter 18), the accurate coding and the specific processing of insurance forms (see Chapters 16 and 17), and the efficient management of collecting on accounts (see Chapter 19). All of these functions are essential to obtaining maximum reimbursement and creating profitability for the practice.

This chapter ties many of these elements together and creates a total picture of their interdependence. Each element is critical to accurate accounting practices in the medical clinic.

BOOKKEEPING AND ACCOUNTING SYSTEMS

Medical practices use a variety of methods to monitor their financial accounts and the total financial operations of the business. Although some clinics still use the single-entry bookkeeping and pegboard systems, the majority prefer double-entry or computerized systems, or a combination.

Financial records should provide the following information at all times:

- Amount earned in a given period
- Amount collected in a given period
- Amount owed in a given period
- Where the expenses were incurred in a given period

The financial records can show these data as often as you like, usually on a monthly, quarterly, or yearly basis. Comparisons can be made with similar periods. Analysis of the financial data can help to determine if some services are not profitable, whether the practice is experiencing healthy growth, or why a loss might be realized. The accounts receivable and accounts payable data are vital to this information.

Single-Entry System

The single-entry system has been used in medical practices for many years. This includes a daily journal or log, patients' statements or accounts, ledgers, checks, and disbursement (expenditure) records. Information is first recorded in the journal, which provides a chronological record of financial transactions. Information from the journal is then transferred to the ledger through the process of posting. All amounts entered in the journal must be posted to the accounts kept in the ledger to summarize the results. This system has been used because of its simplicity and inexpensive nature. However, it is difficult to find errors because there are no internal controls, and financial analysis information is inadequate.

Pegboard System

As discussed in Chapter 18, the pegboard, or "write-it-once," system is easier to use than the single-entry system and has greater internal controls. The pegboard system provides control over collections, payments, and charges. It uses NCR (no carbon required) forms that are layered or shingled on pegs on the left of the board so that both income and disbursement entries need to be written only once. Many pegboard systems include a charge slip (or encounter form), which simplifies third-party payment processing for both the medical practice and the patients. The charge slip is used to record the input needed during the patient's visit, while serving as the patient's receipt for services performed and fees charged. An advantage of the pegboard system is its accuracy, because data are entered at the time of service and not recopied, so fewer errors can creep in.

Double-Entry System

The double-entry system is based on the fact that each transaction has two aspects, that is, a dual effect on the accounting elements. This system is based on the accounting principle that assets equal liabilities plus owner's equity.

Assets = Liabilities + Owner's Equity

Assets are the properties owned by the business (supplies, equipment, accounts receivable, and so on). **Liabilities** include what is owed to creditors. **Owner's equity** is the amount by which the business assets exceed the business liabilities. Net worth, proprietorship, and capital are often used as synonyms for owner's equity.

The double-entry system requires that the two aspects involved in every transaction be recorded on each side of the equation and that the two sides always be in balance. Although this accounting system requires time and skill, it provides a comprehensive financial picture and has built-in accuracy controls. It is orderly, fairly simple, flexible, and accurate, making it impossible for certain types of errors to remain undetected for long. For example, if one aspect of a transaction is properly recorded but the other aspect is overlooked, the records are out of balance. This occurrence may be easily discovered and subsequently corrected.

Practice Management System

The majority of medical practices rely on accounting software packages to prepare financial records, such as ledgers and reports, and to retrieve patient information. An increasing number of practices are using financial management software that is part of a practice management (PM) system. PM is a system of computerizing the entire facility and likely includes:

- Patient information data and scheduling
- Interface with electronic medical records (EMR) and electronic health records (EHR)

- Insurance coding and billing; processing claims electronically
- Management and human resources; payroll, purchases, personnel records
- Bookkeeping and accounting; generation of financial records including business income and expenses

A computerized accounting system is most likely to be based on the principles of either the pegboard (write-it-once) or a double-entry bookkeeping system, or a combination of both.

A computer financial system can be customized to meet the needs of the practice. Most large multi-speciality clinics have a computer system designed particularly for their needs. A PM system has the capability of including the most common procedure and diagnostic codes within a database to be recalled when completing insurance claim forms. The software will assist in matching the charges with the appropriate diagnosis codes.

A PM system has the flexibility of assigning codes in other categories to indicate whether a bill has been paid with cash, with a check, or by a third-party payer. Codes may also be assigned to identify the place of service and the professional performing the service. This facilitates the tracking of payments and also allows for the analysis of specific sources that generate income for the practice. Adjustments to reflect discounts or reduced fees may also be entered into the computer. The software is used in the preparation of billing statements, insurance forms, collection letters, and a number of financial ratios and statements to assist in monitoring the practice's financial stability.

Computer and Billing Service Bureaus

An option for clinics that choose not to purchase accounting software or a PM system in their practice is to use a computer service bureau for billing purposes and the creation of many financial records. In this case, the clinic provides the data, and the bureau provides basic billing and accounting services, furnishing financial statements, completed insurance forms, payroll materials, and checks.

Service bureaus handle accounts from the medical facilities in one of three ways:

1. Through the clinic's own computer terminal, online sharing occurs where the clinic is tied directly to the bureau's mainframe computer
2. Through online servicing, by which the clinic has its own terminal that allows direct communication with the service bureau's computer
3. Through off-line batch processing, where the medical assistant or bookkeeper sends daily batches of data to the bureau to process

Legal

Many facilities, however, prefer to have their own computerized financial or PM system because outsourcing computer services can compromise patient confidentiality and limit control over computer usage. A proper contract should be negotiated and signed with any computer and billing service bureau to ensure confidentiality, HIPAA compliance, and strict privacy of all patient information.

DAY-END SUMMARY

The financial summary at the end of the day is a helpful tool for a quick financial analysis. Computer accounting systems automatically create the day-end summaries in the form of reports. Pegboard systems require the administrative medical assistant to total the summaries that are shown at the bottom of the day sheet.

The first section of the day sheet identifies all the financial transactions of the day. The second section includes the month-to-date totals. This is where today's totals are added to the month-to-date totals; this must be in perfect balance. The third section identifies the year-to-date accounts, which includes all accounts to obtain the year-to-date total. A deposit slip included with most systems enables the assistant to verify the cash receipts with the checks received. This is helpful in preparing the day's bank deposit.

Integrity

When the totals do not balance at the end of the day, the medical assistant must begin the search for errors.

Tips for Finding Errors

Some tips for finding errors are as follows:

- Check the addition of each column, both horizontally and vertically. If a calculator is used, check the tape for entry errors.
- Compute the difference in the totals that are out of balance. Search the day sheet and patient accounts for that exact amount.
- If the amount of the error is divisible by 9, there may be an error in transposition of numbers.
- If the amount of the error is divisible by 2, the amount may have been posted in the wrong column.

- Check your entries when manually carrying forward previous balances. It is quite easy to carry forward an incorrect amount or to place numbers incorrectly. For example, the number $750 might be carried forward as $75.

Anyone who has worked with a manual pegboard system can report horror stories of chasing errors around for several days before finding them. It might be one error in one patient's account that creates the havoc. Also, a search for an error can continue at great length even as the assistant keeps seeing and missing the error. Set the problem aside for a bit, or even a day if you are not pressed with month-end billing deadlines. Have another person check for you. Often that individual sees the error in just a few minutes.

Errors in an electronic financial system can create almost as much havoc but often can be caught earlier. If all data are entered accurately and kept up to date, an error that occurs when keying in certain data will create a warning notice that indicates the data are incorrect. Computers do not automatically update all information when fees for services are changed, reimbursement adjustments are changed, salaries are increased, or new data from the laboratory or clinical area are determined. Any time there is a person who is entering data into the system, errors can occur. All medical professionals entering any data into the system must be reminded not to rush through the process and to carefully check for accuracy.

ACCOUNTS RECEIVABLE TRIAL BALANCE

Before preparing monthly statements, a **trial balance** should be done on the accounts receivable in either a pegboard system or a computer system. The trial balance is created by totaling debit balances and credit balances to confirm that total debits equal total credits. The trial balance will indicate any problem between the daily journal and the ledger. Use the following steps to create the trial balance:

1. Pull all patient accounts that have a balance.
2. Total the balance of those accounts.
3. Create an accounts receivable total.
   a. Enter the accounts receivable at the first of the month.
   b. Add the total charges for the month and subtotal.
   c. Subtract the total payments for the month and subtotal.
   d. Subtract the total adjustments for the month.
   e. The final total is the accounts receivable at the end of the month.

This final total, the end of the month accounts receivable, must be the same as the figure received when adding all the patient account balances. If they match, the accounts are then in balance. If they do not balance, the error must be found (see Procedure 20-1).

ACCOUNTS PAYABLE

Accounts payable are an unwritten promise to pay a supplier for property or merchandise purchased on credit or for a service rendered. Accounts payable are the most common liability or financial obligation in the clinic setting. These include expenses such as medical and office supplies, salaries, equipment, and services. Payments for these expenses are made by check to ensure complete, accurate records of all money received and disbursed.

Supplies and equipment purchased usually come with a packing slip that describes the items purchased and their cost. An invoice may also be enclosed that serves as a bill for the items ordered; however, another invoice is sent to the business later as well. Take time to note on the invoice whether there is a discount for early payment. Some financial managers suggest attaching the invoice and packing slip to the purchase order. File in your tickler file or reminder file on the computer so that payment is made in a timely fashion to receive any discount. Some vendors prefer that payment not be made until a statement (or request for payment) is received from them. This is particularly the case if the practice uses that vendor more than once a month. When the statement arrives, check the invoice for accuracy before sending payment. Prepare the check for the accounts payable as appropriate, either monthly or as necessary to receive a discount (see Chapter 18). Write the check number on the invoice, as well as the amount paid, and place in a file for accounts paid according to the practice's filing system.

Disbursement Records

Computerized accounts payable systems track the disbursements and post to appropriate established accounts similar to a manual system.

PROCEDURE 20-1

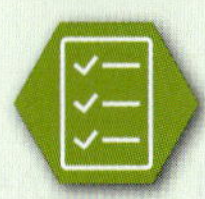

Preparing Accounts Receivable Trial Balance

PURPOSE:

To prepare a trial balance in order to determine if there is any problem between the daily journal and the ledger or patient accounts.

EQUIPMENT/SUPPLIES:

- Patient accounts
- Calculator

PROCEDURE STEPS:

1. Pull all patient accounts that have a balance due. RATIONALE: Provides only amount due information.
2. Enter the balance of those accounts into the calculator.
3. Add the balances and total. (A calculator with tape can make it quicker to check for errors.) RATIONALE: Gives you the total amount due to date.
4. Create an accounts receivable total:
   a. Enter the accounts receivable total from the first of the month into the calculator.
   b. Add total charges for this month and subtotal.
   c. Total the amount of all payments received this month.
   d. Subtract the total of payments from subtotal of b above and subtotal.
   e. Total the amount of the month's adjustments and subtract from the subtotal in d above.
   f. This total is the accounts receivable amount. RATIONALE: The end-of-the month accounts receivable total (f) above must match the total in step 3. If these totals do not match, an error has been made. If they do match, the trial balance is in order.

Computer accounts payable systems have a **check register** that records all checks written and categorizes them into separate columns, such as rent, insurance, office supplies, utilities, and so forth. These categories can be designed to be as general or detailed as preferred. The computer system also can create entries for bank deposits and payroll records.

The computer software has a check-writing file that presents checks on the screen. The information necessary to complete the check is entered at the keyboard; the computer stores it and prints out the check. Printing the checks can be done individually or by batch if several bills are being paid. The amount is automatically subtracted from the account's balance. The computer system also can recall data that need to be entered on the checks each time there is a payment. For example, the name of the company where most supplies are purchased can be recalled from the database; thus the assistant does not have to key in that information again. This feature is a particular timesaver when payroll checks are prepared (see Chapter 21).

The manual or pegboard system uses a check register page to record checks written. The check is aligned on the pegboard over the check register before completion. The pegboard checks have an NCR transfer strip that copies the date, the payee, the check number, and the amount to the check register. Pegboard checks can be designed so that the address is entered beneath the payee line and mailed in a window envelope. This check register has a number of columns to categorize expenses. All entries are totaled on the check register when completed, and these totals are carried forward. A balanced check register provides a way to verify the bank statement when it arrives. The check register can also be used for bank deposits and for payroll records.

THE ACCOUNTING FUNCTION

Accounting is a system of monitoring the financial status of a facility and the financial results of its activities. Accounting may be divided into two major categories: financial and managerial. **Financial accounting** provides information primarily for entities external to the organization such as the government. In contrast, **managerial accounting** generates financial information that can enable more efficient internal management. **Cost accounting** helps to determine what it costs the clinic to perform particular services and is an integral part of managerial accounting. A hospital cost report for Medicare is essentially a part of financial accounting because the report is generated for an external user—the Centers for Medicare and Medicaid Services (CMS), which administers the Medicare program. However, it is also a part of cost accounting because a cost report on Medicare will show what it costs to care for patients on Medicare.

COST ANALYSIS

An important aspect of the practice is **cost analysis**. The purpose of the analysis is to determine the costs of each service. There are two factors to consider: fixed costs and variable costs.

Fixed Costs

Fixed costs are costs that do not vary in total as the number of patients varies. For example, the annual depreciation cost of the equipment is fixed because it will remain the same regardless of the number of patients who use it.

Variable Costs

Variable costs are those that vary in direct proportion to patient volume, such as clinical supplies and laboratory procedures. Average costs to treat patients decline because of fixed costs, not variable costs. The greater the volume, the more widely the fixed costs are spread and the less cost any one unit is responsible for.

Patient cost factors include administrative costs, such as the cost of billing and collections, personnel costs for clinic staff providing patient care, equipment costs, and costs for clinical supplies. The provider cost will include costs for interpreting tests, diagnosing illnesses, and maintaining professional liability insurance.

Calculating and reviewing costs provide the clinic with data to set fees, market the practice, determine profit, and monitor the practice's performance.

FINANCIAL RECORDS

Indicators of the financial status of the medical facility include financial statements that reflect the daily operations of the business. These records comprise an accounting information system that is maintained for numerous reasons, one of which is to provide source data for use in the preparation of various reports. Two financial statements common to the clinic are the income/expense statement and the balance sheet.

Income Statement

Figure 20-1 shows a sample **income statement**, the most commonly generated year-end report. The sample shows the profit and expenses for a given month. The income statement shows the cumulative profit and total expenses by reporting patient income, outside revenue sources, and overhead expenses such as office and medical expenses. Provider's compensation and benefits and employees' compensation, benefits, and withholding taxes can be itemized as well.

Balance Sheet

Sometimes called the statement of financial condition or statement of financial position, the **balance sheet** is an itemized statement of the assets, liabilities, and owner's equity of a medical facility as of a specified date. Its purpose is to provide information regarding the status of these basic accounting elements.

The balance sheet is made possible through the double-entry system of accounting because every transaction is recorded by two sets of entries made in a ledger or journal. Increases in assets are recorded as debits; decreases are recorded as credits. Increases in liabilities and owner's equity are recorded as credits; decreases are recorded as debits.

Debit and credit entries to one or more accounts make up the system. In any recording, the total dollar amount of the debit entries must equal the total dollar amount of the credit entries. Each ledger or journal entry should have the following elements:

1. Date of transaction
2. Journal or ledger account names involved
3. Dollar amount of the charges
4. Brief explanation of the transaction

USEFUL FINANCIAL DATA

A business must determine how and when it will report income earned. There are two systems for doing this. The **accrual basis** reports income at the time charges are generated. This is used mainly in commercial environments. The **cash basis** is most often used in medical practices. In the cash basis, income is recognized when money is collected.

A few financial ratios can help evaluate how the practice is doing. Data from the current year and the previous year's financial statements can be converted into ratios to highlight different financial characteristics. However, ratios should always be viewed in relation to the total financial picture.

INNER CITY HEALTH CARE
INCOME STATEMENT

	Month of , 20XX	Year-to-Date	Budget for Year	Overhead Percentages
A. Revenue:				
1. Office #1	$	$	$	
2. Office #2	$	$	$	
B. Total Revenue:	$	$	$	100%
C. Expenses:				
1. Non–provider (staff) salaries—gross	$	$	$	%
2. Staff fringes:				
– Payroll taxes	$	$	$	
– Empl. benefits	$	$	$	
– Empl. seminars	$	$	$	
– Uniforms	$	$	$	
– Retirement plan	$	$	$	
	$	$	$	%
3. Occupancy costs:				
– Rent—Off. #1	$	$	$	
– Rent—Off. #2	$	$	$	
– Property taxes	$	$	$	
– Insurance	$	$	$	
– Utilities	$	$	$	
– Janitor/Grounds	$	$	$	
	$	$	$	%
4. Medical expenses:				
– Medications	$	$	$	
– Supplies	$	$	$	
– Lab fees	$	$	$	
	$	$	$	%
5. Office expenses:				
– Office supplies	$	$	$	
– Postage	$	$	$	
– Telephone	$	$	$	
	$	$	$	%
6. Malpractice ins.	$	$	$	%
7. Professional expenses:				
– Auto expenses (Providers')	$	$	$	
– Dues/subscriptions	$	$	$	
– Books and videos	$	$	$	
– Dues/memberships	$	$	$	
– Entertainment	$	$	$	
– Professional development	$	$	$	
– Travel	$	$	$	
	$	$	$	%

FIGURE 20-1 A sample income statement that can show profit and expenses for 1 month.

(*continues*)

	Month of ______, 20XX	Year-to-Date	Budget for Year	Overhead Percentages
8. Equipment costs:				
– Depreciation/amortization	$	$	$	
– Rent	$	$	$	
– Service/maintenance	$	$	$	
– Interest (if on equipment purchase loans)	$	$	$	
	$	$	$	%
9. Marketing expenses:				
– Advertising	$	$	$	
– Other fees	$	$	$	
	$	$	$	%
10. Professional expenses:				
– Accounting	$	$	$	
– Legal	$	$	$	
– Consulting	$	$	$	
– Ret. Plan Admin.	$	$	$	
	$	$	$	%
11.				
12.				
13.				
14.				
D. Total Non–Provider Expenses:	$	$	$	%
E. Operating New Income Before Provider's Costs (B minus C)	$	$	$	%
F. Associate Provider's Costs:				
– Salaries—gross:	$	$	$	
– Benefits	$	$	$	
–	$	$	$	
–	$	$	$	
G. Total Non–Owner Provider's Costs	$	$	$	%
H. New Income Available to Owner–Providers (E minus G)	$	$	$	%
I. Owner–Providers' Costs:				
1. Salaries—gross:				
–Dr. A	$	$	$	
–Dr. B	$	$	$	
2. Bonuses—gross:				
–Dr. A	$	$	$	
–Dr. B	$	$	$	
3. Retirement contributions:				
–Dr. A	$	$	$	
–Dr. B	$	$	$	
4. "Semi-personal" expenses:				
–Dr. A	$	$	$	
–Dr. B	$	$	$	
J. Total Owner–Providers' Costs	$	$	$	
K. Net Income (H minus J)	$	$	$	

FIGURE 20-1 *(continued)*

Ratios are not difficult to calculate, but they can be time consuming when using a manual system. They are quick to create in a computer system because all the data are readily available, already totaled, and sometimes created automatically. It is helpful to understand the concept, however, and not rely too heavily on computer-generated reports. Data that have been entered incorrectly at some point will be reflected in reports generated. The user of accounting software must train

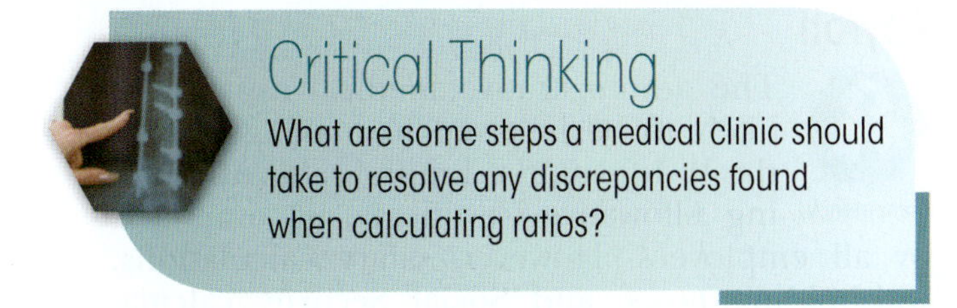

his or her mind to think about the sensibility of the report.

Although two of these ratios were discussed in Chapter 19, some elaboration is in order in the context of this chapter.

Accounts Receivable Ratio

The **accounts receivable (A/R) ratio** formula measures the speed at which outstanding accounts are paid. The accounts receivable ratio provides a picture of the state of collections and probable losses. The longer an account is past due, the less the likelihood is of successfully making the collection.

$$\frac{\text{Total Accounts Receivable}}{\text{Monthly Receipts}} = \text{Turnaround Time}$$

Example:

$$\frac{\$120{,}000}{\$60{,}000} = \text{2 Months Turnaround Time for Payment on an Account}$$

The goal of an efficient billing and collecting policy should be a turnaround time of 2 months or less.

Collection Ratio

The **collection ratio** shows the percentage of out standing debt collected. The goal should be a 90% collection ratio. Total receipts divided by total charges gives the unadjusted collection ratio, but adjustments may include federal and state insurance programs (Medicare and Medicaid, Workers' Compensation), managed care adjustments, and any other adjustments as directed by the provider.

Total Receipts	= $40,000
+ Managed Care Adjustments	$3,000
+ Medicare Adjustments	$2,000
TOTAL	$45,000
Total Charges	$52,000

$$\frac{\text{Total Receipts } \$45{,}000}{\text{Total Charges } \$52{,}000} = \text{86.5\% Collection Ratio after Adjustments}$$

Cost Ratio

The **cost ratio** formula shows the cost of a procedure or service and can help in determining, for instance, the cost effectiveness of maintaining a laboratory in the clinic setting. The ratio is:

$$\frac{\text{Total Expenses}}{\text{Total Number of Procedures for 1 Month}}$$

$$\frac{\text{Total Laboratory Expenses for September}}{\text{Total Number of Procedures Performed for September}}$$

$$\frac{\$48{,}000}{240} = \$200 \text{ per Procedure}$$

A conclusion might be reached that the laboratory is too costly because each procedure is not billed at $200.

LEGAL AND ETHICAL GUIDELINES

It is hoped that a careful hiring process (see Chapter 22) results in the best employees whose credentials, ethics, and personal actions are above reproach. However, embezzlement does occur in medical practices, partly because of the way in which the financial aspect of the practice is designed and managed. To decrease the opportunity for embezzlement:

- The accountant and the managing provider(s) should conduct regular and irregular audits of the practice accounts. Seek an accountant who is available at any time, not just when it is time to report wages or compute the yearly taxes. The accountant also becomes a valuable asset to the practice in providing essential information to the clinic staff.
- Separate duties among several employees. Consider having one employee open the mail and post checks received. A second employee handles all the cash transactions and prepares the deposit slips. A third employee might order the supplies and prepare all the checks. Many providers choose to sign the checks; however, this is

also a task that can be assigned to the office manager.

- Only one person should use the signature stamp; better yet, consider not using a signature stamp at all.
- The signature card on file at the bank must include the names of each individual authorized to sign the checks.
- Seek employees whose personal honesty sets a good example for everyone.

Providers who demonstrate the same personal honesty and integrity expected of their staff are less likely to be victims of embezzlement.

Bonding

There is another recommended step to take. To protect the practice from embezzlement or other financial loss, providers can purchase fidelity bonds. These bonds reimburse the practice for any monetary loss caused by the practice's employees. There are three types of bonds to consider, and it is reasonable to have more than one type. These bonds include:

1. Position-schedule bonds, which cover the position rather than a specific individual. For instance, the bookkeeper, office manager, and receptionist might be covered.
2. Blanket-position bonds, which cover all employees. If the staff members often share duties, cover for one another when there are absences, or work really well together as a team during busy periods, this type of bond might be most beneficial.
3. Personal bonds, which are designed to cover specific individuals by name and generally require a personal background investigation. This type of bond may give the most assurance.

Bonding not only protects the providers and the practice, but it assures employees that they are covered by a bond should there be a problem with the finances during their shift. Bonding service companies will require implementation of certain procedures and security measures as outlined in their contracts. Costs depend on risk levels, but they are well worth the protection.

Payroll

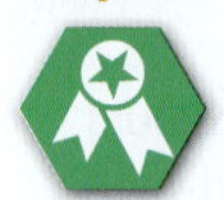
Competency

The administrative medical assistant is likely to be involved in making certain the W-4 form, the Employee's Withholding Allowance Certificate, is completed by all employees. However, salary calculations, withholding taxes, and Social Security calculations are the responsibility of the office manager or, may be outsourced to a payroll service. Payroll tasks usually are assigned to the clinic manager or a service because of the privacy of salary issues, Social Security numbers, and confidentiality of the employees' tax information. Manual systems for managing payroll are available, but the most efficient systems are computerized. The financial management of the payroll responsibilities in the clinic is detailed in Chapter 44.

Utilization Review

In the present health care climate, in which there are many managed care plans, more attention has been focused on how the billing and financial management process should proceed. Because of the influence of governmental mandates in the practice of medicine and because of the growth of the **utilization review (UR)** industry, more accurate record-keeping and documentation in all facets of the clinic have become necessary. There are numerous UR Arms throughout the country. These companies aggressively sell their services to employers and to insurance carriers. UR is actually a review of the patient service required before the actual service may be performed. If the reviewer determines that the procedure or treatment is not needed, then it will not be approved or covered under the patient's insurance plan. Policies that once permitted medical decisions to be made solely by the provider often are now made by other health professionals who are employed by UR Arms. Some clinics may find it beneficial to have one medical assistant whose main responsibility is to present procedures to UR for acceptance or denial. Because of the increasing concern for quality of health care at low cost, more providers also are realizing that they need more documentation of both medical and financial information with more accessible means for retrieval.

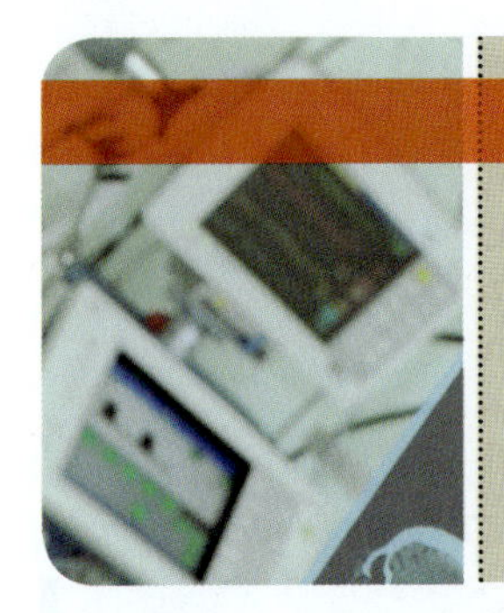

CASE STUDY 20-1

Refer to the scenario at the beginning of the chapter.

CASE STUDY REVIEW

1. Identify the financial records most likely reviewed by Mark King and Marilyn Johnson.
2. What information will be considered when projecting future income?
3. Identify other concerns to consider when hiring an additional medical assistant.

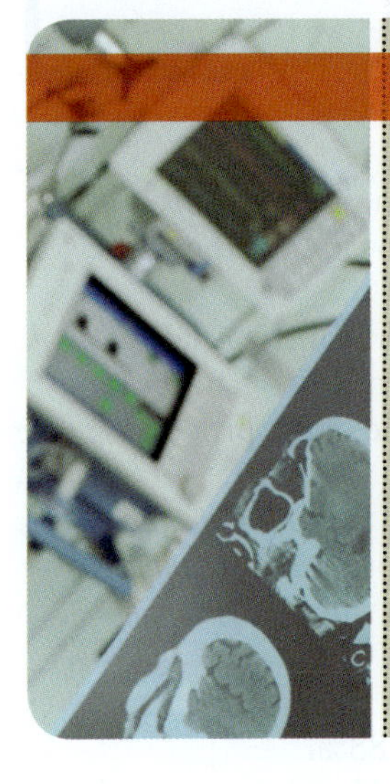

CASE STUDY 20-2

Richard Saxton is a newly licensed acupuncturist who has been in practice for less than a year. He is renting space for his procedures and services with an established doctor of osteopathy. Richard is using a simple pegboard system, makes his own appointments, and collects for most procedures at the time services are rendered unless the patients have medical insurance covering acupuncture. Richard has done fairly well, likes working in the environment the facility offers, and is beginning to show some profit. He would like to purchase a new table, chair, and stool for his acupuncture room.

CASE STUDY REVIEW

1. What facts might Richard want to consider before making the purchases?
2. Consider the variable costs versus the fixed costs of the practice of acupuncture. (You may need to do a little research to determine supplies and other factors.)
3. What information will his pegboard system give him?

Summary

- Accounting is the process of recording financial transactions, including storage, retrieval, report generation for summaries, sorting, and evaluation of clinic information.
- This information serves as a system of monitoring the financial status of a clinic and the specific results of its activities. It provides financial information for decision making at many levels. These functions are essential to obtaining maximum reimbursement and creating profitability for the practice.
- The various methods a clinic may use for accounting and monitoring financial accounts include the single-entry system, the pegboard system, the double-entry system, a practice management (PM) software system, and billing services and bureaus.
- The medical assistant must know how to run a financial analysis by using summary tools in a computer accounting system or manual pegboard systems, including preparing a deposit slip at the end of each day.
- Accuracy is necessary; the medical assistant will use various techniques to find and correct errors should they occur.
- The medical assistant must run and check the trial balance on account receivables before monthly statements are produced. It should be confirmed that total debits equal total credits by producing a final total at the end of each month. This ensures accuracy and that accounts are in balance.
- Collection techniques must be properly used, both by telephone and by letter, following the guidelines of the Fair Debt Collections Practices Act.
- Cost analysis methods include fixed costs and variable costs in order to collect data used to set fees, market the practice, evaluate profits, and monitor the clinic's performance.
- The accounts receivable ratio and cost ratio formulas provide a picture of collections and losses, as well as aiding in the determination of the cost effectiveness of equipment, insurance participation, and other clinic considerations.

Study for Success

To reinforce your knowledge and skills of information presented in this chapter:

- Review the *Key Terms* and *Learning Outcomes*
- Consider the *Critical Thinking* features and *Case Studies* and discuss your conclusions
- Answer the questions in the *Certification Review*

Procedure

- Perform the *Procedure* using the *Competency Assessment Checklists* on the *Student Companion Website*

CERTIFICATION REVIEW

1. What is a tip for finding an error of a transposed number in financial reports?
   a. The error is divisible by 4
   b. The error is divisible by 2
   c. The error is divisible by 9
   d. None of these
2. What is an example of a fixed cost?
   a. Salaries
   b. Cost of supplies
   c. Depreciation of equipment
   d. Cost of treating patients
   e. The monthly utility bill
3. What is the name for the itemized statement of the financial position of a business?
   a. Income statement
   b. Balance sheet
   c. Trial balance
   d. Collection ratio
4. What is the purpose of a check register?
   a. It records all checks and categorizes them into separate columns.
   b. It is used when taking cash from patients.
   c. It is an accounts receivable record.
   d. Both a and c
   e. None of these, it is not necessary.
5. What is the purpose of utilization review?
   a. It looks at the utility of all personnel.
   b. It examines how useful the ambulatory care center is to patients.
   c. It is a review of a procedure before it is performed to determine if it is necessary.
   d. It only affects hospitals.
6. Assets include which of the following?
   a. Equipment and supplies on hand
   b. Building or property
   c. Accounts receivable
   d. All of these
   e. None of these
7. What is a computer billing and service bureau?
   a. It is the service you hire to care for the clinic computer system.
   b. It may compromise patient confidentiality.
   c. It can function through linkage of computers, online servicing, or off-line batch processing.
   d. Both b and c
8. What is true of the collection ratio in a medical facility where the total receipts including any adjustments are $83,500 and the total charges equal $97,750?
   a. It would be great at 94%.
   b. It would be quite good at 88%.
   c. It shows a fair return at 85%.
   d. It shows a modest return at 75%.
   e. None of these
9. When can money be saved with accounts payable?
   a. When bills are paid promptly
   b. When discounts are realized
   c. When supplies are not purchased in bulk
   d. Both a and b
10. Which of the following is true of bonding?
    a. It binds providers to the safe caretaking of their patients.
    b. It protects medical clinic staff and providers if embezzlement occurs.
    c. It can be purchased in three different types.
    d. It is not very costly to the business.
    e. Both b and c

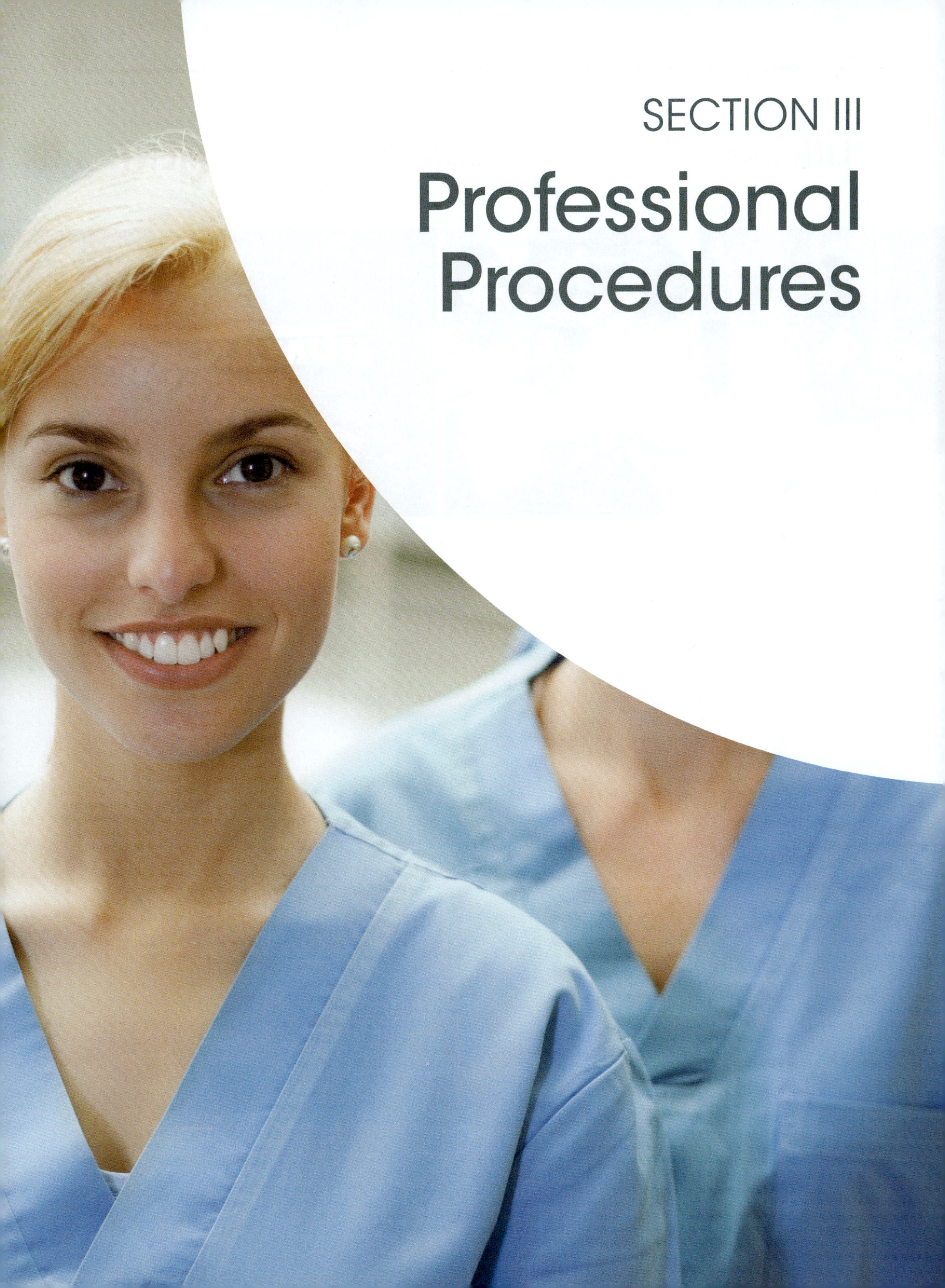

SECTION III
Professional Procedures

UNIT VI
CLINIC AND HUMAN RESOURCES MANAGEMENT

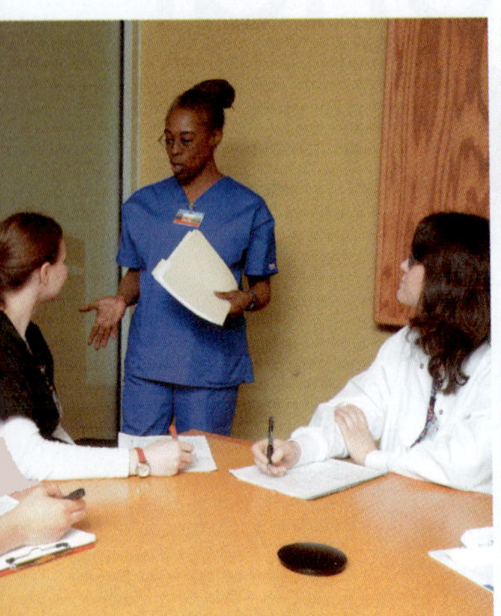
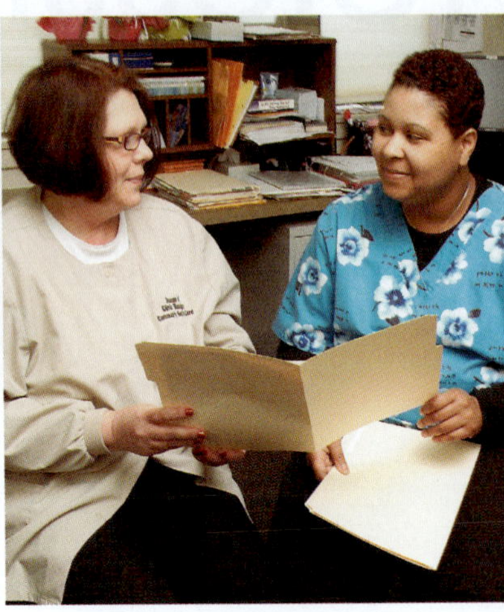
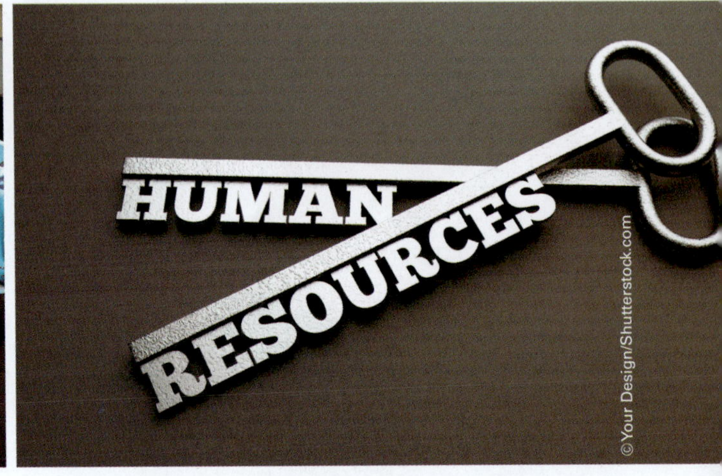

ATTRIBUTES OF PROFESSIONALISM

Many experienced and professional medical assistants find themselves in the role of management, often moving into that position through their clinic employment and familiarity with all aspects of the clinic operation. Management responsibilities mean not only carrying the burden of understanding each facet of the operation, even stepping into the role of an employee when necessary, but also shouldering the responsibility of directing, facilitating, and monitoring employee productivity and patient satisfaction. As a professional manager you will support staff members, carry out the wishes of providers, and treat everyone equitably. Personnel will be fully oriented to their positions, evaluated on a regular and predetermined basis, and provided with opportunities for expansion of their role in the clinic.

Listed below are a series of questions for you to ask yourself, to serve as a professionalism checklist.

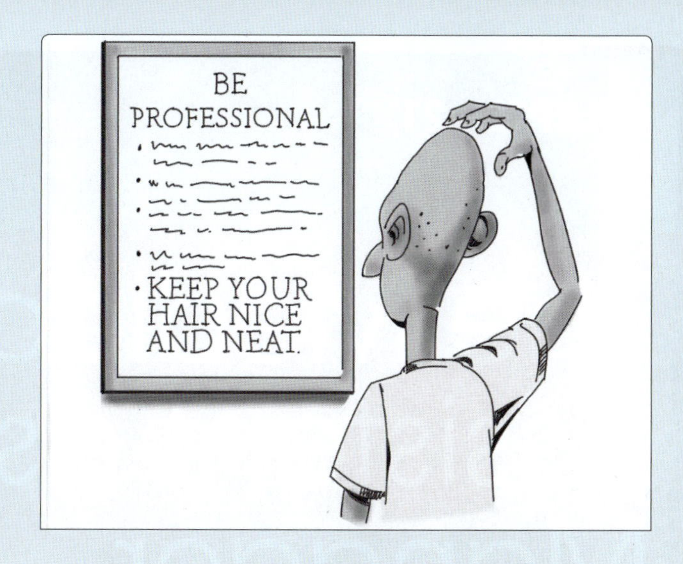

As you interact with patients and colleagues, these questions will help to guide you in the professional behavior that is expected every day from medical assistants.

Ask Yourself

COMMUNICATION

- ☐ Do I apply active listening skills?
- ☐ Do I display professionalism through written and verbal communication?
- ☐ Do I demonstrate appropriate nonverbal communication?
- ☐ Do I display appropriate body language?
- ☐ Does my knowledge allow me to speak easily with all members of the health care team?

PRESENTATION

- ☐ Am I dressed and groomed appropriately?
- ☐ Do I display a positive attitude?
- ☐ Do I display a calm, professional, and caring manner?

COMPETENCY

- ☐ Do I pay attention to detail?
- ☐ Do I ask questions if I am out of my comfort zone or do not have the experience to carry out tasks?
- ☐ Do I display sound judgment?
- ☐ Am I knowledgeable and accountable?

INITIATIVE

- ☐ Do I show initiative?
- ☐ Have I developed a strategic plan to achieve my goals? Is my plan realistic?
- ☐ Do I seek out opportunities to expand my knowledge base?
- ☐ Am I flexible and dependable?

INTEGRITY

- ☐ Do I demonstrate the principles of self-boundaries?
- ☐ Do I work within my scope of practice?
- ☐ Do I demonstrate respect for individual diversity?
- ☐ Do I recognize the impact personal ethics and morals have on the delivery of health care?
- ☐ Do I protect and maintain confidentiality?
- ☐ Do I maintain moral and ethical standards?
- ☐ Do I do the "right thing" even when no one is observing?

CHAPTER 21

The Medical Assistant as Clinic Manager

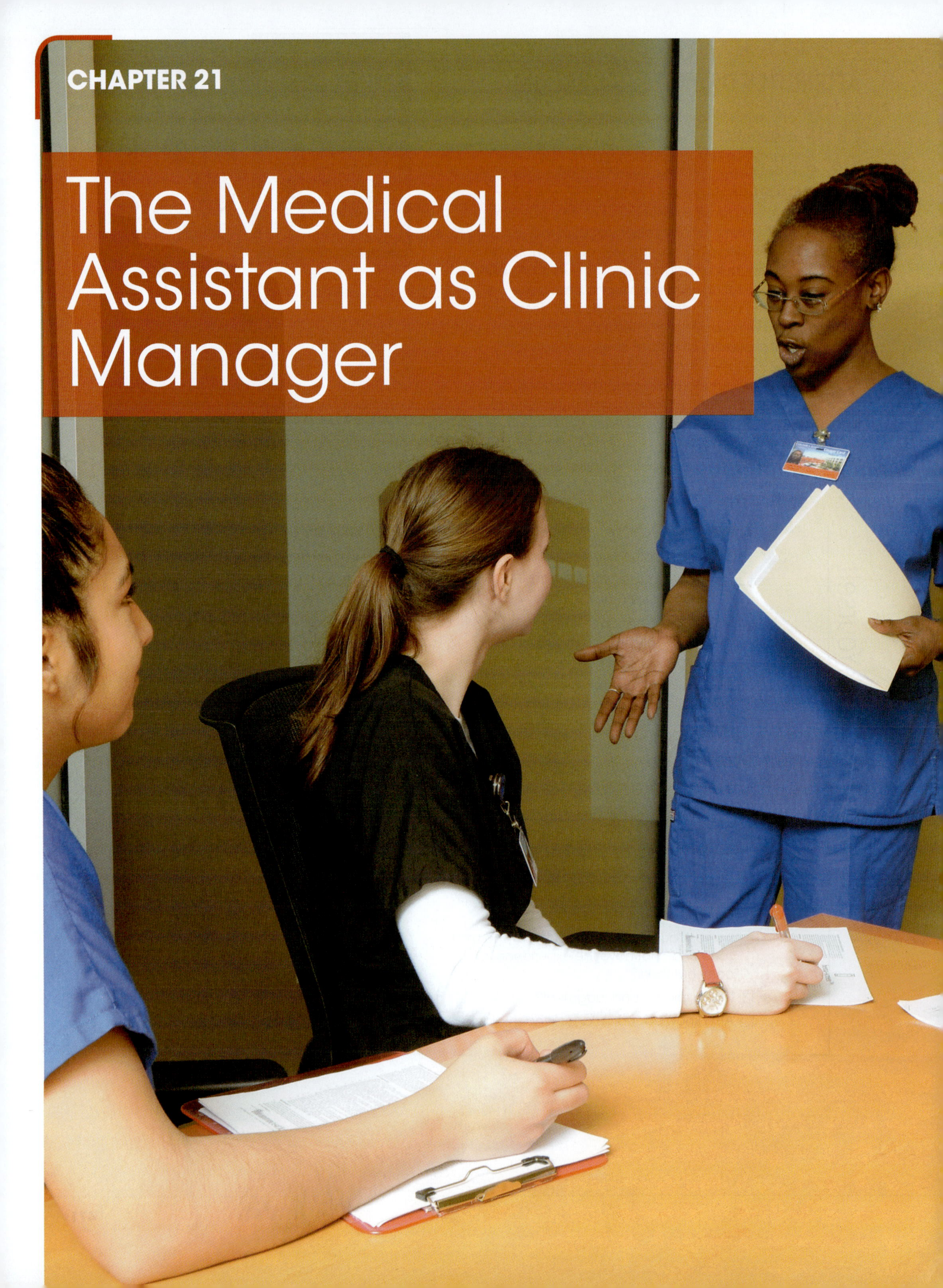

LEARNING OUTCOMES

1. Define and spell the key terms as presented in the glossary.
2. Describe the qualities of a manager.
3. Discuss characteristics of managers and leaders.
4. Differentiate between authoritarian and participatory management styles.
5. Describe management by walking around and its usefulness in ambulatory care settings.
6. Recall a minimum of four common risks and risk-control measures.
7. List three benefits of a teamwork approach.
8. Discuss the importance of a meeting agenda.
9. Describe appropriate evaluation tools for employees.
10. Recall effective methods of resolving conflict.
11. Identify the steps required to make travel arrangements.
12. Define the term *itinerary* and list important information the itinerary should contain.
13. List three methods of increasing productivity and efficient time management.
14. Describe the purpose of a procedure manual.
15. Discuss the impact of HIPAA's privacy policy in ambulatory care settings.
16. Describe the general concept of marketing and recall at least three marketing tools.
17. Discuss the role of social media in the medical clinic.
18. Describe the purpose and benefit of marketing.
19. Discuss the steps involved in the inventory of administrative and clinical supplies and equipment.
20. Discuss the steps involved in administrative and clinical equipment calibration and maintenance.

KEY TERMS

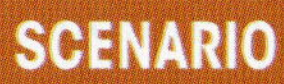

agenda
ancillary services
authoritarian style
benchmark
benefit
blogging
bond
brainstorming
conflict resolution
embezzle
fringe benefits
"going bare"
itinerary
liability
malpractice
management by walking around (MBWA)
marketing
mentor
minutes
negligence
nonretaliation provision
participatory style
practicum
procedure manual
professional liability insurance
profit sharing
risk management
salary review
self-actualization
shadow
social media
subordinate
teamwork
work statement

SCENARIO

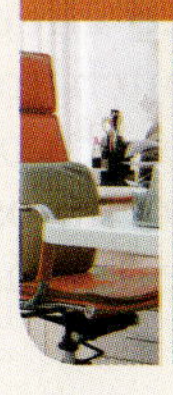

Marilyn Johnson, CMA (AAMA), has been employed by Inner City Health Care for the past 8 years. Three years ago, she was promoted to the position of clinic manager when the facility added a second clinic for its associates in a nearby suburb. Marilyn has a baccalaureate degree in business administration. Her responsibilities at the clinic include various duties involving personnel, finances, and efficiency.

Chapter Portal

The drive to improve the productivity of the medical clinic, precipitated by managed care, Medicare, and insurance limits placed on fees, has broadened the scope of employment options and job marketability for medical assistants. This has created an opportunity for medical assistants to advance to the position of clinic manager.

In small clinics, the position of clinic manager may include the duties of the human resources (HR) representative; in larger clinics, these positions will be independent. This book treats them as separate positions (see Chapter 22). In larger facilities, the clinic manager will coordinate with the HR representative to train and manage administrative and clinical staff.

THE MEDICAL ASSISTANT AS CLINIC MANAGER

The manager of a medical clinic or ambulatory care facility can have vast and diverse responsibilities. This chapter covers the following clinic manager duties:

1. Manage and encourage IT services, relationships, and collaboration, ensuring the clinic EHR and relevant staff are kept updated and are involved in system protocols as appropriate
2. Make travel arrangements and prepare an itinerary
3. Arrange and maintain practice insurance and develop risk management strategies
4. Supervise clinic personnel
5. Approve financial transactions and account disposition; generate financial reports as needed
6. Supervise the purchase and storage of clinic supplies
7. Prepare staff meeting agendas, conduct the meetings, and record minutes
8. Supervise the purchase, repair, and maintenance of clinic equipment
9. Assist in improving work flow and time management
10. Create and update the clinic procedure manual, Material Safety Data Sheets (MSDS), and Health Insurance Portability and Accountability Act (HIPAA) manual
11. Prepare patient education materials and arrange patient/community education workshops as needed

QUALITIES OF A MANAGER

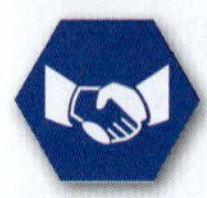
Professional

Your technical skills may be what got you noticed, hired, and ultimately promoted, but that will not be enough as a clinic manager. As a manager, you will also need to have talent with "soft" skills that will help you succeed in working with your staff using different approaches.

A clinic manager should not feel the need to be superior to employees but should strive to develop a synergistic organization. The best manager is like an orchestra conductor. He or she constructively blends together the skills and abilities of diverse people to produce a smooth and efficient team. The result is an organization with greater capability than would be achievable by the individuals acting independently.

The clinic manager should have two overarching goals:

- Get the job done
- Make the process enjoyable

Management styles are expected to change significantly in the forthcoming years. By 2017, there will be five generations in the workforce simultaneously. As Generation Z (born in the 1990s) enters the work force, and with the Baby Boomer generation (born between 1946 and 1964) still working and gradually retiring, the challenges of managing varying ethics and working styles of these generations will become very real.

New approaches to making the most of time management, adapting to different employees, finding ways to enable collaboration across generations, and creatively gapping those bridges will become increasingly important. Clinic managers will need to understand that each individual has his or her own set of skills, and with the potential of up to a 50-year age difference in the work environment, being able to co-mingle and use cross-skills to the benefit of all will emerge as useful tools.

Emerging technologies offer an opportunity for the younger generation to teach how to use these products in the work place effectively. In turn, the older generation has much to offer by instilling the value of interpersonal communication, and building sound relationships with co-workers based on experience and longevity.

There is a unique opportunity for the co-mingling of these skilled generations to mutually benefit each other in the workplace.

A good clinic manager needs to be two persons in one body: manager and leader. The two functions are different, and the good manager will use some of each persona in meeting objectives. Table 21-1 lists the characteristics of a manager and a leader.

Good managers are leaders, providing their coworkers with vision, guidance, and a feeling of ownership in the process. They do these things without threats, usually through the power of their personal charisma. It is also important that managers clearly convey their expectations to their employees. Possibly nothing leads to ill feeling between the manager and an employee more than failure to let the employee know what is expected of him or her. Furthermore, a lack of expectations stifles career growth and organizational vitality. Good leaders need to blend many admirable personality traits of leadership to be successful and still control the resources entrusted to them.

Before proceeding with a listing of qualities of a manager/leader, a rule that defines almost all of the ethical qualities needs to be mentioned. This rule is *Treat others as you would like to be treated.* Commonly known as the Golden Rule, it will make the difference between a manager who is successful and one who fails miserably. The rule needs no explanation and will serve any manager well in any circumstance.

Qualities needed by a manager/leader include the following:

- *Effective communication skills.* Communication skills include written and oral methods. The manager must communicate clearly, diplomatically, tactfully, and with respect for the feelings of others.
- *Fair-mindedness.* It is important to always be fair with co-workers. Decisions that impact one fellow employee create a ripple effect. That is, you may have to make the same decision for another employee at another time. Decisions should be based, as much as possible, on the assumption that what is granted to one employee will be granted to others in similar situations. This approach will decrease the risk for being accused of playing favorites or being unfair.
- *Objectivity.* The clinic manager must be able to view challenges without bias or prejudice. For example, when promotions are made, the clinic manager must be able to focus on the job description criteria and individual qualifications without introducing personal preference.
- *Organizational skills.* Being organized includes being able to prioritize tasks, working efficiently and methodically. Know when and be willing to delegate tasks when others have the expertise and time to complete the task within the timelines.
- *People skills.* The clinic manager must like people in general and enjoy working with them. Building confidence and self-esteem in others and being interested in promoting constructive relationships are essential qualities of the clinic manager. The ability to function as an effective team leader provides a role model for other staff members to emulate.
- *Problem-solving skills.* The clinic manager must be a problem solver. This may include being creative and doing away with old paradigms and traditional approaches to solving a problem. When difficult issues arise, focus on the situation, issue, or behavior, not on the person. A discussion about solving the problem without laying blame is much more productive. Positive solutions may be more readily attained when discussing what was observed rather than what was told by someone else.

TABLE 21-1

DIFFERENCES BETWEEN A MANAGER AND A LEADER

MANAGER	LEADER
Organizes and allocates talent and resources	Provides vision and goals, setting reasonable and clear standards
Plans and budgets using available resources	Communicates direction; promotes teamwork and creativity to reach goals
Controls and solves problems, with the ability to adapt to changes seamlessly	Is an inspiring and motivating influence, able to mentor and direct in ways that keep the team moving forward
Establishes structure by organizing, staffing, and implementing policies and procedures	Overcomes resistance to change and resolves barriers
Consistently achieves goals and targets	Is the role model and go-to for the team

- *Technical expertise.* Have a working knowledge of each procedure performed in the clinic, although it is not necessary to be the acknowledged technical expert. In the medical environment, there are many changes, including updates to laws, insurance guidelines, and various business challenges that occur frequently. A good clinic manager is continually learning and encourages **subordinates** to seek opportunities to continue their education and advance their technical skills.
- *Truthfulness.* Lead by example! If an honest mistake is made, be the first to admit to the error and seek the best solution for preventing it from happening again. Respond honestly to requests. For example, two staff members ask for the same day off. The clinic manager will make the decision that only one member may have the day off and will review the policy manual to determine the appropriate criteria for designating whose request will be granted.

Clinic Manager Attitude

Professional

Many managers share a common enemy—themselves. The part of ourselves that is our enemy is our mind and the outlook we have on the world. People who succeed attribute positive results to their own actions. People who underachieve or fail usually attribute negative results to someone else or to chance, over which they have no control. Because underachievers feel helpless to affect results, psychologists conclude that their motivation to succeed is diminished. A low achiever would be unlikely to have a personal risk management system in place. He or she would feel he or she could not affect events. The more positive person could easily take steps to avoid these problems.

The effect of a negative mindset does not stop with failure to accept responsibility for the things that happen to each of us, it continues on. Unless we change our outlook, we lower our expectations and begin accepting the mediocre. Individuals who feel they are helpless to affect events become afraid of success as well as failure, and they subconsciously find a way to fail to avoid the challenges success will bring.

How do you change your mindset? The following are a few suggestions considered helpful:

- Come to terms with what you would have to change if you are to be successful, and be ready for the change.
- Identify what you really want to achieve.

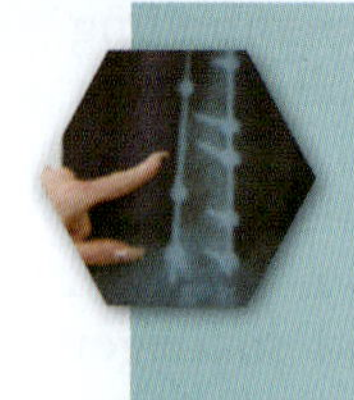

Critical Thinking

How does the clinic manager begin to develop good working relationships with community service organizations to better serve and provide for patients' health care needs? How would this improve the quality of public relations?

- Put your goals in writing using positive terms (say "I will," not "I'll try").
- Begin with small, achievable goals.
- Eliminate poor habits such as procrastination.
- Tune out negative thoughts and focus on positive thoughts.

We are what we think we are. Be careful of your mindset, it can derail you and your job as a manager.

Professionalism

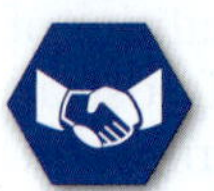
Professional

The medical assistant as clinic manager must exhibit professional behavior at all times. He or she must be courteous and diplomatic and demonstrate a responsible and positive attitude. All verbal and written communications should be accurate and correct and should follow appropriate guidelines. The clinic manager should demonstrate knowledge of federal and state health care legislation and regulations and must perform within legal and ethical boundaries. All documentation must be performed appropriately.

The clinic manager serves as a liaison between the provider, the patient, and other professionals. Therefore, professional demeanor in all respects must be followed. It is not uncommon to be called on to locate community resources and information for patients and employers. A good working relationship with community service organizations fosters the sharing of information vital to your patients' health care needs and promotes quality public relations. Review Procedure 11-5 for specific information on how this is done.

MANAGEMENT STYLES

There are many books written on management styles; however, it is possible to break all of them down into two basic styles, each with an infinite number of variations. Instead of discussing the intricacies of these management styles, for the purpose of this book, we will take a straightforward view and look at only the fundamental styles: authoritarian and participatory. We will also examine a third management technique called, managing by walking around (MBWA), which is, an effective method for keeping abreast of what is going on in an organization and is making a positive comeback in the era of email, texting, and lack of face-to-face interaction due to technology.

Authoritarian Style

A Manager who adopts the **authoritarian style** of management exercises his or her authority over those that report to him or her as a means to achieve goals. Without seeking or considering the input of the staff members, this manager controls the decision making, controls policies, and puts operational plans in place. While this style may seem regimented and inflexible, there are workplace environments where this is beneficial.

For example, in a medical clinic, there is a tendency for there to exist targeted areas of specialty tasks within the support staff. These may be accomplished by just a handful of people, or an extensive group of individuals with focused areas of responsibility. Such is the case in the roles of administrative front desk staff, those working in coding and billing, the clinical staff (including medical assistants, laboratory and diagnostic technicians, physician assistants, and nurse practitioners), in essence, every member that provides a total patient care experience within a clinic. While each member has a specific function, the whole is very much interdependent, and the work flow needs to have a beginning, middle, and end in order for all the parts to be cohesive and accomplish goals for the patient's care, as well as proper reimbursement for the clinic. At the same time, everything must be done within compliance requirements.

Authoritarian management needs to be executed carefully; otherwise, staff may begin to feel resentment and tasks may seem too rote or rigid. This style can foster absenteeism and high turnover, results which can be devastating to the efficient operation of a clinic where every staff member's contribution is of utmost importance. As previously mentioned, each facet of the tasks collectively done by the entire staff are interdependent in the medical environment, creating an opportunity to actually blend management styles to best utilize resources, achieve goals, and maintain a motivated staff.

Participatory Style

A manager who utilizes the **participatory style** of management encourages input and feedback from those that report to him or her. Decision making, policies, and operational plans will at least in part include the suggestions, opinions, and views of those on staff. As an operational whole, each staff member feels that he or she can or has made a contribution, and this increases the sense of value within a team effort. Additionally, the staff can more easily take ownership of the goals, and make adjustments with the assistance of the manager when fine-tuning is necessary. As with any management style, care must be taken with this approach as well. While this style encourages contributions, there will be those that do not contribute, those that are overeager, and in the end, not everyone's ideas can be implemented. Risk of alienating those whose ideas are not used and resentment for others who minimally participate can create unique challenges. However, the opportunity to blend authoritarian and participatory styles can positively influence the needed interdependency in a clinic, where each person's responsibilities have a direct impact on the total care of the patient and smooth operation of the business.

Management by Walking Around

Management by walking around (MBWA) is not really a management style but rather a technique for keeping the manager informed and promoting face-to-face conversations, obtaining feedback, and listening to staff ideas or comments. This style consists of just what the title says—the manager walks around looking at what is going on in the organization and talks with employees. The manager must be careful to make sure his or her motives are not to micromanage and to convey this to the staff.

To this end, some tips are offered here to make the most of using the MBWA technique effectively in the medical clinic.

- *Make this part of a routine, and stay consistent.* When staff see you on a regular basis, and not once a month or only when there is time, the MBWA becomes part of the management

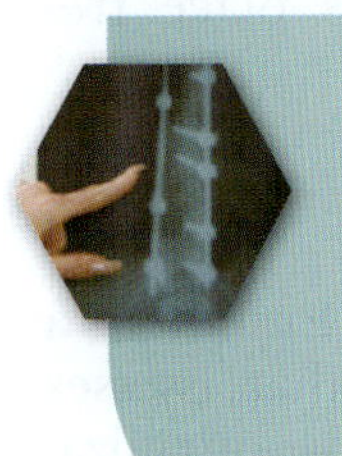

Critical Thinking

How would you make the medical clinic (administrative and clinical space) safe for employees and nonemployees (e.g., patients, venders, visitors)? List as many considerations as possible.

culture in the clinic. This does not mean that a set day and time needs to be adhered to, but rather, simply a consistent habit of stopping by work areas to chat, see how things are going, and gather ideas. You will get more candid and useful information by dropping in unexpectedly, when the staff member was not prepared for your visit.

- *Make it worthwhile.* If you will be stopping by, then make it a point to ask for ideas on improvement, suggestions, and also acknowledge a good idea when presented. When a good idea or suggestion is implemented, give credit where due without showing favoritism. Encourage support from staff that curbs resentment but still allows recognition.
- *Follow up on questions and concerns.* If you are presented with an issue for which you do not have an immediate solution or response, take the time to follow up and get back with an answer in a timely fashion. The staff will appreciate that you have not forgotten or given less than your full attention to a problem they are experiencing.
- *Stick to fact-finding.* Do not utilize MBWA as a means to identify procedures incorrectly done, criticize, or discipline staff if problems are identified by you during the walk around. These should be noted and addressed in a different setting and time, appropriate to the circumstances.

The idea of the MBWA technique is to build rapport and keep on top of the state of the organization through staff feedback. Keep to this objective. Employees are more likely to be engaged and productive when they see the manager and have an opportunity to speak with you frequently than if they do not. We are now in a time where managing people is taking place through email, texting, and formal staff meetings, and the manager can literally be a person always in her office and not easily accessible. Even with an open door policy, most staff are reluctant to initiate a discussion as opposed to having a touch-base visit that takes place frequently in their own work area.

RISK MANAGEMENT

The clinic manager should formulate a **risk management** procedure that assesses risks to which he or she and the organization are exposed and take steps to develop contingencies that minimize probable risks. Some common risks and risk-control measures are:

- *Loss of a critical employee.* Have cross-training of employees to permit them to assume the duties of an employee who is ill or terminates his or her employment.
- *Failure of a supplier or contractor.* Maintain sufficient inventory to permit contracting with a secondary supplier before critical shortages occur. Monitor the status of orders so that you are aware of any failures in delivery before they have a negative impact and so that supplies can be obtained from a second source. Have a list of secondary sources.
- *Accidental disclosure of confidential information through error or unauthorized entry.* Have protocols in place regarding breach of confidentiality and defining steps to be taken in the event information is compromised. Define protocols to patients alerting them to the unlikely but potential possibility of accidental disclosure. Notify patients immediately if confidential information is compromised and work with them for resolution.
- *Computer failure.* Back up the system regularly. Have a secondary system that permits the clinic to operate until repairs are effected. Have a maintenance contract in place with a reputable firm permitting overnight repair.
- *Injury to a staff member or nonemployee.* Continually review safety procedures and conduct safety surveys. Have adequate liability insurance for the medical clinic.
- *Managerial position change.* Continuously network with friends and associates to permit you to rapidly seek a new position before experiencing a job loss. It's always easier to get a job while you still have a job.

Incident reports are required to notify managers of events involving injuries to patients, visitors, or staff; medical errors or omissions; breech of confidential information; and potentially dangerous conditions associated with facilities or equipment. This report signals the risk manager to implement existing protocols to minimize risk. Medical incident reports are confidential and cannot be released to anyone without a signed release of information agreement. The medical incident report form is an administrative document and is not considered part of the medical record. Procedure 21-1 provides steps for completing a medical incident report.

PROCEDURE 21-1

Procedure

Completing a Medical Incident Report

PURPOSE:

To complete an accurate medical incident report providing all legally required information and to submit it in a timely manner.

EQUIPMENT/SUPPLIES:

- Appropriate medical incident report form
- Computer with Incident Report Software
- Notes taken regarding incident

PROCEDURE STEPS:

1. Report situations that were harmful by discussing the incident with the employee(s) involved and read notes of pertinent information. Ask those who witnessed the incident to describe when, where, and what they saw in their own words. RATIONALE: Provides an understanding of what happened and ensures all the information needed is documented.
2. ***Pay attention to detail*** when completing the clinic-approved medical incident report form. A single-sheet, multiple-copy form is best. The form should contain basic patient identification data, a checklist of different incidents, and a space for written comments. RATIONALE: Ensures that all information needed is documented.
3. The person completing the incident report form should be the individual who witnessed the incident, first discovered the incident, or is most familiar with the incident. RATIONALE: This ensures the most accurate recording of the incident.
4. Each section of the form must be completed. The incident description should be a brief narrative consisting of an objective description of the facts but should not draw any conclusions. Quotes should be used when appropriate with any unwitnessed incidents (e.g., "Patient states . . ."). The name(s) of any witnesses should be included on the report as well as employees directly involved in the incident. RATIONALE: To provide unbiased information without making judgments.
5. ***Implement time management principles.*** Incident reports must be submitted in a timely manner to the appropriate administrator or office following protocol identified in the procedure manual for the clinic. RATIONALE: Ensures that appropriate documentation and action is taken for follow-up.

IMPORTANCE OF TEAMWORK

The use of **teamwork** to improve the efficiency of the clinic at first may seem incongruent to your desire to improve clinic efficiency, because it seems that several people are now involved in solving a problem that you as the manager should solve and explain. Teamwork builds morale and actually results in getting more accomplished with the resources you have because the team members develop ownership of the solution to a problem and want to make it work. When it works, it flatters them and builds their esteem.

The efficiency of a team results from collectively working together to plan how to "work smarter" and how to dovetail tasks and support each other so that wasted effort is avoided. To achieve all of these things, a team not only must be given the responsibility and the authority to plan and execute their plan to solve a problem, but they must know your expectations for them. Sometimes this means that you, the clinic manager, must stick your neck out for them. They will reward you handsomely for doing so. For more information on how to build a successful team, see the "Importance of Teamwork" Quick Reference Guide.

QUICK REFERENCE GUIDE

Importance of Teamwork

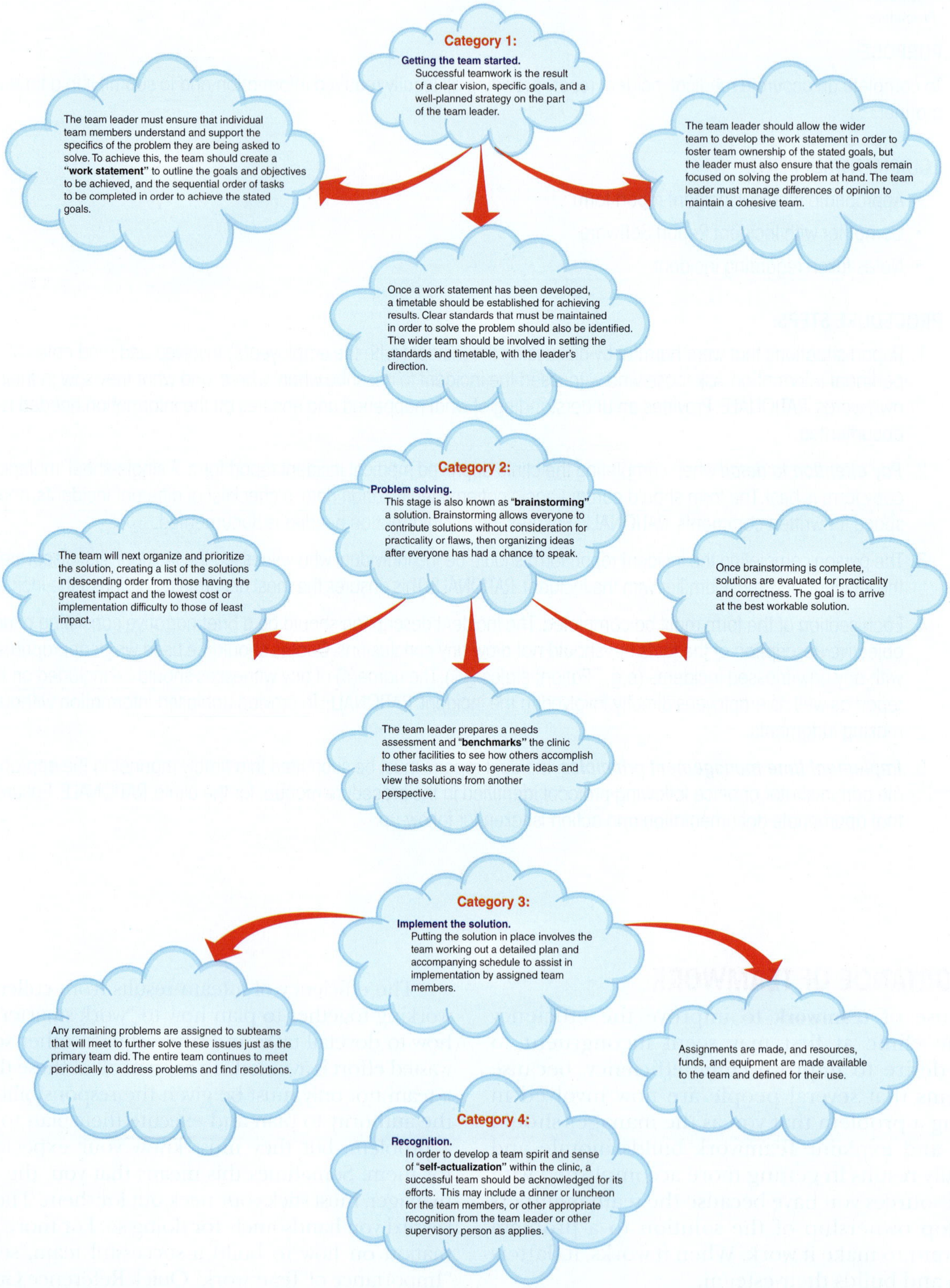

Category 1:

Getting the team started.
Successful teamwork is the result of a clear vision, specific goals, and a well-planned strategy on the part of the team leader.

The team leader must ensure that individual team members understand and support the specifics of the problem they are being asked to solve. To achieve this, the team should create a **"work statement"** to outline the goals and objectives to be achieved, and the sequential order of tasks to be completed in order to achieve the stated goals.

The team leader should allow the wider team to develop the work statement in order to foster team ownership of the stated goals, but the leader must also ensure that the goals remain focused on solving the problem at hand. The team leader must manage differences of opinion to maintain a cohesive team.

Once a work statement has been developed, a timetable should be established for achieving results. Clear standards that must be maintained in order to solve the problem should also be identified. The wider team should be involved in setting the standards and timetable, with the leader's direction.

Category 2:

Problem solving.
This stage is also known as **"brainstorming"** a solution. Brainstorming allows everyone to contribute solutions without consideration for practicality or flaws, then organizing ideas after everyone has had a chance to speak.

The team will next organize and prioritize the solution, creating a list of the solutions in descending order from those having the greatest impact and the lowest cost or implementation difficulty to those of least impact.

Once brainstorming is complete, solutions are evaluated for practicality and correctness. The goal is to arrive at the best workable solution.

The team leader prepares a needs assessment and **"benchmarks"** the clinic to other facilities to see how others accomplish these tasks as a way to generate ideas and view the solutions from another perspective.

Category 3:

Implement the solution.
Putting the solution in place involves the team working out a detailed plan and accompanying schedule to assist in implementation by assigned team members.

Any remaining problems are assigned to subteams that will meet to further solve these issues just as the primary team did. The entire team continues to meet periodically to address problems and find resolutions.

Assignments are made, and resources, funds, and equipment are made available to the team and defined for their use.

Category 4:

Recognition.
In order to develop a team spirit and sense of **"self-actualization"** within the clinic, a successful team should be acknowledged for its efforts. This may include a dinner or luncheon for the team members, or other appropriate recognition from the team leader or other supervisory person as applies.

SUPERVISING PERSONNEL

Creating an atmosphere in which open and honest communication can take place is critical to supervising personnel. This type of communication may be encouraged through the establishment of regular staff meetings, with each staff member sharing ideas for improvement and areas of concern. Eliciting the help of others in problem-solving strategies promotes harmony (Figure 21-1).

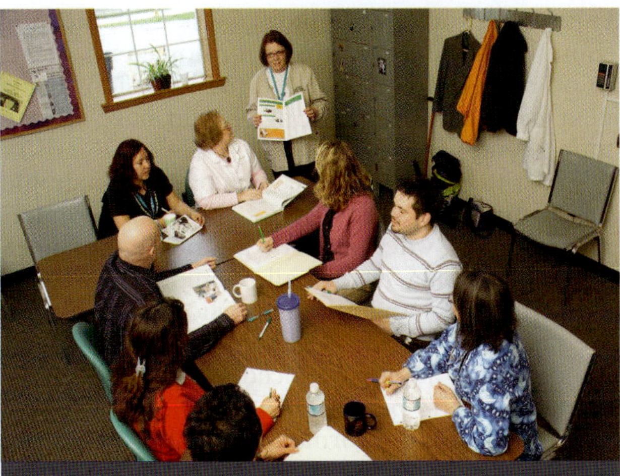

FIGURE 21-1 Consistently scheduled staff meetings promote communication and harmony among the health care team.

Staff and Team Meetings

The clinic manager usually initiates the staff and team meeting idea and should officiate at such meetings. Failure of the clinic manager to be present may convey a message that the meeting is an event not worthy of attention. It is important that the clinic manager be familiar with basic parliamentary procedures. The purchase of books such as *Robert's Rules of Order* or *Parliamentary Procedure at a Glance* is an excellent investment.

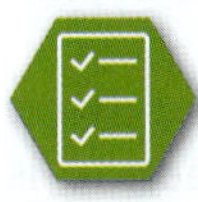

Procedure

Successful staff and team meetings are announced well in advance or on established timelines to enable the majority of clinic personnel to attend. An **agenda** identifying the subjects to be covered during a given meeting should be issued before the meeting so that each attendee arrives prepared with input or questions relevant to the topics. Procedure 21-2 outlines the procedural steps for preparing a meeting agenda.

PROCEDURE 21-2

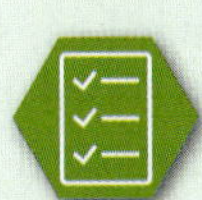

Procedure

Preparing a Meeting Agenda

PURPOSE:

To prepare a meeting agenda, a list of specific items to be discussed or acted on, to maintain the focus of the group and allow business to be transacted in a timely fashion.

EQUIPMENT/SUPPLIES:

- List of participants
- Order of business
- Names of individuals giving reports
- Names of any guest speakers
- Computer and paper to print agendas

PROCEDURE STEPS:

1. ***Paying attention to detail,*** reserve proposed date, time, and place of meeting. RATIONALE: Ensures that the facilities are available for the meeting.
2. Collect information for meeting agenda by previewing the previous meeting's minutes for old business items, checking with others for report items, and determining any new business items. RATIONALE: Ensures that all old and new business items have been identified.
3. Prepare a hard copy of the agenda and have it approved by the chair of the meeting. RATIONALE: Confirmation by the chair of the agenda content ensures that agenda is correct and complete.
4. ***Implementing time management principles,*** send agenda to meeting participants a few days in advance of the meeting. RATIONALE: Permits participants to prepare for the meeting by completing any tasks required and preparing any necessary documentation.

Figure 21-2 shows a sample agenda. Each meeting should end with opportunity for nonagenda items to be discussed or suggested for inclusion in the next meeting. The meeting should have a fixed time to end.

A written record in the form of **minutes** should be maintained and sent to all team members regardless of whether they attended the meeting. This policy keeps all members informed about policy changes and decisions that impact the clinic operations. The minutes also trigger a reminder for any new procedures or revisions to be made in the procedure manual. See Chapter 14 for additional information related to agendas and minutes.

The minutes for a staff and team meeting should record action plans under each agenda topic. Summarize all action items agreed to in the meeting in one section of the minutes. This facilitates easy access to information at a later date should it be required.

The date, time, and place of the next meeting should be included. The person preparing the minutes should always sign them. A copy of the minutes should always be maintained in a book for easy reference.

AGENDA

STAFF MEETING Wednesday, February 16, 20XX
2:00 PM — Conference Room

1. Read and approve minutes of last meeting
2. Reports
   A. Satellite facility — Marilyn Johnson
   B. Patient flow — Joe Guerrero
   C.
3. Discussion of new telephone system
4. Unfinished Business
   A. Review new procedure manual pages
   B.
5. New Business
   A. Appoint committee for design of new marketing brochure
   B.
6. Open discussion and/or topics for next meeting's agenda
7. Set next meeting time
8. Adjourn

FIGURE 21-2 Sample meeting agenda.

Conflict Resolution

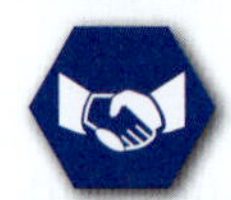

Conflict resolution, or managing conflict in the work place, is a time-consuming and necessary task not only for the clinic manager, but the providers as well. Conflicts can arise between staff members and providers, patient and provider, and even between the health care staff and the patient or patient's family. These conflicts can escalate to litigation or even violent reactions. Conflicts have a direct impact on morale; clinic efficiency; and ultimately, patient care. Without resolution, high turnover and lack of proper work environment will create serious setbacks for the clinic as a whole.

The hostile work environment has been given significant attention in recent years, and action is available for those who feel that they are working in such an environment. Abusive behavior by other employees, managers, supervisors, or even providers may take the form of a condescending attitude, ridicule, inappropriate comments or jokes, sexual harassment, threats, and fear. This type of behavior in the workplace is now less tolerated, if at all, and an organization can be held responsible for allowing the hostile work environment to continue and failing to act.

While volumes of material have been written about successful conflict management, the most helpful preventative measure is to have an office code of conduct in place. By establishing clinic policies for all members of the medical staff, these rules make it easier to correct and administer discipline where necessary. By imposing limits on unacceptable behavior, and delineating the path to discipline through a chain of command, everyone understands the process to resolution, and can often intercept and solve issues at a lower level.

Another useful tip is to recognize how conflict starts in the first place and put preventative measures in place to avoid it. Misunderstandings, lack of communication, favoritism, inequality of any kind, unreasonable expectations, and unfair or inappropriate criticism are just a few of the workplace triggers to watch for. Taking others for granted, not keeping promises, not accepting responsibility for mistakes, and personal issues interfering with work objectives and time management are also areas that can create conflict.

The following are some guidelines that may be helpful in preventing conflicts:

- Listen to your employees. What do they say? What do they communicate non-verbally?
- Manage by walking around and talking to your employees.
- Do not tolerate negative comments or actions among employees.
- Encourage an open-door policy for concerns and complaints.
- Be a role model for all employees. Practice what you preach.
- Keep confidences and treat each person with respect and understanding.

When conflicts arise, do not avoid taking immediate action to resolve the issue even if it appears to be superficially resolved. It will resurface at the first instance of stress between the individuals.

A good manager/leader will stay level and cool headed when confronted with conflict. Listening carefully, avoiding accusations or taking sides, and even repeating the issue in their your own words to show you they are understanding the problem are sound approaches to assisting with the situation. Should the conflict not be easily resolved, allow it to rest for the day, and come back to it when emotions are better able to be controlled, but do so within a day or two at most. Prolonging the issue can exacerbate the situation, with unfavorable results.

When dealing with conflict, the most difficult emotion to control is anger. It is often a self-fueling mood that will cause one to say things that were not meant or take action without thinking of the consequences. Intervening early is the best course of action, and truly understanding the problem is the first and most necessary step to successfully defusing the situation.

When addressing conflict between a provider or a supervisor and an employee, mediation is the only appropriate approach. In all other instances the best approach is to use a confrontational approach. The two persons having a conflict are brought together and asked to express their conflicting opinions without interruption. The purpose is to communicate what each perceives to be the problem. If an obvious solution that is acceptable to both parties does not appear, the manager must insist that the parties come up with an acceptable solution to the conflict. (This latter step is not appropriate for conflicts between an employee and a superior in the organization.) In doing so both parties have ownership of the resolution.

Harassment in the Workplace

Harassment consists of verbal or physical behavior/conduct that is (a) unwelcome; (b) based on a protected class (e.g., race, sex, age, national origin, veteran status, or sexual orientation); (c) severe or pervasive; and (d) has a negative impact or creates a hostile environment. As mentioned previously, as a manager, you are legally responsible for ensuring nondiscrimination and preventing harassment. You, as a manager, may be innocent of any kind of sexual harassment yourself, but if the workplace you manage is construed as hostile by any one of your employees and you do not take appropriate action, you and your clinic can be held liable in a court of law.

Legal

When an employee contacts you or you become aware of harassment, you should immediately contact your Human Resources Equal Opportunity Office (EOO). If your facility does not have an EOO, you should collect facts and confront the offending individuals or group, clearly notifying them that the offensive behavior must stop immediately. A report of the incident should be placed in the file of the offending individuals, with a written warning that a future incident will result in termination.

The manager must carefully evaluate the facts surrounding an incident. It is not uncommon for innocent events to be perceived as harassment. When there is conflict between people who are in some way different from each other, simple misunderstandings can be perceived as harassment. Blatant harassment is far less common than this kind of muddled interaction. Although some situations do involve malicious intent, many are largely the result of poor communication, and it is the manager's responsibility to differentiate between the two.

Every employer needs a written comprehensive policy that prohibits all types of harassment. The policy needs to include a definition of what could constitute harassment or create a hostile work environment, information on who to report to, and a **nonretaliation provision**. A nonretaliation provision provides protection to an employee or applicant from being retaliated against due to participation in filing a complaint regarding discrimination, or participating in an investigation or lawsuit. This would include being fired, demoted, passed up for promotion, or being harassed. For example, it is illegal to refuse to promote an employee based on discrimination charges filed by the individual, even if later it was determined that no such discrimination took place.

The law forbids retaliation when it comes to any aspect of employment, including hiring, firing, pay, job assignments, promotions, layoff, training, fringe benefits, and any other term or condition of employment. The harassment Policies and Procedures must be made available to all employees.

Assimilating New Personnel

The goal in the assimilation of new personnel into the workplace is to make it happen as seamlessly as possible. The clinic manager and HR representative usually assume this task jointly, with the clinic manager being responsible for orientation in medical protocols and procedures, and the HR representative handling orientation regarding medical practice rules and regulations and any legal implications.

New Personnel Orientation. The new personnel orientation process consists of orienting and training new employees in the medical protocols and procedures unique to the practice. If the procedure manual is detailed and accurate, this manual becomes a guide for new employees.

It is important to introduce new employees to other staff members and to assign a **mentor** who can respond to questions that new employees may raise. Sometimes the individual leaving a position still is present and is asked to assist in the orientation process. This is especially beneficial if there is a good working relationship between the employee who is leaving and the management of the practice. Depending on the responsibilities of the new employee, a supervisor may be asked to monitor all procedures for a period for accuracy, safety, and patient protection.

The orientation should clearly present what is expected of new employees and explain that, at the end of their probationary period, their performance will be evaluated to determine if full-time employment will be offered. The same procedures followed for new employees should be followed for student practicums, with the exception that expectations and the evaluation process may vary.

Probation and Evaluation. It is common for a new employee to be placed on probation for 60 to 90 days. During this period, both the employee and supervisory personnel determine if the position is a suitable match for both employer and employee. Near the end of the probation period, the employee should be officially evaluated to determine how competently he or she is performing the assigned tasks/duties. The employee should also be given an opportunity to express his or her personal thoughts relative to job satisfaction. Figure 21-3 shows a sample probationary

PROBATIONARY EMPLOYEE EVALUATION FORM

Name ____________________

Hire Date ____________________

Job Title ____________________

Pay Rate __________ Supervisor __________

Do you recommend the employee continue in employment?

________ Yes ________ No

Please state your reasons for whatever action you recommend. Use the guidelines below to make your decision.

1. Has the employee required more training than is normally needed for the job?
2. Has the employee grasped this job with very little training?
3. Is the employee performing at, above, or below (circle one) the standard for this job?
4. If below, when do you expect the employee to reach the standard?
5. Does the employee get along well with all staff members?
6. Has the employee maintained a good attendance record and a good work attitude?
7. Has the employee expressed any dissatisfactions?

____________________ __________

Supervisor's Signature Date

FIGURE 21-3 Sample probationary employee evaluation.

employee evaluation form. The evaluation becomes part of the employee's personnel record at the end of the probation period.

Supervising Student Practicums. The student **practicum** is a transitional stage that provides opportunities for the student to apply theory learned in the classroom to a health care setting through practical, hands-on experience. Some institutions use the term *externship* or *internship*, and still others operate through a cooperative education program. The number of hours for the practicum are predetermined together with criteria for site selection and tasks to be performed by the student.

The clinic manager should schedule an information interview with the student before the practicum begins. During this time, the expectations of the clinic manager and the student may be established. A tour of the facility and introductions to key personnel aid the student in feeling more comfortable the first day of "work."

Because the student will be writing in medical records where correct spelling is mandatory or may be scheduling appointments and must write telephone numbers without transposition, some pretesting may be offered. By giving a spelling test of 10 commonly used medical terms or verbally stating five telephone numbers for the student to write down, an immediate evaluation is attained.

The clinic manager should directly supervise or identify someone else to supervise the student. During the first few days of the practicum, the student may simply **shadow** the supervisor, learning the routine, provider preferences, and protocols for that particular clinic. As the student begins to feel comfortable in the new environment, minimal tasks should be assigned. Based on the student's ability to follow directions and perform tasks, increased skill–level tasks may be added.

The supervisor will direct and evaluate the student's progress; schedule activities that will provide experience in all aspects of medical assisting, including administrative, clinical, and laboratory procedures; maintain accurate records of attendance and hours "worked"; and communicate the student's progress to the medical assisting supervisor from the educational institution.

When working with students, it is important to remember that they still have much to learn and will need lots of reassuring guidance. When you take time to explain each step and to provide the rationale for each, students will learn more quickly. Demonstrating new or different techniques and approaches helps students by providing them with options that they may find more comfortable.

Remember that this type of learning is stressful. The student is not yet accustomed to communication with a "real" patient, let alone working with a provider. Your role as clinic manager is to reduce as much stress as possible for everyone concerned. Introduce the student to the patient and ask the patient's permission to allow the student to perform a procedure. Many patients will be tolerant when they realize the circumstances and will be quite cooperative.

Employees with Chemical Dependencies or Emotional Problems

Employees with chemical dependencies or emotional problems are ill and are to be treated as such. Approach the situation constructively rather than punitively. Make a commitment to the employee, to the rest of the staff, and to the patients that at no time will patient care be put at risk. Help an employee with a problem to find the support and counseling necessary. No staff member should be permitted to remain on the premise with impaired judgment while under the influence of alcohol or controlled substances. If chemical dependency treatment is necessary, make accommodation as seems appropriate or is warranted. Everyone occasionally feels discouraged and distressed. Hopefully, the provider-employer and the manager are able to recognize problems before they become too serious.

It has been said that one in four individuals will experience some form of a mental health problem during the course of a year. Work-related stress is the base cause of a significant degree of mental strain. Plan for and create a work environment that reduces as much stress as possible. Actions to consider may include the following:

1. Properly educate and train all employees for their positions.
2. Encourage teamwork and reward those who help each other.
3. Mandate "break periods" in the day for each employee.
4. Create a pleasant work environment (plants, water, music, and so on).
5. Establish a blowing off steam place for when employees are especially frustrated.
6. Take everyone out for lunch at least once a quarter.

7. Have regular staff meetings to discuss employee concerns and clinic improvements.
8. Celebrate birthdays and special occasions (e.g., length of service).

Keep in mind that a happy employee who feels valued in his or her position will stay much longer than someone who is unhappy and does not feel valued.

Evaluating Employees and Planning Salary Review

It is important that all employees know whether they are performing their job as expected and know how they can improve their performance if necessary.

Performance Evaluation. Not only is evaluation of employees necessary during the probation period, but it is necessary for current employees as well. Evaluations should be performed no less than once a year on the anniversary of the hire date. Some clinic managers may wish to evaluate an employee more often, especially if a problem has surfaced in an evaluation.

The evaluation may take many forms; it can be formal or informal; it may involve more than one person. The results of the evaluation, however, must be a part of the employee's personnel record. For that reason, a formal evaluation is preferred. Many practices use a written evaluation that requires that the employee evaluate himself or herself before meeting with the clinic manager (Figure 21-4). The clinic manager uses the same form for evaluation. During the meeting, notes are compared as the evaluation is conducted.

The climate of the performance evaluation should be comfortable and provide privacy (Figure 21-5). The meeting should be friendly, but the employee must sense the importance of the evaluation. Do not allow any disagreements to escalate into arguments during the evaluation. Without reading the employee's self-evaluation, ask the employee to tell about the self-assessment. Acknowledge the employee's point of view and identify where you agree or differ from the self-assessment. Be prepared to describe specific examples of positive performance and negative performance.

When negative performance is identified, ask the employee for possible solutions. Then a plan can be determined to alter the negative performance. In this way, a trusting atmosphere is established in that both of you are working together for a solution that will benefit the medical practice. Always look for and seek a win–win situation whenever possible. The action plan determined should then be evaluated at the next performance evaluation.

At the close of the evaluation, always express your confidence in the individual to make any changes necessary, offer assistance where needed, and thank the employee for participating. End any evaluation with a positive statement about some portion of the employee's performance.

There are occasions when reviews are performed more frequently than annually. A review would occur 2 to 3 months after a significant promotion to measure how things are progressing. Reviews occur more often when general performance falls well short of past efforts or a serious error in judgment has been made. This type of review may end with a reprimand; a warning to correct the problem by a given date; or possibly, immediate dismissal. Document any steps to be taken to correct a problem and any reason that is cause for dismissal.

Salary Review. Although the practice is common in some areas, it may be better not to tie salary increases or bonuses with the annual performance evaluation. Conduct the **salary review** at the beginning of the new year separate from performance evaluations.

Salary review is important. Unfortunately, in smaller medical clinic and ambulatory care settings, the review of salary may have to be raised by the employee. Provider-employers tend to forget that their employees have been with them for over a year without a raise or a discussion of financial remuneration. If this is the case, it is perfectly acceptable for the employee to raise the issue on a yearly basis. However, the best approach is for the clinic manager to conduct salary reviews at the beginning or end of each calendar year.

Data should be collected before a salary review. The clinic manager should network with other clinic managers in the local area to determine wages and salaries for comparable individuals with comparable skills. Remember, also, that it is far more cost effective to reward good employees with a salary increase than it is to train a new employee who commands a lesser salary than current employees. Reward employees well and provide benefits that encourage them to stay with the practice. Employees who stay with the practice for a long time not only fully understand

PERFORMANCE REVIEW FORM

______________________________	______________________________
Employee Name	Title
______________________________	______________________________
Supervisor	Department

TYPE OF REVIEW (Check One)

_______ Quarterly

_______ Annual

_______ Probation

_______ Other _____________

Review Period Covered ____________ to ____________

PERFORMANCE DEFINITIONS (To be used for general performance rating and job specific criteria rating)

5 = Outstanding	Performance that is clearly superior, beyond the call of duty, or substantially above standard level. Seldom attained level of performance but achievable.
4 = Above Standard	Very commendable performance; exceeds the norm for the job.
3 = Standard	Competent and consistent performance; expected level of activity and performance for the job. Most often rating received.
2 = Below Standard	Performance needs improvement. This level of performance is unacceptable; needs improvement to meet the standards for the job. **Employee new to the job:** Performance might receive below standard rating due to lack of job knowledge and is expected to improve with experience. **Experienced employee:** Performance is below acceptable level and requires direction and/or counsel.
1 = Unsatisfactory	Performance is unacceptable. Job activity is clearly and substantially lacking in quality, quantity, or timeliness. May also not be meeting cost or budget constraints. Needs much improvement to meet the standards for the job.

(office use only) EVALUATION SUMMARY Total I _____ Total II _____	FINAL RATING: CHECK ONE (clinic use only) _____ Merit Increase Recommended _____ No Merit Increase—Satisfactory Performance/No Growth _____ No Merit Increase (Probationary/Special Evaluation) _____ No Merit Increase (Performance Probation) _____ Re-evaluate in 90 Days for Unsatisfactory or in 180 Days for Needed Improvement

GENERAL PERFORMANCE RATING (PART I)

General Criteria	*Rating*	*Comments Supporting Rating*
1. **Patient Relations:** How well does the employee communicate a "we care" image to the patients, visitors, providers, and fellow employees?		
2. **Work Responsibilities:** Evaluate the employee's work relative to quality, quantity, and timeliness.		
3. **Teamwork:** Does the employee have a team spirit? Does the employee interact well with coworkers/supervisor/manager?		

(continues)

FIGURE 21-4 Sample performance review form.

General Criteria	Rating	Comments Supporting Rating
4. Adaptability: Is the employee open to change and new ideas? Does the employee remain flexible to changes in routine, workload, and assignments?		
5. Personal Appearance: How well does the employee maintain appropriate personal appearance, including proper attire, hygiene?		
6. Communication: Does the employee communicate well? Is information given and received clearly? Does he/she have good verbal and written skills?		
7. Dependability: Can the employee be relied upon for good attendance? Does the employee perform and follow through on work without supervisory intervention or assistance?		

Subtotal I ____________ ÷7 General Criteria = ____________

JOB-SPECIFIC CRITERIA RATING (PART II) (To be used with Job Description attached)

Responsibility and Standard	Rating	Comments Supporting Rating
Complete a section for each responsibility listed on the employee's job description.		

Subtotal II ____________ ÷ ____________ = ____________
job duties

Contributions made since last review:

____

____

____

Education or training received since last review:

____

____

____

Action to be taken based on performance:

____

____

____

Comments:

____

____

____

____________________ ____________
Employee Signature Date

____________________ ____________
Supervisor Signature Date

____________________ ____________
Provider Signature Date

FIGURE 21-4 Sample performance review form. *(continued)*

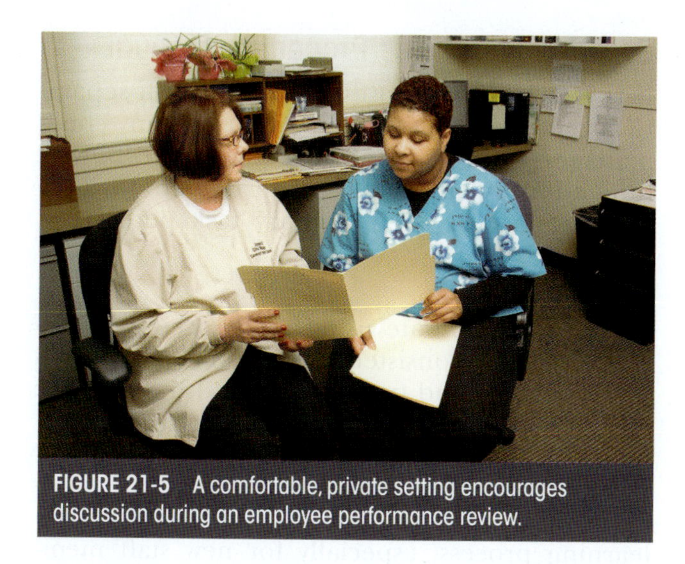

FIGURE 21-5 A comfortable, private setting encourages discussion during an employee performance review.

how best to serve their provider-employers, they have established a relationship with patients that is beneficial.

How much of a raise is to be awarded at the time of salary review is difficult to determine and depends on many factors that might include the profits of the year, the patient load, the workload, and the current cost of living.

The critical shortage of health care employees today is reflected in the shortage of medical assistants across the country. Advertisements for individuals to work in ambulatory care settings tell the story. A consideration worth mentioning is that often the salary does not match the education, experience, and special training required of someone working in the health care field. Educators often hear, "Why would I spend a year or more in education to be paid what I would make working in a fast food restaurant?" Because it is costly in time and resources to replace employees, it is best to invest that cost into a fair and just salary increase for valued employees.

Dismissing Employees

Most clinic/human resource managers do not enjoy rating the performance of other employees, particularly when difficult topics are involved and it may be necessary to dismiss an employee. However, the written performance evaluation actually establishes the format for such a dismissal when necessary and is more likely to remove the emotion from the situation. Involuntary dismissal is still difficult when it is necessary.

Involuntary Dismissal. Involuntary dismissal results from two primary causes: poor performance or serious violation of clinic policies or job descriptions. When it becomes apparent to the clinic manager that the effectiveness of an employee is dropping well below expectations, it will be known in the annual review or a performance review may be called. The review allows the employee to be informed of the shortcomings, to explain any reasons for the present situation, and to determine a plan to alleviate the problem. If the problem is a serious one, probation is usually invoked and any lack of significant improvement in the time provided results in immediate dismissal.

When the problem is a violation of either clinic policy or procedures, both a verbal and a written warning are given to the employee. Involuntary dismissal follows if the situation persists. Dismissal may be immediate if the action is a serious violation of policy. Serious violations depend on the clinic practice, but some causes for immediate dismissal include theft, making fraudulent claims against insurance, placing the patient in jeopardy by not practicing safe techniques, and breach of patient confidentiality.

Some key points to keep in mind when dismissal is necessary are:

1. Make the dismissal in private.
2. Take no longer than 10 minutes for the dismissal.
3. Be direct, firm, and to the point in identifying reasons.
4. Do not engage in an in-depth discussion of performance.
5. Explain terms of dismissal (keys, clearing out area of personal items, final paperwork).
6. Listen to the employee's opinion and emotions; it is not necessary to agree.
7. Accompany the employee to his or her desk to pack his or her belongings.
8. Escort the employee out of the facility; do not allow him or her to finish the work of the day.

Voluntary Dismissal. Other reasons for dismissal may be more pleasant. Changes in personnel occur for many good reasons, and people to voluntarily leave their jobs. They may relocate, seek advancement at another facility, or simply have personal reasons for leaving. These employees will give their manager proper notice and will be able to turn their current projects and duties over to their replacements. They have time to say good-bye to their friends and leave with a good feeling about their employment.

PROCEDURE MANUAL

The **procedure manual** provides detailed information relative to the performance of tasks within the facility in which one is employed. Each procedure manual should be designed for that specific clinic setting and should satisfy its requirements.

The procedure manual serves as a guide to the employee assigned a specific task and may also be useful in evaluating the employee's performance. If a temporary employee is assigned the task, the procedure manual will be invaluable in ensuring that each procedure is completed as outlined.

The provider(s) and the clinic manager should have copies of the procedure manual, and all employees should have access to the procedure manual. Copies of individual sections may be given to the employee responsible for the task; the employee should be instructed to follow these guidelines and told that they may be used as employee evaluation tools. If all employees have access to the clinic computer system, the procedure manual can be made available in electronic format.

Organization of the Procedure Manual

It is best to use a loose-leaf binder with separator pages denoting each procedure. Many clinic managers find it helpful to divide the binder into administrative and clinical sections with subdivisions for each primary task performed (Table 21-2).

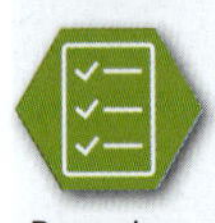

To facilitate using the procedure manual, a consistent format should be developed and used throughout the manual. Each procedure should be a step-by-step outline or list of steps to be taken to complete a task as desired in that facility. Providing the rationale for a step, when appropriate, enhances the learning process, especially for new staff members. Material Safety Data Sheets (MSDS) are required to be maintained in the clinic and available for personnel to reference at any time. MSDS must be compiled for all chemicals considered hazardous and maintained in an appropriate manual. Some clinics opt to maintain these records in a separate tabbed section of the procedure manual. Others choose to maintain a separate MSDS manual. The information must be reviewed and updated on a regular basis. Procedure 21-3 provides steps for developing and maintaining a procedure manual.

TABLE 21-2

ORGANIZING THE PROCEDURE MANUAL

ADMINISTRATIVE SECTION	CLINICAL SECTION	ADMINISTRATIVE/CLINICAL SECTIONS
Personnel Management	Physical Examinations	HIPAA and ADA compliance
Communication (oral and written)	Infection Control	Creating a Safe Environment
Patient Scheduling	Collecting Specimens	Evacuation Procedures
Records Management	Laboratory Procedures	Emergency Codes
Financial Management	Surgical Asepsis	Fire Safety
Facility and Equipment Management	Emergencies	Fire Extinguisher Safety
	Material Safety Data Sheets (MSDS)	Response to National Disaster or Emergency
	OSHA	Medical Assistant Response to Disaster Preparedness
	CLIA '88	

PROCEDURE 21-3

Procedure

Developing and Maintaining a Procedure Manual

PURPOSE:

To develop and maintain a comprehensive, up-to-date procedure manual covering each clinical, technical, and administrative procedure in the clinic, with step-by-step directions and rationales for performing each task.

EQUIPMENT/SUPPLIES:

- Computer (electronic storage allows changes and revisions to be made easily)
- Binder, such as a three-ring binder
- Paper
- Standard procedure manual format

PROCEDURE STEPS:

1. ***Pay attention to detail*** by writing step-by-step procedures and rationales for each clinical, technical, and administrative function. Each procedure is written by experienced employees close to the function and then reviewed by a supervisor and clinic manager. Rationales help employees understand **why** something is done. RATIONALE: Establishes consistent guidelines to be followed.
2. Include regular maintenance instructions and flow sheets for cleaning, servicing, and calibrating of all clinic equipment, both in the clinical and in the administrative areas. RATIONALE: Equipment needs to be cleaned and maintained on a regular basis to ensure it is working properly and that it lasts as long as needed. Some manufacturer guarantees and service contracts require regular cleaning and maintenance, especially on new and leased equipment. Instructions are necessary so that the task can be performed properly. The flow sheets provide documentation of dates the equipment was cleaned, serviced, and/or calibrated and the person who performed the task.
3. Include local and out-of-the-area resources for clinical and administrative staff, providers, and patients. Provide a listing in each area with contact information and services provided. RATIONALE: The procedures and instructions listed in the procedure manual should provide supporting documentation needed for accomplishing each task. For example, if the clinic requires that local public transportation resources be given to each patient who needs transportation, the procedure manual has a listing of transportation available in the area with telephone numbers and schedules. This document could either be printed from the computer or photocopied from the manual and provided to the patient.
4. ***Recognize the importance of local, state, and federal legislation and regulations*** that are related to processes performed in both clinical and administrative areas. RATIONALE: Having a listing of the rules and regulations assists in performing those regulated duties correctly and legally.
5. Include the clinic procedures and flow sheets for taking inventory in each of the areas and instructions on ordering procedures. RATIONALE: When a clinic has processes clearly written for managing inventory and ordering equipment and supplies, the clinic is less likely to run out of needed items and may even be able to take advantage of discounts offered by manufacturers.
6. Collect the procedures into the Clinic Procedure Manual. RATIONALE: Provides a reference guide with step-by-step instructions and examples where appropriate.
7. Store one complete manual in a common library area. Provide a completed copy to the provider-employer and the clinic manager. Distribute appropriate sections to the various departments. RATIONALE: Provides a reference guide with step-by-step instructions and examples where appropriate.
8. Review the procedure manual annually and add any new procedures, delete or modify as necessary, and indicate the revision date (e.g., Rev. 10/12/XX). RATIONALE: Maintains current clinic protocols.

Updating and Reviewing the Procedure Manual

When new procedures are added to the clinic routine, a new procedure page should be developed immediately. The new page is useful as an educational tool or job aid while team members are learning new techniques.

An annual page-by-page review should be done to ascertain if each procedure is still being used and to ensure that each page is correct in each detail and satisfies all criteria established by the staff personnel. This contributes to an efficient clinic and gives all employees a sense of pride and satisfaction that they are performing within the scope of their training and to their greatest potential. The procedure manual should be reviewed by personnel performing the various tasks, and their suggestions should be evaluated and incorporated into the revisions when appropriate. All new procedure pages and revisions should be dated (e.g., Rev. 02/15/XX).

HIPAA IMPLICATIONS

HIPAA regulations require each clinic to develop a separate HIPAA manual that is in either an electronic form or a paper manual. The manual spells out all policies and procedures of the practice and security management measures; identifies the security officer; addresses workforce security issues, information access concerns, security awareness and training, security incidents, and contingency plans; evaluates security effectiveness; and contains copies of all business associate contracts.

The HIPAA manual must be available to all employees and updated on a regular basis. During an audit, the clinic manager will be asked to produce the HIPAA manual for review and to establish compliance with all regulations. All documentation of policies and procedures are to be kept for 6 years even if the wording has changed or a particular policy or procedure has been eliminated. If an incident is under investigation, this allows an investigator to go back to what a policy said 6 years ago.

TRAVEL ARRANGEMENTS

The clinic manager may be asked to make travel arrangements for providers going on vacation or to conventions, symposiums, or out-of-town seminars and continuing medical education (CME) courses. If the providers do a fair amount of travel or if they live in a metropolitan area, they may use the services of a travel agent. Attention to detail is extremely important in preventing travel disruptions.

Read carefully the instructions for completing registration forms, complete them online, or, mail them as quickly as possible to secure reservations to conventions. Next, make hotel and travel arrangements. General information regarding the provider's travel preferences should be maintained in a file and referred to when making travel arrangements. Helpful information to maintain in this file includes:

- Name of travel agents used in the past
- Provider's or clinic credit card numbers (though this information must be properly safeguarded)
- Transportation preferences
- Preferred airline, class of travel, seating choice
- Hotel/motel accommodations (bed size, suite, studio, connecting rooms, price range, amenities)

Next, contact the travel agent and identify the destination, date and time for departure and return, number traveling in party, and seating preference. A travel agent can assist with rental car and hotel accommodations, if needed. Take your time and pay attention to details. When tickets are received, always check to see that all departure and arrival times match what is needed and that a confirmation number has been provided for car rentals and hotel arrangements.

The Internet can be used to search for the lowest-cost air, auto, and lodging reservations. The procedures do not require extensive knowledge of travel and airline reservation protocols. Searching for information on the Internet requires the use of a search engine if you do not already have a list of favorite travel Web sites. Once you refine your search, you may have choices such as Travelocity.com, Expedia.com, or Priceline.com. Select the desired Web sites and follow its instructions.

Procedure

Procedure 21-4 outlines the steps for making travel arrangements via the Internet.

PROCEDURE 21-4

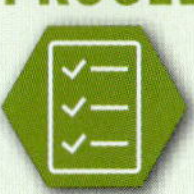
Procedure

Making Travel Arrangements via the Internet

PURPOSE:

To use the Internet to make travel arrangements for the provider.

EQUIPMENT/SUPPLIES:

- Travel plan
- Computer
- Provider's or clinic's credit card to pay for reservations.

PROCEDURE STEPS:

1. ***Paying attention to detail,*** confirm the planned trip: date, time, and place for departure and arrival; preferred mode of transportation (plane, train, bus, car); number of travelers; preferred lodging type and price range; and whether travelers' checks are required. RATIONALE: Confirming pertinent travel details ensures that correct arrangements will be made.
2. Go to the computer and access the Internet.
3. ***Show initiative*** by selecting a search engine to locate Web sites using the key term "air fares." Web sites may provide links to air fares, auto reservations, and hotel/motel reservations. Follow Web site instructions for making arrangements. Review and copy confirmation of your transaction. RATIONALE: The Internet can be a time saver and a cost effective way of securing travel arrangements.
4. Pick up tickets or arrange for their delivery, if necessary. Tickets purchased on the Internet can be mailed or picked up at an airport, or they can be electronic tickets.
5. Make additional copies of the itinerary or create the itinerary. The itinerary should list date and time of departures and arrivals, including flight numbers and seat assignments. Note the mode of transportation to lodging (shuttle, bus, car, taxi). Include name, address, and telephone number of lodgings and meeting places.
6. Maintain one copy of the itinerary in the clinic file.
7. Give several copies of the itinerary to the provider. RATIONALE: Ensures that a copy is on file with the clinic and that there are sufficient copies for the traveler(s) and families.

Itinerary

If you have used a travel agent in making the travel arrangements, the agency most likely will provide several copies of the **itinerary**. An itinerary is a detailed plan for a proposed trip. The clinic should maintain one copy of the itinerary in case the provider must be reached for emergencies. The provider should have one copy to carry with him or her and a copy to leave with family members. You may need to develop the itinerary if you have made the travel arrangements via computer. Figure 21-6 shows a sample travel itinerary.

Important information to be included on any itinerary includes:

- *Air travel.* Departure and arrival date and time, meals, airline name and telephone number, airport
- *Car rental.* Name, telephone number, confirmation number
- *Hotel/motel.* Name, confirmation number, dates, telephone number
- *Meeting location.* Name, address, room number, telephone number

TRAVEL ITINERARY

James Whitney, MD
Inner City Health Care
400 Inner City Way
Seattle, WA 98400

15 Sept 20XX	INVOICE: 880133795				
29 Sept Friday					
USAIR 630	Coach Class	Equip-Boeing 757 Jet			
LV: Seattle	11:55P	Nonstop	Miles-2125		Confirmed
AR: Pittsburgh	7:23A	Elapsed time-4:28		Arrival Date-30Sept	
		Seat-31C			
30 Sept-Saturday					
Alamo		1 Compact 2/4 DR	Drop-101CT		Confirmed
Pickup-Pittsburgh		Pittsburgh Airport	Chg-USD .00		
Rate- 59.98	Base rate	Guaranteed		Extra Hr 10.00-UN	
Phone-412-472-5060					
	Confirmation-1870649				
01 Oct Sunday					
USAIR 1419	Coach Class	Equip-Boeing 737 Jet			
LV: Pittsburgh	3:05P	Nonstop	Miles-2125		Confirmed
AR: Seattle	5:27P	Elapsed time-5:22			
Lunch		Seat-20A			

Ticket Number/s:					
Whitney/James	3570933		BA Card		$461.00
Air Transportation	$416.36	Tax	44.64	TOTAL	$461.00
		Sub Total			$461.00
		Credit Card Payment			$461.00-
		Amount Due			0.00

TICKET IS NON REFUNDABLE. TRIP INSURANCE IS AVAILABLE. RECONFIRM ALL FLTS 24 HRS PRIOR TO DEPARTURE

FIGURE 21-6 Sample travel itinerary.

TIME MANAGEMENT

Time management is an item of critical importance to the manager. You may have upward of 20 staff members putting demands on your time, and added to this are vendors, your superiors, business associates, and a host of others. A manager has not a moment to lose in the day, so managing time makes the difference between a normal 8- or 10-hour day and a 15-hour or more day. The following suggestions are some proven means of managing your time whether in management or as a salaried employee.

- *Handle items once.* Once the mail is opened, sorted, and prioritized, try to handle it only once more, when action is taken with it. Picking it up, reading it, and setting it down again without taking action is a real waste of time.
- *Develop a to-do list.* At the end of each day prepare a list of things you plan to complete the next day and try to work down this list. Prioritize the list by importance or by practical order.
- *Guard your time.* Schedule meetings with personnel and vendors so that they do not

fragment your time, making you have to restart a task and get up to speed over and over again. Although modern management practice is to have an open-door policy with employees, this does not mean you should allow them to come into your office whenever they think about it. Have them schedule time with you. Make them think about what they want to discuss and do not let them monopolize your time. This is also true of meeting with vendors; require vendors to schedule ahead a time to meet with you.

- *Delegate work.* Assign others or a team to perform some of the functions discussed in this chapter. Having a team prepare weekly work schedules and vacation schedules results in less bickering and feelings of favoritism that you would have to spend time defusing if you made the schedules yourself. This does not mean that you do not have to approve them and, in some instances, make the hard decisions, but it results in your people having ownership in the decisions.

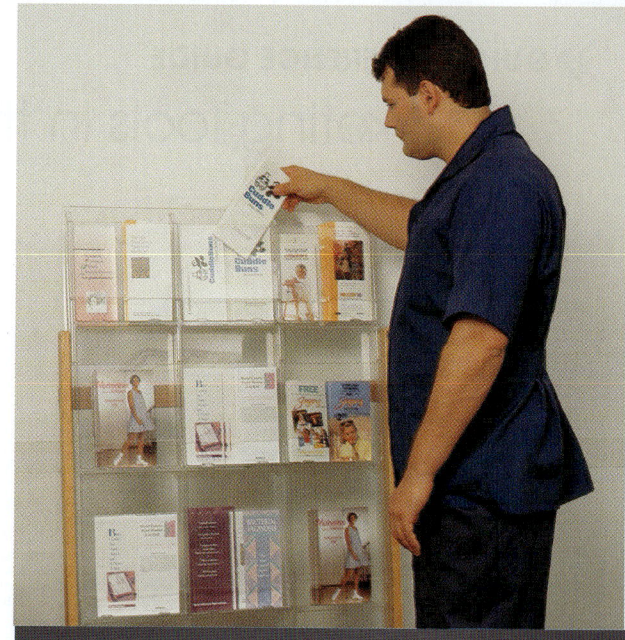

FIGURE 21-7 Brochures and handouts should be accessible and inviting to patients and clinic visitors.

MARKETING FUNCTIONS

Communication

Effective communication skills are essential in the management of the ambulatory care setting. These skills are used by the clinic manager inside the ambulatory care setting to establish friendly, professional relationships with colleagues and patients. Communication is just as critical when relating to external audiences, such as other organizations, potential new patients, and community members. Developing relationships outside the clinic is often called marketing, a concept that clinic managers may use to enhance the image and visibility of an ambulatory care setting while also providing benefits to patients, potential patients, and the neighboring community.

In its broadest sense, **marketing** can be defined as the process by which the provider of services makes the consumer aware of the scope and quality of these services. Although marketing is a tool traditionally used by for-profit organizations to promote and sell products and services, it has become increasingly acceptable among health care organizations, whether they are for- or not-for-profit.

Marketing functions and materials are diverse and can include presence on social media sites, seminars and workshops, patient education brochures (Figure 21-7), brochures that describe the ambulatory care setting and its scope of services, HIPAA policies, newsletters, press releases, and special events such as open houses or participation in community health care events. Depending on the size and resources of the medical clinic, the manager may choose to use all or some of these tools.

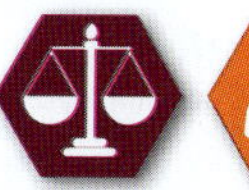
Legal

Diversity

When producing written material and organizing events, it is essential that ethical guidelines be respected at all times. Marketing tools should be appropriate, in good taste, and designed to quietly enhance the reputation of the clinic. Cultural issues should always be considered. For example, patient education brochures for a practice with many Spanish-speaking patients should be produced in bilingual editions, with English on one side and Spanish on the other. Legal issues are important as well; when presenting material of a medical nature, it is extremely important that information be accurate and up to date.

Effective marketing is a valuable tool for the clinic manager, especially as managed care calls on all health care professionals to become more competitive to survive. Marketing can increase visibility and credibility. The effective manager enlists the talents and skills of the entire team in developing a marketing plan. (See the "Marketing Tools in the Medical Environment" Quick Reference Guide.)

QUICK REFERENCE GUIDE

Marketing Tools in the Medical Environment

Category 1:

Internal marketing tools.
Marketing tools specific to the functions of the clinic and services provided are often presented in the form of brochures, seminars, and workshops.

Brochures.
Patient education brochures can address a variety of topics. Specialized procedures, surgeries, and common diseases and syndromes that are explained in simple terms can aid in understanding and patient preparation when needed. This information must always be updated. Clinic brochures describe the clinic, HIPAA policies, insurance and payment information, provider profiles, and scope of services for the patient. Cultural issues should be considered by providing material in multiple languages, as applicable to the practice.

Seminars and workshops.
In clinics where patient education, procedure preparation, or obtaining more information before making medical decisions is important, seminars and workshops are effective tools for providing expert advice. These tools meet patient and community needs by providing a forum for health care professionals and patients to interact. Popular topics include hypertension, diabetes, eating disorders and bariatric surgery, joint replacement, and pain management. Audiovisuals, presentations, handouts, brochures, and anatomical models or samples can elaborate on and enhance seminar content, helping patients remember what was said.

Category 3:

External marketing tools.
Educating the public on various medical topics and procedures often goes hand in hand with the subtle promotion of a clinic when using marketing tools. Whether a clinic specializes in a particular area of medicine, emphasizes preventative measures for better health, or introduces new treatment or surgery options, external marketing provides a platform to accomplish these goals while also giving the community options for local health care professionals providing these services.

Newsletters.
Newsletters are more focused on the individual practice and its philosophies. Newsletters can be sent to the clinic's mailing list, or there are online services that offer newsletter creation and then the newsletters can be sent by email. This is an optimal way to offer health-related articles, including clinic updates such as policy changes, staff introductions, and insurance information. Typically released biannually or quarterly, newsletters can be made available in the waiting room.

Web sites and e-zines.
Having access to clinic information and resources, such as registration forms, portal login, and other clinic-related materials any time of day or night is necessary in our technology-driven world. Web sites also provide a place to present medical information in the form of articles, videos, and interactive tools for current and potential patients. E-zines are online magazines that can be released on Web sites or emailed to a patient base on a regular basis, and can also be archived for future reference.

Special events.
Medicine is a collaborative effort, and special events such as health fairs, community events, and open houses offer an opportunity to join with other organizations to promote wellness. These events are usually well attended and offer the perfect place to discuss clinic services as well as new medical technology and procedures. They're also a great way provide information directly to the community.

Press releases.
Releasing information through local publications and even some online resources requires a press release. The press release follows a particular format for submission, and is almost exclusively accepted in digital form through email or online forms to editors. They are a way to announce clinic expansions, new equipment, providers joining the practice, or add-on services and affiliations with area facilities.

Social media.
Digital forms of communication have made social media such as Facebook, Twitter, and blogging not only necessary marketing tools, but excellent ways to keep information updated and available to patients and visitors seeking information. Video and photo sharing sites, such as Instagram, can be used to present medical information as a tool in patient education. In the clinic, providers often have an archive of videos handy on tablets, smart phones, and on the exam room PC that visually explain diseases, surgeries, and procedure preparation in addition to traditional anatomical models and drawings.

SOCIAL MEDIA AND THE MEDICAL CLINIC

Social media is an instrument of communication enabling communication in both directions. The telephone was an early means of social communication, but its reach to a mass audience was limited. Reading a newspaper or listening to a report on the radio does not allow the user to interact. This is where, on a very basic level, social media stands apart. It does allow a Web site visitor to interact with the site and with other visitors on the site. Social media can take on many different forms. Definitions of some of these social media forms are:

- *Webinar.* A seminar or lecture delivered over the Internet. It can be one-way (webcast) or with audience interaction.
- *Social networking.* Interact by adding friends, commenting on profiles, and joining groups and having discussions. Facebook and LinkedIn are examples of this form of social media, as are Twitter and Instagram on a micro scale.
- *Blogs.* A Web site on which an individual or group of users record opinions and information in a more conversational and informal manner, called blogging.
- *Social photo and video sharing.* Interact by sharing photos or videos and commenting on user submissions. YouTube and Instagram are examples of this form.
- *Wikis.* Interact by adding articles and editing existing articles. Wikipedia is an example of this form.
- *Social news.* Interact by voting on articles and submitting comments. Examples include Reddit and Digg.

The social media revolution has forever carried over to business. A purposeful and carefully designed social media strategy must become an integral part of any modern, complete, and directed business plan or job-seeking strategy.

Social media gives you a voice and a way to communicate with patients and potential consumers, to find qualified employees, and to verify the background of persons seeking employment with your organization. It personalizes the medical clinic and helps you to spread your message in a relaxed and conversational way. Social media projects your clinic as a personality. You want the clinic to become a respected source of information to the patient. According to a study highlighted by the American Academy of Family Physicians' (AAFP) social media guide, more than 70% of primary care physicians and oncologists use social media at least once a month to explore or contribute health information. Purpose, direction, consistent updating, and posting of relevant content will go a long way in making social media sites places where time is well spent by visitors. The main focus should be on providing an source of information for patients, caregivers, and families. As time has proven, many people seek out information on the Internet by searching their symptoms and concerns, and overwhelm themselves and cause anxiety in an effort to self-educate. Social media provides the perfect platform for the medical community to present facts and reasonable data, and encourage the patient to consult with a medical professional in the clinic in order to properly address health concerns.

You must always remember that in no way should social media be a place for offering medical advice. However, the effort to present accurate, valuable information that gently guides the patient to the correct and safest course of action while providing an enjoyable and more personalized experience can be achieved.

The power of social networking as a marketing tool is illustrated by response buttons on Facebook such as the "Like" button. The "Like" button links your Web site to the visitor's Facebook profile if he or she Likes your site. Your site, through his or her profile, becomes a living testimonial to your product or organization. In addition, you have the ability to publish updates to the user. One contact now becomes hundreds.

Many clinic managers are perplexed over whether social networking should be allowed by employees while at work. Many managers have a perception of employees hanging out on cyberspace wasting time. Experts on the subject do not support this perception. They feel that social networking can contribute to team building and can motivate employees, especially in small companies where the staff may be isolated from each other. The result has been increased productivity in most instances. Prohibition of social networking can result in the loss of valued employees. The answer to the question probably lies between total prohibition and uncontrolled use resulting in abuse. If social networking is allowed on the job, protocols should be in place to prevent HIPAA violations, to define where and when social networking is acceptable, and to prohibit bullying of colleagues. A manager must use caution in monitoring employee actions online to avoid overstepping legal boundaries.

RECORDS AND FINANCIAL MANAGEMENT

Providers entrust a great deal of responsibility to their medical clinic managers. The daily payments received through the mail and clinic visits must be processed and prepared for banking. Clinic expenses must be processed and paid in a timely fashion to capitalize on any discounts available. Employee requirements and records such as Social Security records; Withholding Allowance Certificates (W-4 forms) indicating the number of exemptions claimed (Figure 21-8); and Employment Eligibility Verification Forms (Form I-9) ensuring that all persons employed are either U.S. citizens, lawfully admitted immigrants, or citizens of other countries authorized to work in the United States must be completed and filed with the appropriate federal agencies. Also, state and local tax records must be maintained for each employee.

Electronic Health Records and the Clinic Manager

The practice management (PM) system and electronic medical record (EMR) discussed in Chapter 10 is the nerve center for the clinic manager as he or she orchestrates a smooth-running organization. It provides all of the data needed by the clinic manager at the click of a mouse or a few keystrokes. Table 21-3 lists sample data types and the resulting actions by the manager.

TABLE 21-3

CLINIC MANAGER ACTIONS IN RESPONSE TO PM AND EMR DATA

DATA	ACTION BY CLINIC MANAGER
Staffing requirements and appointment schedules	Hire or terminate employees, obtain additional clinic space and equipment, adjust vacation schedules
Equipment and supplies requests, and inventory data	Issue purchase orders, authorize payment of invoices, secure vendors and suppliers, negotiate maintenance contracts
Financial and billing reports	Practice financial status reports, instructions for coding and billing on past due accounts, actions on billing denied due to coding errors
Employee time sheets	Payroll authorization, corrective actions for missed work
Medical records	Review if patient demographics and HIPAA requirements are current
Personnel data	Progress reviews, salary reviews, W-4 forms, corrective actions, licenses, malpractice insurance contracts

Payroll Processing

In some cases, it is the clinic manager's responsibility to prepare payroll checks for each employee and record all deductions withheld. A W-2 form (Figure 21-9) summarizing all earnings and deductions for the year must be prepared for each employee by January 31 of the following year. The Social Security Administration must receive a summary report of W-2 forms each year.

Legal

To comply with all federal, state, and local governmental regulations, it is important that the clinic manager who processes payroll maintain complete, up-to-date records on every employee. This information should be gathered from new employees and updated every year, including any changes in employee status. For more specific information regarding printed and electronic filing forms, consult the Internal Revenue Service Web site (http://www.irs.gov) for detailed instructions. It is a good idea to have employees update their W-4 form each year in case they want to adjust their deductions or make any other change. To accomplish this, many payroll managers include a new W-4 form with the first paycheck at the beginning of each year. Every employee file should contain the employee's Social Security number; number of exemptions claimed on the W-4 form; employee's gross salary; and all deductions withheld for all taxes, including Social Security, federal, state, local, and unemployment tax (where applicable), and disability insurance (where applicable).

Form W-4 (2016)

Purpose. Complete Form W-4 so that your employer can withhold the correct federal income tax from your pay. Consider completing a new Form W-4 each year and when your personal or financial situation changes.

Exemption from withholding. If you are exempt, complete **only** lines 1, 2, 3, 4, and 7 and sign the form to validate it. Your exemption for 2016 expires February 15, 2017. See Pub. 505, Tax Withholding and Estimated Tax.

Note: If another person can claim you as a dependent on his or her tax return, you cannot claim exemption from withholding if your income exceeds $1,050 and includes more than $350 of unearned income (for example, interest and dividends).

Exceptions. An employee may be able to claim exemption from withholding even if the employee is a dependent, if the employee:

- Is age 65 or older,
- Is blind, or
- Will claim adjustments to income; tax credits; or itemized deductions, on his or her tax return.

The exceptions do not apply to supplemental wages greater than $1,000,000.

Basic instructions. If you are not exempt, complete the **Personal Allowances Worksheet** below. The worksheets on page 2 further adjust your withholding allowances based on itemized deductions, certain credits, adjustments to income, or two-earners/multiple jobs situations.

Complete all worksheets that apply. However, you may claim fewer (or zero) allowances. For regular wages, withholding must be based on allowances you claimed and may not be a flat amount or percentage of wages.

Head of household. Generally, you can claim head of household filing status on your tax return only if you are unmarried and pay more than 50% of the costs of keeping up a home for yourself and your dependent(s) or other qualifying individuals. See Pub. 501, Exemptions, Standard Deduction, and Filing Information, for information.

Tax credits. You can take projected tax credits into account in figuring your allowable number of withholding allowances. Credits for child or dependent care expenses and the child tax credit may be claimed using the **Personal Allowances Worksheet** below. See Pub. 505 for information on converting your other credits into withholding allowances.

Nonwage income. If you have a large amount of nonwage income, such as interest or dividends, consider making estimated tax payments using Form 1040-ES, Estimated Tax for Individuals. Otherwise, you may owe additional tax. If you have pension or annuity income, see Pub. 505 to find out if you should adjust your withholding on Form W-4 or W-4P.

Two earners or multiple jobs. If you have a working spouse or more than one job, figure the total number of allowances you are entitled to claim on all jobs using worksheets from only one Form W-4. Your withholding usually will be most accurate when all allowances are claimed on the Form W-4 for the highest paying job and zero allowances are claimed on the others. See Pub. 505 for details.

Nonresident alien. If you are a nonresident alien, see Notice 1392, Supplemental Form W-4 Instructions for Nonresident Aliens, before completing this form.

Check your withholding. After your Form W-4 takes effect, use Pub. 505 to see how the amount you are having withheld compares to your projected total tax for 2016. See Pub. 505, especially if your earnings exceed $130,000 (Single) or $180,000 (Married).

Future developments. Information about any future developments affecting Form W-4 (such as legislation enacted after we release it) will be posted at *www.irs.gov/w4*.

Personal Allowances Worksheet (Keep for your records.)

A Enter "1" for **yourself** if no one else can claim you as a dependent . . . . . **A** ______

B Enter "1" if: { • You are single and have only one job; or • You are married, have only one job, and your spouse does not work; or • Your wages from a second job or your spouse's wages (or the total of both) are $1,500 or less. } . . . **B** ______

C Enter "1" for your **spouse.** But, you may choose to enter "-0-" if you are married and have either a working spouse or more than one job. (Entering "-0-" may help you avoid having too little tax withheld.) . . . . . **C** ______

D Enter number of **dependents** (other than your spouse or yourself) you will claim on your tax return . . . . . **D** ______

E Enter "1" if you will file as **head of household** on your tax return (see conditions under **Head of household** above) . . **E** ______

F Enter "1" if you have at least $2,000 of **child or dependent care expenses** for which you plan to claim a credit . . . **F** ______
(**Note:** Do **not** include child support payments. See Pub. 503, Child and Dependent Care Expenses, for details.)

G **Child Tax Credit** (including additional child tax credit). See Pub. 972, Child Tax Credit, for more information.
- If your total income will be less than $70,000 ($100,000 if married), enter "2" for each eligible child; then **less** "1" if you have two to four eligible children or **less** "2" if you have five or more eligible children.
- If your total income will be between $70,000 and $84,000 ($100,000 and $119,000 if married), enter "1" for each eligible child . . **G** ______

H Add lines A through G and enter total here. (**Note:** This may be different from the number of exemptions you claim on your tax return.) ▶ **H** ______

For accuracy, **complete all worksheets that apply.**
- If you plan to **itemize** or **claim adjustments to income** and want to reduce your withholding, see the **Deductions and Adjustments Worksheet** on page 2.
- If you are **single and have more than one job** or are **married and you and your spouse both work** and the combined earnings from all jobs exceed $50,000 ($20,000 if married), see the **Two-Earners/Multiple Jobs Worksheet** on page 2 to avoid having too little tax withheld.
- If **neither** of the above situations applies, **stop here** and enter the number from line H on line 5 of Form W-4 below.

--- **Separate here and give Form W-4 to your employer. Keep the top part for your records.** ---

Form **W-4** | Department of the Treasury, Internal Revenue Service

Employee's Withholding Allowance Certificate

▶ **Whether you are entitled to claim a certain number of allowances or exemption from withholding is subject to review by the IRS. Your employer may be required to send a copy of this form to the IRS.**

OMB No. 1545-0074 | **2016**

1 Your first name and middle initial	Last name	2 **Your social security number**
Home address (number and street or rural route)	3 ☐ Single ☐ Married ☐ Married, but withhold at higher Single rate. **Note:** If married, but legally separated, or spouse is a nonresident alien, check the "Single" box.	
City or town, state, and ZIP code	4 **If your last name differs from that shown on your social security card, check here. You must call 1-800-772-1213 for a replacement card.** ▶ ☐	

5 Total number of allowances you are claiming (from line **H** above **or** from the applicable worksheet on page 2) | 5 |

6 Additional amount, if any, you want withheld from each paycheck . . . . . | 6 | $

7 I claim exemption from withholding for 2016, and I certify that I meet **both** of the following conditions for exemption.
- Last year I had a right to a refund of **all** federal income tax withheld because I had **no** tax liability, **and**
- This year I expect a refund of **all** federal income tax withheld because I expect to have **no** tax liability.

If you meet both conditions, write "Exempt" here . . . . . ▶ | 7 |

Under penalties of perjury, I declare that I have examined this certificate and, to the best of my knowledge and belief, it is true, correct, and complete.

Employee's signature
(This form is not valid unless you sign it.) ▶ **Date** ▶

8 Employer's name and address (Employer: Complete lines 8 and 10 only if sending to the IRS.)	9 Office code (optional)	10 Employer identification number (EIN)

For Privacy Act and Paperwork Reduction Act Notice, see page 2. Cat. No. 10220Q Form **W-4** (2016)

FIGURE 21-8 Form W-4 indicates the number of exemptions claimed by the employee for income tax purposes.

Deductions and Adjustments Worksheet

Note: Use this worksheet *only* if you plan to itemize deductions or claim certain credits or adjustments to income.

1 Enter an estimate of your 2016 itemized deductions. These include qualifying home mortgage interest, charitable contributions, state and local taxes, medical expenses in excess of 10% (7.5% if either you or your spouse was born before January 2, 1952) of your income, and miscellaneous deductions. For 2016, you may have to reduce your itemized deductions if your income is over $311,300 and you are married filing jointly or are a qualifying widow(er); $285,350 if you are head of household; $259,400 if you are single and not head of household or a qualifying widow(er); or $155,650 if you are married filing separately. See Pub. 505 for details . . . **1** $ ______

2 Enter: { $12,600 if married filing jointly or qualifying widow(er); $9,300 if head of household; $6,300 if single or married filing separately } . . . **2** $ ______

3 **Subtract** line 2 from line 1. If zero or less, enter "-0-" . . . **3** $ ______

4 Enter an estimate of your 2016 adjustments to income and any additional standard deduction (see Pub. 505) **4** $ ______

5 **Add** lines 3 and 4 and enter the total. (Include any amount for credits from the *Converting Credits to Withholding Allowances for 2016 Form W-4* worksheet in Pub. 505.) . . . **5** $ ______

6 Enter an estimate of your 2016 nonwage income (such as dividends or interest) . . . **6** $ ______

7 **Subtract** line 6 from line 5. If zero or less, enter "-0-" . . . **7** $ ______

8 **Divide** the amount on line 7 by $4,050 and enter the result here. Drop any fraction . . . **8** ______

9 Enter the number from the **Personal Allowances Worksheet,** line H, page 1 . . . **9** ______

10 **Add** lines 8 and 9 and enter the total here. If you plan to use the **Two-Earners/Multiple Jobs Worksheet,** also enter this total on line 1 below. Otherwise, **stop here** and enter this total on Form W-4, line 5, page 1 **10** ______

Two-Earners/Multiple Jobs Worksheet (See *Two earners or multiple jobs* on page 1.)

Note: Use this worksheet *only* if the instructions under line H on page 1 direct you here.

1 Enter the number from line H, page 1 (or from line 10 above if you used the **Deductions and Adjustments Worksheet**) **1** ______

2 Find the number in **Table 1** below that applies to the **LOWEST** paying job and enter it here. **However,** if you are married filing jointly and wages from the highest paying job are $65,000 or less, do not enter more than "3" . . . **2** ______

3 If line 1 is **more than or equal to** line 2, subtract line 2 from line 1. Enter the result here (if zero, enter "-0-") and on Form W-4, line 5, page 1. **Do not** use the rest of this worksheet . . . **3** ______

Note: If line 1 is **less than** line 2, enter "-0-" on Form W-4, line 5, page 1. Complete lines 4 through 9 below to figure the additional withholding amount necessary to avoid a year-end tax bill.

4 Enter the number from line 2 of this worksheet . . . **4** ______

5 Enter the number from line 1 of this worksheet . . . **5** ______

6 **Subtract** line 5 from line 4 . . . **6** ______

7 Find the amount in **Table 2** below that applies to the **HIGHEST** paying job and enter it here . . . **7** $ ______

8 **Multiply** line 7 by line 6 and enter the result here. This is the additional annual withholding needed . . **8** $ ______

9 Divide line 8 by the number of pay periods remaining in 2016. For example, divide by 25 if you are paid every two weeks and you complete this form on a date in January when there are 25 pay periods remaining in 2016. Enter the result here and on Form W-4, line 6, page 1. This is the additional amount to be withheld from each paycheck **9** $ ______

Table 1

Married Filing Jointly		All Others	
If wages from **LOWEST** paying job are—	Enter on line 2 above	If wages from **LOWEST** paying job are—	Enter on line 2 above
$0 - $6,000	0	$0 - $9,000	0
6,001 - 14,000	1	9,001 - 17,000	1
14,001 - 25,000	2	17,001 - 26,000	2
25,001 - 27,000	3	26,001 - 34,000	3
27,001 - 35,000	4	34,001 - 44,000	4
35,001 - 44,000	5	44,001 - 75,000	5
44,001 - 55,000	6	75,001 - 85,000	6
55,001 - 65,000	7	85,001 - 110,000	7
65,001 - 75,000	8	110,001 - 125,000	8
75,001 - 80,000	9	125,001 - 140,000	9
80,001 - 100,000	10	140,001 and over	10
100,001 - 115,000	11		
115,001 - 130,000	12		
130,001 - 140,000	13		
140,001 - 150,000	14		
150,001 and over	15		

Table 2

Married Filing Jointly		All Others	
If wages from **HIGHEST** paying job are—	Enter on line 7 above	If wages from **HIGHEST** paying job are—	Enter on line 7 above
$0 - $75,000	$610	$0 - $38,000	$610
75,001 - 135,000	1,010	38,001 - 85,000	1,010
135,001 - 205,000	1,130	85,001 - 185,000	1,130
205,001 - 360,000	1,340	185,001 - 400,000	1,340
360,001 - 405,000	1,420	400,001 and over	1,600
405,001 and over	1,600		

Privacy Act and Paperwork Reduction Act Notice. We ask for the information on this form to carry out the Internal Revenue laws of the United States. Internal Revenue Code sections 3402(f)(2) and 6109 and their regulations require you to provide this information; your employer uses it to determine your federal income tax withholding. Failure to provide a properly completed form will result in your being treated as a single person who claims no withholding allowances; providing fraudulent information may subject you to penalties. Routine uses of this information include giving it to the Department of Justice for civil and criminal litigation; to cities, states, the District of Columbia, and U.S. commonwealths and possessions for use in administering their tax laws; and to the Department of Health and Human Services for use in the National Directory of New Hires. We may also disclose this information to other countries under a tax treaty, to federal and state agencies to enforce federal nontax criminal laws, or to federal law enforcement and intelligence agencies to combat terrorism.

You are not required to provide the information requested on a form that is subject to the Paperwork Reduction Act unless the form displays a valid OMB control number. Books or records relating to a form or its instructions must be retained as long as their contents may become material in the administration of any Internal Revenue law. Generally, tax returns and return information are confidential, as required by Code section 6103.

The average time and expenses required to complete and file this form will vary depending on individual circumstances. For estimated averages, see the instructions for your income tax return.

If you have suggestions for making this form simpler, we would be happy to hear from you. See the instructions for your income tax return.

FIGURE 21-8 Form W-4 indicates the number of exemptions claimed by the employee for income tax purposes. *(continued)*

22222	Void ☐	a Employee's social security number	For Official Use Only ▶ OMB No. 1545-0008	
b Employer identification number (EIN)			1 Wages, tips, other compensation	2 Federal income tax withheld
c Employer's name, address, and ZIP code			3 Social security wages	4 Social security tax withheld
			5 Medicare wages and tips	6 Medicare tax withheld
			7 Social security tips	8 Allocated tips
d Control number			9	10 Dependent care benefits
e Employee's first name and initial	Last name	Suff.	11 Nonqualified plans	12a See instructions for box 12 Code
			13 Statutory employee ☐ Retirement plan ☐ Third-party sick pay ☐	12b Code
			14 Other	12c Code
f Employee's address and ZIP code				12d Code

15 State Employer's state ID number	16 State wages, tips, etc.	17 State income tax	18 Local wages, tips, etc.	19 Local income tax	20 Locality name

Form **W-2** **Wage and Tax Statement** 2016

Department of the Treasury—Internal Revenue Service

For Privacy Act and Paperwork Reduction Act Notice, see the separate instructions.

Cat. No. 10134D

Copy A For Social Security Administration — Send this entire page with Form W-3 to the Social Security Administration; photocopies are **not** acceptable.

Do Not Cut, Fold, or Staple Forms on This Page

FIGURE 21-9 Form W-2 summarizes all earnings and deductions for the year and must be prepared for each employee by January 31 of the following year.

To process payroll, the provider's clinic must have a federal tax reporting number, obtained from the Internal Revenue Service. In some states, a state employer number also is needed.

Preparing Payroll Checks. When preparing payroll checks, it is important to keep a record of all tax and insurance amounts deducted from an employee's earnings. For those clinics that still operate on a manual bookkeeping system, the write-it-once system is one of the most efficient ways to accurately maintain these records. Payroll records should include:

- Employee name, address, and telephone number
- Social Security number
- Date of employment

Each paycheck stub should contain:

- Number of hours worked, including regular and overtime (if hourly)
- Dates of pay period
- Date of check
- Gross salary
- Itemized deductions for federal income tax, Social Security (FICA) tax, state tax, and city or local tax
- Itemized deductions for health insurance and disability insurance
- Other deductions such as uniforms, loan payments, and so on
- Net salary (gross earnings minus taxes and deductions)

Figuring Employee Taxes. When figuring federal income taxes and Social Security taxes, use the "Circular E", also known as Publication 15, which contains federal income tax tables provided by the Internal Revenue Service. Federal tax is based on amount earned, marital status, number of exemptions claimed, and length of pay period. State and city or local taxes are typically a percentage of the gross earnings.

Legal

All federal and state taxes withheld must be paid on a quarterly basis to the appropriate government offices. These monies should be accompanied by the required reporting forms. It is important to observe deposit requirements for withheld income tax and Social Security and Medicare taxes. These requirements, which change frequently, are listed in the Federal Employer's Tax Guide, available from the U.S. Government Printing Office, Internal Revenue Service (or online at http://www.irs.gov).

Additionally, there are third-party providers that offer software and support for payroll preparation, tax filing, and even direct deposit. Examples include ADP and Paychex. Implementing the services of a private book-keeper or accountant to tend to these responsibilities is another solution when performing in-house payroll is not feasible.

Managing Benefits and Other Responsibilities. **Benefits**, or additional remuneration to the salary earned by full-time employees, must be managed and records maintained for each employee. Examples of benefits include paid vacation, paid holidays, health/dental insurance, disability insurance, **profit-sharing** options, and complimentary health care. Some ambulatory care settings may refer to all or some of these benefits as **fringe benefits**.

Other responsibilities of the clinic manager include maintaining a personnel file for each employee, providing his or her history with the facility, application for the current position, evaluations, promotions, problems, awards, entitlements, legal forms required by state and federal agencies, and so on. All Occupational Safety and Health Administration (OSHA) data, hazard material training and documentation, HIPAA training documentation, cardiopulmonary resuscitation (CPR) certifications, immunization records, AIDS education, and confidentiality agreements must be recorded and maintained.

FACILITY AND EQUIPMENT MANAGEMENT

Safety

The physical plant or building must be observed and maintained with safety being a key ingredient. It should be the responsibility of each staff member to report to the clinic manager any facility repairs that require attention and suggest replacement or recommend new pieces of equipment as required by the practice to support the health care needs of its population.

The clinic manager usually is responsible for maintenance of the clinic and may hire **ancillary services** to provide janitorial and laundry services, dispose of hazardous materials, and maintain aquariums or plants that may enhance the environment of the facility. The clinic manager must be cognitive of the importance of patient confidentiality when ancillary services are present. Ancillary services must not view confidential material. A signed business associate agreement must be on file for each ancillary service contracted.

Magazine subscriptions and health-related literature for the reception area are the responsibility of the clinic manager. Selections should be made carefully, keeping in mind the interests of the patients and their cultures. These materials should not be kept once they become dog-eared, torn, or outdated. The use of plastic protectors and appropriate storage shelving aid in keeping the area and materials tidy.

The clinic manager, together with the provider, is responsible for facility improvements, including any necessary repairs, decorating and color scheme, and floor plan suggestions. The wise clinic manager does not make these decisions independently but asks for suggestions from staff members. Remember, the team-building approach adds a cohesive element to any clinic environment.

Administrative and Clinical Inventory of Supplies and Equipment

All administrative and clinical supplies and equipment in the facility must be inventoried. Maintaining a sufficient inventory of administrative and medical supplies requires implementation of a system for taking inventory of supplies frequently enough to permit placing and receiving an order before a shortage occurs. Large facilities frequently use the PM system to inventory items that normally would be billed as part of a procedure, but this will not identify routinely used medical and administrative supplies.

Medical clinics operate on a budget, so comparison shopping is prudent. Many companies have online catalogs with full descriptions and prices of their products. The cost of an item is not the only consideration when purchasing inventory. Consider the following:

- Warranties
- Bulk orders
- Maintenance agreements
- Quality and durability
- Personal preferences
- Cost factors

Online ordering via the Internet can save time and money. When placing orders, select those suppliers with secure Web sites; it is generally safe to use credit cards with these vendors. Supplies also can be ordered through hard copy catalogs. Review Chapter 18 for specifics in completing a purchase order. Benchmarking with other medical clinics nets valuable information in determining reputable vendors.

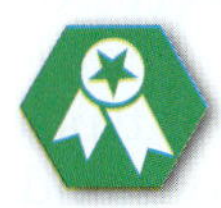
Competency

When an order is received, it must be opened and checked properly. Look first for the packing slip, which lists the items ordered and the items shipped. Verify that no items have been substituted or back-ordered. Each item unpacked must be checked against the packing slip to be sure there are no discrepancies. Write the date the shipment was received, who verified it, and any follow-up information. The new stock should be stored appropriately.

Some items purchased come with a warranty. A warranty usually is activated online at the vendor's Web site or by using a warranty card packaged with the purchased item. Warranty cards are similar to postcards and establish the purchase date and name and address of the purchaser. The returned warranty information provides the vendor with information should it be necessary to notify the buyer of recalls or defective parts. It is also proof of purchase and gives the length of time the warranty is in effect.

Procedure

It is important to create a file or a digital file, such as a spreadsheet, for each piece of equipment in the medical clinic. Information in this file should include:

- Date of purchase and original receipt
- Manufacturer name, address, and telephone number
- Model number and owner's manual
- Technical support information and telephone number
- Warranty information
- Service agreement
- Date last serviced
- Routine maintenance or calibration information

The steps for inventorying supplies and equipment for administrative and clinical needs are given in Procedure 21-5.

PROCEDURE 21-5

Performing an Inventory of Equipment and Supplies

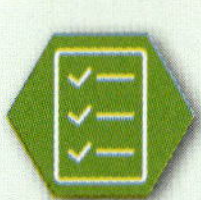
Procedure

PURPOSE:

To develop an inventory of expendable administrative and clinical supplies in a medical clinic.

EQUIPMENT/SUPPLIES:

- Computer
- Printout of most recent inventory spreadsheet, listing items by storage location, name and identification code, number of items, minimum quantity requiring reorder, date and quantity of last reorder, expiration dates of items, if any
- Clipboard, pad of reorder forms, pen or pencil

PROCEDURE STEPS:

1. ***Paying attention to detail,*** compare number of items on hand corresponding to each name or code identification number with the printout, and write in the new inventory number on the printout. RATIONALE: Determines what is on hand and what needs to be ordered.
2. If the number of any item is less than the minimum quantity, fill out a reorder form listing completely the name, identification number, and quantity required.
3. Repeat the previous step for each storage location on the inventory printout sheet.
4. After completing the inventory, enter the new inventory information, including date of inventory, quantity, and date of reorder request, into the computer database. RATIONALE: Determines what needs to be ordered.
5. Forward the reorder forms to the person responsible for purchasing. RATIONALE: Forwards information to the person responsible for reordering supplies and equipment.

   NOTE: If the clinic uses handheld computers on a wireless network, all information can be entered directly into the computer record while doing the inventory, making unnecessary the reentry and preparation of reorder forms. If the handheld computer is not networked, it will be necessary to download or sync the data after completing the inventory.

Administrative and Clinical Equipment Calibration and Maintenance

Administrative and clinical equipment must be cleaned, calibrated, and maintained on a regular basis. Most clinics use a computer spreadsheet or relational-type database, depending on the size of the facility. The database identifies the equipment by name or type, its assigned facility identification number, location in the facility, warranty expiration date, service period, dates when service and calibration were last performed, and when the next service or calibration will be required. The database also may identify service contracts for equipment not maintained or calibrated by facility personnel and information on equipment service contractors such as contacts, phone numbers, and addresses. The database is backed up by a paper file containing operation manuals, warranty information, and service contracts.

Administrative equipment such as computers should be cleaned and maintained regularly. Review Chapter 10 for suggestions on routine maintenance. Telephones as well as any other pieces of administrative equipment should be cleaned and working order checked.

Procedure

Laboratory and clinical equipment must be maintained and quality-control measures utilized. Calibration checks are required for a number of pieces of equipment: sphygmomanometers and centrifuges, to name two. Microscopes and various types of scopes used during physical examinations and specialty procedures contain light sources that must be checked before each use. A replacement supply of bulbs should be available. Assigning a clinical laboratory manager to oversee the equipment is a good idea. Procedure 21-6 provides steps for routine maintenance and calibration of clinical equipment.

The clinic storage areas should be well maintained, and each item should always be put back in its place with lids replaced properly to prevent any accidents. Medication storage requires special attention. Many medications must be stored at certain temperatures, kept dry, or stored in dark, airtight containers. All medications, including samples, must be kept out of patient access areas. Narcotics should always be stored in a separate locked cabinet. A daily inventory should be maintained.

PROCEDURE 21-6

Procedure

Performing Routine Maintenance and Calibration of Clinical Equipment

PURPOSE:

To ensure the operability and calibration of clinical equipment.

EQUIPMENT/SUPPLIES:

- Equipment list with maintenance or calibration requirements
- Clipboard, pen with black ink, maintenance log and service calendar log forms, deficiency tags
- Access to operation and service manuals of equipment to be serviced
- Access to any necessary maintenance tools and supplies

PROCEDURE STEPS:

1. Locate the number assigned by the clinic manager to identify the equipment being serviced, and verify serial number, manufacturer/maker, technical support phone number, warranty information, and last date of service. RATIONALE: Provides medical assistant with all information needed for maintenance and servicing of equipment.
2. ***Paying attention to detail,*** visually inspect each piece of equipment associated with the clinical area.
   - ***Practicing risk management principles,*** check for any frayed electrical cords, loose connections, or safety issues such as tripping hazards associated with electrical cords.
   - Clean each item according to manufacturer specifications, and replace light bulbs and batteries if necessary.

   RATIONALE: Equipment works more efficiently when clean and all parts are working properly.

(continues)

3. Check to ensure the equipment meets operational/calibration standards as defined in the operation and service manual. Recalibrate the equipment following the instructions in the manual if required. RATIONALE: Calibration standards must be maintained for correct results.
4. Follow necessary safety precautions and tag any equipment not meeting operational standards and report the deficiency. RATIONALE: Equipment must be either replaced or repaired to ensure proper results.
5. Fill out and sign the maintenance record sheet if the equipment meets operations standards. RATIONALE: Documents routine maintenance was performed.
6. ***Paying attention to detail,*** complete documentation form by verifying information for each piece of equipment serviced and/or calibrated. Complete the appropriate information for service using the Service Calendar Log form. RATIONALE: Documents what has been done and the date completed.

   NOTE: The equipment list, maintenance records, and deficiency reports may be included in the PM system of many practices.

Documentation Example:

Maintenance Log

Name of Equipment	Serial Number	Mfg/ Maker	Technical Support Phone Number	Purchase Date	Service Plan	Last Serviced	Completed By
EKG #8	80462	HP	xxx-xxx-xxxx	1/20/XX	On file	6/12/xx	bql
Centrifuge #3	79031	HP	xxx-xxx-xxxx	7/20/XX	On file	6/12/xx	bql

Service Calendar Log Form

January	February	March	April	May	June	July	August	September	October	November	December

LIABILITY COVERAGE AND BONDING

Legal

Negligence is performing an act that a reasonable and prudent provider would not perform or failure to perform an act that a reasonable and prudent provider would perform. The common term used to describe professional **liability** or legal responsibility today is **malpractice**. It is much easier to prevent malpractice than to defend it in litigation; therefore every effort should be taken to prevent negligence. Events that could result in a malpractice litigation invariably will occur from time to time in even the best of medical clinics. When such an incident occurs, complete honesty with the patient and insurance carrier is the best policy. Protocols should be implemented or existing ones revised to prevent any future occurrences, and all steps necessary to minimize risk to the patient should be taken.

Insurance policies specifically designed to protect the provider's assets in the event a liability claim is filed and awarded in the patient's favor are available. Any provider not carrying such insurance is said to be **"going bare"** and would personally be responsible for any court costs, damages, and attorney fees if a malpractice suit were lost.

Practicing medical assistants should carry **professional liability insurance** for protection. Medical assistants who are members of the American Association of Medical Assistants (AAMA) have the option of purchasing personal and professional insurance through the organization at corporate rates.

Some providers carry their employees on their policies. If this is the case, always ask to see the policy and verify that your name is printed on the policy—no name indicates no coverage. The manager may need to see that professional liability insurance has been purchased, all appropriate names are listed, and the premiums are paid in a timely fashion.

Professional liability insurance is important if the provider-employer is sued. In this event, the provider and the medical assistant could be named in the suit. If the case were lost, both the provider and the medical assistant could be liable.

Individuals who are responsible for handling financial records and money in the medical clinic may be bonded. A **bond** is purchased for a cash value in an employee's name that ensures that the provider will recover the amount of loss in the event that an employee **embezzles** funds. It is the clinic manager or the HR manager's responsibility to ask prospective employees if they are bondable. Individuals who are not bondable may not be the best candidates for the position.

LEGAL ISSUES

The clinic manager must be aware of and follow all state and federal regulations impacting the practice. Information related to the Clinical Laboratory Improvement Amendments of 1988 (CLIA '88) and the Occupational Safety and Health Administration (OSHA) can be found on the OSHA Web site (http://www.osha.gov). The Centers for Medicare and Medicaid Services Web site also is helpful (http://www.cms.gov).

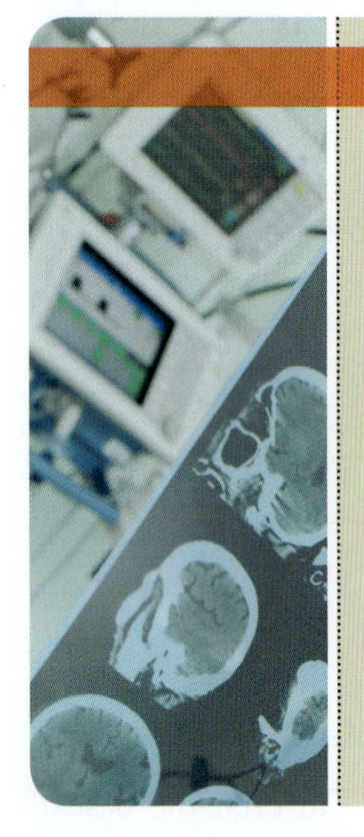

CASE STUDY 21-1

Refer to the scenario at the beginning of the chapter.

Drs. Lewis and King have requested sigmoidoscopy procedures to be scheduled for two different patients. The patients are scheduled. Both patients are put on a strict diet and pretest protocol for several days to prepare for the procedures. The day of the appointments, Marilyn Johnson, CMA (AAMA), and clinic manager, discovers that the two sigmoidoscopy procedures have been scheduled at the same time. The problem is that the clinic has only one sigmoidoscope available.

CASE STUDY REVIEW

1. Form two groups to discuss problem-solving solutions. Assume that rescheduling either of the patients is not an acceptable solution because of the patients' pretest protocol. The patients would be upset if the procedure could not be performed due to a scheduling problem.
2. How could this problem have been avoided?
3. Both patients have been told about the scheduling problem and one is upset and argumentative. What role should the clinic manager assume in this predicament?

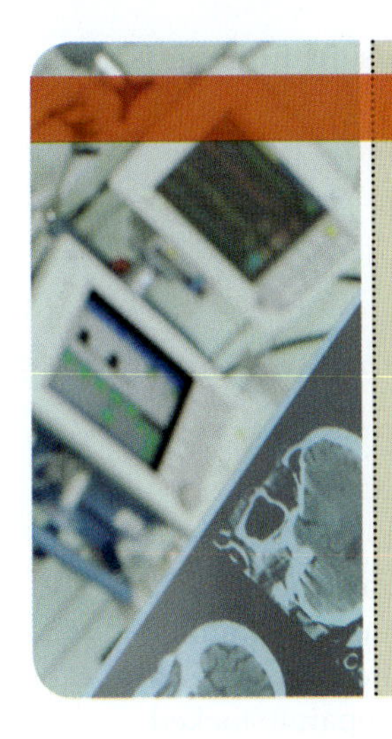

CASE STUDY 21-2

Ellen Armstrong, CMAS (AMT), the clinic administrative medical assistant, speaks privately with Marilyn Johnson, the clinic manager and the person responsible for personnel. Ellen has a suspicious lump in her breast. She has seen both her internist and a surgeon for evaluation. Next week, she will have the lump removed, perhaps even a complete mastectomy. Ellen is concerned about the time she will need to be away from the clinic.

CASE STUDY REVIEW

1. Identify the first and immediate concerns to be addressed.
2. What action might be taken to help both Ellen and the clinic manager address these concerns?
3. Is it helpful to plan for the best results, the worst results, or both?

Summary

- The clinic manager oversees the operations and staff of the clinic and keeps it running smoothly. The role of clinic manager varies greatly depending on the size of the medical practice and the provider's trust in the manager's competency level.
- You should know the qualities of a good manager, including management styles and how to utilize them.
- Formulating risk management procedures to assess and minimize common risks is the duty of the clinic manager.
- The clinical manager must effectively utilize teamwork in the clinic for daily operations, including using recognition as a tool to motivate and develop a team, and using a team for problem solving.
- The clinic manager must use effective supervisory techniques to manage orientation of new personnel as well as discipline and evaluate staff, including proper dismissal methods.
- Time management guidelines that make the most of every work day by increasing productivity should be developed by the clinic manger.
- Marketing strategies for the benefit of the clinic and patients include enhancing the visibility, promotion, and image of the clinic; providing services in the form of patient seminars, support groups, and informational sessions that highlight clinic services and educate the patient; and using social media as a communication and marketing tool.
- The clinic manager is responsible for payroll and managing benefits, or monitoring outsourced payroll services; facility and equipment management, including managing inventory and ordering; and staying current on state and federal regulations that impact the clinic and practice.

Study for Success

To reinforce your knowledge and skills of information presented in this chapter:

- Review the *Key Terms* and *Learning Outcomes*
- Consider the *Critical Thinking* features and *Case Studies* and discuss your conclusions
- Answer the questions in the *Certification Review*

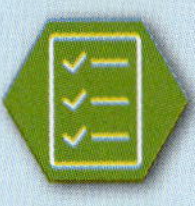

Procedure

- Perform the *Procedures* using the *Competency Assessment Checklists* on the *Student Companion Website*

CERTIFICATION REVIEW

1. What must individual team members do in order for teamwork to be successful?
   a. Do as they are told by the clinic manager
   b. Not ask why they are doing something a certain way
   c. Understand and support the task
   d. Think independently and solve the problem on their own
2. What is the purpose of meeting minutes?
   a. They should address each agenda topic and include a brief summary of discussions, actions taken, name of each person making a motion, the exact wording of motions, and motion approval or defeat.
   b. They are a detailed plan for a proposed trip.
   c. They include information regarding mode of transportation and lodging reservations.
   d. They must follow parliamentary procedures.
   e. They are not important and minutes do not need to be recorded.
3. What is it important to consider when working with practicum students?
   a. They should have expert knowledge about their field.
   b. They do not need supervision when working with a patient.
   c. They are experienced with working on real patients.
   d. They have much to learn.
4. Which of the following statements is *not* correct regarding a student practicum?
   a. It is a transitional stage that provides opportunities for students to apply theory learned in the classroom to a health care setting through hands-on experience.
   b. It assumes that the student is an employee who does not need to be introduced to patients.
   c. It may require the student to shadow another medical assistant for a few days.
   d. It involves an evaluation of the student's progress.
   e. Students gain valuable experience.
5. What is a procedure manual?
   a. It is a detailed plan for a proposed trip.
   b. It provides detailed information regarding mode of transportation and lodging reservations.
   c. It provides detailed information relative to the performance of tasks within the health care facility.
   d. It summarizes action details of staff meetings.
6. Developing relationships outside the clinic is often referred to as what?
   a. Marketing
   b. Benchmarking
   c. Advertising
   d. Sales
   e. A way to find a job
7. Which of the following does *not* involve record and financial management?
   a. Payroll processing
   b. Preparing payroll checks
   c. Figuring taxes
   d. Equipment and supplies maintenance
8. How must controlled substances be handled?
   a. They must be kept separate from other drugs.
   b. They must be stored in a separate locked cabinet.
   c. They are recorded in a book that is maintained daily.
   d. All of these
   e. Only a and c
9. What is the purpose of the procedure manual?
   a. To serve as a guide to the employee assigned a specific task.
   b. It may be used in evaluating the employee's performance.
   c. It is invaluable in assuring that each procedure is completed as outlined.
   d. It should be generic so that any clinic could follow the procedures.
10. What is a benefit of social media in the medical clinic?
    a. It provides another way to communicate with patients and potential consumers.
    b. It provides a way to find employees and to verify the background of persons seeking employment.
    c. It projects your clinic's personality.
    d. It can send notices and reminders to patients on various topics.
    e. All of these

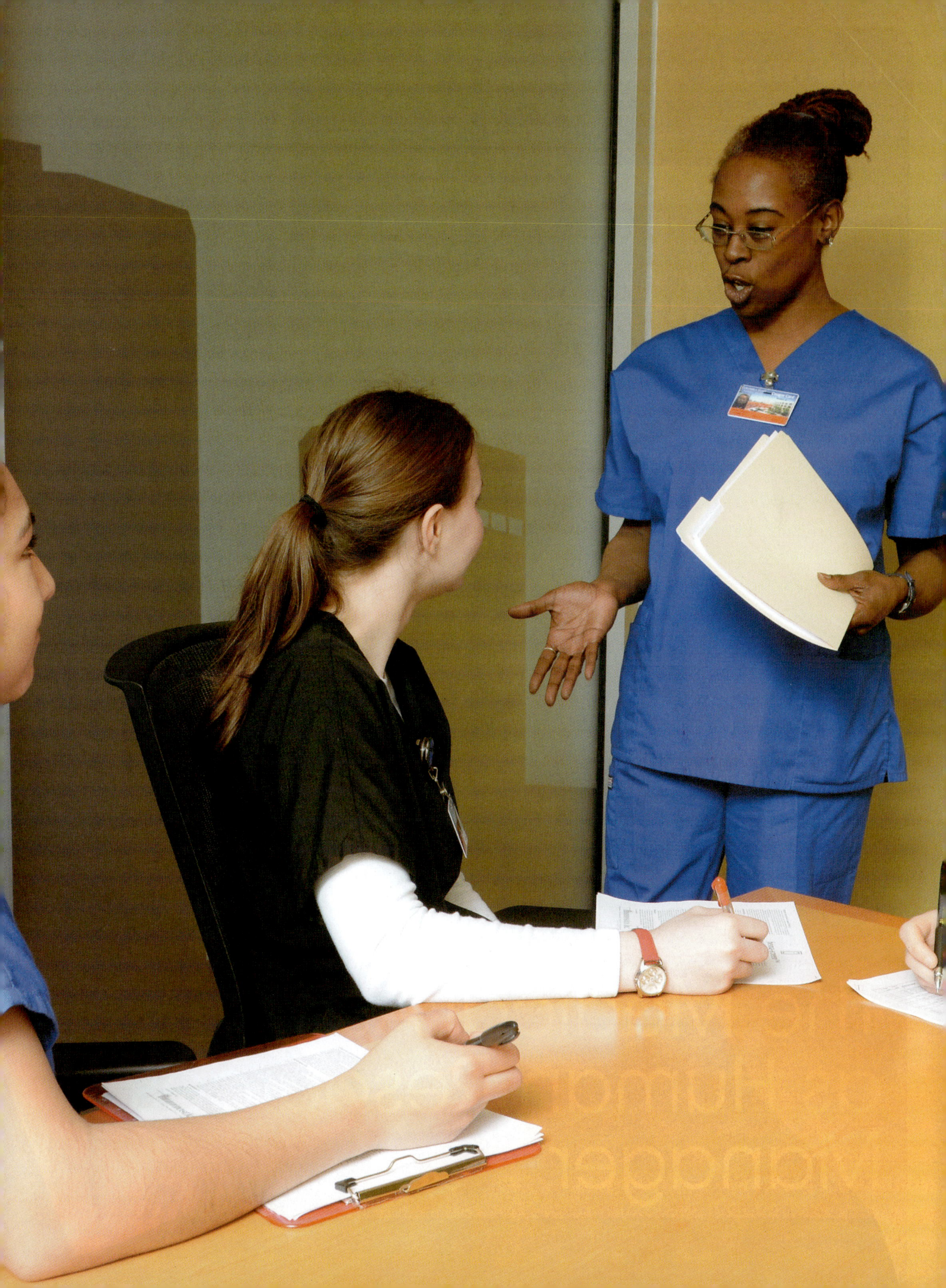

CHAPTER 22

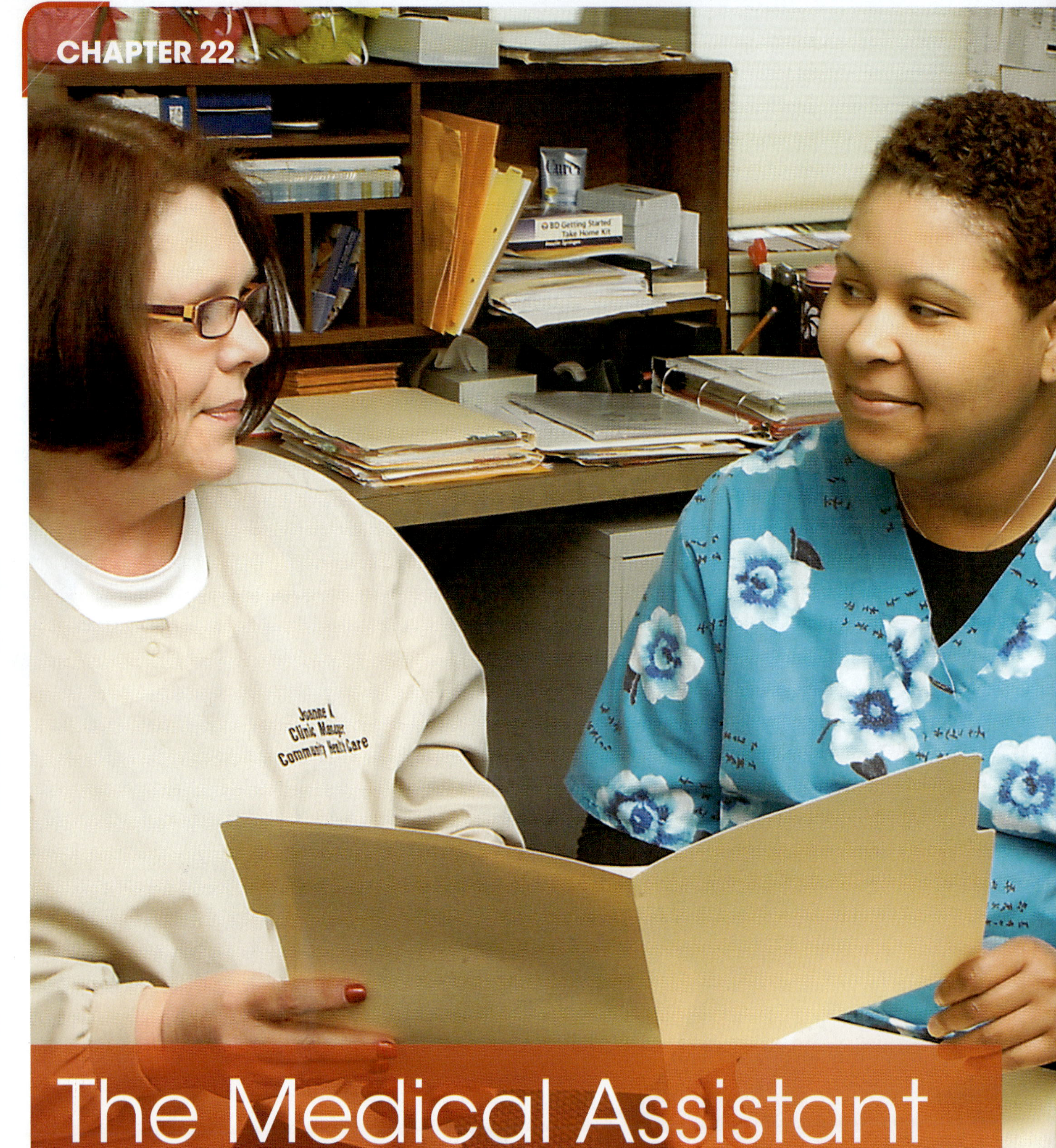

The Medical Assistant as Human Resources Manager

LEARNING OUTCOMES

1. Define and spell the key terms as presented in the glossary.
2. Interpret the role of the human resources manager.
3. Explain the function of the clinic policy manual.
4. Analyze methods of recruiting employees for a medical practice.
5. Conduct an employment interview.
6. Categorize items to keep in an employee's personnel record.
7. List and define a minimum of four laws related to personnel management.
8. Discuss possible methods for evaluating employees.
9. Compare and contrast voluntary and involuntary separations.
10. Recall continuing education possibilities for employees.

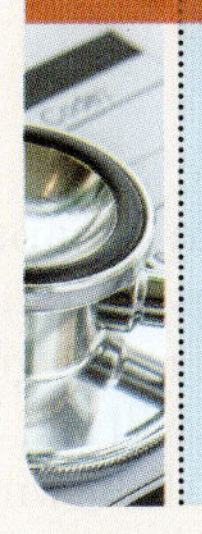

KEY TERMS

- Boomer generation
- exit interview
- Generation X
- Generation Y
- Generation Z
- involuntary dismissals
- letter of resignation
- LGBT (lesbian, gay, bisexual, transgender)
- overtime
- probation

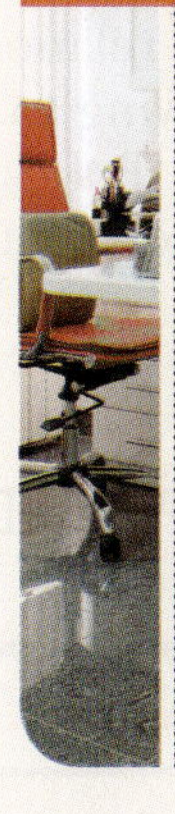

SCENARIO

Inner City Health Care has been open for close to 20 years, and it has seen many changes in the clinic and the neighborhood it serves. A recent and private conference with the clinic manager, the human resources manager, and two of the doctors revealed a conflict. The older of the two doctors has a strong negative opinion about the **LGBT (lesbian, gay, bisexual, transgender)** community. Two men were recently seen in the clinic by this provider. One was quite ill; the other, his partner, was very concerned. While a complete examination was given to the ill patient, the doctor sighed in relief when his blood workup showed suspected probable lymphocytic leukemia and he was able to make a referral to a nearby oncology clinic for the patient's treatment. Because Inner City Health Care practices in a state where there are not laws against discrimination of LGBT patients, it appears that an ethical dilemma must be addressed by the clinic staff.

Chapter Portal

As you near the end of your studies and preparations to enter the field of health care, it is helpful for you to know how human resource managers are likely to function in the hiring process.

The medical assistant's employment responsibilities are many and varied. As you learned in Chapter 21, often they become clinic managers and assume a quite different function in the medical setting once they have been employed in the field and gained sufficient experience. The size of the ambulatory care setting and the number of employees likely determines if a human resources (HR) manager is a part of the practice. Whether the HR manager heads an HR department in a large, corporate medical setting with the title Human Resources Manager, or is a medical assistant/clinic manager who has HR responsibilities, there are some common tasks assigned as specific HR duties.

TASKS PERFORMED BY THE HUMAN RESOURCES MANAGER

A search for employment is likely to involve interactions with individuals with the title of Human Resources Manager. It can be helpful to understand that position and the corresponding responsibilities when applying for a position. Tasks usually assigned to the HR manager include determining job descriptions for, hiring, and orienting employees; maintaining employee personnel records that include credentials and continuing education units (CEUs); and managing employee separations. With today's quest for greater clinic efficiency and the tremendous increase in federal and state regulatory requirements, the skills required of an HR manager have greatly broadened. Former responsibilities have been expanded to include preparing the policy manual, scheduling employee evaluations, preventing and investigating discrimination and harassment claims, and complying with regulatory agencies. The HR manager also assists in providing training and educational opportunities for employees so they are current in all aspects of quality patient care. Today's HR manager must seek to improve employee satisfaction and retention as well as foster accountability. The majority of today's work force will have several positions prior to retirement and are less likely to stay with one practice during their work years than previous workers; therefore, job satisfaction is an important key to retention.

Increasingly, HR managers are expected to be able to support the organization's efforts that focus on productivity, service, and quality. In a climate in which there are too few persons for the positions to be filled and the delivery methods for health care are changing almost daily, productivity, service, and quality are essential to a successful practice. It becomes the responsibility of the HR manager to see that every employee's productivity level is high, that the service is A+, and that quality is at the highest level. Today's customers, the patients, often choose their health care provider, even within their health insurance limitations, on the basis of service and quality.

Competency

Integrity

The position of HR manager now requires a higher level of education and experience to better grasp the legal and regulatory aspects of personnel management. The HR manager also must have excellent people skills, a strong sense of fairness, and the ability to resolve conflicts. None of this is accomplished in a vacuum. It requires working in close cooperation with the clinic manager and the employer(s).

This chapter discusses these responsibilities in the following separate but overlapping functions:

1. Creating and updating the clinic policy manual
2. Recruiting and hiring clinic personnel
3. Orienting new personnel
4. Scheduling salary reviews
5. Conducting exit interviews
6. Maintaining personnel records
7. Complying with all state and federal regulations regarding personnel
8. Planning/providing employee training and education
9. Maintaining records of credentials, licensure, certifications, and CEUs, such as cardiopulmonary resuscitation (CPR)

THE CLINIC POLICY MANUAL

The procedure manual described in Chapter 21 identifies specific methods and steps in performing tasks. The policy manual provides more general guidelines for clinic practices and will be introduced to new employees very quickly following the hiring process. See Table 22-1 for a brief summary of each type of manual. The policy manual identifies clear guidelines and directions required of all employees. It also defines appropriate expectations and boundaries of the employment relationship. Having written policies means not having to determine policy on a case-by-case basis. Policy manuals will vary based on the size of the practice or

TABLE 22-1

POSSIBLE CONTENT OF POLICY AND PROCEDURE MANUALS

POLICY MANUAL	PROCEDURE MANUAL
Mission statement	Details of procedures performed
Employer(s) biographic data	Administrative procedures
Employment issues	Clinical procedures
Wages, salaries, and benefits	Safety issues
Employee conduct	Asepsis
Confidentiality guidelines	Safety Data Sheets
HIPAA compliance	Emergency protocol

problems to be addressed, but some common topics include the mission statement of the practice, biographic data on each provider, employment policies, wage and salary policies, benefits to be awarded, and employee conduct expectations.

Establishing and stating the mission of the practice clearly identifies the goals and objectives to be sought by each employee. Having biographic data of each provider helps employees to respond to queries from patients about a provider's experience, education, and interests.

Employment policies might include statements on equal employment opportunity, job requirements for particular positions and to whom each person reports, recruitment and selection procedures, orientation of new employees, probation, and dismissal. Wage and salary policies should be in writing. How are employees classified? What are the working hours, how is overtime compensated, and how are salary increases determined? What benefits (medical, retirement, vacation, holidays, sick leave, and profit sharing) does the practice have? The answers to such questions are part of the policy manual. A discussion of employee conduct is another component of the policy manual. A statement regarding the strict confidentiality of all information received in the practice is essential in this area of the policy manual and often includes a form requiring a signature from the new hire assuring he or she fully understands the consequences of any breach in confidentiality. Guidelines should be established about uniforms, dress codes, appearance, and personal hygiene. Can an employee hold a second job outside the practice? Are staff members responsible for housekeeping duties? Is updated certification required? If so, what accommodations are made for continuing education requirements?

A computerized policy manual ensures it is an easy task to make any changes and updates. Any changes made are to be shared with employees so that everyone is up to date on policies. Having a policy manual with clearly written directives helps employees understand the expectations and boundaries of the employment relationship. The policy manual is reviewed with each new employee and updated on a regular basis. Procedure 22-1 provides details on developing and maintaining a policy manual.

PROCEDURE 22-1

Developing and Maintaining a Policy Manual

PURPOSE:

To develop and maintain a comprehensive, up-to-date policy manual of all clinic policies relating to employee practices, benefits, clinic conduct, and so on.

EQUIPMENT/SUPPLIES:

- Computer
- Binder, such as a three-ring
- Paper
- Standard policy manual format

PROCEDURE STEPS:

1. Develop precise, written clinic policies detailing all necessary information pertaining to the staff and their positions. The information should include benefits, vacation, sick leave, hours, dress codes, evaluations, rules of conduct, and grounds for dismissal. RATIONALE: Well-defined policies clearly outlined for each employee are necessary for efficient and effective staff operations.
2. Identify procedures for reimbursing overtime, preventing discrimination and harassment, creating a safe working environment, and allowing for jury duty.
3. Include a policy statement related to rules of conduct.
4. Identify steps to follow should an employee become disabled during employment.
5. Determine what employee opportunities for continuing education, if any, will be reimbursed; include requirements for recertification or licensure.

(continues)

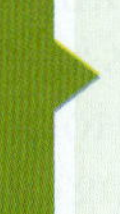

6. Provide a copy of the policy manual for each employee. RATIONALE: Each employee is made aware of facility policies.
7. Review and update the policy manual regularly. Add or delete items as necessary, dating each revised page. RATIONALE: Policy manual will always be current.

RECRUITING AND HIRING CLINIC PERSONNEL

The majority of employees in ambulatory and primary care centers are full-time, part-time, or occasionally independent contractor employees. Full-time employees generally work 30 hours or more per week; part-time employees work less than 30 hours per week. Either may be paid by the hour. Full-time employees may be salaried and exempt from overtime regulations. Most part-time employees are paid by the hour. Benefits are often different between full- and part-time employees. Independent contractors who are employed usually work with the facility to perform specific predetermined tasks at a predetermined rate of pay for the services provided and are not eligible for benefits from the clinic.

Before recruiting and hiring personnel to fill positions within the medical facility, the HR manager and employers must understand exactly what the role and responsibilities of the position are by having a current job description for the position. They must follow a recruiting policy that is effective and fair and that observes all appropriate laws and regulations.

Job Descriptions

Before any position is filled, a job description must be in place. This usually is created cooperatively by the clinic manager and the employer(s). Once the job qualifications are defined, the lead personnel and HR manager can begin efforts to fill the position.

In daily operations, most job descriptions are on file, but if the situation involves a new or greatly expanded clinic, a complete set of job descriptions is needed before recruiting can begin. Even when a written description is on file, it should be reviewed when a new employee is to be hired. The person who is leaving the position is often an excellent resource to assess the accuracy of the current job description and any changes that should be made.

The job description must include basic qualifications necessary for the position and have enough information to provide both the supervisor and the employee with a clear outline of what the position entails (Figure 22-1). Necessary work experience, skills, education, and any special certification or licensure that is expected is to be identified in the job description. Procedure 22-2 provides details on preparing job descriptions.

JOB DESCRIPTION

POSITION TITLE:

Administrative Medical Assistant

REPORTS TO:

Clinic Manager and Provider-Employer(s)

RESPONSIBILITIES AND DUTIES:

- Be a therapeutic and helpful receptionist
  1. Answer telephone as quickly as possible, hopefully by the second ring
  2. Greet all patients warmly and with a helpful attitude
- Manage time efficiently with appropriate scheduling for patients and professional staff
  1. Schedule patients according to their needs, scheduling guidelines, staff availability, and equipment readiness
  2. Call to remind patients of their visit the day before appointment
- Respond to patient requests on the telephone and in person
  1. Ascertain reason for request
  2. Satisfy patient request or refer patient to one who can
- Prepare patient charts for professional staff
  1. Print schedules and encounter forms
  2. Pull patient charts late afternoon the day before appointment; print as necessary
  3. Check charts for completeness
  4. Attach encounter form when patient arrives to check in

AUTHORITY BOUNDARIES:

The Clinic Manager will assist in answering questions. Remember that it is better to ask than to make an error. Screening concerns not identified in a policy/procedure manual also can be directed to the clinical medical assisting staff.

POSITION REQUIREMENTS:

Two years' experience and/or graduate of a medical assistant program. CMA (AAMA), RMA, or CMAS preferred.

FIGURE 22-1 Sample job description for administrative medical assistant.

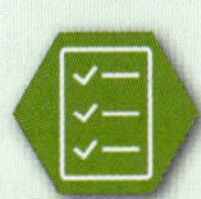

PROCEDURE 22-2

Preparing a Job Description

Procedure

PURPOSE:

To provide a precise definition of the tasks assigned to a job; to determine the expectations and level of competency required; and to specify the experience, training, and education needed to perform the job for purposes of recruiting and performance evaluation.

EQUIPMENT/SUPPLIES:

- Computer
- Paper
- Standard job description format

PROCEDURE STEPS:

1. Describe each task that creates the job. RATIONALE: A detailed job description identifies clear expectations for each employee.
2. List special medical, technical, or clerical skills required.
3. Determine the level of education, instruction, and experience required for the position.
4. Determine where the job fits in the overall structure of the practice.
5. Specify any unusual working conditions (hours, locations, and so on) that may apply.
6. Describe career path opportunities.

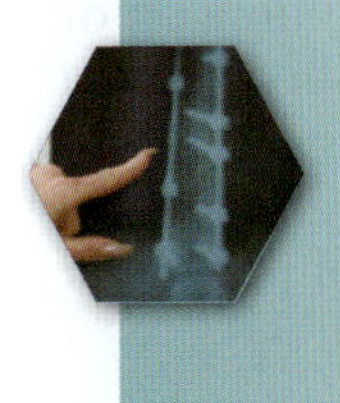

Critical Thinking

Identify proper qualifications for an administrative medical assistant in a fairly large ambulatory care setting. Determine what work experience might qualify versus what work experience is preferred. Identify possible certifications that might be helpful. Explain.

Another important point with respect to the job description is that a review and update of the description should be done every year. Most positions change constantly, whether from a minor shifting of duties or the addition of some new technical procedure or device. Without updating a job description, a person with the wrong qualifications may be recruited to fill a vacancy.

When seeking employment, it is most helpful to understand the job description for the position being sought and to make certain that your qualifications fit that description.

Recruiting

A major challenge facing the HR manager today is recruitment. Medical assisting is among the top 10 occupations where expected employment growth is much faster than average for all occupations. According to the U.S. Department of Labor, Bureau of Labor Statistics, employment for medical assistants is likely to grow 23% from 2014 to 2024. One reason for this demand is the aging of the U.S. population and the demands made upon primary and ambulatory care providers. Medical assistants with formal education, instruction, and appropriate certification will be in high demand. When employers have been unsuccessful in recruiting qualified medical assistants, they have turned to contracting for some work, such as transcription and billing.

Once the hiring need is determined, the HR manager begins the recruitment process. Networking is a highly effective method of finding employees. Networking is a process in which people of similar interests exchange information in social, business, or professional relationships. A survey conducted by Jobvite in 2014 indicated that nearly 75% of companies use social media networks to recruit employees. LinkedIn was the most popular, followed by Facebook. The HR manager may network with members of the American Association of Medical Assistants (AAMA) and express an interest in a new employee for an open position. Current employees are often excellent resources because they may know of a qualified person who is looking for a position. The majority of candidates will come through referrals such as these as well as internal transfers.

The medical assistant departments of nearby colleges are another good resource. Medical assisting students may find employment through their practicum experience near the end of their coursework. Individuals who volunteer to shadow, follow, or work in a facility are often seen as potential employees. Although newspaper advertisements or Craigslist may generate many résumés, they are only marginally effective as search tools. It is often far too time consuming to review the large volume of applications generated by this approach. There are a number of medical employment Internet sites that identify positions for medical assistant personnel, often in specific locales.

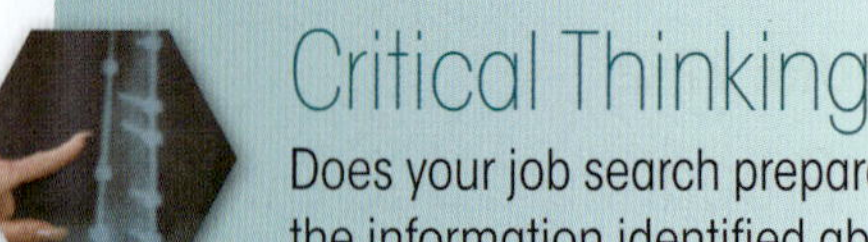

Critical Thinking

Does your job search preparation fit with the information identified above? If not, what might you do now to make a change so that it will fit?

Preparing to Interview Applicants

Once several applicants have expressed interest in the position, preparation for the interview begins. The HR manager is likely to have a number of résumés to consider. Some applicants may have already completed a job application if they dropped off a résumé. The résumés and applications can be reviewed together. Some important points to remember in reading these documents follow.

When considering education, look beyond the degree earned. Look for a good performance record at school and the kinds of supplemental education achieved. Does attendance at seminars and short-course training programs relate to your position needs? When reading a person's work history, make note of any unexplained gaps in employment. You may want to ask specific questions in the interview. Has advancement been gained in each new position? Are the responsibilities and duties of the applicant's positions explained, or will questions need to be asked of the prospective employee?

Look for information that indicates if this candidate really enjoys the kind of work setting you have. Is the applicant comfortable serving the infirm? Can you truly identify the level of skill from the descriptions, or are the applicant's skills descriptions vague? The cover letter, if one is included, should address the specifics required of your position. Does the person display a negative or a positive attitude? Do not excuse any errors or unprofessional appearance in the job application or the résumé. Each should be perfect in all aspects. An individual who is careless in this respect is likely to be careless in the position.

Some applications will be discarded when compared to the preceding guidelines. With the remaining candidates, determine who is to be interviewed and make telephone calls to establish interviews. You may make note of the quality of speaking skills, especially if this person will be using the telephone in the position. Make an interview appointment date with only those who seem truly interested in the position during your telephone conversation.

The Employment Interview

The employment interview is usually conducted by only one person if second interviews are anticipated. The provider-employer, clinic manager, or another employee may be present at either the first or the second interview, however (Figure 22-2). The interviewer(s) will want to review the application and résumé before the interview for particular

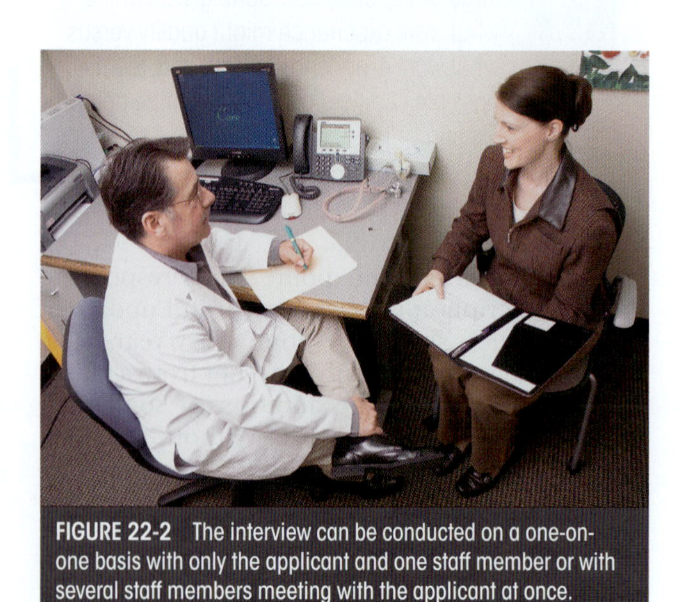

FIGURE 22-2 The interview can be conducted on a one-on-one basis with only the applicant and one staff member or with several staff members meeting with the applicant at once.

points to ask the candidate. Before the interview, those doing the interviewing should establish a set of questions for all of the applicants. These predetermined questions will help avoid one applicant being given advantages over another and will help ensure continuity throughout all the interviews. An interview worksheet is an excellent tool to use to make certain that the interview process is fair and equitable with each candidate. The worksheet should provide enough room for notes taken during the interview.

Suggested items for the interview worksheet are:

- Applicant's name
- Telephone number
- Education and experience
- Work experience
- Special skills
- Professional demeanor
- Voice and mannerisms specific to position
- Questions and responses
- Ability to problem solve when given a scenario
- Any health-related or work-related problems applicant discloses
- Interviewer's personal impressions and recommendations

Conduct interviews in a quiet and private setting. Do not schedule interviews back to back without time to collect your thoughts or to allow you to compare notes with others participating in the interview. Ask job-related questions. For example:

- Describe your last position. What did you like best about it? What did you like least? What is most important to you about a position?
- Describe your administrative and clinical skills.

Refer to Chapter 24 for some more sample questions. Let the applicant do the most of the talking.

Legal

Any questions related to age, sex, race, religion, or national origin are inappropriate. Recall from Chapter 6 that currently 22 states prohibit discrimination based on sexual orientation as well. Inquiries about medical history, drug use, or arrest records may not be made. Keep your questions related to performance on the job. If you may want to bond this employee, you may ask candidates if they have been bonded before or are willing to be bonded. It may be best to leave salary discussions for a second interview, but it can also be helpful to determine if applicants' salary expectations are in line with what you can offer. A question such as "What salary are you expecting?" is appropriate. Do not make a job offer until all the candidates selected for interviews have been interviewed, and do not prejudge someone on any factor other than the person's qualifications presented during or after the interview.

At the close of the interview, let the applicant know when a decision will be made or whether a second interview will be conducted and how notification will be made. A tour of the facility and introduction to key staff members may be offered but are not necessary at the time of the first interview. Finally, thank the applicant for participating in the interview and being interested in the position.

Selecting the Finalists

Shortly after the final interview is completed, the HR manager should talk with all the others involved in the interviews to select the top candidates. This is done by comparing notes and impressions from the interviews and by taking into consideration the ability of a candidate to work with patients and colleagues who might have a variety of problems and cultural backgrounds. The next step is to check references from former employers, supervisors, co-workers, and instructors. A large corporate medical practice may even have a consent form each candidate is asked to sign that gives permission to check references and call former employers and instructors. You may need to recognize, however, that even with a signed release from a potential new employee, many organizations and businesses restrict the release of reference information to only name, dates of employment, and title of position served. Telephone checks for references are an excellent strategy because you receive an immediate response. If you stress confidentiality when you make the contact, it will be more likely that the person will respond candidly to your questions. When possible, always check with more than one reference and former employer to get a more accurate assessment of the candidate. All reference information is to be kept confidential. A sample telephone reference check form is shown in Figure 22-3.

A checklist of questions to ask might include:

1. What were the dates of employment of (name of applicant) at your firm?
2. Describe the position held.
3. Reason for leaving the position?

4. Strong points of the employee?
5. Limitations of the employee?
6. Can you comment on attendance and dependability?
7. Would you rehire?
8. Anything else we should know about this candidate?

TELEPHONE REFERENCE

Name of Applicant ____________________

Person Contacted ____________________

Position and Name of Business ____________________

____

Telephone Number ____________________

Relationship to Applicant ____________________

- May I verify the employment history of (applicant's name) who is applying for a position with our medical clinic?

  ________, ____ to ________, ____

- Describe the responsibilities held by this individual.
- Identify the salary ____________________
- What are this individual's strong points?
- What are this individual's weak points?
- Describe this individual's overall attitude toward the position and toward patients.
- Please comment on dependability and attendance.
- Given the opportunity, would you rehire? Why or why not?
- Why did this individual leave the position?
- Describe personal and professional growth this individual made while in your firm.
- Is there anything else you would like to tell us?

Reference call made by ____________________

Date ____________________

FIGURE 22-3 Sample form to use for telephone references.

Offer the position when a first-choice candidate has been determined and indicate when a response is needed. Be prepared with a second-choice candidate should the preferred candidate respond negatively. At the time of the offer, the candidate should understand the salary offered, the starting date, the practice policies, and the benefits. When a candidate has accepted the position, a confirmation letter should be written that clearly spells out details discussed earlier. Give specific instructions on when and where the new employee should report the first day on the job. If practical, the employee should be given the policy and procedure manuals to read. Employers are required by federal law to verify that all employees are authorized to work. This is done by having the candidate complete an Eligibility Verification (I-9) form (see Case Study 22-1).

For the unsuccessful applicants, send a letter explaining "We have selected another candidate whose qualifications and experience more closely meet our needs at this time. We would like to keep your résumé on file should another suitable position become available." Copies of these letters, as well as the interview checklists, should be kept for a minimum of 6 months should any questions arise regarding your choice of candidate. Procedure 22-3 provides details on interviewing.

ORIENTING NEW PERSONNEL

Orienting new employees is usually the responsibility of both the clinic manager and lead personnel who are most likely to work the closest with the new employee. It is common for a new employee to be placed on **probation** for 30 to 60 days, during which time both the employee and supervisory personnel may determine if the environment and the position are satisfactory for the employee. Procedure 22-4 outlines how to orient personnel.

Elements important to orientation include introducing the new employee to other staff members, assigning a mentor who can respond to questions, and making the employee aware of the procedures to be performed in this new position. If the procedure manual is detailed and accurate, this manual now becomes the daily guide for the new employee. Sometimes the individual leaving a position may still be present and is asked to assist in the orientation process. This is especially beneficial if there is a good working relationship between the employee who is leaving and the management of the practice. Depending on the responsibilities

PROCEDURE 22-3

Procedure

Conducting Interviews

PURPOSE:

To screen applicants for training, experience, and characteristics to select the best candidate to fill the position vacancy.

PROCEDURE STEPS:

1. Review résumés and applications received.
2. Select candidates who most closely match the education and experience being sought.
3. Develop a strategic plan for conducting the interviews by creating an interview worksheet for each candidate listing points to cover.
4. Select an interview team; this team should always include the HR or clinic manager and the immediate supervisor to whom the candidate will report.
5. Call personally to schedule interviews. RATIONALE: This allows you to judge the applicant's telephone manners and voice.
6. Maintain ethical standards by reminding the interviewers of various legal restrictions concerning questions to be asked.
7. Conduct interviews in a private, quiet setting. RATIONALE: Careful interviewing of potential employees is an important step in hiring the best candidate for the position.
8. Put the applicant at ease by beginning with an overview of the practice and staff, briefly describing the job, and answering preliminary questions.
9. Ask questions about the applicant's work experience and educational background using the résumé and interview worksheet as a guide.
10. Provide the most promising applicants additional information on benefits and a tour of the clinic, if practical.
11. Applicant's general salary requirements may be discussed, but avoid discussion of a specific salary until a formal offer is tendered.
12. Inform the applicants when a decision will be made and thank each for participating in the interview.
13. Do not make a job offer until all the candidates have been interviewed.
14. Check references of all prospective employees.
15. Establish a second interview between the provider-employer(s) and the qualified candidate if necessary.
16. Confirm accepted job offers in writing, specifying details of the offer and acceptance. RATIONALE: A written document provides proof of hiring and employment details.
17. Show respect by notifying all unsuccessful applicants by letter when the position has been filled. RATIONALE: Makes a positive statement to those not hired and keeps the doors open for future employment possibilities.

of the new employee, a supervisor may be asked to monitor for a period all the new employee's procedures for accuracy, safety, and patient protection. During the probation period, the employee should be officially evaluated by the clinic manager.

Generational Expectations

Today's HR managers will employ several different generations in their facility and must strive for a cohesive team among the generations. **Generation X** is defined as those born between 1966 and 1976; **Generation Y** (also known as the Millennial generation) was born between 1977 and 1994; and **Generation Z**, which is just now entering the work force, was born between 1995 and 2012. Search for information on Generation X at http://www.pewresearch.org and a summary of the "Gen Y and Gen Z Global Workplace Expectations Study" at http://millennialbranding.com.

Generation Xers are usually more moderate politically and socially than Generations Y and Z. They are fairly comfortable with technology, but

PROCEDURE 22-4

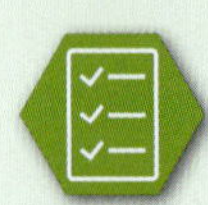
Procedure

Orienting Personnel

PURPOSE:

To acquaint new employees with clinic policies, staff, what the job encompasses, procedures to be performed, and job performance expectations.

PROCEDURE STEPS:

1. Tour the facilities and introduce the clinic staff.
2. Complete employee-related documents and explain their purpose.
3. Explain the benefits program.
4. Present the clinic policy manual and discuss its key elements.
5. Review federal and state regulatory precautions for medical facilities.
6. Review the job description.
7. Explain and demonstrate procedures to be performed and the use of procedure manuals supporting these procedures.
8. Demonstrate the use of any specialized equipment.
9. Assign a mentor from the staff to help with the orientation. RATIONALE: Without proper orientation and training, even the best new employee can fail.

worry about having enough money in retirement. They have learned, however, to be self-reliant, and often loyal to one employer.

It is interesting to note that both Generations Y and Z expect to have a number of job placements before retirement. Money is also not always the driving force in their job-related decisions; generally, these workers seek job advancement and satisfaction over salary. While both Generations Y and Z are quite comfortable in the world of electronic media and production, they increasingly see the value of face-to-face interaction.

The **Boomer generation**, born between 1955 and 1965, may still struggle with the vast advancement of technology in all aspects of their work. They will marvel at how much simpler the modern EKG machine is than what they first used, and are delighted in the bookkeeping and accounting software that keeps track of financial matters so easily. However, while they may seek members of Generations X, Y, and Z for assistance with technology, they likely will have a better understanding of the basic concepts behind these more modern and electronically enhanced methods than either Generation Y or Z.

EVALUATING EMPLOYEES

There are a number of reasons for regular predetermined performance reviews of employees. The review process is an opportunity to check employee compliance with the job description, motivate an employee to a higher level of performance, suggest possible areas of development for an employee, and—perhaps most important—communicate with an employee about job satisfaction and possible changes to be made.

Often, evaluations include a rating scale from 1 to 5 for these and many other qualities to be evaluated. However, there is increasing evidence to discourage such a scale, mostly because many employers tend to score in the middle and because it leaves so much to individual interpretation. To foster communication, motivate, and encourage improvement of employees at the time of evaluation, consider a different piece to add to the guidelines. Both the employer and the employee might be asked to perform an ABC. *A* stands for "What is Awesome about this job or person?" *B* is "What could be Better?" and *C* is "What would you like to Change?" The more standard evaluation format can simply include a straight yes or no—the employee either satisfactorily meets the criteria or does not. However, the ABC method allows for an expansion to include the information an evaluation really hopes to reveal.

DISMISSING EMPLOYEES

The function of employee dismissal or separation falls mostly to the clinic manager; however, in a large facility with an HR representative, discussing dismissal or separation with that individual can be quite beneficial. Such a discussion ensures that all the information necessary is in place before a separation. There are voluntary and involuntary separations or dismissals.

Voluntary separations usually occur when an employee is relocating, advancing to another position elsewhere, retiring, or leaving for other personal reasons. A letter of resignation is usually submitted to both the clinic manager and the HR representative. These employees will give their manager proper notice and may be able to turn current projects and duties over to their replacements. There is also time to say good-bye to their colleagues and have a good feeling about their employment.

Involuntary dismissals or separations usually occur when an employee's performance is poor or there has been a serious violation of the clinic policies or job description. The clinic manager is aware of poor performance through the probationary reviews. Verbal and written warnings must be given to the employee and are to be well documented. Dismissal can be immediate if there is a serious breach of clinic policy. The HR director can provide necessary detail to the clinic manager and/or provider(s) regarding when and if immediate dismissal is recommended. If a clinic manager expects any serious difficulties with an employee during an immediate dismissal, the HR director or another person appointed to assist should be present when the employee is notified (see Chapter 21 for a more detailed discussion).

Exit Interview

An **exit interview** is an excellent opportunity for the employee who voluntarily leaves a practice and the HR manager to discuss the positive and negative aspects of the job and what changes might be made for a new person coming into the facility. A sample exit interview form is shown in Figure 22-4. It also allows the opportunity for the employee to ask for a letter of reference or to view the personnel file before leaving. In a voluntary separation, a **letter of resignation** for the personnel file is necessary.

Any separation process, voluntary or involuntary, must include a statement in the personnel file. For involuntary separation, be certain that the reasons for the dismissal are well documented in an honest, nonjudgmental statement. State only the facts in the personnel file; do not state opinion. Remember that employees have the right to view their personnel file at any time.

Employers are always to be informed of any dismissal as quickly as possible. As indicated above, some may be involved in the actual dismissal process.

EXIT INTERVIEW FORM

1. What did you like and dislike about the work you have been doing?
   (Including: support on the job; opportunity for personal growth; recognition and rewards)
2. What kind of people have you found the providers, your immediate supervisor, and co-workers to be?
   (Including: attitude; fairness; scheduling and assignment of work; work expectations; technical competence; assistance and guidance available; team spirit)
3. What is your view of our management practices and policies?
   (Including: clarity and fairness of practice policies; communications; management and staff)
4. How have you felt about performance appraisals, your salary and benefits?
   (Including: adequacy of salary; regularity and fairness of appraisals)
5. What are your principal reasons for leaving the practice?
   (Including: primary dissatisfactions; job or personal changes)
6. In what areas do you feel we need to improve?

Interviewer signature: ____________ Date ________

Employee signature: ____________ Date ________

FIGURE 22-4 Sample exit interview form.

MAINTAINING PERSONNEL RECORDS

An important aspect of the responsibilities of the HR manager is maintaining personnel records. All documentation and correspondence related to each employee from application to dismissal, ranging from awards to reprimands and including formal reviews, must be kept in the confidential personnel file. Access to this file is limited to certain management personnel and the employee. Not all of these people are allowed to see the entire file. These files are usually kept for a period of 3 to 5 years after employees leave the practice. Some of the personnel files may be maintained electronically on the computer. However, access to those files must be protected so that only those with authorized access are able to open the files or make changes to them.

Such a file also includes the kind of information normally maintained for payroll and business practices. That information includes the name, address, telephone number, and Social Security number of the employee. The position title, date of beginning employment, rate of pay (hourly or otherwise), total overtime pay, deductions or additions to wages, wages paid each pay period, and the date the employee leaves the practice also are included.

COMPLYING WITH PERSONNEL LAWS

Legal

Only a brief introduction to the laws related to the ambulatory care setting are given in this section; therefore, this text is not meant to be a legal guide for an HR manager. The practice attorney should always be contacted if there is any question regarding personnel laws, which may vary in some states depending on the size of the practice.

Overtime must be addressed in each practice. Who is reimbursed for overtime and how is that reimbursement determined? Typically, administrative medical assistants, insurance billers, medical transcriptionists, and clinical medical assistants are likely to be eligible to be paid overtime. Overtime pay at a rate of not less than one and one-half times the regular rate of pay after a 40-hour work week is standard. Each week stands alone and one week cannot compensate for another. If the practice does not want to be involved in contentious overtime situations, require that any overtime be preauthorized in advance.

The Equal Pay Act of 1963 prevents wage discrimination for jobs that require equal skill, effort, and responsibility. The Civil Rights Act of 1964 prevents employers from discriminating against individuals on the basis of race, color, religion, sex, age, or national origin, and a number of states also consider discrimination based on sexual orientation illegal (see Chapter 6). Refer to Case Study 22-1 for an example of this dilemma.

Sexual harassment violates Title VII of the Civil Rights Act. Steps must be taken to ensure that all employees are working in an atmosphere that is not hostile, where sexual gestures, the presence of pornographic or offensive materials, or obscene language are not allowed either from patients or others in the clinic (see Chapter 6).

Safety

Employees have a right to expect safe working conditions. The Occupational Safety and Health Act (OSH Act) was established to prevent injuries and illnesses resulting from unsafe or unhealthy working conditions. Compliance with this law requires that each employee be aware of possible risks associated with chemical hazards and how to protect themselves. Because there are many of these hazards in a medical practice, compliance and protection for employees are extremely important, and training sessions should be held in this area.

The Immigration Reform Act requires employers to verify the right of employees to work in the United States. Documentation acceptable for verification is a Social Security card or birth certificate. The U.S. Citizenship and Immigration Services will provide instructions and a form for employees and employers to complete, commonly referred to as the I-9 or Employment Eligibility Verification form (see Case Study 22-2)

Employers cannot discriminate against or otherwise condemn any full-time employee for jury duty. Although the employer does not have to continue pay during jury duty, the employee cannot lose seniority, insurance, or other benefits. Many employers continue an employee's full pay during the time of service on a jury because the reimbursement from the government for jury service is minimal. This is a way to benefit employees and encourage good citizenship.

The preceding discussion is by no means comprehensive but does include personnel regulations most likely to affect a medical practice. Any concerns should be directed to the practice's attorney.

SPECIAL POLICY CONSIDERATIONS

Several other managerial issues may arise in a medical setting for which the clinic manager and the HR manager will have to plan. These can include policies for temporary employees, rules of conduct, avoiding discrimination, and having a support system in place for employees who need physical or emotional help.

Temporary Employees

Temporary employees who may be employed for 90 days or less include students who are serving an internship or practicum from a local college and are practicing their skills for when they will be on the job. They should be reviewed on a regular basis in cooperation with their college supervisor. Give them as much actual hands-on experience as possible; they are potential future employees. Accommodating students in the practice is a two-way benefit. Students learn what reality is in the ambulatory care setting and are able to practice newly developed skills. Current staff members in the facility are "sharpened" by the students' presence. Teaching and monitoring someone's actions always results in sharpening and rethinking the skills of the current staff. Many HR directors and managers depend on these programs for future job applicants.

Smoking Policy

Smoking on the premises of a health care facility is generally prohibited. Additionally, some states and cities have laws that restrict smoking. When a policy is established, it should cover everyone—employers, employees, *and* patients. The objective is to have a policy that is workable and enforceable, promotes health, encourages employee morale and productivity, and sets examples for patients.

Discrimination

The Americans with Disabilities Act (ADA) and the Americans with Disabilities Act Amendments Act (ADAAA) of 2008 prohibit discrimination against people with disabilities by all private employers with 15 or more employees. Some states may further prohibit discrimination in facilities with a much smaller size workforce. *All* public entities are prohibited from discriminating against qualified individuals with disabilities. The ADA establishes guidelines prohibiting discrimination against a "qualified individual with a disability" in regard to employment. The 2008 Amendment made it easier for an individual to establish a disability. Someone with a disability who satisfies the skills necessary for the job; has the experience, education, and any other job requirements; and who, with reasonable accommodation, can perform the job cannot be discriminated against. Employers often find that persons with disabilities are their finest employees.

Legal

Persons who are HIV positive or have AIDS are included in the guidelines set forth by the ADA. Persons with HIV/AIDS cannot be discriminated against. It can be assumed that if a safe working environment is provided where all employees follow the rules for Standard Precautions, then reasonable accommodation has been made for the person with HIV or AIDS.

An employer cannot refuse a job to a qualified person based on the belief that in the future the employee may become too ill to work. The hiring decision must be based on the individual's ability to perform the functions of the position at the present time. If a current employee reveals to the manager that he or she is HIV positive or has AIDS, that information must be kept confidential and must be kept apart from the general personnel file. The manager may choose to hold a discussion at that time of what accommodations might be needed in the future.

PROVIDING/PLANNING EMPLOYEE INSTRUCTION AND EDUCATION

Health care changes daily—new procedures are established, better techniques are discovered for performing a particular task, and so on. Major changes regularly occur in medical insurance. Computer systems are updated or new software is added. A more sophisticated telephone system is installed to make certain patients are responded to promptly. New state or federal regulations mandate additional education or compliance in safety. New medications become available that providers may prescribe and employees must understand. All this demands that employees receive continuing and constant updates in their area of employment.

Instruction and education may be accomplished within the practice or outside the practice. When an employee is a member of a professional organization such as the American Association of Medical Assistants, many monthly meetings include continuing education opportunities. Recertification of all medical assistants is to be encouraged and supported financially, if required. Numerous seminars and conferences held throughout the country may be beneficial to employees. Local hospitals often have continuing education opportunities that may be beneficial. Managers will keep abreast of these opportunities and encourage employees to attend. Any continuing education opportunity that may benefit the employee on the job and the medical practice hould ideally be paid for by the employ- Credentialed employees will always need ate skills and earn CEUs to maintain their credentials in active status. An important function of HR is to make CEUs opportunities available to employees.

It is often best to provide employee instruction and education within the facility when the necessary instruction is specific to the medical practice. For instance, instruction on new computer software is apt to be specific to the particular setting. When sophisticated new equipment is purchased, companies often provide in-house instruction for the individuals who will be using the equipment. Take advantage of as many of those opportunities as are available and for as many of your employees as possible. When the instruction is quite expensive or time consuming, make certain at least one person receives the instruction. Then have that individual teach others as appropriate. Whenever possible, provide instruction outside of regular hours when patients are not being seen—before the clinic opens or after the clinic closes or during a lunch period. Always pay employees for any time served over their regular working hours. Offer certificates for any in-services.

Careful attention to continuing education and instruction for employees will pay for itself many times over again. The more confident and secure employees feel in the skills they are expected to perform, the more satisfied the practice's patients will be.

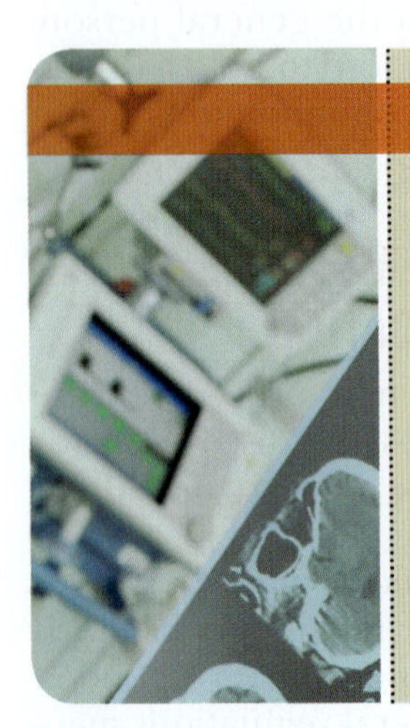

CASE STUDY 22-1

Refer to the scenario at the beginning of this chapter.

CASE STUDY REVIEW

1. Is there a legal issue here, an ethical issue, or both? If so, identify.
2. Should a policy be written to identify how the clinic is to respond to similar patient needs? Explain.
3. Do you agree with the provider's hesitation and relief? Justify your response.
4. If a clinic policy developed is opposite of your beliefs, what will you do? Might the scenario be different if the patient involved was a long-time patient of the clinic whose lifestyle was not known?

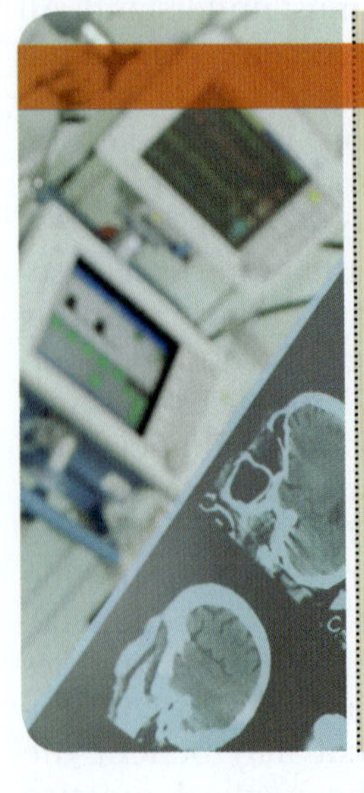

CASE STUDY 22-2

Ellen Armstrong, CMAS (AMT), is an administrative medical assistant at Inner City Health Care. The HR manager has suggested that she might expand her skills and learn some of the procedures related to the hiring process. A new medical assistant who specializes in nutrition is coming on board. Ellen has been asked to make certain his I-9 form is completed appropriately. The HR manager tells Ellen that she will need to download the latest form for the new employee to complete.

CASE STUDY REVIEW

1. Ellen knows that the I-9 is a government form verifying employment eligibility. What keywords might she use in her Internet search to find the form?
2. Once the form has been located, identify the specific rules necessary in completion of the form. What document in List A would a number of prospective employees most likely have?
3. In what area of the clinic might you post the lists of acceptable documents for the I-9 form?
4. With what agency is the form filed on successful completion?

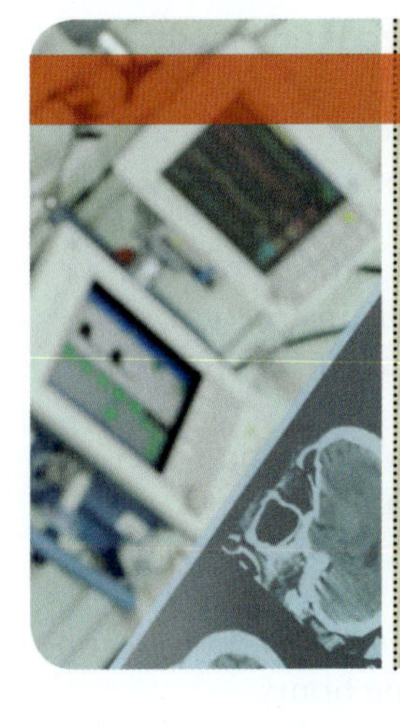

CASE STUDY 22-3

Charles Kensington has just been hired as the HR manager in a large metropolitan clinic. In studying the policy manual, he notes that there is no defined policy for sick leave or bereavement leave. Consider the steps he might take to write such a policy.

CASE STUDY REVIEW

1. To whom should he speak regarding what currently occurs when an employee is ill or when there is a death in the family?
2. What might Charles consider in writing this policy?
3. How should a policy be approved once it is written?
4. What parameters would you suggest for the policy?

Summary

- HR management is a challenge and includes many different tasks.
- Policy manuals assist the management team in recruiting, hiring, and maintaining the employees in the organization.
- The HR manager who is successful will hire the right people for the open positions and monitor employees in a way that enables and encourages them to give the best patient care possible.
- Managing personnel records will include everything from application to dismissal, all reviews, and salary documents.
- HR management must be able to comply with personnel laws, enforce policies, manage temporary employees, prevent discrimination, and provide necessary employee instruction and education.
- The HR manager will always have variety on the job and will have the satisfaction of watching a health care team function smoothly and efficiently.

Study for Success

To reinforce your knowledge and skills of information presented in this chapter:

- Review the *Key Terms* and *Learning Outcomes*
- Consider the *Critical Thinking* features and *Case Studies* and discuss your conclusions
  - Answer the questions in the *Certification Review*
  - Perform the *Procedures* using the *Competency Assessment Checklists* on the *Student Companion Website*

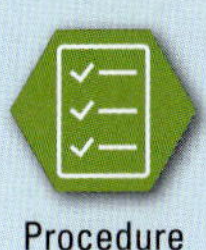
Procedure

CERTIFICATION REVIEW

1. What is a fitting description of HR managers?
   a. They need no special education for the position; experience is sufficient.
   b. They may work longer hours and are responsible for hiring and orienting personnel.
   c. They need legal education to understand labor laws.
   d. Their most important task is to keep the providers out of trouble with employees and patients.
2. Which of the following questions may be asked in an interview?
   a. How old are you?
   b. Have you ever been arrested?
   c. Can you supply a driver's license or a Social Security card?
   d. Do you plan to start a family soon?
   e. Do you have someone to care for your children should they become ill?

3. When a candidate has been accepted for a position, what will the HR manager need to do?
   a. Call the candidate to determine what salary is preferred
   b. Write a letter defining the position details and intent to hire
   c. Check references provided by the candidate
   d. Notify patients of a staff change
4. What is commonly known about overtime hours in the medical facility?
   a. They are to be expected as part of the position.
   b. They do not require prior authorization.
   c. They are usually paid at no less than one and one-half times the regular pay rate.
   d. They are paid only to managers.
   e. They are a sign that the facility is sadly understaffed.
5. Who will the HR manager work with most closely?
   a. The clinic patients and the provider-employer(s)
   b. The clinic manager and county health department
   c. All employees except management
   d. The provider-employer(s), clinic manager, and employees
   e. Only the provider(s) with whom all HR matters are settled
6. Walter, one of the clinic medical assistants has been called to a two-week jury duty assignment. What discussion will he have with HR?
   a. He will be told he cannot serve; the clinic is far too busy.
   b. He will have to find a part-time replacement while he serves.
   c. HR will quickly make plans for a replacement during the days he must serve, pay his full salary, and encourage his participation.
   d. The HR manager will request a hardship excuse from jury duty for Walter.
   e. HR will need to have other employees pick up Walter's duties.
7. What resources are best for recruiting medical employees?
   a. Students in a business college
   b. Newspaper advertisements
   c. Networking sources
   d. The state's unemployment office
8. How will employees receive the instruction/education necessary to remain current in their positions?
   a. They will need to seek that instruction after hours and not expect reimbursement.
   b. They will already be current and up-to-date in the health care field.
   c. They should be paid for any time required and served over regular working hours.
   d. Training is usually done during lunch hours, and hopefully the providers will arrange for lunch.
   e. They will get sufficient updating from their professional associations.
9. Which of the following statements regarding personnel records is accurate?
   a. They are usually kept for 3 to 5 years after employment ends and may include payroll data.
   b. They are available for anyone to view, but are kept locked away.
   c. They will not include any papers related to anything other than employment.
   d. They are available only to HR and the provider(s).
10. Which of the following statements is true regarding dismissal or separation?
   a. It may be voluntary or involuntary and is always documented.
   b. It is always permanent.
   c. It will not require an exit interview.
   d. It requires a letter of referral.
   e. It upsets everyone and is to be kept private.

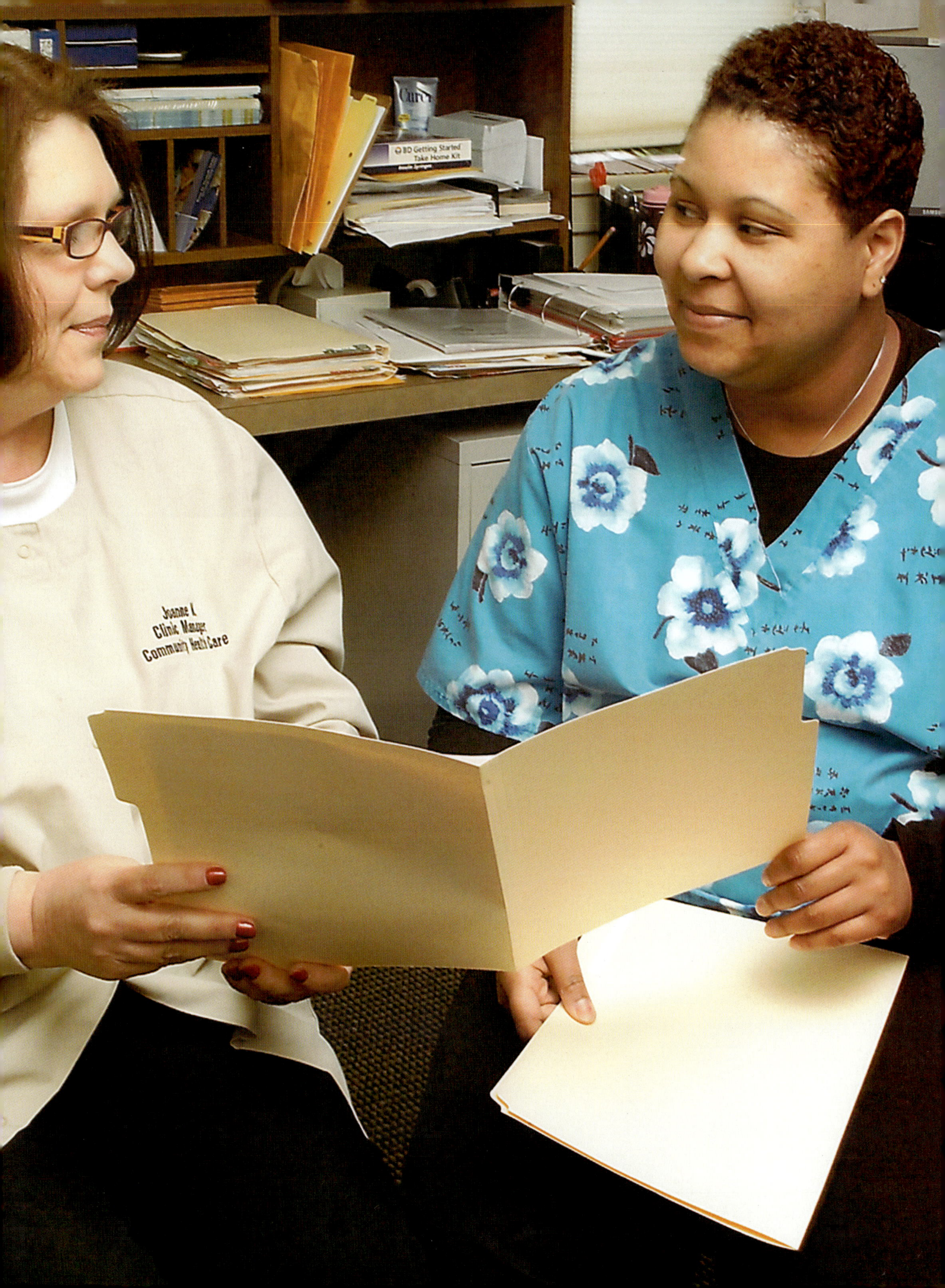
BD Getting Started
Take Home Kit
Joanne K.
Clinic Manager
Community Health Care

UNIT VII

ENTRY INTO THE PROFESSION

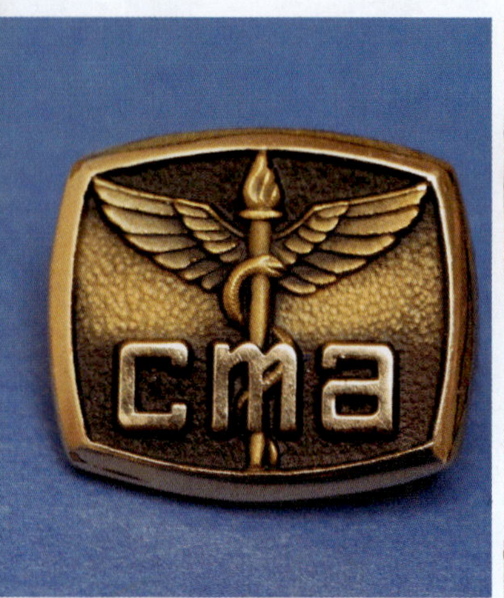

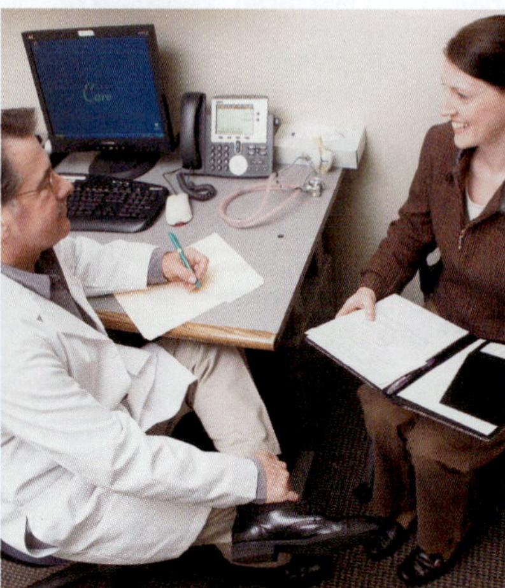

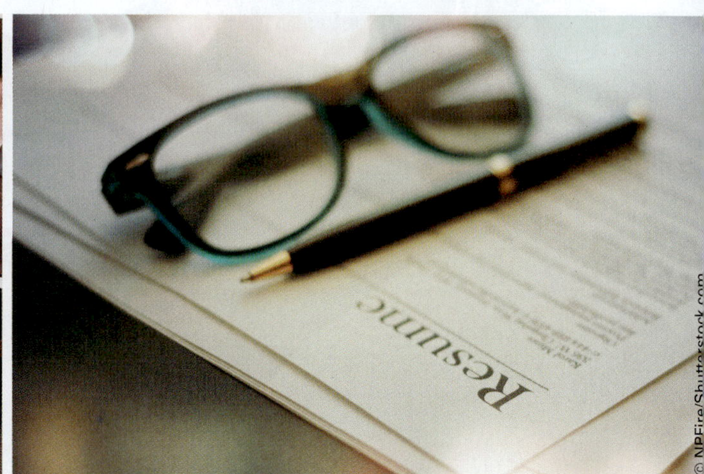

© NPFire/Shutterstock.com

ATTRIBUTES OF PROFESSIONALISM

The medical assisting profession continues to be one of the fastest growing professions in the United States, with increasing numbers of career-oriented candidates entering the profession annually. Therefore, it is important that you develop ways to uniquely present yourself and your skill set to a potential employer. Successfully passing the national certification examination and receiving a medical assisting credential is one way to establish your professionalism. Achieving certification acknowledges that you have standard entry-level knowledge and skills, while continuing to maintain the credential demonstrates a lifelong commitment to professional development.

Securing employment as a certified medical assistant is your first job. Developing a comprehensive job search strategy that includes self-assessment, résumé preparation, interview techniques, and follow-up is a key component to successful employment. Each component of your strategy demonstrates professionalism through communication, presentation, competency, initiative, and integrity.

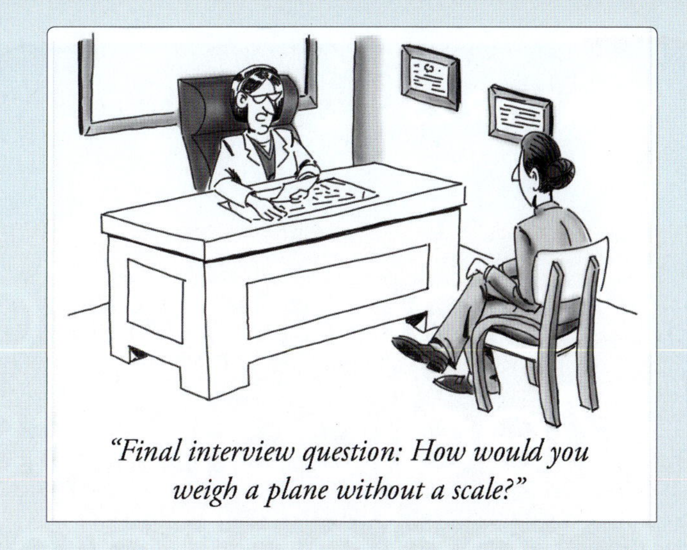
"Final interview question: How would you weigh a plane without a scale?"

Listed below are a series of questions for you to ask yourself, to serve as a professionalism checklist as you prepare for your future career as a medical assistant. As you interact with patients and colleagues, these questions will help to guide you in the characteristics and behaviors that are expected every day from professional medical assistants.

Ask Yourself

COMMUNICATION

- ☐ Do I apply active listening skills?
- ☐ Do I display professionalism through written and verbal communication?
- ☐ Do I demonstrate appropriate nonverbal communication?
- ☐ Do I display appropriate body language?
- ☐ Does my knowledge allow me to speak easily with all members of the health care team?

PRESENTATION

- ☐ Am I dressed and groomed appropriately?
- ☐ Do I display a positive attitude?
- ☐ Do I display a calm, professional, and caring manner?

COMPETENCY

- ☐ Do I pay attention to detail?
- ☐ Do I ask questions if I am out of my comfort zone or do not have the experience to carry out tasks?
- ☐ Do I display sound judgment?
- ☐ Am I knowledgeable and accountable?

INITIATIVE

- ☐ Do I show initiative?
- ☐ Have I developed a strategic plan to achieve my goals? Is my plan realistic?
- ☐ Do I seek out opportunities to expand my knowledge base?
- ☐ Am I flexible and dependable?

INTEGRITY

- ☐ Do I demonstrate the principles of self-boundaries?
- ☐ Do I work within my scope of practice?
- ☐ Do I demonstrate respect for individual diversity?
- ☐ Do I recognize the impact personal ethics and morals have on the delivery of health care?
- ☐ Do I protect and maintain confidentiality?
- ☐ Do I maintain moral and ethical standards?
- ☐ Do I do the "right thing" even when no one is observing?

CHAPTER 23

Preparing for Medical Assisting Credentials

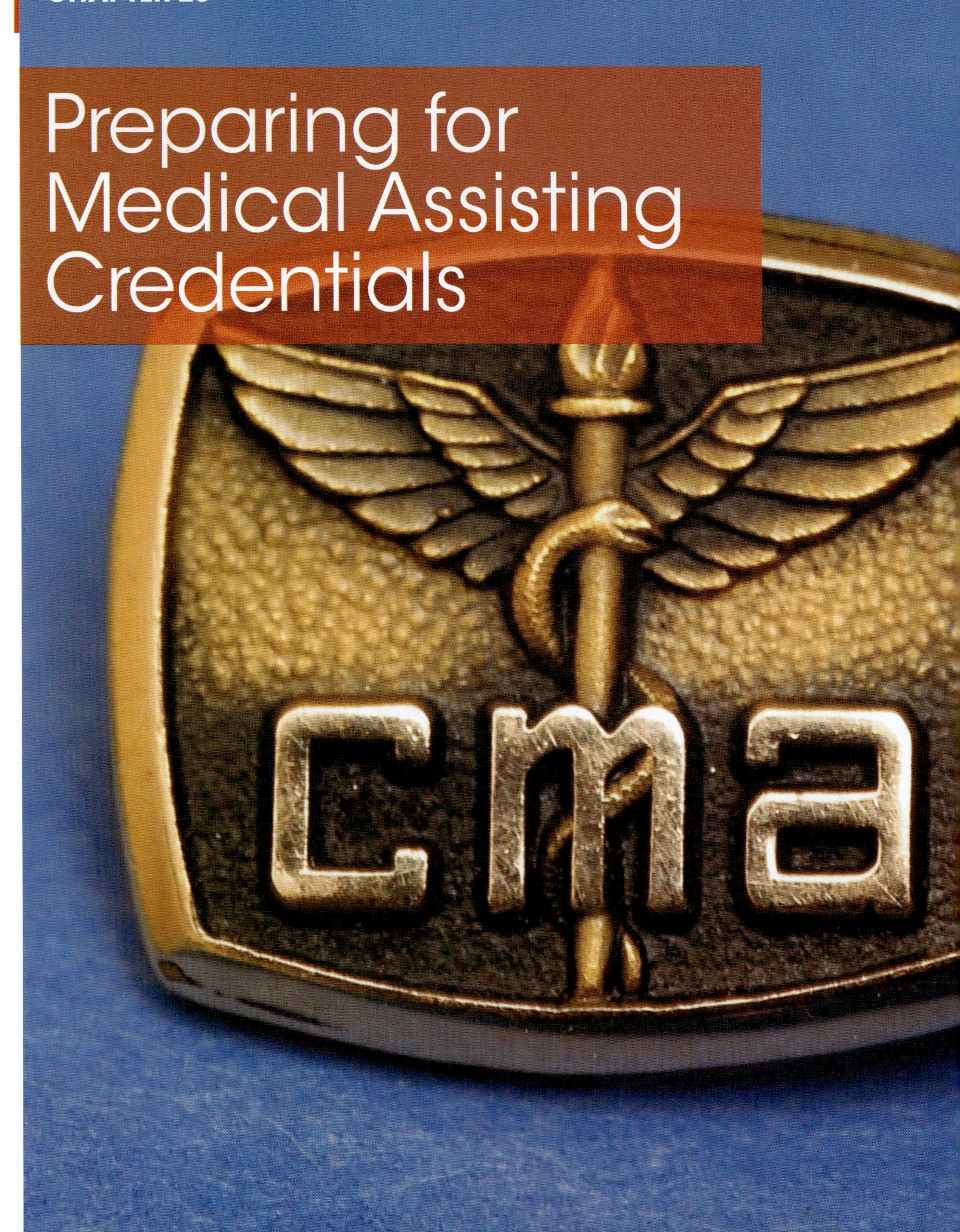

LEARNING OUTCOMES

1. Define and spell all of the key terms as presented in this chapter.
2. Discuss the purpose of certification and the importance of recertification.
3. Develop a plan and study schedule to sit for a medical assistant certification examination.
4. Compare the various agencies providing medical assisting certification.
5. Discuss the role of the Commission on Accreditation of Allied Health Education Programs (CAAHEP), the AAMA Endowment, and the Medical Assisting Education Review Board (MAERB).
6. Analyze the differences between a registered medical assistant and a certified medical administrative specialist.
7. Identify and describe the two medical assisting credentials available through the National Healthcareer Association (NHA).
8. Identify the benefits of medical assistant certification and registration.
9. Describe several methods for pursuing continuing education opportunities through each accrediting agency.
10. Examine professional organizations and the value they offer you as a medical assistant.

KEY TERMS

Accrediting Bureau of Health Education Schools (ABHES)
American Association of Medical Assistants (AAMA)
American Medical Technologists (AMT)
certification
certification examination
Certified Clinical Medical Assistant (CCMA [NHA])
Certified Medical Administrative Assistant (CMAA [NHA])
Certified Medical Administrative Specialist (CMAS [AMT])
Certified Medical Assistant (CMA [AAMA])
Commission on Accreditation of Allied Health Education Programs (CAAHEP)
continuing education units (CEUs)
National Healthcareer Association (NHA)
recertification
Registered Medical Assistant (RMA [AMT])

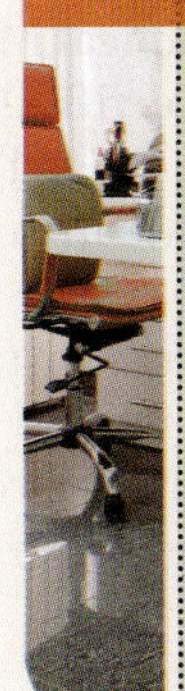

SCENARIO

Dr. Ray Reynolds currently is the senior provider at Inner City Health Care, a multiprovider clinic. When he began his practice years ago, however, he had a private practice and employed one full-time and two part-time medical assistants. Dr. Reynolds felt the practice ran smoothly, except when an assistant had to be replaced. Retraining a new person consumed a great deal of valuable time. Even if the new employee came with experience from another medical practice, the procedures still required retraining.

Dr. Reynolds now finds that when he needs to replace a medical assistant, he looks at the applicants' résumés and interviews only those candidates who are credentialed medical assistants. The practice is too busy to spend time training and retraining new employees.

Chapter Portal

Forty years ago, medical assistants were trained on the job by the practitioner with whom they were employed. With no established criteria for evaluating such training, quality control varied. This chapter will present the purpose of certification, certifying agencies, and preparation for certification examinations.

PURPOSE OF CERTIFICATION

Certification is intended to set a consistent minimum standard for evaluating an individual's professional competence as a medical assistant. The medical assisting profession continues to be one of the fastest growing occupations in the United States. Because of the demand for skilled medical assistants, increasing numbers of career-oriented candidates enter this profession annually. Certification acknowledges the professional has standard entry-level knowledge and skills. The Certifying Board of AAMA recently received accreditation from the International Accreditation Service (IAS). This achievement establishes AAMA as the most respected and credible personnel certification organization for the medical assisting profession.

Successfully passing a certification examination builds personal self-esteem, confidence, and a positive attitude in performing the responsibilities assigned. (See Chapter 1 for more history regarding certification.) Other benefits of certification include help in your career advancement and compensation. Hiring providers view credentialed medical assistants as professionals who have shown proficiency in entry-level skills. Individuals who are competent and interested in continued learning experiences are more apt to be rewarded with promotions and salary increases. Maintaining the credential demonstrates a lifelong commitment to professional development. The graduate medical assistant has a goal and challenge to which to aspire, first by earning the credential and second by maintaining the credential through continuing education and recertification.

Some certifying agencies offer student membership into their organizations. This avenue provides excellent opportunities to network and be mentored by fellow professionals, to enroll in continuing education programs, and to receive many other membership perks. For example, students enrolled as American Association of Medical Assistants (AAMA) members before their graduation date are eligible for reduced student membership rates. Once they are a student member, they may stay at the student rate for 1 year after graduation if they do not choose to be an active or associate member and pay the higher dues amount. The additional year of membership at the reduced rate helps the recent graduate maintain membership while finding a job and becoming established in their career.

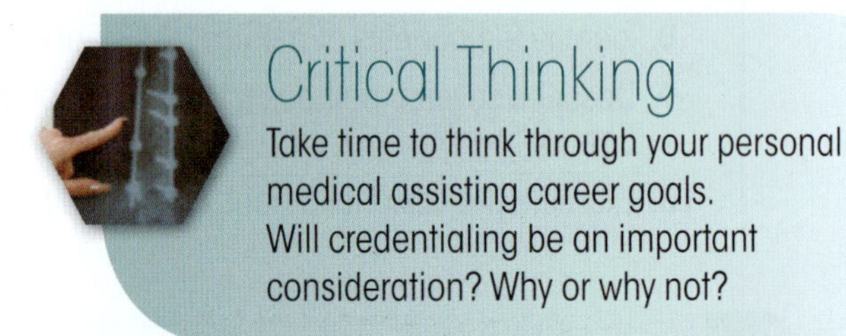

Critical Thinking

Take time to think through your personal medical assisting career goals. Will credentialing be an important consideration? Why or why not?

CERTIFICATION AGENCIES

The **American Association of Medical Assistants (AAMA)** offers examinations to certify the **Certified Medical Assistant (CMA [AAMA])**. The **American Medical Technologists (AMT)** offers examinations to certify the **Registered Medical Assistant (RMA [AMT])** and the **Certified Medical Administrative Specialist (CMAS [AMT])**. The **National Healthcareer Association (NHA)** is another agency offering certification to health care professionals. These professionals include the **Certified Clinical Medical Assistant (CCMA [NHA])** and the **Certified Medical Administrative Assistant (CMAA [NHA])**. See Table 23-1 for a comparison of the various certifying agencies for medical assisting.

When responding to advertisements or during the interview process, "certified medical assistants" are responsible to make clear to prospective employers which credential they have been awarded.

TABLE 23-1

COMPARISON OF AGENCIES PROVIDING MA CERTIFICATION

CERTIFICATION DETAILS			
Certifying agency	American Association of Medical Assistants (AAMA)	American Medical Technologists (AMT)	National Healthcareer Association (NHA)
Credential	CMA (AAMA)	RMA (AMT) or CMAS (AMT)	CCMA (NHA) or CMAA (NHA)
Certification exam	Computer-based national exam; administered through Prometric testing centers (www.prometric.com)	Computer-based national exam offered at Pearson Vue testing centers (www.pearsonvue.com); or paper exam by appointment	National exam; can be taken online or as a paper exam
Exam format	200 multiple-choice questions selected from topics listed on the Content Outline for the CMA (AAMA) Maximum test time is 195 minutes	210 multiple-choice questions covering topics related to clinical, administrative, and general subjects 2.5 hours to complete Immediate pass/fail notification Reschedule within 24 hours if failed Four lifetime attempts allowed	200 multiple-choice questions Separate tests for CCMA and CMAA (exam completion time approximately 90 minutes)
Continuing education	AAMA-approved CEUs: 60 units every five years 10 clinical 10 administrative 10 general 30 discretionary	Certification Continuation Program (CCP): 30 points every three years AMT and AMTIE* offer several CE options for points	Continued Education (CE) Program: 10 NHA-approved continuing education credits every two years

*American Medical Technologists Institute For Excellence (AMTIE)

PREPARING FOR CERTIFICATION EXAMINATIONS

Preparation for the examination requires planning, scheduling, and discipline. It is important to plan well in advance to ensure confidence and a passing score to earn your credential. If you are sitting for the examination immediately upon graduation, your preparation time for the examination may only allow 2 to 3 months. If you have been out of school for some time or your work experience has been very specialized, you may need longer to prepare for the examination.

During the planning stage, determine the date you want to sit for the examination. Check with the appropriate Web site or call the appropriate examination department to obtain the current application form. The application form contains information such as dates, times, and locations of test sites; policies regarding deadlines; incomplete applications; examination verification information; and information regarding study guides.

It is important to consider having a study group or partner. The right study environment can be invaluable to your success for several reasons. First, it is important to select a study partner or group who shares your commitment to a successful outcome and who plans to sit for the examination on or near the same date you have selected. A study partner can also give you some accountability for keeping to the planned schedule.

Once it has been determined when and where you will sit for the examination and who your study partner(s), if any, will be, a meeting should be scheduled to discuss the review/study approach. It may be that your group will decide to review/study each subject provided in the Curriculum Content Outline accompanying the application. Other groups review/study only those areas in which they feel less confident. A plan that meets the needs of each group member and that all can agree to works best.

Meeting once or twice a week helps the group stay focused and on task. Independent study should be done throughout the week. During the independent study time, each group member may be asked to write 10 multiple-choice questions relevant to the week's study topic. Answers to these questions should be on a separate page. Some find it helpful to also provide the rationale or textbook page number that supports their answer. When the group meets, a discussion of the study topic could take place and copies of the questions could be distributed for answering. The questions could then be corrected and discussion of any questionable or missed answers could take place.

Once a schedule has been established and agreed on, discipline is required. It is critical that each group member spend time individually preparing for the next group meeting. Someone should be put in charge of each group meeting to keep the event from turning into a social gathering. To help with this, it is a good idea to set a specific time limit for the study/review session. If individuals want to visit after the session, they are free to do that without disrupting the purpose of the session. All members should be committed to being prepared and attending each scheduled review/study session.

AMERICAN ASSOCIATION OF MEDICAL ASSISTANTS (AAMA)

The AAMA is an organization whose objective is to promote skills and professionalism, protect the medical assistants' right to practice, and encourage consistent health care delivery through professional certification. The AAMA is a sponsoring member of the **Commission on Accreditation of Allied Health Education Programs (CAAHEP)**. CAAHEP establishes the standards for medical assisting programs and is the issuing body of the accreditation for AAMA. (See Chapter 1 for the history of AAMA).

Only graduates of medical assistant programs accredited by CAAHEP and the **Accrediting Bureau of Health Education Schools (ABHES)** may sit for the AAMA Certified Medical Assistant exam. To locate CAAHEP medical assisting information, go to www.aama-ntl.org and follow the drop-down menu for specific information. To locate ABHES registered medical assisting information, go to www.americanmedtech.org and follow the drop-down menu for specific information. The AAMA Endowment is a nonprofit corporation that provides funding for two purposes:

- Awarding of scholarships to students in CAAHEP-accredited medical assisting education programs
- Accrediting medical assisting education programs through CAAHEP

The Medical Assisting Education Review Board (MAERB) operates under the authority of the endowment and evaluates medical assisting programs according to standards adopted by the endowment and CAAHEP. The MAERB recommends programs to CAAHEP for accreditation. The MAERB also reviews standards for medical assisting curricula, conducts accreditation workshops for educators, and provides medical assisting educators with current information about CAAHEP, accreditation laws, policies, and practices.

Certified Medical Assistant (AAMA) Examination Format and Content

The AAMA **certification examination** is a comprehensive test of the knowledge actually used in today's medical clinic. The content is drawn from an in-depth analysis of the numerous tasks practicing medical assistants perform on a daily basis.

Examination questions are formulated by the Certifying Board's Task Force for Test Construction (TFTC). This group is composed of practicing medical assistants, providers, and medical assisting educators from across the United States. The TFTC updates the examination annually to reflect changes in medical assistants' day-to-day responsibilities, as well as the latest developments in medical knowledge and technology.

The three major areas tested include:

1. *General.* Psychology, Communication; Professionalism; Medical Terminology; Medical Law/Regulatory Guidelines; Medical Ethics; and Risk Management, Quality Assurance, and Safety
2. *Administrative.* Medical Reception, Patient Navigator/Advocate, Medical Business Practices, Establish Patient Medical Record, Scheduling Appointments, and Practice Finances
3. *Clinical.* Anatomy and Physiology, Infection Control, Patient Intake and Documentation of Care, Patient Preparation and Assisting the Provider, Nutrition, and Collecting and Processing Specimens

Certified Medical Assistant (AAMA) Application Process

Candidates should read all instructions carefully before completing the application form. Incomplete or incorrect applications will not be processed and will be returned to the candidate. Postmark deadlines for applications, cancellations, and examination location changes are strictly enforced.

Applications are available from the AAMA Certification Department, 7999 Eagle Way, Chicago, IL 60678-1079, or may be downloaded from the AAMA Web site (www.aama-ntl.org) or completed online.

When completing a printed application, it is recommended that the application be sent by certified mail, return receipt requested to verify delivery. The application must be typewritten or printed using black ink only. Be sure the application is signed and dated properly and the eligibility category section is completed appropriately. Applications take up to 45 days after the postmark date to process.

Tear off the application page from the instruction pamphlet. Do not mail the instructions back with the application. Keep this information for future reference together with a copy of everything submitted, including a copy of your completed application and payment check or money order. If you are paying by Visa or MasterCard, provide the requested information at the top of the application.

Certified Medical Assistant (AAMA) Examination Scheduling and Administration

The CMA (AAMA) certification examination is offered via computer-based testing (CBT). Candidates whose applications are accepted will receive a Scheduling Permit containing instructions for making a testing appointment, and will be able to select locations and flexible testing times at Prometric test centers throughout the United States. To schedule examination appointments, candidates go to www.prometric.com and select a test center and appointment test time. Centers are open 9:00 AM to 5:00 PM Monday through Saturday. An email confirming your appointment will be sent to you.

Photo identification is required for admission to the examination. Candidates are not permitted to bring any items except identification into the examination area. All exam candidates will receive an unofficial pass/fail result immediately upon completion of the exam. An official report of your scores will be mailed within 6 to 10 weeks after the exam date.

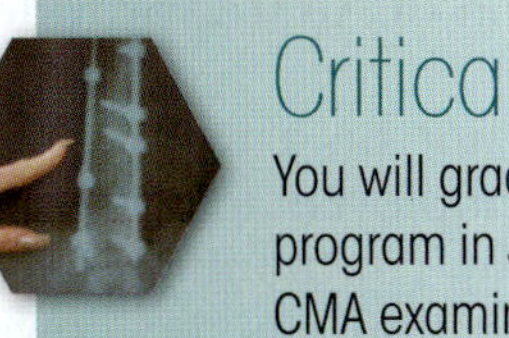

Critical Thinking

You will graduate from a CAAHEP-accredited program in June and want to sit for the CMA examination the last Saturday of June (the same month in which you graduate). Go to the AAMA Web site and determine when your application must be postmarked for acceptance for this test date. What is the date the online application must be completed?

Certified Medical Assistant (AAMA) Recertification

All newly certified and recertifying CMAs (AAMA) will be current through the end of the calendar month of initial certification or most recent recertification for 60 months.

Recertification can be achieved either by reexamination or by **continuing education units (CEUs)**. Recertification units are evaluated on supportive documentation and relevancy to medical assisting as defined by the AAMA *Medical Assistant Role Delineation Study* or the *Content Outline for the Certification/Recertification Examination.*

A total of 60 units is necessary to recertify the CMA (AAMA) credential. A minimum of 10 units is required in each category: general, administrative, and clinical. The remaining 30 units can be accumulated in any of the three content areas or from any combination of the three categories. At least 30 of the required 60 recertification units must be accumulated from AAMA-approved CEUs. If desired, all 60 units may be AAMA CEUs.

Applicants who accumulate all 60 units through AAMA CEUs, and in the correct content areas, can order a recertification over the telephone. Application fees still apply; however, an application form is not required. All CMAs employed or seeking employment must have current certified status to use the CMA (AAMA) credential.

Continuing education courses are offered by local, state, and national AAMA groups. Guided study programs are also available through AAMA's Quest for Excellence program. *CMA Today*, the official bimonthly publication of AAMA, provides articles designated for CEUs.

A CMA (AAMA) need not be a member of the AAMA nor currently employed to recertify. The entire recertification by continuing education instructions and application can be downloaded from AAMA's Web site (www.aama-ntl.org). Review of recertification applications can take up to 90 days. If all criteria are met, recertification is granted. The date that the application was postmarked to the AAMA Executive Office will be the date of recertification.

CEU Documentation. On successfully passing the certification examination and earning the CMA (AAMA) credential, one should begin to document all CEUs earned. It is important to have the following information for CEU documentation:

- Complete date of the activity
- Sponsor (group or organization issuing the credit for the continuing education activity)
- Program title
- Amount and type of credit earned (e.g., CEU, CME, contact hour or college credit)
- Recertification units (AAMA CEUs or other credit)
- Units per content area (general, administrative, clinical)

A copy of the handbook *Recertify your CMA (AAMA) Credential* may be downloaded from www.aama-ntl.org. A sample continuing education verification form as well as a blank form is included for your convenience. Recertification is made much easier when this form is documented completely and kept up to date.

AMERICAN MEDICAL TECHNOLOGISTS (AMT)

The American Medical Technologists (AMT) awards the registered medical assistant RMA (AMT) credential to individuals graduating from ABHES-accredited medical assisting programs who successfully pass their examination. ABHES is recognized by the U.S. Department of Education for accreditation of postsecondary schools offering traditional instruction as well as instruction by distance delivery.

The AMT also offers certification for the certified medical administrative specialist (CMAS). The CMAS (AMT) is employed primarily in the administrative area of provider clinics or hospitals. They must understand and use medical terminology properly and be skilled in all administrative tasks performed in health care settings. Each individual state decides the scope of practice for the CMAS (AMT), with most states not requiring licensure.

Additional information regarding CMAS (AMT) education requirements, duties performed, working conditions, employment outlook, and estimated earnings can be found online at www.americanmedtech.org.

Registered Medical Assistant (AMT) Examination Format and Content

AMT certification examinations are intended to evaluate the competence of entry-level practitioners. The Education, Qualifications, and Standards Committee of American Medical Technologists develops registered medical assistant RMA (AMT) examinations. The medical assistant committee writes test questions and reviews questions submitted from other sources (e.g., instructors, experts, practitioners, and other individuals associated with the medical assistant profession). The medical assistant committee also determines certification requirements and addresses standard-setting issues related to the credential. Once test construction has been completed, the examination is reviewed and approved by the AMT Board of Directors.

Examinees are required to select the single best answer; multiple answers for a single item are scored as incorrect. Test questions may require examinees to recall facts, interpret graphic illustrations and information presented in case studies, analyze situations, or solve problems. The approximate percentage of questions in each content area is as follows:

1. General Medical Assisting Knowledge—41.0%
    - Anatomy and Physiology
    - Medical Terminology
    - Medical Law
    - Medical Ethics
    - Human Relations
    - Patient Education
2. Administrative Medical Assisting—24.0%
    - Insurance
    - Financial bookkeeping
    - Medical secretarial-administrative medical assistant

3. Clinical Medical Assisting—35.0%
    - Asepsis
    - Sterilization
    - Instruments
    - Vital signs
    - Physical examinations
    - Clinical pharmacology
    - Minor surgery
    - Therapeutic modalities
    - Laboratory procedures
    - Electrocardiography
    - First aid

Registered Medical Assistant (AMT) Application Process

The following criteria have been established for applicants sitting for the RMA (AMT) examination:

1. Applicant shall be of good moral character and at least 18 years of age.
2. Applicant shall be a graduate of an accredited high school or acceptable equivalent.
3. Applicant must meet one of the following requirements:
    a. Applicant shall be a graduate of a:
        - Medical assisting program that holds programmatic accreditation by (or is in a postsecondary school or college that holds institutional accreditation by) the ABHES or the CAAHEP.
        - Medical assisting program in a postsecondary school or college that has institutional accreditation by a Regional Accrediting Commission or by a national accrediting organization approved by the U.S. Department of Education. That program must include a minimum of 720 clock hours (or equivalent) of training in medical assisting skills (including a clinical practicum of no less than 160 hours).
        - Formal medical services training program of the U.S. Armed Forces.

    b. Applicant shall have been employed in the profession of medical assisting for a minimum of 5 years, no more than 2 years of which may have been as an instructor in a postsecondary medical assisting program.
4. Applicants applying under criteria 3 a or b *must* take and pass the AMT certification examination for RMA.

The AMT Board of Directors has further determined that applicants who have passed a generalist medical assistant certification examination offered by another medical assisting certification body (provided that examination has been approved for this purpose by the AMT Board of Directors), who have been working in the medical assisting field for 3 of the past 5 years, and who meet all other AMT training and experience requirements may be considered for RMA (AMT) certification without further examination. Applications and a useful handbook for the AMT candidate can be downloaded from AMT's Web site at (www.americanmedtech.com).

Registered Medical Assistant (AMT) Examination Scheduling and Administration

All applications must be completed online or printed clearly except for the signatures required. All ancillary documentation must also be submitted (e.g., application fee; proof of high school graduation or equivalent; and official final transcripts stating graduation from medical assistant school, college, or training program [with school seal affixed or notarized]).

When the AMT registrar has received the application and all required information, an authorization letter containing a toll-free number is mailed to you. You can then contact Pearson Vue locations at www.pearsonvue.com/amt to schedule a date and time to take the examination. Two forms of valid identification are required, both bearing your signature and at least one bearing your photo. Photo identification is limited to a driver's license, state-issued identification card, military identification, or passport.

All AMT registration examination tests are available in paper-and-pencil format or in computerized formats at over 200 locations in the United States, its territories, and Canada. Tests can be scheduled daily except Sundays and holidays. Both formats are identical in length; however, experience has shown the computerized test takes less time to complete. Your computerized test score is displayed moments after you complete your test. A paper copy of your result is provided to you before you leave the testing center.

Registered Medical Assistant (AMT) Recertification

The AMT has established the Certification Continuation Program (CCP) for continuing education points. Certification will be suspended following a 30-day grace period if proper documentation is not submitted. Each RMA (AMT) is required to accumulate 30 points, which must be turned in every 3 years for recertification. You can use the AMTrax mobile app to record and track your activities for submission. You may view and print your record at any time using date ranges. Retaking the RMA examination is not an option for reinstatement or recertification.

NATIONAL HEALTHCAREER ASSOCIATION (NHA)

The National Healthcareer Association (NHA) also offers national certification examinations for health care professionals. Certified programs are accredited by the National Commission for Certifying Agencies (NCCA), a division of the Institute for Credentialing Excellence (ICE). NHA works with educational institutions throughout the country on curriculum development, competency testing, and preparation and administration of their examination and offers a continuing education (CE) program.

Certified Clinical Medical Assistant and Certified Medical Administrative Assistant Examination Format and Content

The NHA certifies the Certified Clinical Medical Assistant (CCMA [NHA]) and the Certified Medical Administrative Assistant (CMAA [NHA]) among other health career professions. Criteria for taking NHA certification examinations include one of the following: The applicant must have a high school diploma and have recently successfully completed an NHA-approved training program or the applicant must have either a high school diploma or equivalency and have recently worked in the field of certification for a minimum of 1 year as a full-time employee. Work experience must be documented in writing and signed by the director or employer.

The NHA offers several methods to help prepare candidates for their national certification examination. All students applying for NHA certification examination receive NHA study guides. The examination is offered in traditional pencil-and-paper formats or can be taken online at any of the approved locations.

Certified Clinical Medical Assistant and Certified Medical Administrative Assistant Application Process

There are four ways to apply for the NHA national certification examination:

- Online using www.nhanow.com. Go directly to the secured registration page and submit the registration form using Visa, MasterCard, Discover, American Express, or school voucher.
- The registration form can be downloaded and printed. Once it is filled out completely, it can be mailed along with payment. Address and mail to:

  National Healthcareer Association
  7 Ridgedale Avenue, Suite 203
  Cedar Knolls, NJ 07927
- The completed registration form can be faxed to the NHA with credit card information or school voucher. The fax number is 1-973-644-4797.
- Telephone the Customer Service Department at 1-800-449-9092. You can then complete the registration over the phone. You will need your credit card number and expiration date or school voucher accessible for payment information.

Certified Clinical Medical Assistant and Certified Medical Administrative Assistant Examination Scheduling and Administration

The NHA examination can be scheduled at any of the approved locations:

- *Training schools/colleges.* Check with your school for details.
- *Testing sites.* There are more than 550 PSI/LaserGrade testing sites nationwide.
- Experienced individuals can take examinations at their place of employment.

NOTE: All examinations are required to have an exam proctor present.

Certified Clinical Medical Assistant and Certified Medical Administrative Assistant Recertification

NHA offers a Continuing Education (CE) Program to make the process of continuing education more convenient for the health care professional. Courses in this program can be taken at your convenience at home. New industry standards require that each NHA-certified health care professional complete 10 CE credits every 2 years.

In the event that certification expires, reinstatement is permitted within a year of the expiration date. If reinstatement is initiated within a year of the expiration date, the individual must submit evidence of 15 completed CE credits and pay a renewal and reinstatement fee. After a year from the expiration date, reinstatement is not permitted and the individual must apply and take the certification examination again to become recertified.

Applicants who pass the examination will be nationally certified as recognized by the NHA. They will receive a certification certificate suitable for framing and a wallet-size ID certification card containing their national certification number. CE credits will be reviewed by NHA, and a sticker to apply to the certification ID card will be mailed if the credits are accepted.

PROFESSIONAL ORGANIZATIONS

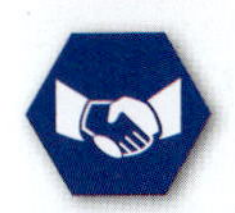
Professional

Professional organizations have evolved to establish standards by which medical assistants and medical assisting programs are evaluated. Programs accredited by agencies must meet certain criteria, and students must pass national examinations to become certified. Medical assistants are not licensed and need not be certified to meet employment requirements; however, those certified are viewed as professionals with entry-level skills and a commitment to continuing education.

American Association of Medical Assistants (AAMA)

The AAMA was instrumental in defining the scope of training required for the profession and developed standards and guidelines by which programs could become accredited and the medical assistant credentialed. Membership in the AAMA offers many benefits, including the following:

- Medical assisting news and health care information through the bimonthly magazine *CMA Today*
- CEUs for AAMA activities entered in the Continuing Education Registry and access to your transcript online
- Educational events provided by local chapters, state societies, and national meetings
- Answers to legal questions regarding job-related issues
- If eligible, application for the prestigious CMA examination at a reduced fee
- Discounts on car rentals, conventions, workshop and seminar fees, and self-study courses
- Opportunity to network with other practicing medical assistants

American Medical Technologists (AMT)

The AMT is another nonprofit certification agency and professional membership association representing allied health care individuals. It certifies medical assistants by awarding the RMA (AMT) national credential to those candidates successfully satisfying requirements. AMT has many local chapters, state societies, and a Uniform Services Committee. Each of these societies meets regularly and annually for a national convention.

AMT benefits and services include:

- Continuing education through the *Journal of Continuing Education Topics & Issues*, which is published three times a year
- AMT's Institute for Excellence (AMTIE), which monitors continuing education credits and sends a "report card" each year
- Four scholarships available to members who want to return to school and five scholarships for current students enrolled in allied health care programs
- State societies that offer opportunities for continuing education, activities, and networking
- Peer recognition through AMT's prestigious RMA (AMT) credential
- Personal discount programs

National Healthcareer Association (NHA)

The NHA serves as a reliable resource for up-to-date information on health career opportunities, training programs, education opportunities, and industry forecasts. The NHA newsletter *The NHA Today* is well respected and provides current trends, articles, and information regarding the health care field.

NHA benefits and services include:

- National certification
- Continuing education opportunities
- Collaboration with educational institutions in curriculum development and competency testing
- Annual Continuing Education Program
- Elite Membership Program that puts you in touch with a team of placement specialists to expand job opportunities

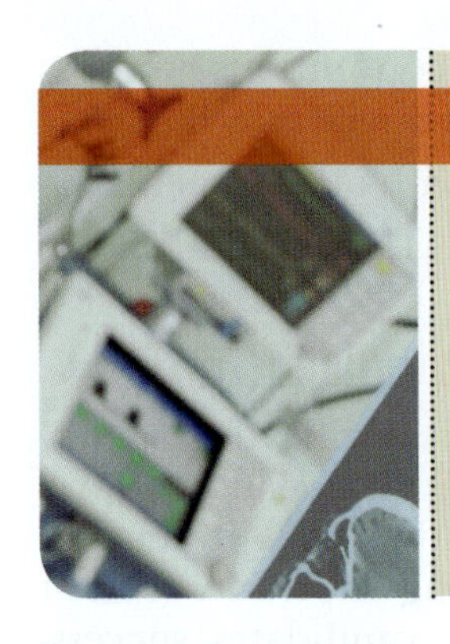

CASE STUDY 23-1

Refer to the scenario at the beginning of the chapter.

CASE STUDY REVIEW

1. Discuss the advantages of certification to the medical assistant.
2. Discuss the advantages of certification to the provider.
3. How does certification set a consistent minimum standard for evaluating professional competence as a medical assistant?

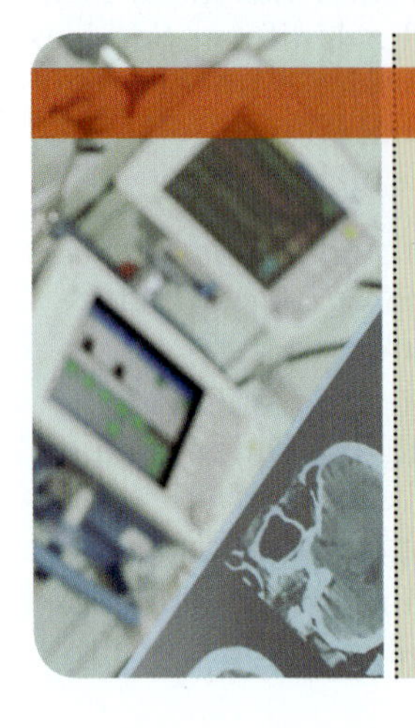

CASE STUDY 23-2

It is May, and Nancy McFarland, who graduated from an ABHES-accredited program 4.5 years ago, is beginning to research the procedures and requirements for taking the RMA (AMT) examination. Nancy completed her internship at Inner City Health Care and was hired to work there full time (35 hours per week) when she graduated.

CASE STUDY REVIEW

1. If Nancy wants to take the examination in January, what is the procedure for applying?
2. Nancy is setting up a study schedule. She plans to review course textbooks and tests, purchase a study guide, and set up a study group. Develop a simple study schedule.
3. What criteria should Nancy consider when asking people to join her study group?

Summary

- The purpose of certification is to establish a minimum standard for evaluating an individual's professional competence and acknowledges standard entry-level knowledge and skills as a medical assistant.
- Strategies for preparing for the certification examination include determining the date to sit for the examination, completing the application process, selecting study partner(s), establishing a meeting schedule and itinerary, and appointing a meeting facilitator.
- The objective of AAMA is to promote skills and professionalism, protect medical assistants' right to practice, and encourage consistent health care delivery through certification. CAAHEP establishes the standards for medical assisting programs, and is the issuing body of accreditation for AAMA. The Endowment is a nonprofit corporation that provides funds for scholarships and accreditation of medical assisting education programs through CAAHEP. MAERB operates under the authority of the Endowment and evaluates medical assisting programs and recommends programs for CAAHEP accreditation. It also reviews standards for medical assisting curricula; conducts accreditation workshops for educators; and provides educators with current information regarding accreditation laws, policies, and practices.
- Candidates sitting for CMA (AAMA) credentialing must pass a computer-based national test administered through Prometric testing centers. Sixty CEUs in specific categories are required every 5 years to maintain accreditation.
- Candidates sitting for the RMA (AMT) and the CMAS (AMT) credentials must pass a computer-based national test administered through Pearson Vue testing centers. Thirty points every 3 years are required to maintain certification.
- Candidates sitting for the CCMA (NHA) and the CMAA (NHA) credentials must pass an online test. Ten NHA-approved credits every 2 years are required to maintain certification.
- Professional organizations offer current news and health information; continuing education options; local, state and nation chapters; discount programs; and networking and employment opportunities.

Study for Success

To reinforce your knowledge and skills of information presented in this chapter:

- Review the *Key Terms* and *Learning Outcomes*
- Consider the *Critical Thinking* features and *Case Studies* and discuss your conclusions
- Answer the questions in the *Certification Review*

CERTIFICATION REVIEW

1. What should the goal and challenge of each graduating medical assistant be?
   a. Find employment
   b. Have a good benefit package
   c. Possess entry-level skills
   d. Earn the CMA/RMA credential and maintain it
2. Which statement is true of the certification examination?
   a. It is a comprehensive test based on tasks medical assistants perform daily.
   b. It contains all true/false questions.
   c. It is developed by the AMTIE.
   d. It is developed by the NBME.
   e. It is developed by CAAHEP.
3. Which of the following is *not* a benefit of membership in a professional organization such as AAMA or AMT?
   a. Answers to legal questions regarding job-related issues
   b. Legal advice regarding divorce
   c. Nationwide networking opportunities
   d. Professional journal publications
4. Which of the following is valid for recertification of the CMA (AAMA) credential?
   a. Submitting work experience
   b. Reexamination or CEU method
   c. Submitting on-the-job training
   d. Submitting military training
   e. Submitting practicum experience
5. To keep the RMA (AMT) credential current, an individual must complete which of the following?
   a. 10 credits every 2 years
   b. 30 points every 3 years
   c. 30 points every 5 years
   d. 60 points every 5 years
6. The RMA was established by which of the following organizations?
   a. ABHES
   b. CAAHEP
   c. AMT
   d. AAMA
   e. NHA
7. The NHA offers medical assisting certification for which of the following?
   a. CMA
   b. RMA
   c. CCMA and CMAA
   d. CMAS
8. Which answer is true of the RMA examinations?
   a. They are offered at Pearson Vue locations.
   b. They are offered twice a year.
   c. They are offered three times a year.
   d. They are offered six times a year.
   e. They are offered at Prometric locations.
9. Which credential may *only* graduates of CAAHEP- and ABHES-accredited medical assisting programs earn?
   a. CCMA (NHA)
   b. CMAS (AMT)
   c. CMA (AAMA)
   d. CMAA (NHA)
10. To retain certification, industry standards require that each NHA-certified health care professional complete which of the following?
    a. 10 credits every 2 years
    b. 30 points every 3 years
    c. 30 points every 5 years
    d. 10 credits every 5 years
    e. 10 credits every 3 years

CHAPTER 24

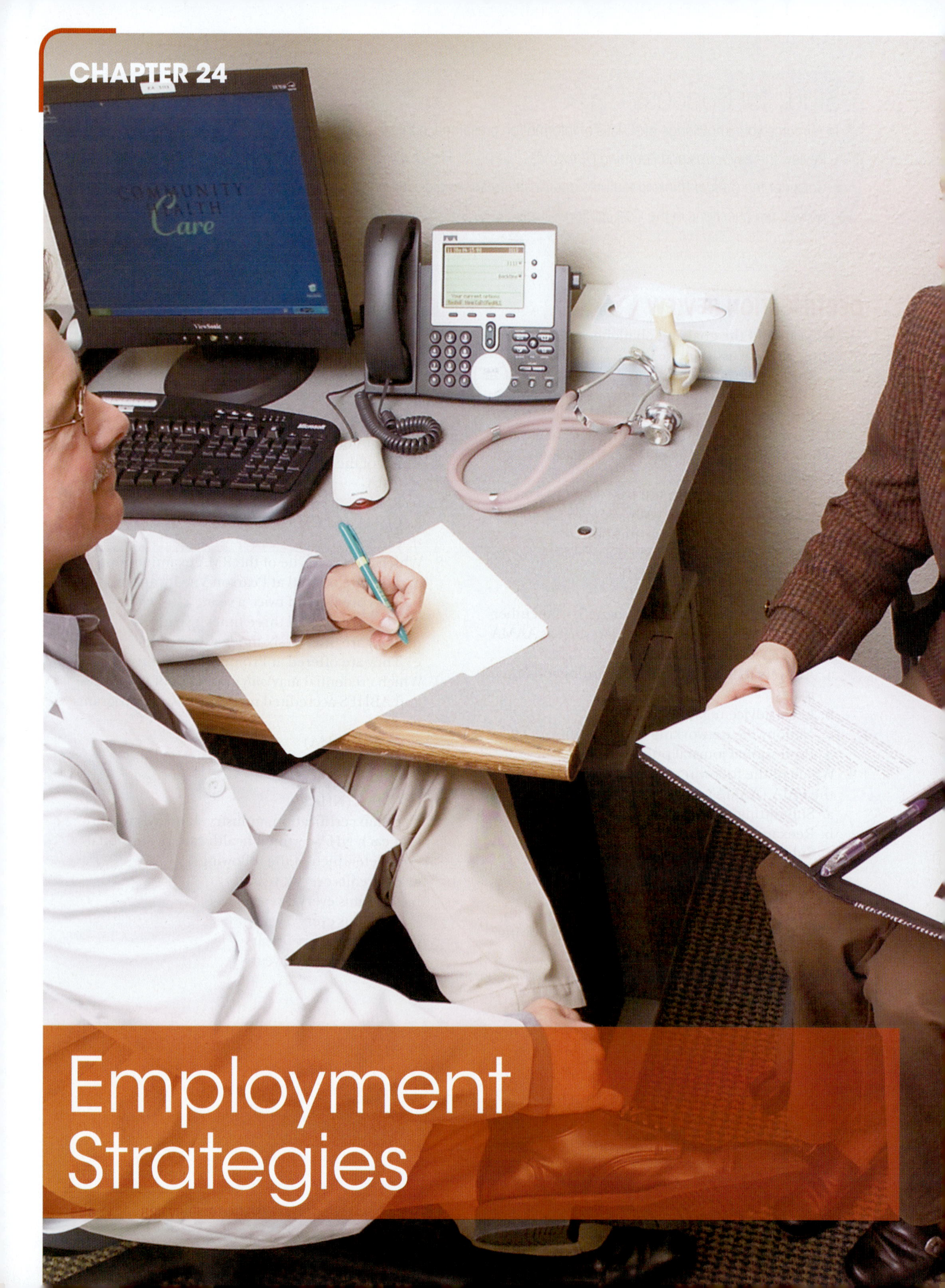

Employment Strategies

LEARNING OUTCOMES

1. Define and spell the key terms as presented in the glossary.
2. List the steps involved in job analysis and research.
3. Describe a contact tracker and its usefulness.
4. Formulate three examples of accomplishment statements.
5. Differentiate chronologic, functional, targeted, online profile, and e-résumé.
6. Identify the purpose and content of a cover letter.
7. Demonstrate effective ways to anticipate and respond to an interviewer's questions.
8. Describe appropriate overall appearance and dress for an interview.
9. Identify the benefits of writing a follow-up letter.

KEY TERMS

accomplishment statements
application/cover letter
application form
career objective
chronologic résumé
contact tracker
direct skills
e-résumé
functional résumé
headline
Internet blogs
interview
keywords
networking
profile
references
résumé
social media
targeted résumé
transferable skills

SCENARIO

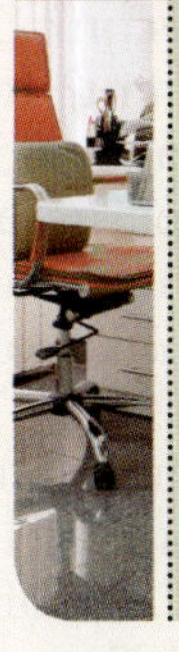

Eun Mee Soo, RMA (AMT), is a graduate of an accredited medical assisting program and recently passed the national certification examination. While attending school, Eun Mee was employed part-time as a sales representative in one of the city's prestigious clothing stores. She has no medical work experience except her practicum at Inner City Health Care. She is now preparing her résumé and beginning her job search. Eun Mee plans to move out of state (she always dreamed of moving north), so she will also be looking for a new apartment. All of these changes are a bit unsettling for Eun Mee. She is beginning to wonder if she should defer relocating at this time and stay close to home until she feels more secure.

Chapter Portal

The work-a-day world is very different from what you have experienced in school. In the work world, your success or failure will not be determined by passing tests at the completion of an instructional course. Success will be based upon your attitude and performance on a day-to-day basis, sometimes under difficult and stressful conditions. This chapter will focus on helping you plan a job search strategy and prepare a résumé that presents you as a qualified candidate for the job, and it will walk you through the steps to a successful interview.

DEVELOPING A STRATEGY

It is best to begin developing your job search strategy early in your training as a medical assistant. If you have not started this phase, determine to begin today by developing a strategy that is realistic, recognizing that you and a hundred other medical assistants may be applying for the same job. How are *you* different from every other person applying for this job? The following sections will help make *you* stand out, be different, and hopefully be successful in your job search.

Attitude and Mindset

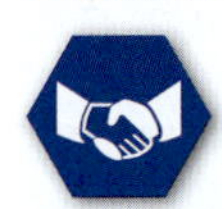

One important quality an employer looks for in employees is their attitude. Your attitude is not something you turn on and off or learn in school. It is the result of your innate personality combined with the events that mold you during your life. Your instructors and acquaintances have a significant impact over who you are. Your attitude is reflected by how you react to:

1. Taking direction
2. Seeking excellence or doing just enough to get by
3. Meeting your employer's needs, not just looking forward to payday
4. Assuming responsibility for your actions versus considering your problems to be someone else's fault

An employer will zero in on a negative attitude and eliminate you as a candidate almost immediately. While formal training is important and you can be retrained to do things the way a new employer desires, your attitude takes time to change and requires a willingness to make the change. Develop a strategy to cultivate a positive attitude while you are still in school. This is a time when you will have professional guidance and resources, as well as excellent role models to emulate.

Self-Assessment

Before starting to explore employment opportunities that are right for you, focus on yourself and build a picture of your strengths and weaknesses, what motivates you, how you relate to other people in the workplace, and how you cope with stress. The assessment should not be totally based on your own conclusions, but will require obtaining the opinions of your peers, instructors, and friends as well.

What are your strengths and weaknesses? Review your work or prior employment experience, academic studies, and outside interests as well as those things you have found difficult or challenging. Ask yourself—would I be willing to do that all day every working day? Could I obtain additional training to make myself more competent in a given task where I am weak?

What do I enjoy? Starting with the items you noted as strengths, rank them in order of how much you like doing them. Do a similar ranking of the items that are weaknesses. Make a separate list of the recreational activities you enjoy. From your list of strengths and weaknesses, build a job description for your ideal job. From your list of recreational activities, evaluate where you would like to live to continue those activities. Repeat this procedure to create a list of several jobs and locations you would enjoy.

Evaluate your working style. As part of the self-assessment, you should evaluate what direct and transferable skills you have that will make you a contributing member of the medical team. **Direct skills** are the medical skills and procedures you have acquired in school and developed proficiency in during the practicum experience. **Transferable skills** are those skills that would be useful in a wide variety of professions and may have been perfected during the education process or learned in employment settings. Leadership, communication, writing, computer literacy, keyboarding, linguistics, and spelling are some examples of transferable skills.

Think about what work environment you find most suited to your personality. Do you enjoy working with people or working alone? Are you a self-starter or do you require supervision? Do you perform well in a stressful environment? Identify what motivates you. What type of manger do you want to work for: authoritarian or participatory? When you interview, you need to interview your potential employer to determine the style of management you will encounter.

What is your salary requirement? The salary of a medical assistant varies with location, proficiency in skills, credentials, and experience. As of 2016, the national median salary is $30,135 per year, ranging from $20,021 to $41,900. As part of your preparation for seeking a position, assess your salary needs and the salary schedule in your location. You may be asked as part of the interview what salary you expect. You also need to consider the benefits offered by the employer. If your employer does not provide medical coverage, for example, this will be an expense you will need to take into consideration. Likewise, while retirement may be a long way off, an IRA plan is part of the salary compensation requiring consideration.

Research clinic profile. Is this a specialty clinic and would you enjoy working in this specialty? Evaluate what the clinic does and compare that with your moral and ethical standards. For example, if the clinic performed abortions or certain types of birth control procedures, would you be comfortable assisting?

Is there opportunity for advancement in the future? Consider where you want to be in your career in 5 or 10 years. Evaluate the opportunity for advancement at a particular clinic, or what the current and future job market looks like in a specific geographic location.

Initiative

Your employment strategy does not end with landing a position. Once hired, continue to prepare for the next step in your career. Be active in technical organizations and professional groups that help you develop future contacts. Most job opportunities are developed through **networking** or personal referrals. Prepare yourself for a more responsible position by broadening your skills. Interview for positions that advance your career even when you are currently satisfied. The key is to gain as much exposure as possible, as you may need it in the future.

THE JOB SEARCH

Many of your instructors may have contacts with prospective employers through practicum sites, and your school may have an employment office that posts employment opportunities. Take advantage of every opportunity to let people know you are looking for a job. Consider speaking with your primary care provider, your dentist, and other professionals such as your hair and nail specialists. You never know where a good lead will come from. Personal networking and **social media** will be critical to your job search.

Person-to-person networking is the linking together of individuals who, through trust and relationship-building that is genuine and authentic, advertise for one another. It should be a major part of your job search and should begin during your practicum experience. Let your practicum supervisor know your employment availability and ask if there are current or future job openings for which you might qualify. During the practicum experience, take full advantage of every opportunity to demonstrate your skills, to learn new skills, and to be a team member.

Networking also develops through student memberships and participation in AAMA, AMT, or other professional organizations. Student membership discounts are offered by these organizations and opportunities to participate in leadership roles, continuing education sessions, and observing professional behaviors are just a few of the benefits of membership. Professional organizations provide exposure through local, state, and national functions. (See Chapter 23 for additional information about professional organizations.)

Social media is currently used by more than 95% of employers seeking to fill positions with qualified applicants. Employers use social media to post positions and check the background and attitude of applicants. In today's technological setting, the first thing recruiters and employers will do is investigate you online. Be aware of any and all postings online, as they are there for the entire world to view.

LinkedIn is probably the number one site for professional networking and job search, used by over 94% of recruiters. Facebook, used by 65% of recruiters, is the largest social network and can be used to network with city, school, or workplace associates to make your position availability public knowledge. Twitter, used by 55% of recruiters, is another networking option. Participation in professional **Internet blogs** such as LinkedIn discussion groups is yet another social media avenue to explore during your job search. By establishing your own Web site, you can post your résumé, portfolio, and letters of recommendation. This platform can also be used to highlight specific skills such as critical thinking, communication, and professionalism. You will want to be sure that all information is accurate and well supported.

In order to effectively use social media, you will need to establish a professional profile and participate intelligently in group activities to establish a business-like online presence for yourself. Your online **profile** should demonstrate professional experience, tenure, and accomplished skills. It should include a summary that highlights the qualities and personal attributes that make you a good fit for the companies and organizations you are targeting. The summary can include real situations from your classroom experiences or related jobs and should include keyword-rich content. See the "Keyword Descriptors" Quick Reference Guide for a list of effective keywords that can be used in your professional profile.

QUICK REFERENCE GUIDE

KEYWORD DESCRIPTORS

Awards and Affiliations

- Accrediting Bureau of Health Education Schools (ABHES)
- American Association of Medical Assistants (AAMA)
- American Medical Technologists (AMT)
- Associate in Applied Science degree (AAS)
- Cardiopulmonary resuscitation (CPR)
- Certification examination
- Certified Clinical Medical Assistant CCMA ((NHA)
- Certified Medical Administrative Assistant CMAA (NHA)
- Certified Medical Administrative Specialist CMAS (AMT)
- Certified Medical Assistant CMA (AAMA)
- Commission on Accreditation of Allied Health Education Programs (CAAHEP)
- Continuing education units (CEUs)
- National Healthcareer Association (NHA)
- Registered Medical Assistant RMA (AMT)

Sample: After earning an associate in applied science (AAS) degree, sat for the certification examination and was awarded the Certified Clinical Medical Assistant (CCMA) credential from the National Healthcareer Association.

Direct Skills

Bilingual	First aid	Patient navigator/ advocate	Safety issues
Charting	Infection control	Patient preparation	Scheduling
Coding	Injections	Pharmacology	Surgical asepsis
Communication	Insurance	Processing specimens	Telephone techniques
Data entry	Interpersonal skills	Quality assurance	Valued
Diagnostic testing	Laboratory	Reception	Venipuncture
Documentation of care	Medical asepsis	Regulatory guidelines	Vital signs
EKGs	Medical terminology	Risk management	X-rays
Emergency management	Patient intake		

Sample: Utilized bilingual skills to aid diverse populations to feel valued and understood during medical encounters.

Power Verbs

Assembled	Communicated	Expedited	Increased
Assessed	Compiled	Evaluated	Integrated
Assigned	Computed	Exhibited	Interpreted
Attended	Contributed	Facilitated	Justified
Budgeted	Created	Formalized	Logged
Catalogued	Delegated	Generated	Maintained
Classified	Developed	Greeted	Measured
Charted	Documented	Headed	Modified
Coded	Established	Identified	Negotiated
Collected	Evaluated	Implemented	Observed

(continues)

- Operated
- Organized
- Participated
- Perfected
- Prepared
- Procured
- Proofread
- Recommended
- Reconciled
- Regulated
- Requested
- Responsible for
- Retrieved
- Revised
- Scheduled
- Selected
- Served as
- Solicited
- Streamlined
- Summarized
- Supervised
- Taught
- Telephoned
- Trained
- Transferred
- Verified

Sample: Streamlined procedure-scheduling through the use of computer technology, decreasing patient wait time from 6 to 2 days.

Transferrable Skills

- Analyzed
- Accommodated
- Bilingual skills
- Brainstormed
- Communication skills
- Conducted
- Demonstrated
- Displayed
- Enumerated
- Established
- Evaluated
- Facilitated
- Implemented
- Improvised
- Incorporated
- Instituted
- Inventoried
- Maximized
- Mobilized
- People skills
- Processed
- Quantified
- Realized
- Rejuvenated
- Specified
- Solicited
- Summarized
- Time management skills
- Validated
- Verified
- Welcomed

Sample: Implemented time management skills learned while working as a server in my last position.

As part of a serious job search, you should contact many individuals and will need some means of recording the contacts, their responses, and your actions. Figure 24-1 shows a helpful sample **contact tracker**. It should be used to prevent confusion and to keep track of valuable information and action

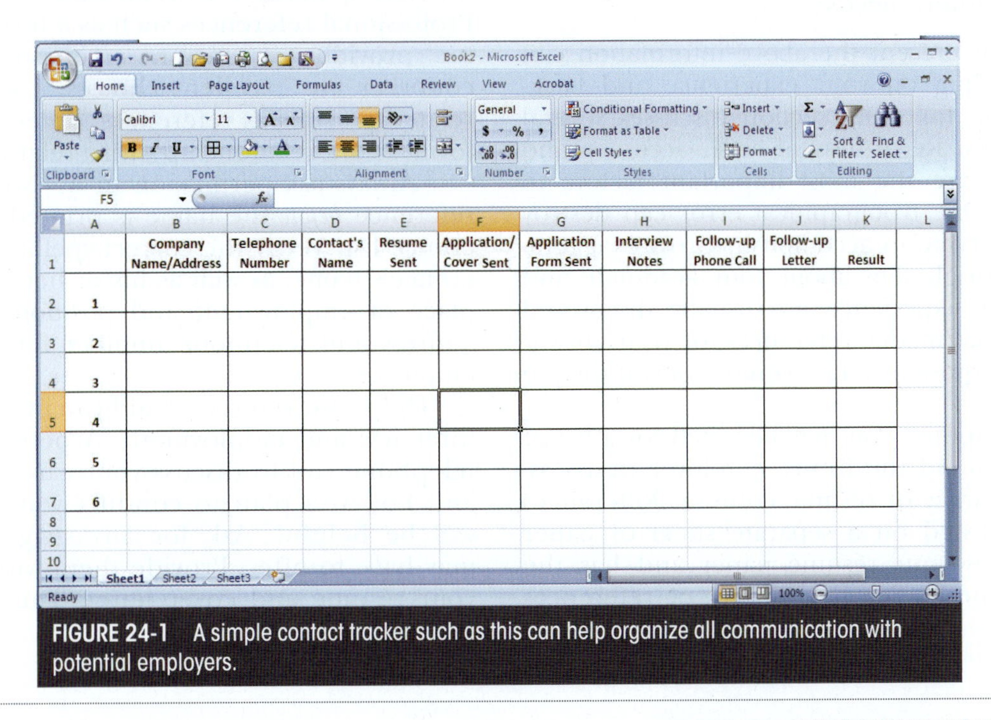

FIGURE 24-1 A simple contact tracker such as this can help organize all communication with potential employers.

items. Copy or design your own contact tracker form and document all pertinent information regarding your job search contacts.

RÉSUMÉ PREPARATION OR ONLINE PROFILE

A **résumé** is a brief presentation of your qualifications and experience in your chosen career. You need to capture in words the most important qualities and characteristics to communicate a clear vision both online and offline of who you are. Your message should be tailored to your target audience. Try to answer the following questions:

- What is your vision for the job that you are seeking?
- What are your guiding principles? (Being all you can be, decisive, driven, enjoy challenges, team-worker, etc.)
- What are your short and long-range goals?
- What are your job-specific attributes? (Use keyword-rich content.)
- What are your core technical strengths and accomplishments?
- Who is your target audience and what they are looking for in a candidate?
- What will differentiate you from your competition?
- Did you emphasize your value to the organization and position yourself as a good fit to meet the employers' needs?

How you present the above information can vary depending on your experience and background. The following section discusses several résumé styles. Regardless of style, accuracy and truthfulness are the most important factors to remember. One typographical error can destroy all you are trying to accomplish. Gross exaggerations or outright lies about your academic and employment experience are usually discovered through social media, references, or your answer to interview questions. Lies could cost you the job (see Table 24-1).

At some point, you may be asked for a list of **references** to aid the future employer in assessing the accuracy of résumé content. References should be listed on a separate sheet of paper that matches your résumé paper and has the same letterhead. Select a variety of references to be included with your résumé. An individual who knows you well or has worked with you long enough to make an honest assessment and recommendation regarding your employment history and qualifications is an excellent reference. Professional references such as a former instructor, provider, practicum supervisor, or fellow coworker are excellent choices. Use only nonrelated persons as references, unless you have a formal work relationship with a relative.

TABLE 24-1

TOP 10 LIES ON RÉSUMÉS

TOP 10 SERIOUS LIES ON RÉSUMÉS	TOP 10 WHITE LIES ON RÉSUMÉS
School awarding degree	Communication skills
Foreign language fluency	Job duties in former positions
Degree received	Presentation skills
College major	Research skills
GPA	References
Work history	Computer skills
Recognition	Salary
Portfolio of projects	Graduation year
Position held (job title)	Professional memberships
College minor	Career growth

Source: http://fortune.com/2014/09/10/resume-lies-are-on-the-rise/

Always ask permission to use someone as a reference *before* the name is printed on the reference list. Verify the correct spelling of the reference's name, as well as his or her correct title, place of employment and position, and email address and telephone number for prospective employers.

Help your references aid you in obtaining an interview and employment. A personal visit or telephone call to discuss your career objectives and how you plan to conduct your job search will be helpful. Ask for any suggestions they may have to offer. Provide them with a copy of your résumé and cover letter. This helps your references visualize the position for which you are applying and picture how you may benefit that employer.

Keep in touch with references. Check back to see what prospective employers have called and types of questions asked. Add information or notes to your contact tracker. Knowing what questions employers ask of your references may produce some valuable pointers for your next letter, résumé, or interview. Finally, thank your references. They will appreciate knowing how you are doing and that you value their assistance.

Résumé Styles

Various résumé styles have been developed, each having specific advantages and disadvantages. Choose the style or combination of styles that best describes your strengths and ability to do the job. It may be advantageous to check with the human resource department of the facility to which you are applying to determine if they have a résumé style preference. Many facilities accept only online résumés and have specific guidelines to be followed. The objective of an online résumé or online profile is different from a paper résumé. The online résumé is not tailored to a specific job, but is designed to tell who you are and to sell your personality and general qualifications. The paper résumé is designed to sell what you can do for a potential employer. If you obtain an interview from an online résumé or profile, you should also have a job-specific paper résumé and reference list available to leave with the interviewer if requested. See Procedure 24-1 for steps to prepare a résumé.

Chronologic Résumé. Your **chronologic résumé** should be organized so that the most important information you want to share is the first thing the reader sees. If your job experience is your greatest asset and may set you apart from other applicants, put your work history and job skills first. If your education and training is your best professional feature, put your education and training first. Some medical managers and human resources directors take only 10 seconds to scan a résumé. You want them to see clearly and quickly what you have to offer.

The chronologic résumé is advantageous when:

- The position is in a highly traditional field, such as teaching, law, or health care, where specific employers are of paramount interest
- You are staying in the same field as prior jobs
- Job history shows real growth and development
- Prior titles are impressive

The chronologic résumé is *not* advantageous when:

- Your work history is spotty
- You are changing career goals
- You have been in the same job for many years
- You are looking for your first job

Figure 24-2 illustrates a chronologic résumé.

Functional Résumé. The **functional résumé** highlights specialty areas of accomplishment and strengths. It allows you to organize them in an order that supports your work objective.

The functional résumé is advantageous when:

- Your experience can be sorted into areas of function, for example, administrative, clinical, supervisory
- You are changing careers
- You are reentering the job market after an absence
- Your career path or growth is not clear from a chronologic listing
- You have had a variety of different, apparently unconnected, work experiences
- Much of your work has been volunteer, freelance, or temporary
- You want to eliminate repetition of descriptions of job duties
- You have extensive specialized experience

The functional résumé is *not* advantageous when:

- You want to emphasize a management growth pattern
- Your most recent employers are highly prestigious and the specific employers are of paramount interest

A sample of a functional résumé for a person reentering the job market is shown in Figure 24-3.

Targeted Résumé. The **targeted résumé** is best for focusing on a clear, specific job target. It should contain a **career objective** and list your skills, capabilities, and any supporting accomplishments related

ASHLEY JACKSON, CMA (AAMA)
2031 Craig Street ~ Renton, Washington 98055
Work: 206-878-1545 Cell: 206-835-9879
Home: 253-838-6690 email: asjack@pinetree.com

WORK EXPERIENCE

September, 20XX–Present GROUP HEALTH COOPERATIVE
Directed support for a dermatology/surgery practice.
Patient preparation.
Medical and surgical asepsis.
Assist with sterile procedures.
Patient follow-up.

June, 20XX–August, 20XX VALLEY INTERNAL MEDICINE
Clinical responsibilities.
Assisted with surgeries in ambulatory care setting.
Patient preparation.
Medical and surgical asepsis.
Assisted with sterile procedures.

March, 20XX–June, 20XX VALLEY INTERNAL MEDICINE
Medical Assistant Practicum
Administrative duties and clinical responsibilities utilizing all medical assisting skills, including patient induction, chief complaint, vital signs, patient preparation, EKGs, medical and surgical asepsis, and sterile procedures.

EDUCATION/CERTIFICATION

Associate in Applied Science degree, June, 20XX, Highline Community College, Des Moines, Washington 98198-9800.

Certified Medical Assistant (AAMA), June, 20XX.

FIGURE 24-2 Sample chronologic résumé.

to that objective. **Accomplishment statements** begin with power verbs and give a brief description of what you did and the demonstrable results that were produced. The targeted résumé style enables graduating students to list classes related to their career objective, grade point average, student awards, and achievements. This information adds substance to a résumé when work experience is minimal and should be at the beginning of the résumé because it is your most significant asset.

The targeted résumé is advantageous when:

- You are very clear about your job target
- You have had a variety of experiences that appear unrelated to each other but that include skills that you can use in a skills list related to your job target
- You can go in several directions and want a different résumé for each
- You are just starting your career and have little experience but know what you want, and are clear about your capabilities

The targeted résumé is *not* advantageous when:

- You want to use one résumé for several different applications
- You are not clear about your abilities and accomplishments

JOAN BISHOP, RMA (AMT)
4320 Sprig Street
Renton, Washington 98055

Work: 206-878-1545 Cell: 206-835-9879
Home: 253-838-6690 email: jbishop@abc.net

TEACHING:

Instructed community groups on issues related to child abuse.

Taught volunteers how to set up community program for victims of domestic violence.

Conducted workshops for parents of abused children.

Instructed public school teachers on signs and symptoms of potential and actual child abuse.

COUNSELING:

Consulted with parents for probable child abuse and suggested courses of action.

Worked with social workers on individual cases, in both urban and suburban settings.

Counseled single parents on appropriate coping behaviors.

Handled pre-take interviewing of many individual abused children.

ORGANIZATION/COORDINATION:

Coordinated transition of children between original home and foster home.

Served as liaison between community health agencies and schools.

Wrote proposal to state for county funds to educate single parents and teachers.

WORK HISTORY:

20XX–20XX Community Mental Health Center, Tacoma, Washington
Volunteer Coordinator—Child Abuse Program

20XX–20XX C.A.R.E.—Child-Abuse Rescue-Education, Trenton, New Jersey
County Representative

EDUCATION:

20XX B.S. Sociology, Douglass College, New Brunswick, New Jersey

FIGURE 24-3 Sample functional résumé. This style is useful for a person reentering the job market.

Figures 24-4A and 24-4B show samples of targeted résumés.

Online Profile. An online profile may have to follow specified rules. For example, a LinkedIn profile should employ the following tips to appear more professional:

- Establish a custom LinkedIn URL.
- Use a clear, friendly, and appropriate professional action photo of yourself. Written permission will be required if a patient is included in your action photo such as the photo used in the example.
- Make your **headline** promote your skills like a news headline. As an example, "Medical Assistant" is common and does not separate you from the other job seekers. A more exciting and enticing headline might be "Patient Friendly and Proactive Paraprofessional."

ASHLEY JACKSON, CMA (AAMA)
2031 Craig Street ~ Renton, Washington 98055

Work: 206-878-1545 Cell: 206-835-9879
Home: 253-838-6690 email: asjack@pinetree.com

CAREER OBJECTIVES: To obtain a position as a medical assistant in an ambulatory care/surgery facility that allows use and development of clinical skills.

ACHIEVEMENTS:

Certified Medical Assistant.
Graduate of an accredited medical assistant program accredited by the Commission on Accreditation of Allied Health Education Programs (CAAHEP).
Experienced in providing assistance with surgeries in an ambulatory care setting.
Excellent communication and interpersonal skills.

SKILLS AND CAPABILITIES:

Post-surgery patient follow-up.
Patient induction.
Vital signs.
Patient preparation.
EKGs.
Medical and surgical asepsis.
Sterile procedures.

WORK HISTORY:

September, 20XX to present	Group Health Cooperative, Seattle, WA Surgical Medical Assistant.
June, 20XX–August, 20XX	Valley Internal Medicine, Renton, WA Clinical Medical Assistant.
March 20XX–June, 20XX	Valley Internal Medicine, Renton, WA Practicum Student/Trainee.

EDUCATION/CERTIFICATION:

Associate in Applied Science Degree, Highline Community College.
Certified Medical Assistant (AAMA).

AFFILIATIONS:

American Association of Medical Assistants.

FIGURE 24-4A Sample targeted résumé. This style is useful when focusing on a specific job target.

- Use action words in your target job description to show your passion for the job you are seeking.
- Your work summary should be around three to five short paragraphs, preferably with a bulleted section in the middle. It should walk the reader through your work passions, key skills, and unique qualifications. It should also list the various facilities you have had exposure to over the years. Highlight past results in your summary.
- Avoid buzzword such as *experienced* (say in what), *team player* (more specific language would be *led a team to develop office protocols*), *references available on request* (it is obvious they are). Be specific and personable.
- Highlight your achievements

Ashley Jackson, CMA (AAMA)
1321 Craig Street
Renton, Washington 98055
(253) 838-6690
Cell (206) 835-9879
Asjackson@pinetree.com

Professional Profile

Eager to utilize my medical assisting knowledge and skills in an ambulatory/surgery facility that allows further development of clinical skills.

- Dedicated to meeting the needs of individual patients at their level of need.
- Committed team member approach to care delivered to patients.

What People Say:

"Ashley's positive attitude is a strong asset as it helps guide her actions, thoughts, and words. Ashley uses her strong knowledge base to make critical thinking choices."
Stephanie Young, CMA (AAMA)
Group Health Cooperative

"Ashley builds strong relationships with her co-workers, supervisors, providers, and patients. She shows interest in their lives and models respect, kindness, and empathy. She truly cares about people."
Martha Marshall, RN
Valley Internal Medicine

"Ashley's clinical critical thinking skills are excellent. She is competent and works well with others to see that quality care is provided to each patient in an efficient and timely manner."
Donald Blackburn, PA
Valley Internal Medicine

Education, Honors, and Certification

Associate in Applied Science
Highline Community College, Des Moines, Washington
Overall GPA: 3.9
Dean's List
Current Red Cross First Aid and CPR cards
Certified Medical Assistant (AAMA)
President SeaTac Chapter of AAMA

Work Experience

Group Health Cooperative Seattle, Washington
September, 20XX to present

- Post-surgery patient follow-up
- Patient induction
- Vital signs
- Patient preparation
- EKGs
- Medical and surgical asepsis
- Sterile procedures

Valley Internal Medical, Renton, Washington
June, 20XX to August, 2011

- EKGs
- Patient preparation
- Medical and surgical asepsis
- Surgical procedures

FIGURE 24-4B Sample of a more creative targeted résumé.

- Do not leave the current job entry blank. Put something like *Full-Time Student/Medical Assistant* in the current job block, and in the company block use something like *In Transition* or *Seeking Opportunity*. Many search engines will skip you if you leave a blank.
- Use the additional profiles section to showcase outside activities that are appropriate.
- Request LinkedIn recommendations from people who have complimented you on your work. As appropriate, have them highlight your skills. (See Figure 24-5.)

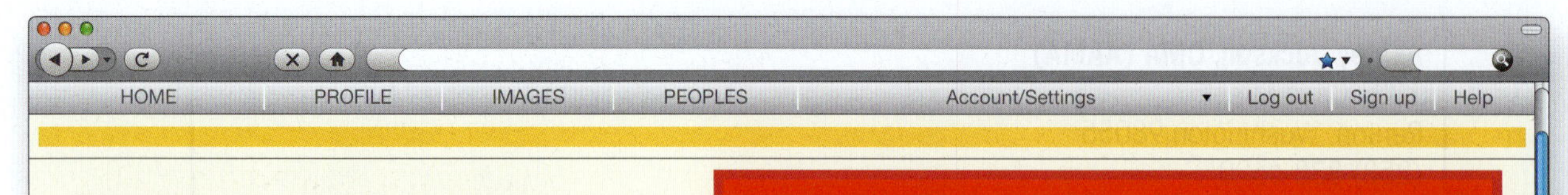

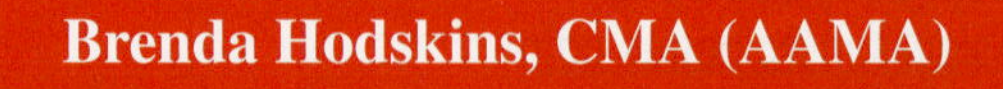

Making the Medical Office Encounter a Pleasant Experience

Brenda Hodskins, CMA (AAMA)

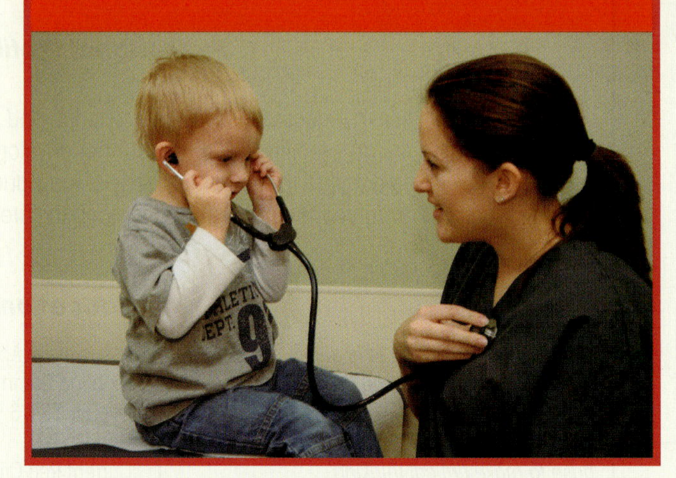

Current:

Full Time MA Student/In Transition, Practicum Experience at Pediatrics NorthWest

Education:

Highline College, AAS degree awarded

Summary:

I am a very outgoing person who enjoys working with children of all ages. My career goal is to create an environment that supports the medical team while helping the patient feel more comfortable and less stressed.

I enjoy working in both Administrative and Clinical Areas. I am proficient in the following skills:

- Reception
- Scheduling
- Therapeutic communication
- Coding and billing
- Patient induction
- Vital signs
- Setting up a sterile field
- Assisting with surgical procedures
- Injections
- Venipuncture

Additional Profiles:

I have been actively working in our local community homeless shelter preparing and serving meals on Saturday evenings, and counseling clients on health care needs and availability of resources.

FIGURE 24-5 Sample online profile.

E-Résumé. An electronic résumé, also known as an **e-résumé**, is electronically delivered via email, submitted to Internet job boards, or placed on Web pages. When employers post jobs on their own Web sites, they generally expect job seekers to respond electronically.

Special care must be taken when preparing the e-résumé, as many employers place résumés directly into searchable databases. The following points should be considered:

- Formatting must be removed before the résumé can be placed in a database. Submitting a formatted résumé may cause it to be eliminated.
- Submit a text résumé, also known as a text-based résumé, plain-text résumé, or ASCII

text résumé. These variations are preferred when submitting résumés electronically.

- The e-résumé is not visually appealing. Eye appeal is not required because its main purpose is to be placed into a keyword-searchable database.
- The text résumé is not vulnerable to viruses and is compatible across computer programs and platforms.
- The text résumé is versatile and can be used for:
  - Posting on job boards
  - Pasting piece-by-piece into the profile forms of job boards, such as Monster.com
  - Pasting into the body of an email to be sent to prospective employers
  - Converting to a Web-based HTML résumé
  - Sending as an attachment to prospective employers
  - Converting to a scannable résumé

Employers are often inundated with résumés from job seekers each time they advertise a position opening. Therefore, in an effort to save time and to determine the best-qualified candidates for the position, employers digitize the résumés to create an electronic résumé. Using software to search for specific **keywords** that relate to the position, the number of candidates can quickly be narrowed. If you apply for a job with a company that searches databases for keywords and your résumé does not conform, you may not be considered for the position.

How do you determine keywords? Begin scrutinizing employment ads and list keywords repeatedly mentioned in association with jobs that interest you. Nouns that relate to the skills and experience the employer is looking for will quickly surface. Keywords may include job-specific skills/profession-specific words, technologic terms and descriptions of technical expertise, job titles, certifications, types of degrees, awards received, and professional organization memberships.

Keywords should be used throughout the résumé, but they should be front loaded. Front loaded means to use as many keyword descriptors as possible in the first 100 words of the résumé. A good goal is to aim for 25 to 35 keyword descriptors. This may be achieved by using synonyms, various forms of the keyword, and both the spelled-out and acronym versions of common terms. If a person reviews the résumé, he or she will see enough keywords to process it through the software search. (Refer back to the "Keyword Descriptors" Quick Reference Guide for suggested keywords.)

PROCEDURE 24-1

Preparing a Résumé

PURPOSE:

To prepare a résumé that presents you as a uniquely qualified candidate for a specific employment opportunity. The résumé should document your education, experience, and skills for the position to which you are applying.

EQUIPMENT /SUPPLIES:

- Computer and printer
- High-quality paper and matching envelope
- Dictionary and thesaurus
- Names, titles, addresses, telephone numbers, and email addresses of educational institutions and past employers

PROCEDURAL STEPS:

1. Check with the human resource department of a prospective employer to see if they have a résumé style preference. Many accept only online resumes.

(continues)

2. Select the résumé style, or combination of styles, that best showcases your experience and skills to a prospective employer. RATIONALE: Demonstrates your professionalism and competence level.
3. Create a letterhead that includes your legal name, address, telephone number, cell number, work telephone number, email address, and social media contact information (e.g., LinkedIn). RATIONALE: Provides all of the pertinent information a prospective employer needs to contact you.
4. Itemize your educational experience beginning with the most recent or present date, following the format for the résumé style selected.
5. List all significant employment experience beginning with the most recent or present date following the format for the résumé style selected.
6. Include other relevant information such as certifications; first aid, CPR, AIDS, or AED training; achievements; GPA and awards; memberships in professional organizations such as AAMA, AMT, NHA; community service; and volunteer programs. RATIONALE: Steps 4 through 6 provide an overall picture of the competence, skills, and professionalism you have to offer to your future employer. Be sure to front load your résumé with as many keyword descriptors as possible. Mention all direct and transferrable skills and use accomplishment statements in your narrative. This provides a clear picture of what you have to offer an employer and demonstrates your professionalism and communication skills.
7. Proofread carefully for any errors or omissions. Be sure the information is accurate and truthful. RATIONALE: Check to be sure that the grammar, spelling, punctuation, and capitalization are correct. Review the résumé carefully to ensure you have been honest and not misled an employer. Proofread several times and ask a trustworthy person that knows you well to read your résumé for accuracy and correctness in all respects.
8. Print résumé on good quality paper, at least 20- to 24-pound stock with a watermark. Choose a shade of white, cream, or gray bond paper. RATIONALE: To distinguish yourself from other candidates and to present a professional image.
9. Convert your résumé into PDF format to ensure formatting remains consistent with the printed version of your résumé.
10. Update your contact tracker. RATIONALE: To maintain current status on any and all employment opportunities.

APPLICATION/COVER LETTERS

The **application/cover letter** is a means of introducing yourself and submitting your résumé to a potential employer in response to an unsolicited application or job posting, with the goal of obtaining an interview. A well-written cover letter highlights your qualifications and experience for employment and enhances the information contained within your résumé. It should reflect how your skills satisfy the employer's needs. The letter should follow a standard business style and should not be more than one page in length. (Review Chapter 14.) It should be printed on the same type of paper as the résumé.

Because this may be your first contact with a potential employer, the letter should sell you and describe your intentions regarding employment, display your personality, and create interest in reading your enclosed résumé.

Some guidelines to follow in writing the application/cover letter include:

1. Address your letter to a specific individual whenever possible. You may need to make a telephone call to obtain the name, title, and correct spelling.
2. Keep the letter concise, use correct grammar and spelling, and follow standard business letter format (formality is key).
3. The first paragraph should state your reason for writing and focus the reader's attention. It should not give as a reason "in response to a help wanted ad" or "referral from a network contact."
4. The second paragraph should identify how your education, experience, and qualifications relate to the job and refer to the enclosed résumé.

5. The last paragraph should close with a request for an interview.
6. Have someone with management experience review your cover letter. This could be your practicum supervisor, an instructor, a friend, or an acquaintance who is in a supervisory position.
7. Do not reproduce cover letters. An original letter should be sent to each individual.
8. The cover letter should be placed on top of the résumé and mailed in a business-size envelope that matches its contents or in an 8½-by-11 manila envelope containing your return address.
9. Do not staple the cover letter to the résumé.

A sample of an application/cover letter is shown in Figure 24-6A.

An alternate example of an application/cover letter using Information Mapping® to highlight and draw attention to specific information in your letter is shown in Figure 24-6B. This format is considered easier to read because the focus is on specific blocks of information. In addition, its uniqueness draws attention to your letter and may result in your being selected when competition is keen.

2031 Craig Street
Renton, Washington 98055
August 22, 20XX

Sarah Molles, Manager
Seattle Group Health Cooperative
304 Fourth Avenue
Seattle, Washington 98124-1716

Dear Ms. Molles:

I am interested in the medical assistant position to assist in a dermatology surgery practice. I meet the qualifications and would like to be considered for the position.

I am currently a certified clinical medical assistant certified through the National Healthcareer Association (NHA). I have experience as a clinical assistant in an internal medicine clinic and have excellent communication and interpersonal skills.

I will be available for an interview Tuesday and Thursday afternoons from 1:00 p.m. to 4:00 p.m. I will call you next Thursday to set up an appointment for an interview.

Yours truly,

Porscha Dolan, CCMA (NHA)

Enclosure, Résumé

FIGURE 24-6A Sample application/cover letter.

2031 Craig Street
Renton, Washington 98055
August 22, 20XX

Sarah Molles, Manager
Seattle Group Health Cooperative
304 Fourth Avenue
Seattle, Washington 98124-1716

SUBJECT: SURGICAL MEDICAL ASSISTANT POSITION

Background	I am interested in the medical assistant position to assist in a dermatology surgery practice. I meet the qualifications and would like to be considered for the position.
Qualifications	I am currently a certified medical assistant graduated from a 2-year program accredited by the Commission on Accreditation of Allied Health Education Programs (CAAHEP). I have experience as a clinical assistant in an internal medicine clinic and have excellent communication and interpersonal skills.
Requested Action	I will be available for an interview Tuesday and Thursday afternoons from 1:00 p.m. to 4:00 p.m. I will call you next Thursday to set up an appointment for an interview.

Yours truly,

Ashley Jackson, CMA (AAMA)

Enclosure, Résumé

FIGURE 24-6B Sample information mapped application/cover letter.

COMPLETING THE APPLICATION FORM

Sooner or later during the job search you will be asked to complete an **application form**. In most cases this will be an online activity. How well you complete this task may be a key factor in obtaining an interview and that first job.

Reading through the application form questions, you may be tempted to write "See résumé" rather than repeat pertinent information already contained within your résumé. Do not fall into this pitfall. Answer every item completely. The application is organized in the manner that suits the clinic, whereas individual résumés are organized in a variety of ways. Finding specific information on a résumé is more time consuming for the clinic, whereas finding the same information on the job application is easy and quick because they know where to look for it. Read all the directions carefully. Look for seemingly insignificant directions placed at the top or bottom of the page that state "Print Carefully," "Complete in Your Own Hand-writing," or "Please Type." Employers may use this to assess your ability to read and follow directions and pay attention to detail.

If the application is to be handwritten, use black ink to complete the form. Black ink is considered legal, often is an indelible (permanent) ink, and is more legible if the form must be duplicated. Concentrate when completing the form and be sure to print clearly and make no errors. When possible, copy the application before beginning in case an error is made.

The current trend is toward online application forms. These forms are prepared by keying information into the appropriate spaces or blocks by using a computer. The completed forms are printed and mailed to the prospective employer or sent electronically. Sending electronically is increasingly the preferred method. All of the concerns relative to care in following instructions, providing complete and accurate information, and proofreading the application for any errors before sending are applicable.

If you are asked to list experience but the application does not specify "paid experience," be sure to list any volunteer or practicum experience that relates to the position you are seeking. Volunteer work can be important as an indicator of your willingness to work, your ability to serve the public, and your organizational skills.

You may be asked to complete the application form "on the spot." Plan ahead for this event and carry a completed copy of your résumé, reference list, and application/cover letter with you. These documents should provide all the information needed to complete the application form and may be submitted with the application form. This demonstrates to the potential employer your seriousness and preparedness for finding a job. Also carry with you information not included in your résumé, such as which years you attended high school and your salary history. A pocket spelling wordbook or dictionary may be a useful tool to carry for those who find spelling challenging.

THE INTERVIEW PROCESS

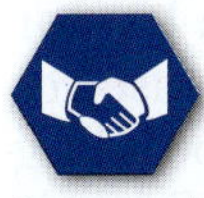
Professional

If your application/cover letter, résumé, and application form have made a favorable impression with the organization, you may be invited for an interview. An **interview** is a meeting in which you and the interviewer discuss the employment opportunities within that particular organization. It is the interviewer's responsibility to determine if you are the right fit to be a part of the team. The interviewer uses the interview process to assess appearance, attitude, and dependability. The interviewer also tries to verify that you have been honest in the skills you claim to have mastered. You, on the other hand, are selling your qualifications and assessing if this is an organization in which you want to be employed.

Being well prepared for the interview will increase your self-confidence and ability to focus during the actual interview. Knowing that your application/cover letter, résumé, and references all support your career goal and objectives allows you time to concentrate on interview preparation and presentation.

The Look of Success

The look of success begins with the outward appearance. First impressions are lasting, so strive for a favorable, professional look from head to toe. Appropriate conservative attire is important. Remember, your goal is to sell your professional abilities.

Hair should be clean and healthy looking, and worn in an appropriate style for the ambulatory care setting. Long hair should be worn off the collar in perhaps a French braid or twist. Strive for a neat, professional style.

The skin should have a healthy glow. Consultation with a cosmetician may prove helpful in solving skin problems or may provide an opportunity for trying new products. A basic understanding of your personal skin type and selection of cosmetics that complement your skin tone aid in the presentation of a professional appearance. The natural look is most appropriate for the medical clinic.

A daily shower and use of personal hygiene products is advised. Remember to use caution where perfumes and scents are concerned because many magnify when the body is under stress and the scent may be offensive or cause allergic reactions in others. Smokers should be aware that smoke odor carries in their hair, skin, and clothing. This odor may not be acceptable in health care settings.

Fingernails should be short and oval shaped or have rounded corners. Only clear nail polish should be worn in the ambulatory care setting if you are not working in the clinical area. Nail polish that is chipped or cracked must be removed or replaced immediately because it creates crevices in which pathogens may hide, multiply, and spread.

First impressions are lasting, so make yours professional in all respects. Smart casual attire is appropriate for both men and women. This consists of a skirt and blouse or a tailored pantsuit for women and slacks and dress shirt with or without a tie for men. Pay attention to details such as your accessories and shoe selection. Accessories should be small and tasteful. Shoes should be clean, polished, and in good repair. They should fit properly and be comfortable and easy to walk in (Figure 24-7). Women may carry a small purse if necessary. Be sure that your cell phone is turned off before entering the clinic.

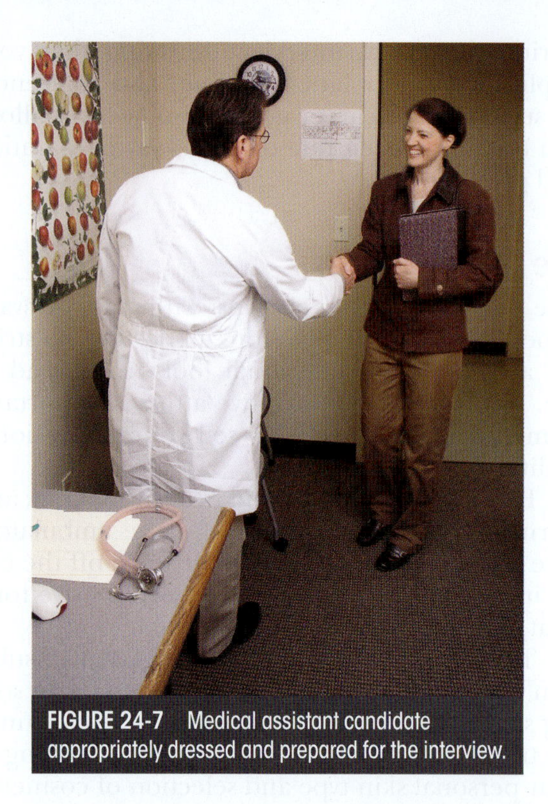

FIGURE 24-7 Medical assistant candidate appropriately dressed and prepared for the interview.

When you feel well and know that you look good, you project a confident and professional appearance. In other words, you are professionally poised. *Webster's Dictionary* defines *poise* as balance and stability; ease and dignity of manner. Personal poise combines all of the previously mentioned body appearances plus smoothness of movement and physical flexibility.

Preparing for the Interview

Before the interview takes place, carefully research the organization offering the position. Study the organization's mission statement, financial reports, future projections, and any other information available. Be prepared to relate your skills and interests to the needs of this organization. In other words, what can you contribute and why should they hire you? The interview is your opportunity to sell yourself and identify ways in which you can benefit the employer.

A portfolio is recommended in which to keep an extra copy of your résumé, reference list, application, and cover letter. An interviewer may ask for these documents especially if you have applied online. You should also have copies of letters of recommendation, a copy of your transcript from the schools you attended, and copies of any certificates such as AIDS training, first aid, CPR, and AED training. These items should not be presented unless dictated by events that take place during the interview. You might also have with you the name of the interviewer and a copy of any questions you plan to ask the interviewer. A last-minute review will refocus your thoughts before you go into the interview. Keep your list available for quick reference in the event your mind goes blank when you are asked if you have questions.

To arrive 5 to 10 minutes early, check a map for directions or make a trip the day before your interview. Try to travel about the same time as you would for the interview so you have an idea of the time it takes, traffic flow, construction areas encountered, and parking availability. Plan for inclement weather (raincoat, umbrella, shoes). It is a good idea to make a quick trip to the restroom on arrival to change shoes or recheck your appearance.

Introduce yourself confidently to the administrative medical assistant and identify by name the person you wish to see and the time of your appointment. Always arrive alone. The employer wants to see you and sense your self-reliance and responsibility. While you wait, try to relax and observe the clinic setting, other employees, what they are wearing, and their manner of conducting business. This may be helpful to you during the interview and in making a decision to work there.

The following Quick Reference Guide lists reasons employers do not hire applicants.

The Actual Interview

When you enter an interviewer's office, think of yourself as a guest and take your cues from him or her. Most interviewers will introduce themselves and extend a hand. A firm handshake, responding by introducing yourself, and smiling confidently convey a positive professional image. Remain standing until you are invited to be seated. Keep

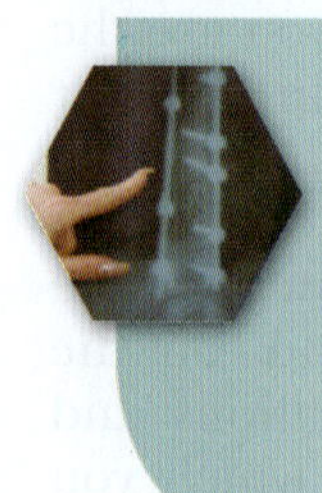

Critical Thinking

If you are a smoker, how can you minimize the smoke odor carried on your person before you go on a job interview? Make a list and prioritize each suggestion into a plan of action.

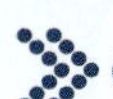 **QUICK REFERENCE GUIDE**

Reasons for Employers Not Hiring

Employers in business were asked to list reasons for not hiring a job seeker. Given in rank order (from most unwanted to least unwanted), the 15 biggest gripes are as follows:

1. Poor appearance (not dressed properly, poorly groomed)
2. Acting like a know-it-all
3. Cannot express self clearly; poor voice, diction, grammar
4. Lack of planning for work—no purpose or goals
5. Lack of confidence or poise
6. No interest in or enthusiasm for the job
7. Not active in school extracurricular programs
8. Interested only in the best dollar offer
9. Poor school record (academic, attendance)
10. Unwilling to start at the bottom
11. Making excuses, hedges on unfavorable record
12. No tact
13. Not mature
14. No curiosity about the job
15. Critical of past employers

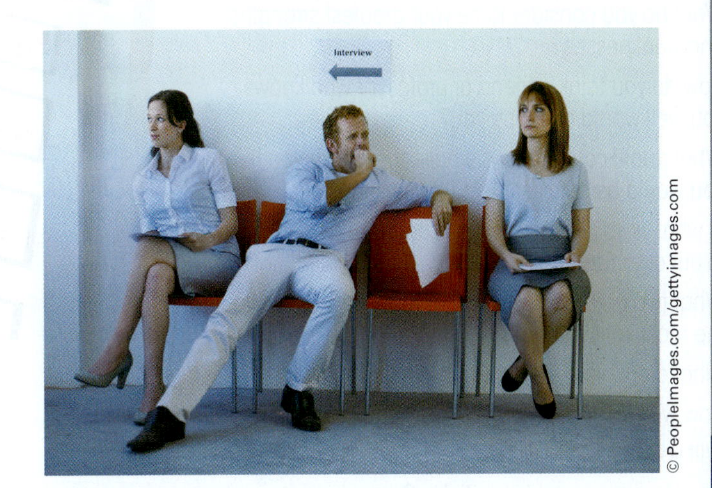

your personal items on your lap or place them on the floor near your chair. Do not invade the interviewer's territory by placing your things on the desk.

Sit erect in the chair with your feet flat on the floor or cross only your ankles. Avoid nervous mannerisms while you speak and maintain good eye contact, but do not stare the interviewer down. Be natural and positive about the position, organization, and yourself. Present a professional image by using medical terminology when responding to questions or providing information. Observe the interviewer carefully for cues. Respond to questions completely, trying not to repeat yourself or give more information than was requested.

Be prepared for the kinds of questions that may be asked during the interview process. Ask yourself, "If I were the employer, what would I want to know about the applicant?" Examples of standard questions asked by most employers are provided in the following Quick Reference Guide. Consider how you would respond to each question.

Remember that the interviewer is asking questions to determine if you are qualified for the position and if you are the kind of person who will fit into the organization. *Think* before answering questions; try to provide the information requested in a positive and professional manner. Do not respond with slang terms. *Listen* carefully so that you understand what information the question is requesting. *Ask* for clarification if you are uncertain. This demonstrates your ability to be open enough to ask questions when in doubt.

QUICK REFERENCE GUIDE

Typical Questions Asked During An Interview

- I see from your résumé you graduated from ___ college. What did that college have to offer that others didn't?
- What subjects did you enjoy the most and why?
- What do you see yourself doing 5 years from now?
- What salary do you expect and what do you think it will be in 5 or 10 years?
- What do you consider to be your greatest strengths and weaknesses?
- How do you think a friend or professor who knows you well would describe you?
- What qualifications do you have that make you think you would be successful in this position?
- In what ways do you think you can make a contribution to our organization?
- What two or three accomplishments have given you the most satisfaction?
- What didn't you like about your last employer?
- How well do you work under pressure?
- Will you be able to work overtime occasionally?
- How do you respond to criticism?
- How would you respond if a patient or coworker made advances toward you?
- How would you handle following procedures with which you do not agree?
- Describe a specific medical procedure.
- Do you have any questions you would like to ask?
- How would you establish credibility quickly with our team?
- What attracted you to this clinic?
- What is the last book you read?
- Why should we hire you?
- What is your personal mission statement?

Interviewing the Employer

The worst thing that can happen to an entry-level employee is to be hired and then have to quit or be fired because of a conflict with the employer. The interview process is a two-way street. You, the interviewee, should also interview the potential employer. The following are danger signs of an employer who could make your work life very difficult:

- Disrespectful behavior during the interview toward other staff members or you
- Signs of insecurity by the manager
- Lack of enthusiasm toward the organization
- Signs of being highly stressed
- Negative attitude in statements
- Arrogance or answers own questions
- Uses the pronoun *I* excessively

You have to "read" the interviewer because some of the signs listed could be attributed to a "bad day." If too many signals are showing or, after prudent questioning on your part, you still have concerns, perhaps you should look for employment elsewhere to avoid the possibility of damaging your future career.

Following are a few questions you might ask the interviewer to resolve some of these concerns raised by observations:

- How would you describe the clinic culture?
- How do you handle differing opinions on how best to accomplish tasks?
- How are employee accomplishments recognized?
- What is the leadership style at the clinic?
- What is the attitude toward professional growth and educational opportunities?

Answers to these questions will help you determine if the clinic culture is one you can embrace.

Closing the Interview

By observing the interviewer and listening carefully, you will be able to determine when the interviewer feels he or she has enough information about you to make a decision. Usually during the closing the interviewer asks if you have any additional questions. This is your opportunity to collect information helpful in making a decision to accept or decline an offer. Your questions provide another opportunity to sell yourself, show that you have done your homework about the organization, and have listened carefully during the interview. Select three or four questions that will help you the most.

Questions about the organization are excellent choices. Examples are:

- What are the opportunities for advancement with this organization?
- I read that your organization has educational benefits. Could you explain briefly how that program works?
- You mentioned in-house training programs for employees. Could you give one or two examples?

You may also have some questions about the job itself. Examples of these types of questions are:

- Is this a newly created position? If so, what results are you hoping to see?
- Was the last person in this position promoted? What contributed to his or her advancement?
- What do you consider the most difficult task on this job?
- What are the lines of authority for this position?

Do not use this question time to ask about salary, sick leave, vacations, or retirement benefits. At this point, your focus should be on the value and skills you can contribute to the organization. These questions may be asked during a second interview or when a position is offered.

Before you leave, thank the interviewer for taking time to discuss the position with you. If you definitely are interested in the position, ask to be considered as a candidate for the position. If follow-up procedures have not been explained, now is the time to ask when the final selection will be made and how you will be notified. A firm handshake as you leave, a pleasant smile, and confidence as you exit will leave a professional picture in the interviewer's mind.

INTERVIEW FOLLOW-UP

Following up after the interview is essential. Remember to update your contact tracker with the date and method of your follow-up. If a question caught you off-guard, formulate a response for future interviews. It is now time to telephone your references to let them know the name of the organization and the person's name with whom you interviewed, something about the position, and your qualifications. Share any information that will help your references support you in obtaining the position.

Follow-Up Letter

Procedure

Take time to write a follow-up letter or handwritten note to the interviewer a day or two after your interview to thank him or her for the time spent interviewing you. The handwritten note should be a simple professional-looking thank you blank note card used to express your appreciation for the interview. Handwriting should neat and aligned evenly. A request to be considered for the position may be reiterated if you truly are interested in the position. The follow-up letter should be written in standard business format and printed on the same paper as your application/cover letter, references, and résumé. Be sure that all spelling and grammar are correct (see Procedure 24-2).

The follow-up letter provides another opportunity to express your interest in the organization and the position. You can briefly emphasize the experience and skills you have to offer and again request to be considered a candidate for the position.

Record the mailing date on your contact tracker and keep a copy of the letter in a file with other

PROCEDURE 24-2

Procedure

Prepare an Interview Follow-Up Letter

PURPOSE:

To write an error-free follow-up letter or handwritten thank you note in appreciation for a job interview and to express continued interest in the position posted.

EQUIPMENT/SUPPLIES:

- Computer and printer
- High-quality paper and envelope
- Addressee's name, title, and address
- Dictionary and thesaurus

PROCEDURAL STEPS:

1. Collect the needed equipment and information required to write the letter.
2. Follow standard business format for writing the letter. If handwriting a note, be sure to use good penmanship. RATIONALE: Following up after an interview provides yet another opportunity to express your interest in the position, to briefly emphasize the experience and skills you can contribute, and to request being considered for the position.
3. Proofread carefully to be sure that the grammar, spelling, punctuation, and capitalization are correct. RATIONALE: To present a professional image and an error-free résumé.
4. Print the letter on good quality paper, at least 20- to 24-pound stock with a watermark. Choose a shade of white, cream, or gray bond paper. RATIONALE: To distinguish yourself from other candidates and to present a professional image.
5. Sign the letter and place the original in the addressed envelope to be mailed.
6. Update your contact tracker and maintain a copy of the letter in your file. RATIONALE: To maintain current status on any and all employment opportunities.

information about the organization. Figure 24-8 shows a sample follow-up letter.

Follow Up by Telephone

Allow a few days for your follow-up letter to reach the interviewer. If you do not hear from the interviewer within a week or by the designated time established during the interview, you may call to ask if you are still being considered for the position or if a decision has been made.

Speak directly into the mouthpiece of the telephone using good diction and voice volume. Identify yourself and provide some information to aid the interviewer in recalling who you are. Perhaps mentioning the date you interviewed will suffice. Be polite and professional, and remember to thank the individual for speaking with you. At the end of the conversation say good-bye and wait until the other person hangs up before you break the connection. Log the telephone call and its response on your contact tracker for future reference.

AFTER YOU ARE EMPLOYED

You are now a newly employed medical assistant. What do you do now to advance your career? Following are some suggestions:

- Make sure your workstation is set up and you have what you need to do the job.
- Practice good time management skills.
- Try to allow time for emergencies, which will occur.
- Do not be a know-it-all; ask other employees how they do things around here.
- Get to know colleagues and be part of the team.
- Seek feedback on how you are doing your job.
- Create a professional image.

Dealing with Difficult People

Sooner or later you will encounter co-workers who could be described as just plain "jerks." Jerks may

2031 Craig Street
Renton, Washington 98055
August 28, 20XX

Sarah Molles, Manager
Seattle Group Health Cooperative
304 Fourth Avenue
Seattle, Washington 98124-1716

Dear Ms. Molles,

Thank you for scheduling a personal interview with me last Wednesday, August 26, at 9:45AM. I enjoyed discussing the medical assistant position open in one of your dermatology surgery practices. I would like to be considered for the position.

After talking with you, I feel my qualifications match closely with those you requested. My communication and interpersonal skills are excellent and a necessary ingredient for any medical assistant.

I look forward to hearing from you September 5 as you mentioned during the interview. If there are any questions I may answer, please telephone me.

Sincerely,

Ashley Jackson, CMA (AAMA)
(206) 255-1365

FIGURE 24-8 Sample follow-up letter.

be defined as persons who use power to belittle and ridicule people who work under them. These people may be foul-mouthed, power hungry, bullies, uncouth, or unethical. There are several ways to free yourself from jerks:

- Check out emotionally (attempt to ignore the comments); indifference is an underrated virtue.
- Try to move to a different position within the organization.
- If all else fails, change jobs.

Getting a Raise

One of the main reasons people do not get a raise is because they do not ask. This is particularly true of professional women. It has been reported that less than half ask for a raise or promotion within the first 12-month working period. Of those that ask, almost three quarters received a raise or promotion. After taking into consideration the wages of persons with similar job descriptions and experience, if your salary appears to be lagging, you should not feel uncomfortable asking for a raise at your next favorable performance review.

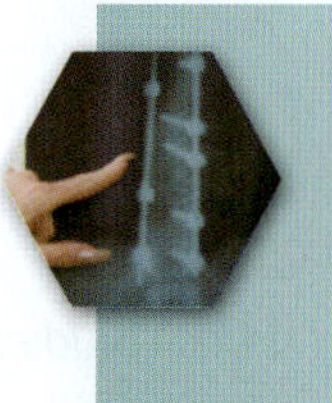

Critical Thinking

As you begin to prepare for a job interview, how can you prepare yourself to reflect a professional image, attitude, and demeanor, and verbal and nonverbal communication skills, as well as articulately describe your skills and abilities to fit the position to which you are applying? Develop a complete written checklist and review it before each interview.

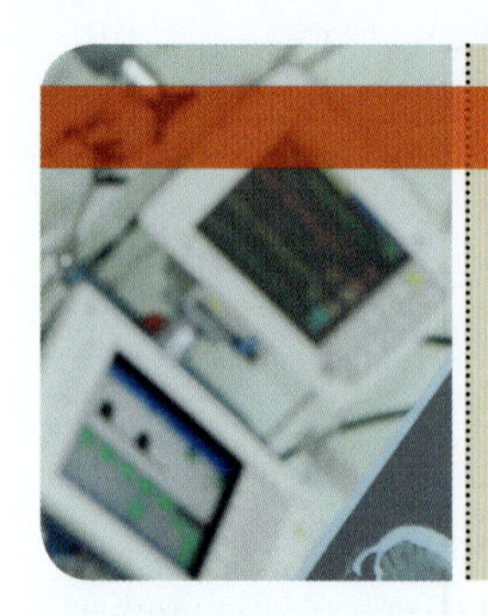

CASE STUDY 24-1

Refer to the scenario at the beginning of the chapter.

CASE STUDY REVIEW

1. Which résumé style represents Eun Mee best and why?
2. List transferable skills that Eun Mee may want to include in her résumé.
3. What is the purpose of an accomplishment statement? Provide examples Eun Mee might use.

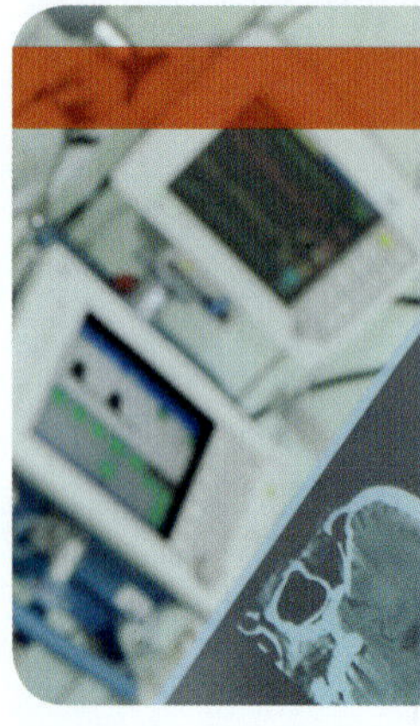

CASE STUDY 24-2

Drs. Lewis and King are part of a multi-provider family practitioner clinic. They are in need of a new medical assistant to take the place of one who will be leaving at the end of the month. They have scheduled interviews with five applicants. Eun Mee Soo is the first candidate to be interviewed.

CASE STUDY REVIEW

1. Eun Mee wants to bring some papers to the interview. What is the best way to do this? What paperwork would be appropriate to bring with her?
2. Why should Eun Mee arrive 5 to 10 minutes early for the interview?
3. How should Eun Mee enter the room?

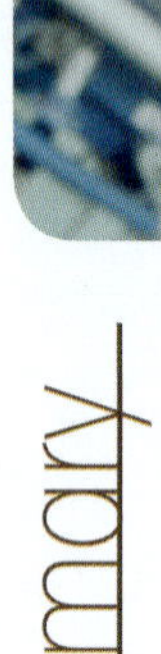

Summary

- Begin the job search while still in school and look for ways to distinguish yourself from other applicants.
- Remember that attitude and mindset are important qualities employers look for.
- Self-analysis aids in the overall picture of who you are and what you are looking for in an employment package. In addition, it helps with résumé and interview techniques.
- Choose the résumé style that best reflects what you have to offer a future employer. Use keyword descriptors to describe the skills and attributes you possess.
- Your employment package should include a well-written, accurate résumé, reference sheet, and application/cover letter. Complete the application form if requested to do so. Include copies of any pertinent awards, certifications, and letters of recommendation in your employment package.
- Dress for success for the interview and be prepared by preplanning answers to questions that may be asked or that you may want to ask.
- Interview follow-up may include a thank you letter and/or a telephone call.

Study for Success

To reinforce your knowledge and skills of information presented in this chapter:

- Review the *Key Terms* and *Learning Outcomes*
- Consider the *Critical Thinking* features and *Case Studies* and discuss your conclusions
- Answer the questions in the *Certification Review*

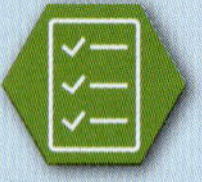

Procedure

- Perform the *Procedures* using the *Competency Assessment Checklists* on the *Student Companion Website*

CERTIFICATION REVIEW

1. Which response best describes a résumé?
   a. It is a summary or brief account of your qualifications and progress in your career.
   b. It is also known as a contact tracker.
   c. It always includes references.
   d. It is known as an e-résumé.
2. Which of the following statements is true of references?
   a. References must always be listed on the résumé.
   b. A reference should be a relative.
   c. A reference should be someone who likes you and your work but may not be a good communicator.
   d. A reference should be someone who knows you or has worked with you long enough to make an honest assessment of your capabilities and integrity.
   e. References must only be persons with whom you have worked.
3. When is it advantageous to use the targeted résumé style?
   a. When prior titles are impressive
   b. When reentering the job market after an absence
   c. When you are just starting your career and have little experience
   d. When you have extensive specialized experience
4. Which of the following is true of the application/cover letter?
   a. It is a detailed data sheet describing your vital information, education, and experience.
   b. It introduces you to a prospective employer and captures their interest in you as a candidate for the position.
   c. It lists individuals who can vouch for you.
   d. It should be lengthy and detailed.
   e. It thanks the employer for reviewing your résumé.
5. Which of the following is true of the interview?
   a. It does not require much thought or preparation.
   b. It requires you to think before answering questions, listen carefully, and ask for clarification if uncertain of the question.
   c. It provides time to ask questions about salary, vacation, and benefits.
   d. It does not require any follow-up.
6. Which task is *not* involved in self-assessment?
   a. Compiling a list of potential employers
   b. Identifying your strengths and weaknesses
   c. Listing things you enjoy
   d. Researching the clinic profile
   e. Evaluating your work style
7. What is the purpose of a résumé?
   a. To sell yourself
   b. To provide references
   c. To assist in maintaining your contact tracker
   d. To provide an opportunity to use social media
8. Which social media avenue is the number one networking site for the job search?
   a. The Internet
   b. Internet blogs
   c. Facebook
   d. LinkedIn
   e. Twitter
9. Which of the following best describes the term *accomplishment statement*?
   a. It is comprised of keywords descriptors that give a brief description of what you did and the results produced.
   b. It is a list of contacts and their responses and your actions.
   c. It is a list of who you know or have worked with.
   d. It is a brief account of your qualifications and progress in your career.
10. Which of the following responses is not included in follow-up after the interview?
    a. Telephoning references to update them
    b. Sending a follow-up letter to the interviewer
    c. Asking references to call the interviewer and put in a good word for you
    d. Following up with the interviewer by telephone
    e. Updating contact tracker information

APPENDIX A

Common Health Care Abbreviations and Symbols

Abbreviation	Meaning
AAMA	American Association of Medical Assistants
AAP	American Academy of Pediatrics
AAPC	American Academy of Professional Coders
ab	abortion
abd	abdomen
ABE	acute bacterial endocarditis
ABG	arterial blood gases
ABHES	Accrediting Bureau of Health Education Schools
ABO	blood grouping system
ac	acute
	before meals (ante cibum)
AC	alternating current
ACA	Affordable Care Act
ACAP	Alliance of Claims Assistance Professionals
ACIP	Advisory Committee on Immunization Practices
ACO	Accountable Care Organization
ACOG	American Congress of Obstetricians and Gynecologists
ACS	American Cancer Society
ACTH	adrenocorticotropic hormone
ADA	Americans with Disabilities Act
ADAAA	Americans with Disabilities Act Amendments Act of 2008
ADAD	autosomal dominant Alzheimer's disease
ADHD	attention deficit hyperactivity disorder
ADL	activities of daily living
ad lib	as desired
adm	admission
ADR	alternative dispute resolution
AED	automated external defibrillator
AES	Advanced Encryption Standard
Afib	atrial fibrillation
AFP	alpha-fetoprotein
AHA	American Heart Association
AHD	arteriosclerotic heart disease
	atherosclerotic heart disease
AHDI	Association for Healthcare Documentation Integrity
AHIMA	American Health Information Management Association
AIDS	acquired immunodeficiency syndrome
AIIR	airborne infection isolation room
Alb	albumin
ALP	alkaline phosphatase
ALT	alanine aminotransferase
	argon laser trabeculoplasty
AM	before noon (ante meridiem)
AMA	against medical advice
	American Medical Association
AMBA	American Medical Billing Association
AMI	acute myocardial infarction
amt	amount
AMT	American Medical Technologists
AMTIE	American Medical Technologists Institute for Excellence
ant	anterior
ante	before
AP	anterior/posterios
A&P	anatomy and physiology
	anterior and posterior
	auscultation and palpation
	auscultation and percussion
APC	ambulatory payment classifications
APGAR	appearance, pulse, grimace, activity, and respiration
Apps	applications
Aq	water (aqua)
A/R	accounts receivable
ARDS	acute (or adult) respiratory distress syndrome
ARRA	American Recovery and Reinvestment Act
ARU	automated routing unit
ASA	acetylsalicylic acid
ASAP	as soon as possible
ASC	atypical squamous cell
ASCAD	arteriosclerotic coronary artery disease
	athrosclerotic coronary artery disease
ASC US	atypical squamous cell of uncertain significance
ASCVD	arteriosclerotic cardiovascular disease
	atherosclerotic cardiovascular disease
ASD	autism spectrum disorder
ASRT	American Society of Radiologic Technologists
AST	aspartate aminotransferase
AV	atrioventricular
A&W	alive and well
Ax	axillary

Ba	barium
BaE	barium enema
BBB	bundle branch block
BC	birth control
BC/BS	Blue Cross/Blue Shield
BCP	birth control pills
BE	bacterial endocarditis
BHRT	bioidentical hormone replacement therapy
bid	twice a day
bil	bilateral
BM	basal metabolism bowel movement
BMI	body mass index
BMR	basal metabolism rate
BNA	budget neutrality adjuster
BNP	B-type natriuretic peptide
BP	blood pressure
B/P	blood pressure
BPH	benign prostatic hypertrophy
BRCA1	breast cancer susceptibility protein mutations 1
BRCA2	breast cancer susceptibility protein mutations 2
BS	blood sugar bowel sounds breath sounds
BSA	body surface area
BSE	bovine spongiform encephalopathy breast self-exam
BSL	blood sugar level
BSN	bowel sounds normal
BSO	bilateral salpingo-oophorectomy
BSR	blood sedimentation rate
BUN	blood urea nitrogen
BW	birth weight blood work body weight
Bx	biopsy
C	Celsius Centigrade cup
C1	first cervical vertebra
Ca	calcium
CA	cancer carcinoma
CAAHEP	Commission on Accreditation of Allied Health Education Programs
CAD	computer-aided detection coronary artery disease
CAHD	coronary arteriosclerotic heart disease coronary athersclerotic heart disease
CAM	complementary and alternative medicine
caps	capsules
CARE	Consistency, Accuracy, Responsibility, and Excellence in Medical Imaging and Radiation Therapy Act of 2013
CAT	computerized axial tomography
cath	catheterization
CBC	complete blood count
CBT	computer-based testing
CC	chief complaint
CCA	Certified Coding Associate
CCHIT	Certification Commission for Health Information Technology
CCMA (AMT)	Certified Clinical Medical Assistant through American Medical Technologists
CCP	Certification Continuation Program
CCR	continuity of care record
CCS	Certified Coding Specialist
CCS-P	Certified Coding Specialist–Physician-Based
CCT	cardiac computerized tomography
CCU	coronary care unit
C&D	cystoscopy and dilation
CDC	U.S. Centers for Disease Control and Prevention
CE	continuing education
CEA	carcinoembryonic antigen
cerv	cervical cervix
CEU	continuing education unit
CF	conversion factor
CHAMPVA	Civilian Health and Medical Program of the Department of Veterans Administration
CHD	childhood disease congenital heart disease congestive heart disease coronary heart disease
CHEDDAR	chief complaint, history, examination, details of problems, drugs and dosages, assessment, return visit if applicable
CHF	congestive heart failure
CHO	carbohydrate
CHP	Chemical Hygiene Plan
CIN	cervical intraepithelial neoplasia
CJD	Creutzfeldt-Jakob disease
ck	check
Cl	chlorine
cldy	cloudy
CLIA	Clinical Laboratory Improvement Amendments
cm	centimeter
CMA (AAMA)	Certified Medical Assistant through the American Association of Medical Assistants
CMAA (NHA)	Certified Medical Administrative Assistant through the National Healthcareer Association
CMAS (AMT)	Certified Medical Administrative Specialist through American Medical Technologists
CME	continuing medical education
CMR	cardiac magnetic resonance
CMS	Centers for Medicare and Medicaid Services
CMT	Certified Medical Transcriptionist
CNS	central nervous system
C/O	complains of
CO_2	carbon dioxide
COB	coordination of benefits
COPD	chronic obstructive pulmonary disease
COW	Certificate of Waiver
CPAP	continuous positive airway pressure
CPC	Certified Professional Coder
CPC-A	Certified Professional Coder–Apprentice

CPC-H	Certified Professional Coder–Hospital
CPC-HA	Certified Professional Coder–Hospital Apprentice
CPE	complete physical exam
CPR	cardiopulmonary resuscitation
CPT	Current Procedural Terminology
CPU	central processing unit
CR	computed radiography
CRB	Curriculum Review Board
crit	hematocrit
CRP	C-reactive protein
CS	cerebrospinal cesarean section
C&S	culture and sensitivity
CSF	cerebrospinal fluid
CT	computerized tomography
CVA	cerebrovascular accident
CVE	capsule video endoscopy
CVP	central venous pressure
CVS	chorionic villus sampling
cx	cervix
CXR	chest X-ray
cysto	cystoscopic examination cystoscopy
DACUM	developing a curriculum
DARP	data, assessment, response, plan
d/c	discharge discontinue
DC	doctor of chiropractic discontinue discharge
D&C	dilation and curettage
DDS	doctor of dentistry
DEA	U.S. Drug Enforcement Agency
DEERS	Defense Enrollment Eligibility Reporting System
del	delivery
DES	diethylstilbestrol
DHHS	U.S. Department of Health and Human Services
diab	diabetic diabetes
diag	diagnosis
diff	differential white blood cell count
dil	dilute
Disp	dispense
dL	deciliter
DM	diabetes mellitus
DNA	deoxyribonucleic acid does not apply
DNR	do not resuscitate
DO	doctor of osteopathy
DOA	dead on arrival
DOB	date of birth
DOD	date of death
DOE	dyspnea on exertion
dos	dosage
DPI	dry powder inhaler
DPM	doctor of podiatric medicine
DPT	diphtheria, pertussis, and tetanus
Dr	doctor
DR	delivery room
DRGs	diagnosis-related groups
DS	discharge summary
DSD	dry sterile dressing
dsg	dressing
DT	delirium tremens
DTaP	diphtheria and tetanus toxoids and acellular pertussis vaccine, pediatric formulation
DTR	deep tendon reflex
D&V	diarrhea and vomiting
DW	distilled water
D/W	dextrose in water
dx	diagnosis
DXA	dual-energy X-ray absorptiometry
ea	each
EAP	extensible authentication protocol
EBV	Epstein–Barr virus
ECC	emergency cardiac care
ECG	electrocardiogram
echo	echocardiogram echoencephalogram
E. coli	*Escherichia coli*
ECT	electroconvulsive therapy electronic claims transmission
ED	erectile dysfunction emergency department
EDB	expected date of birth
EDC	estimated date of confinement expected date of confinement
EDD	estimated date of delivery expected date of delivery
EEG	electroencephalogram
EENT	eyes, ears, nose, and throat
e.g.	for example
EGD	esophagogastric duodenoscopy
EHR	electronic health record
EKG	electrocardiogram
elix	elixir
email	electronic mail
EMG	electromyography
EMR	electronic medical record
EMS	emergency medical service
ENT	ear, nose, and throat
EO	ethylene oxide
EOB	explanation of benefits
eos	eosinophil
EPA	Environmental Protection Agency
EPCA-2	early prostate cancer antigen-2
EPO	Exclusive Provider Organization
eq	equivalent
ER	emergency room
ERCP	endoscopic retrograde cholangiopancreatography
ERT	estrogen replacement therapy
ERV	expiratory reserve volume

ESR	erythrocyte sedimentation rate
ESRD	end-stage renal disease
EST	electroshock therapy
exam	examination
ext	extract
F	Fahrenheit
FAM	fertility awareness methods
FAS	fetal alcohol syndrome
FAST	face drooping, arm weakness, speech, time to call 911
fax	facsimile
FBS	fasting blood sugar
FDA	U.S. Food and Drug Administration
Fe	iron
FECA	Federal Employees Compensation Act Program
FEF	forced expiratory flow
FEV	forced expiratory volume
FGM	female genital mutilation
FH	family history
FHR	fetal heart rate
FHS	fetal heart sound
fl	fluid
fl oz	fluid ounce
FLMA	Family and Medical Leave Act
FMP	first menstrual period
FP	family practice
freq	Frequent
FSH	follicle-stimulating hormone
ft	foot
FTA	fluorescent treponemal antibody
FTP	file transfer protocol
FTT	failure to thrive
FVC	forced vital capacity
fx	fracture
g	gram
G	Gravida
	gauge
gal	gallon
GB	gallbladder
GC	gonococcus
	gonorrhea
GERD	gastroesophageal reflux disease
GGT	gamma glutamyltransferase
GI	gastrointestinal
GIFT	gamete intrafallopian transfer
Gm	gram
GP	general practice
GPCI	Geographic Practice Cost Index
gr	grain
grav	pregnancy
GTH	gonadotropic hormone
GTT	glucose tolerance test
gtt(s)	drop (drops)
GU	genitourinary
GYN	gynecology
h	hour
HAART	highly active antiretroviral therapy
HAI	health care–associated infection
HAV	hepatitis A
HBIG	hepatitis B immune globulin
HBP	high blood pressure
HBV	hepatitis B
HCFA	U.S. Health Care Financing Administration
hCG	human chorionic gonadotropin
HCl	hydrochloric acid
HCP	health care provider
HCPCS	Healthcare Common Procedure Coding System
Hct	hematocrit
HCV	hepatitis C
HCVD	hypertensive cardiovascular disease
HDL	high-density lipoprotein
HDV	hepatitis D
HEENT	head, eyes, ears, nose, and throat
HEPA	high-efficiency particulate air
HEV	hepatitis E
Hgb	hemoglobin
HGP	Human Genome Project
H&H	hemoglobin and hematocrit
Hib	*haemophilus influenza* type b
HIC number	the identification number of a Medicare beneficiary issued by CMS or the RRB
HIDA scan	hepatobiliary iminodiacetic acid scan
HIPAA	Health Insurance Portability and Accountability Act
HIV	human immunodeficiency virus
HITECH	Health Information Technology for Economic and Clinical Health Act
HMO	health maintenance organization
H/O	history of
H_2O	water
H&P	history and physical
HPI	history of present illness
HPV	human papillomavirus
HR	human resources
HRS	Healthcare Reimbursement Specialist
HRT	hormone replacement therapy
HSV1	herpes simplex virus 1
HSV2	herpes simplex virus 2
ht	height
HT	hormone therapy
hx	history
Hz	Hertz
IBS	irritable bowel syndrome
ICCU	intensive coronary care unit
ICD	implantable cardioverter-defibrillator
ICD-9-CM	International Classification of Diseases, 9th revision, Clinical Modification
ICD-10-CM	International Classification of Diseases, 10th revision, Clinical Modification
ICU	intensive care unit

ID	intradermal
I&D	incision and drainage
IDDM	insulin-dependent diabetes mellitus
IDS	integrated delivery system
IIS	immunization information system
IM	internal medicine
	intramuscular
	infectious mononucleosis
imp	impression
IN	intranasal
inf	infusion
Inj	injection
INR	international normalization ratio
I&O	intake and output
IOM	Institute of Medicine
IP	inpatient
IPA	independent provider association
IPV	inactive poliovirus
	intimate partner violence
IPPB	intermittent positive pressure breathing
IPPS	inpatient prospective payment systems
ISMP	Institute of Safe Medicine Practices
ISP	Internet service provider
IT	information technology
IUD	intrauterine device
IV	intravenous
IVF	in vitro fertilization
IVP	intravenous pyelogram
JAAMT	*Journal of the American Association for Medical Transcription*
JAMA	*Journal of the American Medical Association*
JCAHO	Joint Commission on Accreditation of Healthcare Organizations
K	potassium
kg	kilogram
KOH	potassium hydroxide
KUB	kidney, ureter, and bladder
kV	Kilovolt
KVO	keep vein open
l	length
L	liter
LA	left atrium
	lactic acid
	left arm
L&A	light and accommodation
lab	laboratory
lac	laceration
LAC	long arm cast
LAN	local area network
lap	laparotomy
LASIK	laser-assisted in-situ keratomileusis
lat	lateral
lb	pound
LBBB	left bundle branch block
LDH	lactate dehydrogenase
LDL	low-density lipoprotein
LE	lupus erythematosus
LEEP	loop electrosurgical excision procedure
LGBT	lesbian, gay, bisexual, transgender
LHRH	luteinizing hormone-releasing hormone
Liq	liquid
LL	left leg
LLQ	lower left quadrant
LMP	last menstrual period
LP	lumbar puncture
LRQ	lower right quadrant
LUQ	left upper quadrant
L&W	living and well
lymphs	lymphocytes
M	male
m	meter
MA	medical allowable
Mac	Macintosh (Apple computer)
MBCD	management by coaching and development
MBCE	management by competitive edge
MBDM	management by decision models
MBP	management by performance
MBS	management by styles
MBWA	management by wandering around
MBWS	management by work simplification
mcg	microgram
MCHC	mean corpuscular hemoglobin and red cell indices
MCO	managed care organization
MCV	mean corpuscular volume and red cell indices
MD	doctor of medicine
	muscular dystrophy
MEF	mean expiratory flow
MDI	metered dose inhaler
MDR	minimum daily requirement
med	medicine
mEq	milliequivalents
MFS	Medicare fee schedule
mg	milligram
MH	marital history
	medical history
	menstrual history
MHT	menopausal hormonal therapy
MHx	medical history
MI	maturation index
	myocardial infarction
MICE	motion, ice, compression and elevation
mL	milliliter
mm	millimeter
mm^3	cubic millimeter
MMA	Medicare Prescription Drug Improvement and Modernization Act
mm Hg	millimeters of mercury
MMR	measles, mumps, and rubella
MOM	milk of magnesia
mono	mononucleosis
MP	menstrual period
MRC	Medical Reserve Corps

MRI	magnetic resonance imaging
MRIA	magnetic resonance imaging angiography
MRSA	methicillin-resistant *Staphylococcus aureus*
MS	mitral stenosis
	multiple sclerosis
MSAFP	mother's serum alpha-fetoprotein
MSHA	Mine Safety and Health Administration
MT	medical technologist
	medical transcriptionist
multip	multipara
MVP	mitral valve prolapse
MVV	maximum voluntary ventilation
NA	not applicable
NaCl	sodium chloride
NACP	National Association of Claims Assistance Professionals
NAPPSI	National Alliance for the Primary Prevention of Sharps Injuries
narc	narcotic
NB	newborn
NBSTSA	National Board of Surgical Technology and Surgical Assisting
N/C	no complaints
NCAI	National Coalition for Adult Immunization
ND	doctor of naturopathy
NDC	National Drug Code
NEBA	National Electronic Billers Alliance
NEC	not elsewhere classified
neg	negative
NG	nasogastric
NGU	nongonococcal urethritis
NHA	National Healthcareer Association
NIDA	National Institute on Drug Abuse
NIDDM	noninsulin-dependent diabetes mellitus
NIH	National Institutes of Health
NL	normal limits
NLNA	National League for Nursing Accrediting
NMP	normal menstrual period
noct	at night
Non-PAR	nonparticipating provider
NOS	not otherwise specified
NPI	national provider identification
NPO	nothing by mouth
NR	no refill
	nonreactive
	normal range
	nonspecific
NS	normal saline
	not significant
	not sufficient
NSAID	nonsteroidal anti-inflammatory drug
N&T	nose and throat
N&V	nausea and vomiting
NVD	nausea, vomiting, and diarrhea
O	oral
O_2	oxygen
OB	obstetrics
OB-GYN	obstetrics-gynecology
OC	office call
	on call
	oral contraceptive
occ	occasionally
OCR	Office of Civil Rights
	optical character reader
OGTT	oral glucose tolerance test
OM	office manager
OOB	out of bed
OP	outpatient
O&P	ova and parasites
OPD	outpatient department
OPIM	other potentially infectious material
OPPS	a system that classifies all hospital outpatient services into Ambulatory Payment Classifications for reimbursement
	outpatient prospective payment systems
OPV	oral polio vaccine
OR	operating room
	operative report
ortho	orthopedics
os	mouth
OSHA	U.S. Occupational Safety and Health Administration
OT	occupational therapist
	occupational therapy
OTC	over the counter
OURQ	outer upper right quadrant
OV	office visit
OWCP	Office Workers' Compensation Programs
oz	ounce
P	phosphorus
	pulse
PA	physician's assistant
	posteroanterior
P&A	percussion and auscultation
PAC	phenacetin, aspirin, and codeine
	premature atrial contraction
PACS	picture archiving and communications systems
Pap	Papanicolaou (smear, test)
PAR	participating provider
para	number of pregnancies
para I	primipara
PAT	paroxysmal atrial tachycardia
path	pathology
PBI	protein-bound iodine
pc	after meals
PC	personal computer
PCA	patient-controlled analgesic
PCC	Poison Control Center
PCMH	patient-centered medical home
PCN	penicillin
PCP	primary care provider
PCR	polymerase chain reaction
PCV	packed cell volume

PDA	personal digital assistant
PDR	*Physician's Desk Reference*
PE	physical examination
peds	pediatrics
PEG	percutaneous endoscopic gastrostomy
	pneumoencephalography
Peg-IFN	pegylated interferon
per	by or with
PERF	peak expiratory flow rate
PERRLA	pupils equal, round, regular, react to light, and accommodation
PET	positron emission transmission or tomography
PFT	pulmonary function testing
pH	hydrogen in concentration
PH	past history
	personal history
	public health
PHI	protected health information
PHO	physician-hospital organization
PI	present illness
	pulmonary infarction
PID	pelvic inflammatory disease
PKU	phenylketonuria
PM	after noon (post meridiem)
	post mortem (after death)
PMN	polymorphonuclear neutrophils
PMP	past menstrual period
PMS	premenstrual syndrome
PNC	penicillin
PRNT	plague reduction neutralization test
PO	postoperative
po	by mouth (per os)
POB	place of birth
POCT	point of care testing
POL	physician office laboratory
POLST	Physician Orders for Life-Sustaining Treatment
POMR	problem-oriented medical record
pos	positive
POS	point-of-service
postop	postoperative
PP	present problem
	postprandial
PPB	positive pressure breathing
PPBS	postprandial blood sugar
PPD	purified protein derivative
PPE	personal protective equipment
PPO	preferred provider organization
preop	preoperative
primip	woman bearing first child
prn	as the occasion arises, as necessary
procto	proctoscopy
prog	prognosis
PROM	premature rupture of membranes
pro-time	prothrombin time
PRSP	penicillin-resistant *Streptococcus* pneumonia
PSA	prostate-specific antigen
PSDA	Patient Self-Determination Act
PSRO	Professional Standards Review Organization
pt	patient
	pint
PT	physical therapy
	prothrombin time
PTA	prior to admission
PTCA	percutaneous transluminal coronary angioplasty
PTT	partial thromboplastin time
PUBS	percutaneous umbilical blood sampling
pulv	powder
PVC	premature ventricular contraction
PVP	photoselective vaporization of the prostate
px	physical examination
	prognosis
QA	quality assurance
q AM	every morning
qh	every hour
q (2, 3, 4)h	every 2, 3, or 4 hours
qid	four times a day
QISMC	Quality Improvement System for Managed Care
qns	quantity not sufficient
qt	quart
R	right
	respirations
	rectal
RA	right arm
RAM	random access memory
RBC	red blood cell
RBC/hpf	red blood cells per high power field
RBCM	red blood cell mass
RBCV	red blood cell volume
RBRVS	Resource-Based Relative Value Scale
REM	rapid eye movement
resp	respiration
Rh	rhesus (factor)
Rh−	rhesus negative
Rh+	rhesus positive
RHD	rheumatic heart disease
RICE	rest, ice, compression, and elevation
RL	right leg
RLQ	right lower quadrant
RMA (AMT)	Registered Medical Assistant through American Medical Technologists
RNA	ribonucleic acid
R/O	rule out
ROA	received on account
ROM	range of motion
	read-only memory
ROS	review of systems
ROTA	rotavirus
RPR	rapid plasma reagin test
RSV	respiratory syncytial virus
RT	radiation therapy

RUQ	right upper quadrant
RV	residual volume
RVUs	relative value units
Rx	prescription
S	subjective data (POMR)
SA	sinoatrial
S&A	sugar and acetone (urine)
SAC	short arm cast
SARS	severe acute respiratory syndrome
SBE	shortness of breath on exertion
	subacute bacterial endocarditis
SDS	safety data sheet
SE	standard error
sed rate	sedimentation rate
segs	segmented neutrophils
seq	sequela
SF	scarlet fever
	spinal fluid
SG	specific gravity
SH	social history
SIDS	sudden infant death syndrome
sig	instructions, directions
sigmoid	sigmoidoscopy
SIL	squamous interepithelial lesion
SMA 12/60	Sequential Multiple Analyzer (12-test serum profile)
SOAP	subjective data, objective data, assessment, and plan
SOAPER	subjective, objective, assessment, plan, education, response
SOAPIER	subjective, objective, assessment, plan, implementation, evaluation, response
SOB	shortness of breath
SOF	signature on file
sol	solution
solv	solvent
SOMR	source-oriented medical record
SOP	standard operating procedure
SOS	if necessary
spec	specimen
sp gr	specific gravity
spont ab	spontaneous abortion
SQ	subcutaneous
SR	sedimentation rate
SS	signs and symptoms
SSI	Supplemental Security Income
SSL	service sockets layer
Staph	*Staphylococcus*
stat	immediately
STD	sexually transmitted disease
Strep	*Streptococcus*
subq	subcutaneous
supp	suppository
surg	surgery
sx	signs
	symptoms
sym	symptoms
syr	syrup
T	temperature
T3	tri-iodothyronine
T4	thyroxine
TA	temporal artery
T&A	tonsillectomy and adenoidectomy
tab	tablet
TB	tuberculin
	tuberculosis
Tbs	tablespoon
TC	throat culture
	tissue culture
	total capacity
	total cholesterol
Td	tetanus and diphtheria immunization
TDD	telecommunication device for the deaf
TDM	therapeutic drug monitoring
temp	temperature
TENS	transcutaneous electrical nerve stimulator
TESE	testicular sperm extraction
TFTC	Task Force for Test Construction
ther	therapy
therap	therapeutic
TIA	transient ischemic attack
tid	three times a day
TIG	tetanus immune globulin
tinct	tincture
TKO	to keep open
TLC	tender loving care
	total lung capacity
TLS	transport layer security
TMJ	temporomandibular joint
top	topically
TOPV	trivalent oral poliovirus vaccine
TP	total protein
tPA	tissue plasminogen activator
TPI	treponema pallidum immobilization test
TPMS	Total Practice Management System
TPN	total parenteral nutrition
TPR	temperature, pulse, and respiration
tr	tincture
trig	triglycerides
TSH	thyroid-stimulating hormone
tsp	teaspoon
TSS	toxic shock syndrome
TTY	teletype communications
TUNA	transurethral needle ablation
TURBT	transurethral resection of bladder tumor
TURP	transurethral resection of prostate
tus	cough
Tx or tx	treatment
T&X	type and cross match
Tym	tympanic
UA	urinalysis
UB04	Uniform Bill 04
UCG	urinary chorionic gonadotropin
UCHD	usual childhood diseases
UCR	usual, customary, reasonable
ULQ	upper left quadrant

ung	ointment
UNICEF	United Nations International Children's Emergency Fund
UR	utilization review
urg	urgent
URI	upper respiratory infection
URL	Uniform Resource Locator
urol	urology
URQ	upper right quadrant
URT	upper respiratory tract
URTI	upper respiratory tract infection
USB	universal system bus port
USDA	United States Department of Agriculture
USDE	United States Department of Education
USMLE	United States Medical Licensing Examination
USP	United States Pharmacopoeia
UT	urinary tract
UTI	urinary tract infection
UV	ultraviolet
Vac	vaccine
VAERS	Vaccine Adverse Event Reporting System
vag	vagina vaginal
VD	venereal disease
VDRL	Venereal Disease Research Laboratory
VIS	vaccine information statement
vit	vitamin
vit cap	vital capacity
VoIP	voice over Internet protocol
vol	volume
VRE	vancomycin-resistant enterococcus
VRS	voice recognition software
VS	vital signs
VSED	voluntarily stop eating and drinking
VT	tidal volume
V tach	ventricular tachycardia
WAN	wide area network
WBC	white blood cell
WCE	wireless capsule endoscopy
WDWN	well developed, well nourished
WHI	Women's Health Initiative
WHO	World Health Organization
WN	well nourished
WNF	well-nourished female
WNL	within normal limits
WNM	well-nourished male
WO	written order
w/o	without
wt	weight
WVE	wireless video endoscopy
x	multiply by
XDR TB	extensively drug-resistant tuberculosis
XR	X-ray
XRA	X-ray angiography
X-ray	radiograph or radiogram
YOB	year of birth
yr	year
ZIG	zoster immunoglobulin

Symbols

*	birth
†	death
♂	male
♀	female
+	positive
−	negative
±	positive or negative, indefinite
÷	divide by
=	equal to
>	greater than
<	less than
×	multiply by
#	number, pound
'	foot, minute
"	inch, second
ā	before
c̄	with
Δ	change
°	degree
Ⓛ	left
p̄	after
q̄	each; every
®	registration
s̄	without
s̄s̄	one-half
x̄	except without

GLOSSARY OF TERMS

Note: The equivalent Spanish word follows in parentheses in blue.

abrasion (abrasión) a superficial scraping of the epidermis (Ch. 8).

abuse (abuso) misuse; excessive or improper use, especially of narcotics or psychoactive drugs (Ch. 16).

accession record (numeric system) (registro de entrada [sistema de ordenación por número]) logbook used to assign numbers to correspondence or patients (Ch. 13).

accomplishment statements (declaraciones de logros) statements that begin with a power verb and give a brief description of what you did, and the demonstrable results that were produced (Ch. 24).

accountable care organization (ACO) a group of health care providers (doctors, other primary care providers, clinics, and hospitals) that voluntarily organize in order to provide coordinated and high-quality care to their Medicare patients (Ch. 2).

accounting (contabilidad) system of monitoring the financial status of a facility and the financial results of its activities, providing information for decision making (Ch. 20).

accounts payable (cuentas por pagar) sum owed by a business for services or goods received (Ch. 18); also unwritten promise to pay a supplier for property or merchandise purchased on credit or for a service rendered (Ch. 20).

accounts receivable (cuentas por cobrar) amount owed to a business for services or goods supplied (Ch. 18).

accounts receivable (A/R) ratio assets (relación de cuentas por cobrar a activos) outstanding accounts receivable divided by the average monthly gross income for the past 12 months (Ch. 19, 20).

accreditation (acreditación) process whereby recognition is granted to an educational program for maintaining standards that qualify its graduates for professional practice; to provide with credentials (Ch. 1).

Accrediting Bureau of Health Education Schools (ABHES) (Junta de Acreditación de Escuelas de Educación en Salud [ABHES]) entity accrediting private, postsecondary institutions in the United States which offer allied health education programs as well as programmatic accreditation of medical assistant, medical laboratory technician, and surgical technology programs (Ch. 23).

accrual basis accounting (contabilidad según el principio del devengo) reports income at the time charges are generated (Ch. 20).

active listening (escucha activa) received message is paraphrased back to the sender to verify the correct message was decoded (Ch. 4).

acupuncture (acupuntura) treatment to relieve pain and disease by puncturing the skin with thin needles at specific points (Ch. 2).

acute stress (estrés agudo) the most common form of stress; occurs with rapid onset. It comes from demands and pressures of the recent past and anticipated demands and pressures in the future. It is thrilling and exciting in small doses, but too much is exhausting (Ch. 3).

adjustments (ajustes) increases or decreases to patient accounts not due to charges incurred or payments received (Ch. 16, 18).

administer (administrar) to give a medication (Ch. 6).

administrative law (derecho administrativo) establishes agencies that are given the power to make laws and enact regulations (Ch. 6).

Affordable Care Act (ACA) act signed into law in March 2010 by President Barack Obama with the goal of placing individuals, families, and small businesses in control of their health care (Ch. 1).

agenda (orden del día) printed list of topics to be discussed during a meeting, sometimes giving time allocation (Ch. 14, 21).

agent (agente) person representing another (Ch. 6).

alternative dispute resolution (ADR) (resolución alternativa de conflictos [RAC]) an alternative to trial that encourages the parties to settle their differences out of court (Ch. 6).

ambulatory care setting (entorno de atención ambulatoria) health care environment where services are provided on an outpatient basis. *Ambulatory* is from Latin and means "capable of walking." Examples include the solo provider's office, the group practice, the urgent care center, and the health maintenance organization (Ch. 1, 2).

American Association of Medical Assistants (AAMA) (Asociación Estadounidense de Asistentes Médicos [AAMA]) professional organization dedicated to serving the interests of Certified Medical Assistants (Ch. 23).

American Medical Technologists (AMT) (Tecnólogos Médicos Estadounidenses [AMT]) national organization which credentials health care professionals, including Registered Medical Assistants (RMA) and Certified Medical Administrative Specialists (CMAS) (Ch. 23).

anaphylaxis (anafilaxia) hypersensitive state of the body to a foreign protein or drug (Ch. 8).

ancillary services (servicios auxiliares) professional companies hired to complete a specific job (Ch. 21).

answering services (servicios de respuesta) services employed to answer the calls of an ambulatory care setting after hours; unlike an answering machine, a live operator answers the call and forwards it appropriately (Ch. 11).

application/cover letter (solicitud/carta de presentación) letter used to introduce yourself and your résumé to a prospective employer with the goal of obtaining an interview (Ch. 24).

application form (formulario de solicitud) form devised by a prospective employer to collect information relative to qualifications, education, and experience in employment (Ch. 24).

application software (software de aplicación) software that performs a specific data-processing function (Ch. 10).

arbitration (arbitraje) a form of dispute resolution that allows a neutral party to settle the dispute (Ch. 6).

articulating (elocuente) expressing oneself clearly and distinctly (Ch. 11).

assets (activos) properties of value that are owned by a business entity (Ch. 20).

assignment of benefits (asignación de beneficios) signing over of benefits by the beneficiary to another party (Ch. 16).

associate's degree (Título de técnico) a degree granted by a junior college at the end of a two-year course (Ch. 1).

Association for Healthcare Documentation Integrity (AHDI) (Asociación para la Integridad de la Documentación del Cuidado de la Salud [AHDI]) professional organization in the field of medical transcription/editing (Ch. 15).

assumptive coding (suposición de codificación) assuming a positive lab value can be coded as a disease or condition (Ch. 17).

attributes (atributos) inherent characteristics (Ch. 1).

auditor (auditor) a person responsible for determining the final content of a document and the document's correctness in every aspect (Ch. 15).

authoritarian style operates on the premise that most workers cannot make a contribution without being directed (Ch. 21).

automated external defibrillator (AED) (desfibrilador externo automatizado [DEA]) portable, self-contained, automatic device with voice instructions on how to use for individuals in cardiac arrest. It is used externally to electronically "shock" the myocardium into contracting again. Same as cardioversion (Ch. 8).

automated routing unit (ARU) (enrutador automático [ARU]) telephone system that answers a call and uses a recorded voice to identify departments or services (Ch. 11).

autopsy report (informe de autopsia) also called an autopsy protocol, a necropsy report, or a medical examiner report. Autopsies are performed to determine the cause of death or to ascertain and confirm disease presence (Ch. 15).

avulsion (avulsión) an open wound in which the skin is torn off and bleeding is profuse (Ch. 8).

bachelor's degree (licenciatura) four-year academic degree conferred by colleges and universities (Ch. 1).

balance (balancear) amount owed (N); to verify posting accuracy (V); records difference between debit and credit columns (Ch. 18).

balance sheet (balance general) itemized statement of assets, liabilities, and equity; a statement of financial condition (Ch. 20).

bandages (venda) nonsterile gauze or other material applied over a sterile dressing to protect and immobilize (Ch. 8).

benchmark (comparador de rendimiento) making a comparison among different organizations relative to how they accomplish tasks, such as office computerization, file system organization, and employee remuneration (Ch. 21).

beneficiary (beneficiario) person under a policy eligible to receive benefits (Ch. 16).

benefit (beneficio) remuneration that is in addition to salary (Ch. 21).

benefit period (período de beneficios) the specified time during which benefits will be paid under certain types of health insurance coverages (Ch. 16).

bias (sesgo) slant toward a particular belief (Ch. 4).

bioethics (bioética) branch of medical ethics concerned with moral issues resulting from high technology and sophisticated medical research. Social issues such as genetic engineering, abortion, and fetal tissue research raise important bioethical questions (Ch. 7).

birthday rule (regla del cumpleaños) method to determine which of two or more health insurance policies covering a dependent child will be primary; that parent with the birthday falling first in the calendar year has the primary policy (Ch. 16).

blind copy (copia oculta) protects the privacy of email. Other recipients cannot identify who else may have received the transmitted message (Ch. 14).

blogging (blogging) using a digital platform for expressing thoughts, ideas, experiences, or observations (Ch. 21).

body language (lenguaje corporal) nonverbal communication that includes wordless clues and unconscious body movements, gestures, and facial expressions that accompany verbal messages (Ch. 4).

bond (fianza) binding agreement with an employee ensuring recovery of financial loss should funds be stolen or embezzled (Ch. 21).

bond paper (papel bond) durable, strong paper usually used for correspondence (Ch. 14).

Boomer generation (generación de Boomer) individuals born from 1955–1965 (Ch 22).

brainstorming (tormenta de ideas) process of developing ideas through a synergistic interaction among participants in an environment free of criticism (Ch. 21).

buffer words (palabras de relleno) expendable words used while answering the telephone (Ch. 11).

bundled codes (códigos agrupados) a grouping of several services that are directly related to a specific procedure and are paid as one (Ch. 17).

burnout (agotamiento profesional) a state of fatigue or frustration brought about by a devotion to a cause, a way of life, or a relationship that failed to produce the expected reward (Ch. 3).

capitation (capitación) use of the number of members enrolled in a plan to determine salary of the provider; the provider is paid a fixed fee for each member no matter how many times that member is seen by the provider (Ch. 16).

caption (leyenda) method of designation used on file guides (Ch. 13).

cardiogenic (cardiogénico) a type of shock in which the cardiac muscle is unable to contract and adequately provide blood to the body (Ch. 8).

cardiopulmonary resuscitation (CPR) (reanimación cardiopulmonar [RCP]) combination of rescue breathing and chest compressions performed by a trained individual on a patient experiencing cardiac arrest (Ch. 8).

cardioversion (cardioversión) conversion of a pathological cardiac rhythm (arrhythmia), such as ventricular fibrillation, to normal sinus rhythm (Ch. 8).

career objective (objetivo profesional) expresses your career goal and the position for which you are applying (Ch. 24).

cash basis accounting (contabilidad de caja) reports income at the time money is collected (Ch. 20).

cashier's check (cheque de caja) bank's own check drawn against the bank's account (Ch. 18).

Centers for Medicare and Medicaid Services (CMS) (Centros de Servicios de Medicare y Medicaid [CMS]) formerly known as HCFA. CMS is a federal agency within the U.S. Department of Health and Human Services (DHHS). The agency administers Medicare, Medicaid, and the State Children's Health Insurance Program (SCHIP). CMS also administers the Health Insurance Portability and Accountability Act of 1996 (HIPAA) and Clinical Laboratory Improvement Act of 1988 (CLIA '88) (Ch. 16).

central processing unit (CPU) (unidad de procesamiento central [CPU]) brain of the computer that performs instructions defined by software (Ch. 10).

certification (certificación) guarantees something or someone as being true or as represented by or as meeting a standard (Ch. 1, 23).

certification examination (examen de certificación) standardized means of evaluating medical assistant competency (Ch. 23).

certified check (cheque certificado) depositor's own check that the bank has indicated with a date and signature to be good for the amount written (Ch. 18).

Certified Clinical Medical Assistant (CCMA [NHA]) (Asistente Clínico Médico Certificado [CCMA]) an NHA certification for a clinical medical assistant (Ch. 1, 24).

Certified Medical Administrative Assistant (CMAA [NHA]) (Asistente Administrativo Médico Certificado [CMAA]) an NHA certification for a medical administrative assistant (Ch. 1, 23).

Certified Medical Administrative Specialist (CMAS [AMT]) (Especialista Administrativo Médico Certificado [CMAS]) an AMT certification for a medical administrative specialist (Ch. 23).

Certified Medical Assistant (CMA [AAMA]) (Asistente Médico Certificado [CMA (AAMA)]) a medical assistant who has successfully completed the AAMA's national certification examination (Ch. 1, 23).

Certified Medical Transcriptionist (CMT) (Transcriptor Médico Certificado [CMT]) one who has completed a two-part certification examination administered by the Association for Healthcare Documentation Integrity (AHDI) (Ch. 15).

chart notes (notas clínicas) (also called progress notes) provider's formal or informal notes about presenting problem, physical findings, and plan for treatment for a patient examined in the office, clinic, acute care center, or emergency department (Ch. 15).

check register (registro de cheques) record of checks written; categorized into separate and identified columns (Ch. 20).

chief complaint (CC) (queja principal [QP]) specific symptom or problem for which the patient is seeing the provider today (Ch. 15).

chronic stress the response to emotional pressure for a prolonged period over which an individual perceives he or she has no control. Chronic stress can have a serious impact on physical and psychological health (Ch. 3).

chronologic résumé (curriculum vitae cronológico) résumé format used when you have employment experience (Ch. 24).

civil law (derecho civil) law related to actions between individuals (Ch. 6).

claim register (registro de reclamaciones) diary or register of claims submitted to each insurance carrier. When payment is received, the date and amount of payment is entered in the register (Ch. 17).

closed questions (preguntas cerradas) questions answered with a yes or no (Ch. 4).

cloud computing (computación en la nube) storing program software on servers at a hosting company so that software download is available on demand (Ch. 10).

cluster scheduling (programación de cluster) a method of appointment scheduling which involves grouping or categorizing similar types of visits or procedures on particular days or blocks of time. Also known as specialty scheduling or practice-based scheduling (Ch. 12).

clustering (agrupación) a grouping together of nonverbal messages into statements or conclusions (Ch. 4). Can also be used to describe a scheduling system where patients with similar complaints/conditions are scheduled consecutively (example is scheduling all the allergy injections for 3:00 PM to 4:00 PM every Tuesday and Thursday) (Ch. 12).

CMS 1500 (02/12) (CMS 1500 [02/12]) formerly known as the HCFA 1500 form; the office health insurance claim form for Medicare and Medicaid (Ch. 17).

coach (entrenador de) one responsible for helping patients gain the knowledge, skills, tools, and confidence to become an active participant in the management of their health care. Health coaches may act as advocates or intermediaries in the patient–provider relationship (Ch. 4).

coinsurance (coseguro) that percentage paid by either the insured party, or the insured's employer (Ch. 16).

collection ratio (relación de cobranza) gross income divided by the amount that could have been collected less disallowances (Ch. 19, 20).

Commission on Accreditation of Allied Health Education Programs (CAAHEP) (Comisión de Acreditación de Programas Educativos Asociados a la Salud [CAAHEP]) entity accrediting over 2,000 educational programs in 20 health sciences professions (Ch. 23).

common law (derecho consuetudinario) refers to laws developed in England and France and brought to the United States by the early settlers; sometimes referred to as judge-made law (Ch. 6).

compensation (compensación) overemphasizing of characteristics to make up for a real or imagined failure or handicap (Ch. 4).

competency (competencia) demonstrating mastery of a task, the skill or ability to perform a task (Ch. 1).

complementary and alternative medicine complementary medicine complements or is used with traditional or mainstream medicine. Alternative medicine is used in place of traditional or mainstream medicine. When health care providers cooperate in offering both types of care, the term *integrative medicine* is used (Ch. 2).

compliance (cumplimiento) conformity in fulfilling official requirements (Ch. 1).

confidentiality agreement (acuerdo de confidencialidad) when signed, the agreement signifies that the medical transcriptionist is committed to keeping all patient information confidential (Ch. 15).

conflict resolution (resolución de conflictos) solving problems between co-workers or any two parties (Ch. 21).

congruency (congruencia) occurs when the verbal message and the nonverbal message agree (Ch. 4).

constitutional law (derecho constitucional) consists of laws that are made by the constitution of the United States or individual states (Ch. 6).

consultation report (informe de consulta) document that reports the findings and advice of another provider requested to see a patient by the attending provider (Ch. 15).

contact tracker (seguidor de contactos) form used to keep track of employment contact information such as name of employer, name of contact person, address and telephone number, date of first contact, résumé sent, interview date, follow-up information (Ch. 24).

continuing education units (CEU) (unidades de educación continua [UEC]) method for earning points toward recertification (Ch. 23).

contract law (derecho contractual) law that refers to agreements between individuals and entities that are binding (Ch. 6).

coordination of benefits (COB) (coordinación de beneficios [COB]) the provision of an insurance contract that limits benefits to 100% of the cost (Ch. 16).

co-payment (copago) payment required when a patient is seen by the provider (Ch. 16).

cost accounting (contabilidad de costos) helps to determine what it costs the ambulatory care setting to perform particular services and is an integral part of managerial accounting (Ch. 20).

cost analysis (análisis de costos) procedure that determines the costs of each service (Ch. 20).

cost ratio (relación de costos) formula that shows the cost of a procedure or service and helps determine the financial value of maintaining certain services (Ch. 20).

crash cart or tray (bandeja o carro de parada) tray or portable cart that contains medications and supplies needed for emergency and first aid procedures (Ch. 8).

credentialed (acreditado) a document or certificate proving a person's qualifications (Ch. 1).

credit (crédito) decreases balance due; column used for entering payments (Ch. 18).

crepitation (crepitación) grating sound heard on movement of ends of a broken bone (Ch. 8).

criminal law (derecho penal) law related to wrongs committed against the welfare and safety of society as a whole (Ch. 6).

crossover claim (reclamación de crossover) A claim that is billed to the supplemental insurer by the regional Medicare fiscal intermediary for providers PAR with Medicare, after Medicare pays its portion (Ch. 16).

cross-reference (referencia cruzada) notation in a file to direct the reader to a specific record that may be filed under more than one name/subject (e.g., married name/maiden name or foreign names) where the surname is not easily recognizable (Ch. 13).

cryopreservation (crioconservación) storage of biologic materials (sperm, embryo, tissue, plasma) at extremely cold temperature for use at a later time (Ch. 7).

culture (cultura) the attitudes and behavior that are characteristic of a particular social group or organization (Ch. 4).

Current Procedural Terminology (CPT) (Terminología Actual sobre Procedimientos [TAP]) standard codes for procedures and services. Used by most ambulatory care settings in encoding the claim form and recognized by most insurance carriers (Ch. 17).

current reports (informes actuales) reports such as history and physical examinations that should be complete within 24 hours (Ch. 15).

data backup (backup de datos) storage of all files, programs, and the operating system necessary to restore the computer in the event of a major failure (Ch. 10).

day sheet (hoja diaria) form used with pegboard system to record daily patient transactions (Ch. 18).

debit (debe) used for entering charges and description of services; column is on the left (Ch. 18).

decode (decodificar) to translate into language that is easily understood; to interpret (Ch. 4).

deductible (deducible) that amount of incurred medical expenses that must be met before the insurance policy will begin to pay (Ch. 16).

defendant (demandado) person who defends action brought in litigation (Ch. 6).

Defense Enrollment Eligible Reporting System (DEERS) (Sistema de Informes de Elegibilidad para la Inscripción en Defensa [DEERS]) a system operated by the Department of Defense and used by TRICARE contractors to determine and confirm the eligibility of beneficiaries (Ch. 16).

defense mechanisms (mecanismo de defensa) behaviors that protect the psyche from guilt, anxiety, or shame (Ch. 4).

defragmentation (desfragmentación) reorganization of information on a hard disk to store files as continuous units rather than as small packets. A computer with little fragmentation of files will operate at a higher speed (Ch. 10).

denial (rechazo) rejection of or refusal to acknowledge (Ch. 4).

deposition (declaración) oral testimony given by an individual with a court reporter and attorneys for both sides present; often used as part of the discovery process (Ch. 6).

dexterity (destreza) skill and ease in using the hands (Ch. 1).

diagnosis (diagnóstico) determination of disease or condition (Ch. 17).

diagnosis-related groups (DRGs) (grupos relacionados de diagnóstico) these designations ensure that all given diagnoses are as specific as possible and also justify the length of a patient's stay in the hospital (Ch. 16).

diploma (diploma) a document bearing record of graduation from or of a degree conferred by an educational institution (Ch. 1).

diplopia (diplopia) the subjective complaint of seeing two images instead of one; also known as double-vision (Ch 8).

direct skills (habilidades directas) skills that are job specific. Skill in taking a blood pressure reading would be specific to the medical field (Ch. 24).

discharge summary (DS) (resumen de alta médica [DS]) medical reports that document the hospitalization history of a patient (Ch. 15).

discovery (exhibición de pruebas) the time in which both parties are allowed access to all information and evidence related to a legal case; follows the subpoena process (Ch. 6).

dislocation (luxación) displacement of a bone or joint from its normal position (Ch. 8).

dispense (dosificar) prepare and give out a medication to be taken at a later time (Ch. 6).

displacement (desplazamiento) displacing negative feelings onto something or someone else with no significance to the situation (Ch. 4).

disposition (temperamento) temperament, character, personality (Ch. 1).

documentation (documentación) written material that accompanies purchased software containing the information necessary for using the software appropriately; sometimes known as the manual (Ch. 10)

donut hole (período sin cobertura) within the Medicare Part D prescription drug program, the donut hole is the phase of coverage in which all costs are covered by the enrollee rather than CMS (Ch. 16).

double-booking (doble-reserva) a method of appointment scheduling where two or more patients are given a particular appointment time (Ch. 12).

down-code (baja de codificación) insurance carriers down-code if documentation or codes are ambiguous and reimburse for the lowest possible fee (Ch. 17).

dressing (apósito) sterile gauze or other material applied directly to a wound to absorb secretions and to protect (Ch. 8).

durable power of attorney for health care (poder legal duradero para atención médica) legal form that allows a designated person to act on another's behalf in regard to health care choices (Ch. 5, 6).

editor (corrector) see auditor (Ch. 15).

EHR (RSE) see electronic health record (Ch. 10).

electrocautery (electrocauterización) control of bleeding using an instrument that is electrically heated (Ch. 8).

electronic check (cheque electrónico) electronic version of a paper check, used to make payments online (Ch. 18).

electronic health record (EHR) (registro de salud electrónico [RSE]) a patient's electronic medical records from multiple sources combined into one master database (Ch. 10).

electronic mail (email) (correo electrónico) the process of sending, receiving, storing, and forwarding messages in digital form over computer networks (Ch. 11).

electronic medical record (EMR) (registro médico electrónico [RME]) patient medical record from a single medical practice, hospital, or pharmacy (Ch. 10, 15).

emancipated minors (menor emancipado) persons under age 18 years who are financially responsible for themselves and free of parental care (Ch. 6).

embezzle (malversar) appropriate fraudulently to one's own use (Ch. 21).

emergency medical services (EMS) (servicios médicos de emergencia [SME]) a local network of police, fire, and medical personnel trained to respond to emergency situations. In many communities, the system is activated by calling 911 (Ch. 8).

empathy (empatía) ability to be objectively aware of and have insight into another's feelings, emotions, and behaviors, and to be aware of the significance and meaning of these to the other person (Ch. 1).

EMR (RME) see electronic medical record (Ch. 10).

encode (encoding) (codificar [codificación]) creating a message to be sent (Ch. 4).

encounter form (formulario de visita) formerly known as a charge slip or superbill. A copy of the encounter form is given to the patient after seeing the provider. It identifies the procedures performed, diagnoses, charges, and when to return (Ch. 17, 18).

encryption (cifrado) the process of coding email to render the transmission essentially secure (Ch. 11).

encryption technology (tecnología de cifrado) converts information into code; used to protect privacy and confidentiality of individuals in computer software (Ch. 12).

enunciation (dicción) speaking clearly; articulating (Ch. 11).

epinephrine (epinefrina) used to treat allergic reactions (Ch. 9); also known as adrenaline.

episodic stress (tensión episódica) occurs when individuals take on too many tasks, becoming overwhelmed by all of the demands, and are unable to satisfy all of the demands (Ch. 3).

e-résumé (curriculum vitae electrónico) electronic résumés may be delivered electronically via email, submitted to Internet job boards, or placed on Web pages (Ch. 24).

ergonomics (ergonomía) scientific study of work and space, including factors that influence worker productivity and that affect workers' health (Ch. 10).

Ethernet (Ethernet) references the networking of computers using metallic conductors or hard wires (Ch. 10).

ethics (ética) defined in terms of what is morally right and wrong; ethics will differ from person to person; often defined by a code or creed as in the Code of Ethics from the American Association of Medical Assistants (AAMA) (Ch. 7).

euthanasia (la eutanasia) causing death of someone who is suffering from an incurable and painful disease or who is in an irreversible coma (Ch. 7).

exclusion (exclusión) specific disease or condition listed in an insurance policy for which the policy will not pay (Ch. 16).

exclusive provider organization (EPO) (organización de proveedor exclusivo [EPO]) a closed-panel preferred organization (PPO) plan where enrollees receive no benefits if they opt to receive care from a provider who is not in the EPO (Ch. 16).

exit interview (entrevista de salida) opportunity for departing employees to provide their positive and negative opinions of the position and facility (Ch. 22).

expert witness (testigo experto) individual with highly specialized knowledge and skills in a particular area who testifies to a standard of care (Ch. 6).

explanation of benefits (EOB) (explicación de beneficios [EDB]) insurance report that is sent with claim payments explaining the reimbursement of the insurance carrier (Ch. 16, 17).

explicit (explícito) fully revealed or expressed without ambiguity or vagueness, leaving no question as to intent (Ch. 8).

expressed consent (consentimiento expreso) permission given either verbally or in writing (Ch 6).

expressed contract (contrato explícito) written or verbal contract that specifically describes what each party in the contract will do (Ch. 6).

externship (práctica laboral) transition stage between the classroom and actual employment; may also be referred to as internship or practicum (Ch. 1).

facilitate (facilitar) to make an action or process easier (Ch. 1).

Fair Debt Collection Practice Act (FDCPA) (Ley sobre Prácticas Justas para el Cobro de Deudas) 1977 federal law that outlines collection practices (Ch. 19).

fax (facsimile) (fax [facsímilx]) machine that sends documents from one location to another by way of telephone lines (Ch. 11).

felony (delito mayor) a serious crime such as murder, larceny (thefts of large sums of money), assault, and rape (Ch. 6).

female genital mutilation (FGM) (mutilación genital femenina) Partial or complete removal of the clitoris; partial or total removal of the labia minora and/or labia majora; narrowing the vaginal opening by creating a covering seal; and the pricking, piercing, or cauterizing of genitals (Ch. 7).

financial accounting (contabilidad financiera) provides information primarily for entities external to the organization such as the government (Ch. 20).

firewall (cortafuegos) hardware device or software program designed to prevent unauthorized access to a computer system (Ch. 10).

first aid (primeros auxilios) immediate (or first) care provided to persons who are suddenly ill or injured; first aid is typically followed by more comprehensive care and treatment (Ch. 8).

fiscal intermediary (intermediario fiscal) local administrator for Medicare (Ch. 16).

fixed cost (costo fijo) cost that does not vary in total as the number of patients vary (Ch. 20).

flag (indicador de mensaje) method of identifying a blank space or a question regarding dictator's meaning by attaching a note or marker to indicate the question (Ch. 15).

form letter (carta tipo) letter containing the same content in the body but sent to different individuals (Ch. 14).

fracture (fractura) break in a bone. There are several types of fractures, but all are classified as either open or closed fractures (Ch. 8).

fraud (fraude) deliberate misrepresentation of facts (Ch. 16).

fringe benefits (beneficio complementario) benefits above and beyond salary to which an employee may be entitled. Examples include health and life insurance, paid vacation, sick days, personal days, and tuition reimbursement for courses related to employment (Ch. 21).

full block letter (carta de bloque completo) major letter style in which all lines begin flush with the left margin. This style is suggested for offices desiring a contemporary-looking, efficient letter (Ch. 14).

functional résumé (curriculum vitae funcional) résumé format used to highlight specialty areas of accomplishment and strengths (Ch. 24).

Generation X (Generación X) individuals born from 1966 to 1976 (Ch. 22).

Generation Y (Generación Y) Individuals born from 1977 to 1994; also known as the Millennial generation (Ch. 22).

Generation Z (Generación Z) Individuals born from 1995 to 2012 (Ch. 22).

genetic engineering (ingeniería genética) alteration, manipulation, replacement, or repair of genetic material (Ch. 7).

goal (meta) result or achievement toward which effort is directed (Ch. 3).

"going bare" ("estar desprotegido") said of a provider who does not carry professional liability insurance (Ch. 21).

Good Samaritan laws (leyes del Buen Samaritano) laws designed to protect individuals from legal action when rendering emergency medical aid, without compensation, within the areas of their training and expertise (Ch. 8, 11).

gross examination (examen macroscópico) viewing specimens with the naked eye (Ch. 15).

guarantor (garante) the person identified as responsible for payment of the bill (Ch. 18).

hardware (hardware) physical equipment used by the computer system to process data (Ch. 10).

headline (titular) The words or phrases used in a profile that promote qualifications and skills that distinguish an application from others (Ch. 24).

Healthcare Common Procedure Coding System (HCPCS) (Sistema de Códigos de Procedimientos Comunes de la Atención Médica [HCPCS]) a coding system consisting of the CPT, national codes (level II), and local codes (level III); previously known as HCFA Common Procedure Coding System (Ch. 17).

health care directive (directiva salud) A document that allows a patient to appoint an agent to make health care decisions in the event the patient is unable to do so (Ch. 5).

Health Insurance Portability and Accountability Act (HIPAA) (Ley de Portabilidad y Responsabilidad de Seguros de Salud [HIPAA]) government rules, regulations, and procedures resulting from legislation designed to protect the confidentiality of patient information (Ch. 6, 15).

health maintenance organization (HMO) (organización de mantenimiento de la salud [HMO]) type of managed care operation that is typically set up as a for-profit corporation with salaried employees. HMOs "with walls" offer a range of medical services under one roof; HMOs "without walls" typically contract with providers in the community to provide patient services for an agreed-upon fee (Ch. 2, 16).

HIC number (número HIC) The identification number of a Medicare beneficiary issued by CMS or the RRB (Ch. 16).

Hierarchy of Needs (jerarquía de necesidades) needs that are arranged in a specific order or rank; sequential arrangement. Associated with Abraham Maslow (Ch. 4).

high-context communication (comunicación de alto contexto) communication style that involves great reliance on body language, reference to objects in the environment, and culturally relevant phraseology to convey an idea. Relies on the listener knowing related events through close association with the speaker or culture (Ch. 4).

history and physical examination report (H&P) (informe de historia clínicay examen físico [H&P]) report of patient's history and physical examination to document reason for visit (Ch. 15).

history of the present illness (HPI) (antecedentes de enfermedad actual [AEA]) the chronologic description of the development of the patient's illness (Ch. 15).

homeopathy (homeopatía) a healing modality that uses diluted doses of certain substances to create an "energy imprint" in the body to bring about a cure (Ch. 2).

hospital outpatient prospective payment system (OPPS) (sistema de pago prospectivo de hospital para pacientes ambulatorios) A system that classifies all hospital outpatient services into Ambulatory Payment Classifications for reimbursement (Ch. 16).

hyperglycemia (hiperglucemia) increased levels of blood glucose. Hyperglycemia does not necessarily mean that the patient is diabetic but may be an indication of prediabetes (Ch. 8).

hyperthyroidism (hipertiroidismo) an overactive thyroid gland which causes an increase in thyroid hormone being released.

hypoglycemia (hipoglucemia) state of having a lower than normal blood glucose level (Ch. 8).

hypothermia (hipotermia) extremely dangerous cold-related condition that can result in death if the individual does not receive care and if the progression of hypothermia is not reversed. Symptoms include shivering, cold skin, and confusion (Ch. 8).

hypothyroidism (hipotiroidismo) an underactive thyroid gland which causes a decrease in thyroid hormone being released.

hypovolemic (hipovolémico) a type of shock in which the body has lost blood or fluid volume to such an extent that there is not enough circulating volume to fill the ventricles. The heart attempts to compensate by increasing the heart rate (Ch. 8).

hypoxia (hypoxia) oxygen deficiency (Ch. 8).

implicit (implícito) capable of being understood from something else though unexpressed; implied (Ch. 8).

implied consent (consentimiento implícito) consent assumed by the health care provider, typically in an emergency that threatens the patient's life. Implied consent also occurs in more subtle ways in the health care environment; for example, when a patient willingly rolls up the sleeve to receive an injection (Ch. 6).

implied contract (contrato implícito) contract indicated by actions rather than words (Ch. 6).

improvise (improvisar) to make, invent, or arrange in an unplanned or spontaneous manner (Ch. 1).

incision (incisión) a surgical cut made into the skin or tissue (Ch. 8).

income statement (estado de resultados) financial statement showing net profit or loss (Ch. 20).

incompetence (incompetencia) a legal term indicating a person who is not able to manage his/her affairs due to a low I.Q., mental deterioration, illness or psychosis, or it may sometimes indicate physical disability (Ch. 6).

independent provider association (IPA) (Asociación Independiente de Médicos [IPA]) independent network of physicians in private practice who contract with the association to treat patients for an agreed-upon fee (Ch. 2, 16).

indexing (indexar) selecting the name, subject, or number under which to file a record and determining the order in which the units should be considered (Ch. 13).

indirect statements (declaraciones indirectas) means of eliciting a response from a patient by turning a question into a statement of interest (Ch. 4).

informed consent (consentimiento informado) consent given by the patient who is made aware of any procedure to be performed, its risks, expected outcomes, and alternatives (Ch. 6).

inner-directed people (personas con autodeterminación) people who decide for themselves what they want to do with their lives (Ch. 3).

input device (dispositivo de entrada) a device used to input data into a computer (Ch. 10).

integrated delivery system (IDS) (sistema de prestación de servicios médicos integrado [IDS]) a health care organization of affiliated provider sites combined under a single ownership that offers the full spectrum of managed health care (Ch. 16).

integrative medicine (medicina integradora) brings together two or more treatment modalities so they function as a harmonious whole, as seen in alternative forms of health care (Ch. 2).

***International Classification of Diseases, 9th Revision, Clinical Modification* (ICD-9-CM) (Clasificación Internacional de Enfermedades, 9.ª Revisión, Modificación Clínica [CIE-9-MC])** standard diagnosis codes used to identify a patient's medical problem. Used by most ambulatory care settings in encoding the claim form and recognized by most insurance carriers (Ch. 17).

***International Classification of Diseases, 10th Revision, Clinical Modification* (ICD-10-CM) (Clasificación Internacional de Enfermedades, 10.ª Revisión, Modificación Clínica [CIE-10-MC])** a classification system developed by the National Center for Health Statistics (NCHS) as a clinical modification to the ICD-10 system developed by the World Health Organization (WHO), primarily as a unique system for use in the United States for morbidity and mortality reporting (Ch. 17).

***International Classification of Diseases, 10th Revision, Procedure Coding System* (ICD-10-PCS) (Clasificación Internacional de Enfermedades, 10.ª Revisión, sistema de codificación de procedimiento)** developed by the United States as mandated by the Health Insurance Portability and Accountability Act for reporting inpatient procedures (Ch. 17).

Internet (Internet) a worldwide publicly accessible network of networks and computers (Ch. 10).

Internet blog (blogs de Internet) A Web site or web page updated regularly by one person or a small group. It is often written in conversational style and discusses one or more specific topics. The blog is usually interactive, allowing visitors to leave comments (Ch. 24).

internship (pasantía) transition stage between classroom and employment (Ch. 1).

interrogatory (interrogatorio) a written set of questions that must be answered, under oath, within a specific time period; part of the discovery process (Ch. 6).

interview (entrevista) meeting in which you and the interviewer discuss employment opportunities and strengths you can contribute to the organization (Ch. 24).

intimate partner violence (IPV) (violencia de pareja [IPV]) refers to violence or abuse between a spouse or former spouse; boyfriend, girlfriend or former boyfriend/girlfriend; and same-sex or heterosexual intimate partner or former same-sex or heterosexual intimate partner (Ch. 6, 7).

in vitro fertilization (IVF) (fertilización in vitro [IVF]) the ovum is fertilized in a culture dish, allowed to grow, and then implanted into the uterus (Ch. 7).

involuntary dismissals (despido involuntario) termination of employment based on poor job performance or violation of office policies (Ch. 22).

itinerary (itinerario) detailed written plan of a proposed trip (Ch. 21).

jargon (jerga) words, phrases, or terminology specific to a profession (Ch. 11).

ketoacidosis (cetoacidosis) accumulation of ketones in the body, occurring primarily as a complication of diabetes mellitus; if left untreated, it could cause a coma (Ch. 8).

key (keyed) (mecanografiar) to input data by keystrokes on a computer keyboard (Ch. 14).

key unit (unidad clave) first indexing unit of the filing segment (Ch. 13).

keywords (palabras clave) words that relate to a job-specific position. Keywords may be job-specific skills or profession-specific words (Ch. 24).

kinesics (cinésica) study of body language (Ch. 4).

laceration (laceración) tears or splits in the skin or tissues caused by trauma (Ch. 8).

ledger (libro mayor) record of charges, payments, and adjustments for individual patient or family (Ch. 18).

letter of resignation (carta de renuncia) letter informing the current employer of the employee's decision to resign from a current position (Ch. 22).

LGBT (LGBT) common abbreviation to refer to individuals who are lesbian, gay, bisexual, or transgender (Ch. 22).

liability (pasivo) debts and financial obligations for which one is responsible (Ch. 20); legal responsibility (Ch. 21).

libel (calumnia) false and malicious writing about another constituting a defamation of character (Ch. 6).

license (licencia) permission by competent authority (the state) to engage in a profession; permission to act (Ch. 1); permission statement authorizing the use of copyrighted computer software (Ch. 10).

licensure (matrícula) granting of licenses to practice a profession (Ch. 1).

limiting charge (limitación de carga) The dollar amount up to 115% of the Medicare allowed amount that can be charged to the patient by a Medicare non-PAR provider (Ch. 16).

litigation (litigio) court action (Ch. 6).

long-range goals (metas a largo plazo) achievements that may take three to five years to accomplish (Ch. 3).

low-context communication (comunicación de bajo contexto) communication style that uses few environmental or cultural idioms to convey an idea or concept. Ideas are spelled out explicitly (Ch. 4).

macroallocation (macroasignación) of scarce medical resources; decisions are made by Congress, health systems agencies, and insurance companies (Ch. 7).

major medical (médicos mayores) Insurance that covers catastrophic expenses resulting from illness or injury (Ch. 16).

malfeasance (fechoría) conduct that is illegal or contrary to an official's obligations (Ch. 6).

malpractice (mala praxis) professional negligence (Ch. 6, 21).

managed care operation (establecimiento de atención administrada) any health care setting or delivery system that is designed to reduce the cost of care while still providing access to care (Ch. 2).

managed care organization (MCO) (organización de atención administrada [MCO]) a health insurance organization that adheres to the principles of strong dependence on selective contracting with providers, the use of primary care physicians, prospective and retrospective utilization management, use of treatment guidelines for high cost chronic disorders, and an emphasis on preventive care, education, and patient compliance with treatment plans (Ch. 16).

management by walking around (MBWA) (gestión itinerante [MBWA]) a technique for keeping managers informed about the health of their organization (Ch. 21).

managerial accounting (contabilidad administrativa) generates financial information that can enable more efficient internal management (Ch. 20).

marketing (comercialización) process by which the provider of services makes the consumer aware of the scope and quality of those services. Marketing tools might include public relations, brochures, patient education seminars, and newsletters (Ch. 21).

masking (ocultamiento) attempt to conceal or repress true feelings or the message (Ch. 4).

matrix (matriz) to establish an appointment matrix, a provider's unavailable time slots are marked with an *X*. Patients are not scheduled during those times (Ch. 12).

mature minor (menor maduro) a person, usually younger than 18 years, who is able to understand and appreciate the consequences of treatment despite his or her young age (Ch. 6).

meaningful use (uso significativo) a Centers for Medicare and Medicaid (CMS) program that awards incentives for using certified electronic health records (EHR) to improve patient care (Ch. 13).

mediation (mediación) dispute resolution that allows a facilitator to help the two parties settle their differences and come to an acceptable solution (Ch. 6).

medical necessity (necesidad médica) the likelihood that a proposed health care service will have a reasonable beneficial effect on the patient's physical condition and quality of life at a specific point in his or her illness or lifetime. The concept that procedures are eligible for reimbursement only as a covered benefit when they are performed for a specific diagnosis or specified frequency (Ch. 17).

medical transcriptionist (transcriptor médico) A specialist that listens to voice recordings dictated by health care providers and create medical records in the proper format for the type of document (Ch. 15).

medically indigent (médicamente indigente) refers to those individuals unable to pay for their own medical coverage (Ch. 6).

Medicare Part A (Medicare Parte A) benefits covering inpatient hospital and skilled nursing facilities, hospice care, and blood transfusion (Ch. 16).

Medicare Part B (Medicare Parte B) benefits covering outpatient hospital and health care provider services (Ch. 16).

Medicare Part C (Medicare Parte C) commonly referred to as Medicare advantage plans. These plans are approved by Medicare and are run by private companies (Ch. 16).

Medicare Part D (Medicare Parte D) prescription drug coverage by Medicare (Ch. 16).

Medigap policy (póliza de Medigap) an individual plan covering the patient's Medicare deductible and co-pay obligations that fulfills the federal government standards for Medicare supplemental insurance (Ch. 16).

memorandum (memorándum) interoffice correspondence, usually referred to as a memo (Ch. 14).

memory (memoria) refers to storage of computer data. Memory can be volatile (lost when computer is turned off) or nonvolatile (permanently written to storage device) (Ch. 10).

mentor (mentor) person assigned or requested to assist in training, guiding, or coaching another (Ch. 21).

mHealth (mHealth) a term that stands for mobile health, which refers to the practice of medicine supported by mobile devices (Ch. 11).

microallocation (microasignación) of scarce medical resources; decisions are made by providers and individual members of the health care team (Ch. 7).

microscopic examination (examen microscópico) viewing a specimen with the aid of a microscope (Ch. 15).

minor (menor) person who has not reached the age of majority, usually 18 years (Ch. 6).

minutes (actas) written record of topics discussed and actions taken during meeting sessions (Ch. 14, 21).

misdemeanor (contravención) a lesser crime; misdemeanors vary from state to state in their definition. Punishment is usually probation or a time of public service and a fine (Ch. 6).

misfeasance (irregularidad) a civil law term referring to a lawful act that is improperly or unlawfully executed (Ch. 6).

modified block letter, indented (carta estilo bloque modificado, con sangría) modified letter style with indented paragraphs. Paragraphs in this style of letter may be indented five spaces (Ch. 14).

modified block letter, standard (carta estilo bloque modificado, estándar) major letter style where all lines begin at the left margin with the exception of the date line, complimentary closure, and keyed signature. The exceptions usually begin at the center position or a few spaces to the right of center (Ch. 14).

modified wave scheduling (planificación en olas modificada) system where multiple patients are scheduled at the beginning of each hour, followed by single appointments every 10 to 20 minutes the rest of the hour (Ch. 12).

modifiers (modificador) additional codes that may be added to a five-digit CPT code to further explain the service provided (Ch. 17).

modulated (modulado) speech that varies in pitch and intensity (Ch. 11).

money market savings accounts (cuentas de ahorro del mercado monetario) bank accounts that pay a higher interest rate (money market rate) than standard savings accounts and permit writing a limited number of checks (Ch. 18).

morbidity (morbilidad) number of cases of disease in a specific population (Ch. 17).

mortality (mortalidad) the ratio of the number of deaths to a given population (Ch. 17).

motherboard (tarjeta madre) printed circuit containing the inner connections of a digital computer including the CPU, RAM and ROM memory, and other support systems. It provides connectivity to input and output systems (Ch. 10).

myocardial infarction (infarto de miocardio) a heart attack; usually caused by a blockage of one or more of the coronary arteries (Ch. 8).

National Healthcareer Association (NHA) (Asociación Nacional de Profesiones de Salud [NHA]) an association that offers national certification examinations for health care professionals. NHA works with educational institutions on curriculum development, competency testing, and preparation and administration of their examination for certification (Ch. 23).

navigator (navigator) works in conjunction with the medical home health care team (Ch. 4).

negligence (negligencia) failure to exercise a certain standard of care (Ch. 6, 21).

networking (conexión en red) connecting two or more computers together to share files and hardware. The system is called a network (Ch. 10); process in which people of similar interests exchange information in social, business, or professional relationships (Ch. 24).

neurogenic (neurogénico) a type of shock in which there is injury or trauma to the nervous system causing the loss of tone in the vessels resulting in massive dilation of arterioles and venuoles. This results in a dramatic drop in blood pressure (Ch. 8).

nomenclature systems (sistemas de nomenclatura) provide terms that follow preestablished naming conventions; a disease nomenclature is a listing of the proper name for each disease entity with its specific code number (Ch. 17).

noncompliant (inobservancia) describes one who fails to follow a required command or instruction (Ch. 6).

nonfeasance (omisión) a civil law term referring to the failure to perform an act, official duty, or legal requirement (Ch. 6).

nonretaliation provision (disposición de no represalias) provides protection to an employee or applicant from being retaliated against due to participation in filing a complaint regarding discrimination, or participating in an investigation or lawsuit (Ch. 21).

normal saline (solución salina normal) a solution of sodium chloride (salt) and distilled water. It has the same osmotic pressure as blood serum. It is also known as isotonic or physiologic saline (Ch. 8).

notary (notary public) (escribano público) someone with the legal capacity to witness and certify documents; can take depositions (Ch. 18).

occlusion (oclusión) closure of a passage (Ch. 8).

old reports (informes anteriores) reports such as a discharge summary that should be completed within 71 hours (Ch. 15).

open-ended questions (preguntas abiertas) questions that encourage verbalization and response; questions that seek a response beyond a simple yes or no (Ch. 4).

operating system (OS) (sistema operativo [SO]) software used to control the computer and its peripheral equipment. Also referred to as system software (Ch. 10).

operative report (OR) (informe quirúrgico [OR]) medical report that chronicles the details of a surgical procedure (Ch. 15).

optical character recognition (OCR) (reconocimiento óptico de caracteres) U.S. Postal Service's computerized scanner that reads addresses printed on letter mail. If the information is properly formatted, then the OCR will find a match in its address files and print a bar code on the lower right edge of the envelope (Ch. 14).

outer-directed people (personas influenciables) people who let events, other people, or environmental factors dictate their behavior (Ch. 3).

out guide or sheet (señalador o marcador) card, folder, or slip of paper inserted temporarily in the files to replace a record that has been retrieved from the files (Ch. 13).

output device (dispositivo de salida) a device used to output data from a computer. Includes printers, faxes, data storage drivers, screens, and plotters (Ch. 10).

outsourcing (subcontratación) the practice of contracting with a service outside of the clinic or hospital to a company where the task can be accomplished at a lower cost and with a faster turnaround time (Ch. 15).

overtime (horas extra) money paid at a rate of not less than one and one-half times the regular rate of pay after a 40-hour work week is completed (Ch. 22).

palliative (paliativa) refers to measures taken to relieve symptoms of disease (Ch. 5).

parasympathetic nervous system (sistema nervioso parasimpático) part of the autonomic nervous system that returns the body to its normal state after stress has subsided (Ch. 3).

participatory style operates on the premise that the worker is capable and wants to do a good job (Ch. 21).

patch (parche) modification to software to fix deficiencies in the software. Frequently downloaded from the software supplier's Web site or from floppy disks provided by the supplier (Ch. 10).

pathology report (informe de patología) medical reports generated to describe the gross and microscopic examinations performed during a surgical procedure (Ch. 15).

patient-centered medical home (PCMH) (hogar médico centrado en el paciente) a model of care that responds to each patient's unique needs through: (1) making a personal and coordinating physician available for care; (2) providing comprehensive care at all stages of life; (3) practicing culturally sensitive, integrated and coordinate care while focusing on quality and safety; and (4) enhancing patients' access to care. As of 2016, PCMH recognition and accreditation is not available in all states (Ch. 2).

patient portal system (sistema de portal del paciente) secure Web sites or applications combined with other software, such as an EMR, that allow patients to have convenient 24-hour access to interact and communicate with their health care providers (Ch. 11).

Patient Self-Determination Act (PSDA) (Ley de Autodeterminación del Paciente [PSDA]) the Act that includes the advance directive giving patients the right to be involved in their health care decisions (Ch. 6).

payee (beneficiario) person named on a check who is to receive the amount indicated (Ch. 18).

pegboard system (sistema de tablero de clavijas) most commonly used manual medical accounts receivable system (Ch. 18).

petty cash (caja chica) small sum kept on hand for minor or unexpected expenses (Ch. 18).

phishing (suplantación de identidad) a practice where the recipient of email is directed to go to a Web site to provide information to his or her bank, the IRS, or other official organization. The Web site is actually a fake made to resemble the real thing, and when information is given, it goes to the consumer fraud criminal (Ch. 10).

plaintiff (demandante) person bringing charges in litigation (Ch. 6).

point-of-service (POS) device (dispositivo de punto de servicio [POS]) device allowing direct communication between a medical office and the health care plan's computer (Ch. 17).

point-of-service (POS) plan (plan de punto de servicio [POS]) a plan that allows direct communication between a medical office and the health insurance company (Ch. 16).

portfolio (cartera) notebook or file containing examples of materials commonly used (Ch. 14).

posting (asiento) recording financial transactions into a bookkeeping or accounting system (Ch. 18).

practice-based scheduling (programación basada en la práctica) see cluster scheduling (Ch. 12).

practice management (prácticas de gestión) type of health care software, often intertwined with EMR and used in the day-to-day financial and administrative operations of a medical clinic (Ch. 10).

practicum (práctica) transitional stage providing opportunity to apply theory learned in the classroom to a health care setting through practical, hands-on experience (Ch. 1, 21).

preauthorization (autorización previa) obtaining an insurance carrier's consent to proceed with patient care and treatment. Unless authorization is obtained, insurance carriers may not pay benefits for specific problems (Ch. 16).

precedents (precedentes) refers to rulings made at an earlier time and include decisions made in a court, interpretations of a constitution, and statutory law decisions (Ch. 6).

preferred provider organization (PPO) (organización de proveedor preferido [PPO]) organization of providers who network together to offer discounts to purchasers of health care insurance (Ch. 2, 16).

prejudice (prejuicio) opinion or judgment that is formed before all the facts are known (Ch. 4).

prescribe (recetar) to order or recommend the use of a drug, diet, or other form of therapy (Ch. 6).

present problem (PP) (problema presente [PP]) see chief complaint (CC) (Ch. 15).

primary care provider (PCP) (médico de atención primaria [PCP]) primary care provider for a patient; all care is coordinated through the PCP (Ch. 16).

privileged (privilegiada) confidential information that may only be communicated with the patient's permission or by court order (Ch. 15).

probate court (tribunal sucesorio) court that administers estates and validates wills (Ch. 19).

probation (período de prueba) period during which the employee and supervisory personnel may determine if both the environment and the position are satisfactory for the employee (Ch. 22).

problem-oriented medical record (POMR) (historia clínica orientada al problema [POMR]) a type of patient chart recordkeeping that uses a sheet at a prominent location in the chart to list vital identification data. Patient medical problems are identified by a number that corresponds to the charting; for example, bronchitis is #1, a broken wrist is #2, and so forth (Ch. 13).

procedure manual (manual de procedimientos) manual providing detailed information relative to the performance of tasks within the job description (Ch. 21).

professionalism (profesionalismo) the qualities that characterize or distinguish a professional person who conforms to the technical and ethical standards of the profession (Ch. 1).

professional liability insurance (seguro de responsabilidad profesional) insurance policy designed to protect assets in the event a claim for damages resulting from negligence is filed and awarded (Ch. 21).

profile (perfil) a brief written description providing information describing your personality, qualifications, and skills for an employment position (Ch. 24).

profit sharing (participación en las ganancias) sharing in the financial profits, gains, and benefits of an organization (Ch. 21).

progress notes (notas de evolución) also called chart notes. Provider's formal or informal notes about presenting problem, physical findings, and plan for treatment for a patient examined in the office, clinic, acute care center, or emergency department (Ch. 15).

projection (proyección) act of placing one's own feelings on another (Ch. 4).

proofread (revisar) to read a document to verify the accuracy of content and that correct grammar, spelling, punctuation, and capitalization were used (Ch. 14).

proprietary (empresa de propiedad privada) privately owned and managed facility, a profit-making organization (Ch. 1).

puncture (punción) a wound caused by an object piercing the skin and underlying soft tissues that creates a small hole (Ch. 8).

purging (purga) method of maintaining order in files by separating active from inactive and closed files (Ch. 13).

quality assurance (QA) (aseguramiento de calidad [QA]) process to provide accurate, complete, consistent health care documentation in a timely manner while making every reasonable effort to resolve inconsistencies, inaccuracies, risk management issues, and other problems (Ch. 15).

RACE (RACE) an acronym that stands for Remove patients from area, activate Alarm, Contain the fire and smoke, and Extinguish if safe to do so (Ch. 9).

radiology and imaging reports (informes de radiología y de diagnóstico por imágenes) medical reports that describe the findings and interpretations of the radiologist (Ch. 15).

rationalization (racionalización) act of justification, usually illogically, that one uses to keep from facing the truth of the situation (Ch. 4).

reception (recepción) the area of a medical clinic where patients are received and greeted. It should never be referred to as a "waiting area" (Ch. 9).

recertification (nueva certificación) documentation submitted to support continued education for maintaining a professional credential (Ch. 23).

references (referencias) during the job application process, individuals who have known or worked with a person long enough to make an honest assessment and recommendation regarding the person's employment history (Ch. 24).

referral (remisión) term used by managed care facilities for authorization for someone other than the patient's primary care provider to treat the patient (Ch. 16).

Registered Medical Assistant (RMA [AMT]) (Asistente Médico Matriculado [RMA]) credential awarded for successfully passing the AMT examination (Ch. 1, 23).

Registered Medical Transcriptionist (RMT) (transcriptor médico registrado [RMT]) credential awarded following completion of a two-part certification examination administered by the Association for Healthcare Documentation Integrity (AHDI) (Ch. 15).

regression (regresión) moving back to a former stage to escape conflict or fear (Ch. 4).

remittance advice (aviso de pago) summarizes all of the benefits paid to a provider within a particular period of time; includes all of the patients covered by a specific insurance company for the time period (Ch. 16).

repression (represión) occurs when one copes with an overwhelming situation by temporarily forgetting it; temporary amnesia (Ch. 4).

rescue breathing (respiración de rescate) performed on individuals in respiratory arrest, rescue breathing is a mouth-to-mouth (using appropriate protective equipment) or mouth-to-nose procedure that provides oxygen to the patient until emergency personnel arrive (Ch. 8).

resource-based relative value scale (RBRVS) (escala de valores relativos basada en recursos [RBRVS]) basis for the Medicare fee schedule (Ch. 16).

résumé (curriculum vitae) written summary data sheet or brief account of qualifications and progress in your chosen career (Ch. 24).

review of systems (ROS) (revisión de sistemas [ROS]) inquires about the system directly related to the problems identified in the history of the present illness (Ch. 15).

risk management (gestión de riesgos) techniques adhered to in the ambulatory care setting that keep the practice, its environment, and its procedures as safe for the patient as possible. Proper risk management also reduces the possibility of negligence that leads to torts and malpractice suits (Ch. 6, 8, 15, 21).

roadblock (obstáculo) Any barrier that blocks therapeutic communication (Ch. 4).

salary review (revisión de salario) process by which the employee is informed of his or her revised base pay rate (Ch. 21).

scope of practice (ámbito de práctica) the range of clinical procedures and activities that are allowed by law for a profession (Ch. 1).

screening (prueba de detección) evaluating patient symptoms to determine emergent needs. Sometimes used to determine the next best course of action when assisting a provider in giving appropriate patient care (Ch. 11, 12).

Secure Sockets Layer (SSL) (capa de sockets seguros) a protocol designed to allow secure Web-based transfer of data using encryption (Ch. 10).

self-actualization (autorealización) being all that you can be; developing your full potential and experiencing fulfillment (Ch. 3, 21).

self-insurance (autoseguro) insurance carried by large companies, nonprofit organizations, and government to reduce costs and gain more control of their finances. Each plan differs in coverage and claim filing requirements (Ch. 16).

septic (sepsis) Overwhelming infection that occurs most often in critically ill patients. Chemicals are released into the bloodstream that cause vasodilatation and other organic products that are harmful to the organs and tissues. The vasodilation and decreased ability of the cells and tissues to utilize oxygen is the basis for this type of shock (Ch. 8).

server (servidor) computer with massive hard drive capacity that is used to link other computers together so that data can be shared by multiple users. A computer system in an ambulatory care facility is likely to be linked or networked with a central server (Ch. 10).

shadow (aprendizaje por observación) follow a supervisor or delegated subordinate to learn facility protocol (Ch. 21).

shock (shock) potentially serious condition in which the circulatory system is not providing enough blood to all parts of the body, causing the body's organs to fail to function properly (Ch. 8).

short-range goals (metas a corto plazo) created when long-range goals are dissected and reassembled into smaller, more manageable time segments (Ch. 3).

simplified letter (carta simplificada) major letter style recommended by the Administrative Management Society that omits the salutation and complimentary closure. All lines are keyed flush with the left margin. In medical offices, this style is most often used when sending a form letter (Ch. 14).

slander (calumnia) false and malicious words about another constituting a defamation of character (Ch. 6).

smartphone (teléfono inteligente) a mobile device that is used as a phone and has many functionalities of a computer (Ch. 11).

SOAP/SOAPI/SOAPER/SOAPIER a form of medical documentation that includes all or a portion of the following:

- **S** Subjective data; patient's complaint in his or her own words
- **O** Objective, observable, measurable findings
- **A** Assessment, probable diagnosis based on subjective and objective factors
- **P** Plan for treatment, medications, instructions, return visit information
- **I** Implementation, or how the actions were carried out
- **E** Education for the patient
- **R** Response of patient to education and care given or Revision of the plan (Ch. 13).

social media (medios sociales) forms of electronic communication such as Web sites or blogs that enable users to share content or to participate in social networking, sharing ideas, and personal messages (Ch. 21, 24).

source-oriented medical record (SOMR) (historia clínica orientada a la fuente [SOMR]) a type of patient chart record-keeping that includes separate sections for different sources of patient information, such as laboratory reports, pathology reports, and progress notes (Ch. 13).

splint (férula) any device used to immobilize a body part. Often used by EMS personnel (Ch. 8).

sprain (esguince) injury to a joint, often an ankle, knee, or wrist, that involves a tearing of the ligaments. Most sprains are minor and heal quickly; others are more severe, include swelling, and may not heal properly if the patient continues to put stress on the affected joint (Ch. 8).

Standard Precautions (Precauciones Estándar) precautions developed in 1996 by the Centers for Disease Control and Prevention (CDC) that augment Universal Precautions and body substance isolation practices. They provide a wider range of protection and are used any time there is contact with blood, moist body fluid (except perspiration), mucous membranes, or nonintact skin. They are designed to protect all health care providers, patients, and visitors (Ch. 8).

stat report (informe de tendencia) a medical report requested of medical transcription that should be returned within 2-4 hours (Ch. 15).

status epilepticus (estado epiléptico) a continuous seizure that is prolonged, or two or more seizures without a recovery period between them. Status epilepticus is associated with significant morbidity and mortality (Ch. 8).

statute of limitations (ley de prescripción) statute that defines the period in which legal action can take place (Ch. 19).

statutory law (derecho estatutario) refers to the body of laws established by states (Ch. 6).

strain (distensión) injury to the soft tissue between joints that involves the tearing of muscles or tendons. Strains often occur in the neck, back, and thigh muscles (Ch. 8).

stream scheduling (programación ininterrumpida) system where patients are seen on a continuous basis throughout the day (e.g., at 15-, 30-, or 60-minute intervals), with each patient having a distinct appointment time (Ch. 12).

stress (estrés) body's response to change; can be manifested in a variety of ways, including changes in blood pressure, changes in heart rate, and onset of headache (Ch. 3).

stressors (factores estresantes) demands to change that cause stress (Ch. 3).

sublimation (sublimación) occurs when a socially unacceptable impulse is redirected into one that is socially acceptable (Ch. 4).

subordinates (subordinado) in an organization, people under the direction of (reporting to) a person of greater authority (Ch. 21).

subpoena (citación) written command designating a person to appear in court under penalty for failure to appear (Ch. 6).

subscriber (suscriptor) A term used by some insurance plans to describe the policyholder or insured (Ch. 16).

superbill (superbill) see encounter form (Ch. 17).

suppression (supresión) occurs when one deliberately refuses to acknowledge something that causes mental pain or suffering (Ch. 4).

surge protection (protección contra sobretensiones) protection of the fragile electronics from spikes in electrical voltage that occur on electric distribution lines (Ch. 10).

surrogate (sustituto) substitute; someone who substitutes for another (Ch. 7).

symbols (símbolos) instructional guides assisting with the coding process (Ch. 17).

sympathetic nervous system (sistema nervioso simpático) large part of the autonomic nervous system that prepares the body for fight or flight (Ch. 3).

syncope (síncope) fainting (Ch. 8).

system software (software de sistema) see operating system (Ch. 10).

targeted résumé (curriculum vitae dirigido al objetivo) résumé format utilized when focusing on a clear, specific job target (Ch. 24).

teamwork (trabajo en equipo) persons synergistically working together (Ch. 21).

telemedicine (telemedicina) the remote delivery of health care by means of telecommunication (Ch. 11).

therapeutic communication (comunicación terapéutica) use of specific and well-defined professional communication skills to create a feeling of comfort for patients even when difficult or unpleasant information must be exchanged (Ch. 4).

tickler file (archivo de recordatorios) system to remind of action to be taken on a certain date (Ch. 13).

time focus (enfoque en el tiempo) defines the period of time that is important and to which an individual's actions are directed or oriented (Ch. 4).

tonic-clonic phase (fase tónico clónica) muscular stiffening followed by the rapid and rhythmic jerking of the extremities during a seizure (Ch. 8).

tort (agravio) wrongful act that results in injury to one person by another (Ch. 6).

tort law (derecho de responsabilidad civil) law that stems from torts, or wrongful acts that cause harm to one person, by another (Ch. 6).

tourniquet (torniquete) device used to facilitate vein prominence (Ch. 8).

traditional indemnity insurance (seguro de responsabilidad civil tradicional) A type of insurance that provides coverage on a fee-for-service basis (FFS). There is usually a deductible and a co-payment or co-insurance (Ch. 16).

transferable skills (habilidades transferibles) skills that would be used in a host of different and unrelated occupations. Keyboarding skill is an example of a transferable skill. It could be used by a secretary, data entry clerk, medical assistant, or clothing manufacturer (Ch. 24).

triage (triage) screening to determine which patient is treated first when two or more patients present with emergencies simultaneously (Ch. 8).

trial balance (saldo de comprobación) created by totaling debit balances and credit balances to confirm that total debits equal total credits (Ch. 20).

TRICARE (TRICARE) formerly the Civilian Health and Medical Program for Uniformed Services (CHAMPUS). TRICARE offers HMO, PPO, and fee-for-service medical insurance for dependents of active duty and retired military personnel and dependents of personnel who died while on active duty (Ch. 16).

triple option plan (plan de opción triple) a managed care model allowing enrollees the option of traditional, HMO, or PPO health plans (Ch. 16).

Truth-in-Lending Act (Ley de Veracidad en los Préstamos) also known as the Consumer Credit Protection Act of 1968; an act requiring providers of installment credit to state the charges in writing and to express the interest as an annual rate (Ch. 19).

tubal ligation (ligadura de trompas) female surgical sterilization procedure that severs and seals the female fallopian tubes (Ch 7).

turnaround time (TAT) (plazo de entrega) specific time limit established for completion of medical reports (Ch. 15).

ulcer (úlceras) gradual disturbance of the skin and underlying tissues due to an underlying process; for example, prolonged pressure that interrupts tissue oxygenation or the pressure that occurs from increased venous pressure in vascular disease (Ch. 8).

unbundling (desagregación) refers to separating the components of a procedure and reporting them as billable codes with charges to increase reimbursement rates (Ch. 17).

undoing (reparación) partaking in actions designed to make amends to cancel out inappropriate behavior (Ch. 4).

Uniform Bill 04 (UB04) (Factura Uniforme 04 [UB04]) unique billing form used extensively by acute care facilities for processing inpatient and outpatient claims (Ch. 17).

URL (uniform resource locater) (localizador uniforme de recursos [URL]) the address that defines the route to a file on the Web or any other Internet facility (Ch. 11).

unit (unidad) each part of a name (business or person), words, or numbers that will be indexed and coded for filing (Ch. 13).

universal emergency medical identification symbol (símbolo universal de identificación médica para emergencias) identification sometimes carried by individuals to identify health problems they have (Ch. 8).

up-coding (sobrecodificación) also known as code creep, overcoding, and overbilling. Up-coding occurs when the insurance carrier deliberately bills a higher rate service than what was performed to obtain greater reimbursements (Ch. 17).

usual, customary, and reasonable (UCR) (usual, acostumbrado y razonable [UCR]) fee schedule often used by Medicare and some insurance carriers. *Usual* refers to the fee typically charged by a provider for certain procedures; *customary* is based on the average charge for a specific procedure by all providers practicing the same specialty in a defined geographic region; and *reasonable* refers to the mid-range of fees charged for this procedure (Ch. 16).

utilization review (UR) (revisión de utilización [RU]) review of medical services to determine they are necessary before they can be performed (Ch. 20).

variable cost (costo variable) cost that varies in direct proportion to volume (Ch. 20).

vasectomy (vasectomía) male surgical sterilization procedure that severs and cuts each vas deferens (Ch. 7).

Voice over Internet Protocol (VoIP) (protocolo de voz por Internet [VoIP]) the real-time transmission of voice signals over the Internet or Internet Protocol (IP) network (Ch. 11).

voice recognition software (VRS) (software de reconocimiento de voz) software that translates voice commands and is used in place of a mouse and keyboard (Ch. 15).

voucher check (cheque con comprobante) check with detachable form used to detail reason check is drawn; commonly used for payroll checks (Ch. 18).

watermark (sello de agua) design incorporated in paper during the papermaking process that is visible when the paper is held up to the light (Ch. 14).

wave scheduling (planificación en olas) system where patients are scheduled for the first half hour of every hour and then are seen throughout the hour (Ch. 12).

Workers' Compensation insurance (seguro de indemnización por accidentes de trabajo) medical and paycheck insurance for workers who sustain injuries associated with their employment (Ch. 16).

work statement (declaración de trabajo) concise description of the work you plan to accomplish (Ch. 21).

wound (herida) a break in the continuity of soft parts of body structures caused by violence or trauma to tissues. In an open wound, skin is broken, as in a laceration, abrasion, avulsion, or incision. In a closed wound, skin is not broken, as in contusion, ecchymosis, or hematoma (Ch. 8).

ZIP+4 (ZIP+4) standard zip code plus four additional digits that identify a postal delivery area. Mail will be processed more efficiently and effectively with the use of the ZIP+4 code in the address (Ch. 14).

REFERENCES/BIBLIOGRAPHY

GENERAL REFERENCES

Acello, B., & Hegner, B. R. (2016). *Nursing assistant: A nursing process approach* (11th ed.). Clifton Park, NY: Cengage Learning.

Altman, G. B. (2004). *Delmar's fundamentals and advanced nursing skills* (2nd ed.). Clifton Park, NY: Cengage Learning.

Blesi, M. (2017). *Medical assisting: Administrative and clinical competencies* (8th ed.). Clifton Park, NY: Cengage Learning.

Delaune, S. C., & Ladner, P. K (2011). *Fundamentals of nursing standards and practice* (4th ed.). Clifton Park, NY: Cengage Learning.

French, L. L. (2018). *Administrative medical assisting* (8th ed.). Clifton Park, NY: Cengage Learning.

Green, M. A. (2016). *3-2-1 Code It!* (5th ed.) Clifton Park, NY: Cengage Learning.

Ingenix. (2003). *HIPAA tool kit.* Salt Lake City, UT: St. Anthony's Publishing/Medicode.

Josephson, D. L. (2004). *Intravenous infusion therapy for nurses: Principles and practices* (2nd ed.). Clifton Park, NY: Cengage Learning.

Krager, D., & Krager, C. (2005). *HIPAA for medical clinic personnel.* Clifton Park, NY: Cengage Learning.

Lewis, M. A., Tamparo, C. D., & Tatro, B. (2012). *Medical law, ethics, and bioethics for health professions* (7th ed.). Philadelphia: F. A. Davis.

Moisio, M. A. (2014). *A guide to health insurance billing* (4th ed.). Clifton Park, NY: Cengage Learning.

Rice, J. (2017). *Principles of pharmacology for medical assisting* (6th ed.). Clifton Park, NY: Cengage Learning.

Simmers, L. (2014). *DHO health science* (8th ed.). Clifton Park, NY: Cengage Learning.

Spratto, G. R., & Woods, A. L. (2016). *PDR nurse's drug handbook.* Clifton Park, NY: Delmar Cengage Learning.

Tamparo, C. D. (2016). *Diseases of the human body* (6th ed.). Philadelphia: F. A. Davis.

Tamparo, C. D., & Lindh, W. Q. (2017). *Therapeutic communications for health care professionals.* (4th ed.) Clifton Park, NY: Cengage Learning.

Venes, D. (2013). *Taber's cyclopedic medical dictionary* (22nd ed.). Philadelphia: F. A. Davis.

Walters, N. J., Estridge, B. H., & Reynold, A. P. (2012). *Basic Clinical Laboratory Techniques* (6th ed.) Clifton Park, NY: Cengage Learning.

SECTION I: GENERAL PROCEDURES

UNIT I: INTRODUCTION TO MEDICAL ASSISTING AND HEALTH PROFESSIONS

Chapter 1: The Medical Assisting Profession

American Association of Medical Assistants. http://www.aama-ntl.org

American Medical Technologists. http://www.americanmedtech.org

Balasa, D. (2000, January/February). Securing the future for medical assistants to practice. Professional Medical Assistant, 6–7.

Balasa, D. (2003). Vigilance is key to protecting practice rights. CMA Today, 36(4). Retrieved May 4, 2016 from http://www.aama-ntl.org/cmatoday/archives

Balasa, D. (2005). CARE bill gains momentum in Congress. CMA Today, 38(4). http://www.aama-ntl.org/cmatoday/archives

Balasa, D. (2012). Frequent questions about medical assistant's scope of practice. CMA Today, 45(2). http://www.aama-ntl.org/CMAToday/archives/publicaffairs/details.aspx?ArticleID=886

Bureau of Labor Statistics, Occupational Employment Statistics. Medical assistants. Retrieved May 10, 2016 from http://www.bls.gov/oes/current/oes319092.htm

Carli, L. L., LaFleur, S. J., Loeber, C. C., Connell, F., & Geiser, R. (1995). Nonverbal behavior, gender, and influence. Journal of Personality and Social Psychology, 68(6), 1030–1041.

Congress.gov. H.R.1146: Consistency, Accuracy, Responsibility, and Excellence in Medical Imaging and Radiation Therapy Act of 2013. Retrieved May 12, 2016 from https://www.congress.gov/bill/113th-congress/house-bill/1146/all-actions?overview=closed

McCarty, M. (2003, March). The lawful scope of a medical assistant's practice. AMT Events. http://hws.hrsa.gov/default.aspx? category=Auxiliary+Health&occu=Medical+Assistants http://www.bls.gov/oco/ocos164.htm
National Healthcareer Association. http://www.nhanow.com

Chapter 2: Health Care Settings and the Health Care Team

American Board of Medical Specialties & Subspecialties. (2016). Approved ABMS specialty & subspecialty certificates. http://www.abms.org/
Commonwealth Fund. (2015, August). Primary care providers' views of recent trends in health care delivery and payment. http://www.commonwealthfund.org/publications/issue-briefs/2015/aug/primary-care-providers-views-delivery-payment
National Center for Complementary and Integrative Health. (2010). Credentialing: Understanding the education, training, regulation, and licensing of complementary health practitioners. http://nccam.nih.gov/health/decisions/credentialing.htm
Creswell, J. (2014). Race is on to profit from rise of urgent care. New York Times Business Day. http://www.nytimes.com/2014/07/10/business/race-is-on-to-profit-from-rise-of-urgent-care.html?_r=0
American Medical Association. (2013). Health care careers directory, 20129–20130. Chicago: Author.
Miles, C. J. (2014, June). Concierge medicine: An alternative to insurance. Association of Mature American Citizens. http://amac.us/concierge-medicine-alternative-insurance/
National Committee for Quality Assurance (NCQA). The future of patient-centered medical homes: Foundation for a better health care system. http://www.ncqa.org/Portals/0/Public%20Policy/2014%20Comment%20Letters/The_Future_of_PCMH.pdf
Urgent Care Association of America. (2015). Industry FAQs. http://www.ucaoa.org/?page=IndustryFAQs

UNIT II: THE THERAPEUTIC APPROACH

Chapter 3: Coping Skills for the Medical Assistant

About.com. (n.d.). What you need to know about stress management. http://stress.about.com
American Institute of Stress. Stress effects. Retrieved April 4, 2016 from http://www.stress.org/stress-effects/
HelpGuide.org. (2016, June). Preventing burnout. http://www.helpguide.org/articles/stress/preventing-burnout.htm
HelpGuide.org. (n.d.). Understanding stress. Retrieved April 4, 2016 http://www.helpguide.org/mental/stress.htm
Mayo Clinic. (n.d.). Job burnout: How to spot it and take action. Retrieved April 4, 2016 http://www.mayoclinic.org/healthy-lifestyle/adult-healt/in-depth/burnout/art-20046642
Milliken, M. E., & Honeycutt, A. (2012). *Understanding human behavior: A guide for health care providers* (8th ed.). Clifton Park, NY: Cengage Learning.

Chapter 4: Therapeutic Communication Skills

EuroMed Info. (n.d.). Doing a cultural assessment. http://www.euromedinfo.eu/doing-a-cultural-assessment.html
EuroMed Info. (n.d.). How culture influences health beliefs. http://www.euromedinfo.eu/how-culture-influences-health-beliefs.html/
Humes, K. R., Jones, N. A., & Ramirez, R. R. (2011, March). Overview of race and Hispanic origins: 2010. 2010 Census Briefs. Washington, DC: U.S. Census Bureau. http://www.census.gov/prod/cen2010/briefs/c2010br-02.pdf
Luckmann, J. (2000). *Transcultural communication in health care.* Clifton Park, NY: Cengage Learning.
Novickas, R. (2014, January/February). Helping hands: Reach out to deaf and hearing-impaired patients. CMA Today.
Pew Research Center. (2013). 45% say Muslim Americans face "a lot" of discrimination: After Boston, little change in views of Islam and violence. http://www.people-press.org/files/legacy-pdf/5-7-13%201Islam%20Release.pdf
Purnell, L. D. (2014) *Culturally competent health care.* Philadelphia: F.A. Davis.

Chapter 5: The Therapeutic Approach to the Patient with a Life-Threatening Illness

Back, A., Arnold, R., & Tulsky, J. (2010). *Mastering communication with seriously ill patients.* New York: Cambridge University Press.
Callinan, K. (2016). End-of-life care. Are we ready for real reform? Compassion & Choices. https://www.compassionandchoices.org/2016/01/28/end-of-life-care-are-we-ready-for-real-reform/
Kübler-Ross, E., & Kessler, D. (2005). *On grief and grieving.* New York: Scribner.

Purnell, L., & Paulanka, B. (2008). *Transcultural health care: A culturally competent approach.* Philadelphia: F. A. Davis.

WebMD. (2016, February). HIV & AIDS: How they're different. http://www.webmd.com/hiv-aids/difference_between_hiv_aids

UNIT III: RESPONSIBLE MEDICAL PRACTICE

Chapter 6: Legal Considerations

Centers for Disease Control and Prevention. (2016). 2016 Nationally notifiable conditions. http://wwwn.cdc.gov/nndss/conditions/notifiable/2016/

Centers for Medicare and Medicaid Services. (n.d.). Patient's bill of rights. https://www.cms.gov/CCIIO/Programs-and-Initiatives/Health-Insurance-Market-Reforms/Patients-Bill-of-Rights.html

Compassion & Choices. (2016, February 2). Durable power of attorney for health care: How to make the selection. https://www.compassionandchoices.org/durable-power-of-attorney-for-healthcare-how-to-make-the-selection/

Drug Policy Alliance. (2013, May). Removing marijuana from the Controlled Substances Act. http://www.drugpolicy.org/sites/default/files/DPA_Fact%20sheet_Marijuana%20Reclassification_May%202013.pdf

MedlinePlus. (2015, May 1). Reportable diseases. https://www.nlm.nih.gov/medlineplus/ency/article/001929.htm

National Healthcare Decisions Day (NHDD). (n.d.). Advance care planning resources. http://www.nhdd.org/public-resources/#where-can-i-get-an-advance-directive

Physician Orders for Life-Sustaining Treatment Paradigm. (n.d.). What is POLST? http://www.polst.org/about-the-national-polst-paradigm/what-is-polst/

U.S. Department of Health and Human Services. (2015, August 28). About the law, health care. http://www.hhs.gov/healthcare/about-the-law/read-the-law/index.html

U.S. Department of Labor. (n.d.). Family and Medical Leave Act. http://www.dol.gov/whd/fmla/spouse/

Washington State Medical Association (WSMA). (2007). Durable power of attorney for health care, health care directive, and POLST. http://www.wsma.org

World Health Organization. (n.d.). Understanding and addressing violence against women. http://www.who.int/reproductivehealth/topics/violence/vaw_series/en/

Chapter 7: Ethical Considerations

Aliesch, S. (ed.). (2016, Spring). Document and discuss. Compassion and Choices Magazine, 4–5.

American Medical Association. (2016, April 10). Code of medical ethics: Current opinions of the council on ethical and judicial affairs. http://www.ama-assn.org; http://www.ama.assn.org/ama/pub/physician-resources/medikcal-ethics/code-medical-ethics.page

Blanchard, K., & Peale, N. V. (1988). *The power of ethical management.* New York: William Morrow and Company, Inc.

Collins, S., Gunja, M., & Beutel, S. (2015, September). New U.S. Census data show the number of uninsured americans dropped by 8.8 million. Commonwealth Fund Blog, Commonwealth Fund. U.S. Census Bureau, 2013 and 2014 Current Population Survey Reports.

Covey, S. R. (2015). The 7 habits of managers. Audio CD. Franklin Covey on Brilliance Audio.

Covey, S. R. (1991). *Principle-centered leadership.* New York: Simon & Schuster.

Gold, J. (2014, January 29). In cities, the average doctor wait-time is 18.5 days. Wonkblog, Washington Post.

Patient Bill of Rights and Responsibilities. (2012, October). John Hopkins Medicine, John Hopkins Hospital, Baltimore, MD. http://www.hopkinsmedicine.org/the_johns_hopkins_hospital/

Planned Parenthood. (2016, April). The U.S. Supreme Court: Your boss can now decide if you can have access to birth control coverage. https://www.plannedparenthoodaction-org/blog/supreme-court-bosses-can-deny-birth-control-coverage-employees

Smith, S. (2014, April). Happening now. CNN. http://www.cnn.com/2014/04/10/health/tissue-engineering-success/

Stewart, K. (2015, October 8). At Catholic hospitals, a "right to life" but not a right to death. Retrieved April 18, 2016 from http://www.thenation.com/.../at-catholic-hospitals-a-right-to-life-but...

World Health Organization. (2011). An update on WHO's work on female genital mutilation (FGM) progress report. Retrieved from WHO_11.18_eng.pdf, April 14, 2016.

Chapter 8: Emergency Procedures and First Aid

American Heart Association. (2016). Hands only CPR. http://cpr.heart.org/AHAECC/CPRAndECC/Programs/HandsOnlyCPR/UCM_473196_Hands-Only-CPR.jsp

American Heart Association. (2015). Adult Basic Life Support. https://ebooks.heart.org//epubreader/bls-provider-manual-ebook#

American Heart Association. (n.d.). Advanced Cardiovascular Life Support. http://www.heart.org/HEARTORG/CPRAndECC/HealthcareTraining/AdvancedCardiovascularLifeSupportACLS/Advanced-Cardiovascular-Life-Support-ACLS_UCM_001280_SubHomePage.jsp

American National Red Cross. (2001). *Staywell.* St. Louis, MO: Mosby.

American Red Cross. (2005). CPR and emergency cardiac care: New CPR guidelines for professionals and nonprofessionals. http://www.redcross.org/cpr.html

Emergency Nurses Association. (n.d.). Use of tourniquets for control of extremity bleeding. Retrieved May 16, 2016 from https://www.ena.org/practice-research/Practice/Documents/TIPSTourniquets.pdf.

Epilepsy Foundation. (2013, July). What is a tonic-clonic seizure? http://www.epilepsy.com/learn/types-seizures/myoclonic-seizures

Medical Reserve Corps. (2008). Emergency medical care. http://www.medicalreservecorps.gov

MedlinePlus. (2015, January 11). Gastrointestinal bleeding. http://www.nlm.nih.gov/medlineplus/ency/article/003133.htm

National Institutes of Health. (2008). New CPR guidelines. http://www.health.nih.gov

SECTION II: ADMINISTRATIVE PROCEDURES

UNIT IV: INTEGRATED ADMINISTRATIVE PROCEDURES

Chapter 9: Creating the Facility Environment

Azoulay, R. (2009). *Music, the breath and health: Advances in integrative music therapy.* New York: Satchnote Press.

Barker, J., Pocock, E., Huber, C., & Black Associates. The future of ambulatory care. American Institute of Architects. http://www.aia.org/practicing/groups/kc/AIAB086508

Cama, R. (2009). *Evidence-based healthcare design.* New York: John Wiley & Sons.

Centers for Disease Control and Prevention. (n.d.). Emergency preparedness and response. http://emergency.cdc.gov/preparedness/kit/disasters/

Healthcare Designed. (n.d.). Interior design + architecture for healthcare. https://healthcaredesigned.wordpress.com/category/healthcare-design-architecture/

Purnell, L. D. (2014) *Guide to culturally competent health care.* Philadelphia: F. A. Davis Publishers.

TGBA Architects. (n.d.). Medical office building and clinic design. www.tgbarchitects.com/medical-clinic-architects.php

U.S. Department of Labor, Occupational Safety and Health Administration. (n.d.). Fire extinguisher basics. https://www.osha.gov/SLTC/etools/evacuation/portable.html

U.S. Department of Labor, Occupational Safety and Health Administration. (n.d.). How to plan for workplace emergencies and evacuations. http://www.osha.gov/Publications/osha3088.html

Chapter 10: Computers in the Medical Clinic

American Medical Association. (2015). E-5.07 confidentiality: Computers. http://www.ama-assn.org

Centers for Disease Control and Prevention. (2012, September 1). Self-study modules on tuberculosis measures to protect patient confidentiality. http://www.cdc.gov/tb/education/ssmodules/module7/ss7reading4.htm

GFI Blog. (2015, February 18). Most vulnerable operating systems and applications in 2014. http://www.gfi.com/blog/most-vulnerable-operating-systems-and-applications-in-2014/

Heller, M. (2017). *Clinical medical assisting: A professional, field smart approach to the workplace* (2nd ed.). Clifton Park, NY: Cengage Learning.

Storage Craft. (n.d.). Data storage lifespans: How long will media really last? https://www.storagecraft.com/blog/data-storage-lifespan/

U.S. Department of Health and Human Services. (2014, August 7). More physicians and hospitals are using EHRs than before. http://www.hhs.gov/about/news/2014/08/07/more-physicians-and-hospitals-are-using-ehrs-than-before.html

Chapter 11: Telecommunications

Administrative Arts. (n.d.). How to be a great assistant. http://administrativearts.com/welcome-to-administrative-arts/

HiMSS. (n.d.). Using patient portals to achieve meaningful use. http://www.himss.org/using-patient-portals-achieve-meaningful-use-ep-edition?ItemNumber=35966

HIPAA Journal. (n.d.). FCC confirms rules regarding HIPAA and patient telephone calls. http://www.hipaajournal.com/fcc-confirms-rules-regarding-hipaa-and-patient-telephone-calls-8048/

Chapter 12: Patient Scheduling

See General References

Chapter 13: Medical Records Management

Burt, C. W., Hing, E., & Woodwell, D. (2005). *Electronic medical record use by office-based physicians: United States, 2005.* Hyattsville, MD: U.S. Department of Health and Human Services, Centers for Disease Control and Prevention.

Centers for Medicare and Medicaid Services. (2016, June). Ensuring proper use of electronic health record features and capabilities. https://www.cms.gov/Medicare-Medicaid-Coordination/Fraud-Prevention/Medicaid-Integrity-Education/Downloads/ehr-decision-table.pdf

Hansen, D. (2008). Congress considers mandate for Medicare e-prescribing. http://www.ama-assn.org/amednews/2008/01/07/gvsb0107.htm

Healthcare IT News. (2015, January 15). 12 tips for better EHR usability. http://www.healthcareitnews.com/news/12-tips-better-ehr-usability

HealthIT.gov. (2014, August 29). Benefits of EHRs. https://www.healthit.gov/providers-professionals/why-adopt-ehrs

Medical Economics. (2015, December 10). Last word: Medical records. Creation vs. control. http://medicaleconomics.modernmedicine.com/medical-economics/news/last-word-medical-records-creation-vs-control

Chapter 14: Written Communications

Humphrey, D. D. (2004). *Contemporary medical office procedures* (3rd ed.). Clifton Park, NY: Cengage Learning.

Reed Tinsley. (n.d.). Forms & checklists. http://www.rtacpa.com/forms-checklists

Robert, H. M., III, Evans, W. J., Honemann, D. H., & Balch, T. J. (2000). *Robert's rules of order newly revised* (10th ed.). Cambridge, MA: Perseus.

Terryberry, K. (2005). *Writing for the health profession.* Clifton Park, NY: Cengage Learning.

Villemarie, D., & Villemarie, L. (2005). *Grammar and writing skills for the health professional.* Clifton Park, NY: Cengage Learning.

Chapter 15: Medical Documents

American Association for Medical Transcription. (1990). *AAMT model job description: Medical transcriptionist.* Modesto, CA: American Association for Medical Transcription.

Burns, L., & Maloney, F. (2003). *Medical transcription and terminology: An integrated approach* (2nd ed.). Clifton Park, NY: Cengage Learning.

Conerly-Stewart, D. L., & Ireland, P.A. (2015). *Forrest general medical center: Advanced medical transcription course* (4th ed.). Clifton Park, NY: Cengage Learning.

Ireland, P. A., & Stein, C. (2018). *Hillcrest medical center: Healthcare documentation and medical transcription* (8th ed.). Clifton Park, NY: Cengage Learning.

Tossey, K. L. (1998). The integration of digital photographs into medical transcription. Journal of the American Association for Medical Transcription, 17(6), 19–21.

UNIT V: MANAGING FACILITY FINANCES

Chapter 16: Medical Insurance

Green, M. A., & Rowell, J. C. (2017). *Understanding health insurance: A guide to billing and reimbursement* (13th ed.). Clifton Park, NY: Cengage Learning.

Chapter 17: Medical Coding

American Medical Association. (2016). *Current procedural terminology.* Chicago: American Medical Association.

American Medical Association. (2011). *International classification of diseases, clinical modifications (ICD-9)* (2nd ed., 9th rev.). Chicago: American Medical Association.

Bowie, M. J. (2017). *Understanding ICD-10-CM and ICD-10-PCS: A worktext* (3rd ed.). Clifton Park, NY: Cengage Learning.

Ingenix. (2011). *HCPCS level II.* Salt Lake City, UT: St. Anthony Publishing/Medicode.

Office of Inspector General, U.S. Department of Health and Human Services. (2000). Compliance program guide for individual and small group physician practices. http://oig.hhs.gov/authorities/docs/physcian.pdf

Optum360. (2016). *ICD-10-CM professional for physicians, 2016* (2016 ed.). Providence, RI: Optum360.

Papazian-Boyce, L. M. (2016). *Comprehensive medical coding.* Boston: Pearson.

Sayles, N. B. (2017). *Health information management technology: An applied approach.* Chicago: American Health Information Management Association.

Chapter 18: Daily Financial Practices

Beehive. (n.d.). How to write a personal check. http://www.thebeehive.org

Centers for Medicare and Medicaid Services. (2007). CMS clarifies guidelines for national provider identifier (NPI) deadline implementation. http://www.cms.hhs.gov

Electronic prescriptions. (n.d.). http://www.medisoft.com

Chapter 19: Billing and Collections

Dana Neal's Best Credit. (n.d.). Summary of the Fair Debt Collection Practices Act. http://www.bestcredit.com/summary-of-the-fair-debt-collection-practices-act/

Free Advice Legal. (n.d.). How are estate creditors handled? http://law.freeadvice.com/estate_planning/probate/estate_creditors.htm

IC System. (n.d.). Medical collections services. http://www.icsystem.com/medical-collections-services/

Johnson, J. (1994). *Basic filing procedures for health information management.* Clifton Park, NY: Cengage Learning.

NOLO. (n.d.). What is the difference between Chapter 7 and Chapter 13 bankruptcy? http://www.nolo.com/legal-encyclopedia/what-is-the-difference-between-chapter-7-chapter-13-bankrutpcy.html

Shatzman, B. (n.d.). Medical billing resources: Use better collection techniques to increase patient payments. http://www.mbrbilling.com/blog/bid/138985/Use-Better-Collection-Techniques-To-Increase-Patient-Payments

Chapter 20: Accounting Practices

Droms, W. G. (2003). *Finance and accounting for nonfinancial managers* (2nd ed.). Cambridge, MA: Perseus.

SECTION III: PROFESSIONAL PROCEDURES

UNIT VI: CLINIC AND HUMAN RESOURCES MANAGEMENT

Chapter 21: The Medical Assistant as Clinic Manager

Colbert, B. J. (2006). *Workplace readiness for health occupations* (2nd ed.). Clifton Park, NY: Cengage Learning.

Facebook. (n.d.). "Like" button. http://developers.facebook.com/docs/opengraph/

Nations, D. (n.d.). What is social media? What are social media sites? http://webtrends.about.com/od/web20/a/social-media.htm

Sobell, S. (2011, June). Social networking @ work: The costro connection.

Chapter 22: The Medical Assistant as Human Resources Manager

Schawbel, D. (2014). Comparing Gen Y and Gen Z workplace expectations: Millennial Branding and Randstad US release first worldwide study. http://millennialbranding.com/2014/geny-genz-global-workplace-expectations-study/

Smith, B. E., & Ricci, C. Healthcare trends 2015: White paper. https://www.besmith.com/thought-leadership/white-papers/healthcare-trends-2015

UNIT VII: ENTRY INTO THE PROFESSION

Chapter 23: Preparing for Medical Assisting Credentials

American Association of Medical Assistants. (2015). Recertify your CMA (AAMA) credential. http://www.aama-ntl.org

American Association of Medical Assistants. (n.d.). FAQs on CMA (AAMA) certification. http://www.aama-ntl.org

American Medical Technologists. (n.d.). AMT certification: A guide to allied health certification. http://www.americanmedtech.org

National Healthcareer Association. (n.d.). NHA national certification examination. http://www.nhanow.com

Chapter 24: Employment Strategies

CBS News. (2011, September 1). The best career strategy ever. http://www.cbsnews.com/news/the-best-career-strategy-ever/

Daily Muse. (n.d.). The 31 best LinkedIn profile tips for job seekers. https://www.themuse.com/advice/the-31-best-linkedin-profile-tips-for-job-seekers

Fletcher, L. (n.d.). How to write a LinkedIn profile. http://www.blueskyresumes.com/free-resume-help/article/how-to-write-a-linkedin-profile/

Imperial College London Business School. (n.d.). Career strategy. http://www3.imperial.ac.uk/pls/portallive/docs/1/50325698.PDF

Job-Hunt. (n.d.). Guide to Facebook for job search. http://www.job-hunt.org/social-networking/facebook-job-search/facebook-job-search.shtml

Job-Hunt. (n.d.). Guide to using LinkedIn for job search. http://www.job-hunt.org/social-networking/LinkedIn-job-search/LinkedIn-job-search.shtml

Job-Hunt. (n.d.). Personal branding makes your LinkedIn summary dazzle. http://www.job-hunt.org/personal-branding/branded-linkedin-summary.shtml

Job-Hunt. (n.d.). 10-step personal branding worksheet. http://www.job-hunt.org/personal-branding/personal-branding-worksheet.shtml

PayScale. (n.d.). Medical assistant salary (United States). http://www.payscale.com/research/US/Job=Medical_Assistant/Hourly_Rate

Schawbel, D. (2016, April). 7 secrets to getting your next job using social media. http://mashable.com/2009/01/05/job-search-secrets/

Social Media Defined. (2016, April). LinkedIn defined. http://www.socialmediadefined.com/2009/01/30/linkedin-defined/

INDEX

Note: Page references in **bold type** refer to boxes, procedures, figures, and tables.

A

B

C

D

E

F

G

H

I

J

K

L

M

N

O

P

T

U

V

W

Z